CRITICAL CARE PRACTICE

John W. Hoyt, M.D.

Clinical Professor of Anesthesiology and Critical Care Medicine
University of Pittsburgh School of Medicine
Chairman, Department of Critical Care Medicine
St. Francis Medical Center, Pittsburgh, Pennsylvania

Alan S. Tonnesen, M.D.

Professor of Anesthesiology, School of Medicine
University of Texas Health Science Center
Medical Director, Shock Trauma Intensive Care Unit
Hermann Hospital, Houston, Texas

Steven J. Allen, M.D.

Associate Professor of Anesthesiology, School of Medicine
University of Texas Health Science Center
Medical Director, Respiratory Therapy and Neurologic Critical Care Unit
Hermann Hospital, Houston, Texas

Foreword by **Peter Safar, M.D.**

Distinguished Professor; Director,
International Resuscitation Research Center; and
Past Chairman, Department of Anesthesiology and
Critical Care Medicine, University of Pittsburgh
Co-founder and Past President, Society of Critical Care Medicine
Past Chairman, Committee on Acute Medicine,
American Society of Anesthesiologists

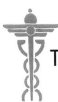 The American Society of Critical Care Anesthesiologists

1991

W. B. SAUNDERS COMPANY
Harcourt Brace Jovanovich, Inc.
Philadelphia • London • Toronto • Montreal • Sydney • Tokyo

W. B. SAUNDERS COMPANY
Harcourt Brace Jovanovich, Inc.

The Curtis Center
Independence Square West
Philadelphia, PA 19106

Critical care practice / [edited by] John W. Hoyt, Alan S. Tonnesen,
Steven J. Allen ; American Society of Critical Care
Anesthesiologists.
    p. cm.
  ISBN 0-7216-4701-4
    1. Critical care medicine.   I. Hoyt, John W.   Tonnesen, Alan
S.   III. Allen, Steven J.   IV. American Society of Critical Care
Anesthesiologists.
  [DNLM: 1. Critical Care.   WX 218 C9364]
RC86.7.C75 1991
616´.028 – dc20
DNLM/DLC   90-9159
for Library of Congress   CIP

Editor: Richard Zorab

CRITICAL CARE PRACTICE   ISBN   0-7216-4701-4

Printed in the United States of America

Last digit is the print number: 9   8   7   6   5   4   3   2   1

Contributors

STEVEN J. ALLEN, MD
Associate Professor,
Department of Anesthesiology,
The University of Texas Health Science Center;
Medical Director, Respiratory Therapy and Neurologic Critical Care Unit,
Hermann Hospital,
Houston, Texas
Advanced Respiratory Life Support; Advanced Neurologic Life Support; Respiratory Failure

MORRIS BROWN, MD
Associate Professor of Anesthesiology,
Wayne State University School of Medicine;
Vice-Chairman, Department of Anesthesiology,
and Director, Critical Care Services,
Sinai Hospital,
Detroit, Michigan
Infectious Disease

GRAZIANO C. CARLON, MD
Professor of Clinical Anesthesiology,
Cornell University Medical College;
Acting Chairman, Department of Anesthesiology and Critical Care Medicine,
Memorial Sloan-Kettering Cancer Center,
New York, New York
Psychologic Stress in the Intensive Care Unit; Administration of the Intensive Care Unit

DONALD CHALFIN, MD
Heyward Fellow in Critical Care Medicine,
Memorial Sloan-Kettering Cancer Center,
New York, New York
Administration of the Intensive Care Unit

BART CHERNOW, MD
Professor of Medicine, Anesthesia, and Critical Care,
The Johns Hopkins University School of Medicine;
Physician-in-chief, Sinai Hospital,
Baltimore, Maryland
Endocrinology in Critical Care

SIDNEY DEVINS, MD
Clinical and Research Fellow in Critical Care,
Department of Anesthesia,
Massachusetts General Hospital, Harvard Medical School,
Boston, Massachusetts
Endocrinology in Critical Care

NORIG ELLISON, MD
Professor of Anesthesia,
University of Pennsylvania School of Medicine;
Vice Chairman, Department of Anesthesia,
Hospital of the University of Pennsylvania;
Senior Anesthesiologist,
Children's Hospital of Philadelphia,
Philadelphia, Pennsylvania
Coagulation

I. ALAN FEIN, MD
Associate Professor of Surgery, Assistant Professor of Medicine, and
Director, Division of Critical Care Medicine,
Department of Surgery, Albany Medical College
Albany, New York
Administration of the Intensive Care Unit

WILLIAM R. FURMAN, MD
Assistant Professor, Anesthesiology and Critical Care Medicine,
The Johns Hopkins University School of Medicine;
Chairman, Department of Anesthesiology,
Francis Scott Key Medical Center,
Baltimore, Maryland
Burns

GORDON L. GIBBY, MD
Assistant Professor, Departments of Anesthesiology
and Medicine, University of Florida College of Medicine
Gainesville, Florida
Technology of Intensive Care Unit Monitors

V. RANDOLPH GLEASON, JD
Adjunct Faculty, University of Houston Law Center and
University of Texas Medical School at Houston;
Member, Institutional Ethics Committee, and
Vice President and General Counsel,
Hermann Hospital;
Member, Bioethics Committee,
Houston Northwest Medical Center,
Houston, Texas
Legal and Ethical Issues in the Intensive Care Unit

AKE GRENVIK, MD
Professor of Anesthesiology, Medicine, and Surgery, University of
Pittsburgh School of Medicine;
Director, Multidisciplinary Critical Care Medicine Training Program,
University of Pittsburgh Medical Center,
Pittsburgh, Pennsylvania
Postoperative Intensive Care of Transplantation Patients

ALVIN HACKEL, MD
Professor of Anesthesia and Pediatrics, Stanford University Medical
School;
Medical Director, Medical Transport Program,
Stanford University Hospital,
Stanford, California
Transport

ROBIN J. HAMILL, MD
Assistant Professor of Anesthesiology,
University of Virginia School of Medicine;
Associate Director, Surgical Intensive Care Unit, and
Staff Anesthesiologist, Pain Management Center,
University of Virginia Health Sciences Center,
Charlottesville, Virginia
Pain Management in the Intensive Care Unit

ELOISE M. HARMAN, MD
Professor of Medicine, Pulmonary Division,
Department of Medicine,
University of Florida College of Medicine;
Medical Director, Medical Intensive Care Unit and Coronary Care Unit,
Shands Hospital at the University of Florida,
Gainesville, Florida
Acquired Immunodeficiency Syndrome in the Intensive Care Unit

KENNETH HASPEL, MD
Clinical and Research Fellow in Critical Care and
Clinical Instructor of Anesthesia,
Department of Anesthesia,
Massachusetts General Hospital,
Harvard Medical School,
Boston, Massachusetts
Endocrinology in Critical Care

JOY L. HAWKINS, MD
Associate Professor of Anesthesiology and Obstetrics and Gynecology,
Department of Anesthesiology
Baylor College of Medicine and Ben Taub Hospital,
Houston, Texas
Critical Care of Obstetric Patients

JOHN W. HOYT, MD
Clinical Professor of Anesthesiology and Critical Care Medicine,
University of Pittsburgh School of Medicine;
Chairman, Department of Critical Care Medicine,
St. Francis Medical Center
Pittsburgh, Pennsylvania
Advanced Cardiovascular Life Support; Cardiovascular Disorders

SHARON M. IRVING
Lead Technical Writer,
Nellcor Incorporated.
Hayward, California
Clinical and Technical Issues in Pulse Oximetry and Capnometry

ANDREW JACKIW, MD
Department of Emergency Medicine,
Sinai Hospital,
Detroit, Michigan
Infectious Disease

MONICA M. JONES, MD
Assistant Professor of Anesthesiology and Obstetrics and Gynecology,
Department of Anesthesiology,
Baylor College of Medicine and Ben Taub Hospital,
Houston, Texas
Critical Care of Obstetric Patients

THOMAS H. JOYCE III, MD
Professor of Anesthesiology and Obstetrics and Gynecology,
Department of Anesthesiology,
Baylor College of Medicine and Ben Taub Hospital,
Houston, Texas
Critical Care of Obstetric Patients

ROBERT A. KILROY, PharmD
Clinical Supervisor, Intensive Care Unit,
Shands Hospital at the University of Florida,
Gainesville, Florida
Acquired Immunodeficiency Syndrome in the Intensive Care Unit

DAVID J. KRAMER, MD
Assistant Professor, Anesthesiology and Critical Care Medicine, Medicine, and Surgery,
University of Pittsburgh School of Medicine;
Co-Director, Liver Transplant Intensive Care Unit Service,
Presbyterian University Hospital,
Pittsburgh, Pennsylvania
Postoperative Intensive Care of Transplantation Patients

A. JOSEPH LAYON, MD
Assistant Professor of Anesthesiology and Medicine,
Department of Anesthesiology
(Division of Critical Care) and Medicine (Pulmonary Division),
University of Florida College of Medicine;
Director, Preoperative Evaluation Clinic,
Shands Hospital at the University of Florida,
Gainesville, Florida
Acquired Immunodeficiency Syndrome in the Intensive Care Unit

PHILIP D. LUMB, MB, BS
Professor of Anesthesiology and Surgery and
Chairman, Department of Anesthesiology, Albany Medical College;
Anesthesiologist in Chief and
Co-Director, Surgical Intensive Care Unit,
Albany Medical Center, Albany, New York
Multiple Organ System Failure

NIELS LUND, MD, PhD
Associate Professor of Anesthesiology,
University of Rochester;
Director, Critical Care Medicine and Critical Care Fellowships, and
Co-Director, Surgical Intensive Care Unit,
University of Rochester Medical Center,
Rochester, New York
Overdoses, Ingestions, and Intoxications

COLIN F. MACKENZIE, MD
Associate Professor of Anesthesiology and Physiology,
University of Maryland, School of Medicine;
Attending Anesthesiologist, University of Maryland Medical Systems,
Baltimore, Maryland
Critical Care Management of Traumatized Patients

MICHAEL J. MURRAY, MD, PhD
Assistant Professor, Mayo Medical School;
Director, Critical Care Service,
Chairman, Division of Intensive Care and Respiratory Therapy, and
Consultant, Department of Anesthesiology and Nutrition Support Service,
St. Mary's Hospital and Rochester Methodist Hospital,
Rochester, Minnesota
Nutritional Support in the Critically Ill

CHARLES W. OTTO, MD
Professor of Anesthesiology and
Associate Professor of Medicine,
University of Arizona College of Medicine;
Director, Critical Care Medicine,
University Medical Center,
Tucson, Arizona
Cardiopulmonary Resuscitation

BRIAN D. OWENS, MD

Staff Anesthesiologist,
Virginia Mason Clinic,
Seattle, Washington
Selected Red and White Blood Cell Disorders

PETER J. PAPADAKOS, MD

Senior Instructor in Anesthesiology,
The University of Rochester;
Attending Physician,
Surgical Intensive Care Unit,
University of Rochester Medical Center,
Rochester, New York
Overdoses, Ingestions, and Intoxications

RONALD G. PEARL, MD, PhD

Assistant Professor of Anesthesia, Stanford University Medical School;
Associate Director, Medical Transport Program and
Intensive Care Unit,
Stanford University Hospital,
Stanford, California
Transport

DONALD S. PROUGH, MD

Associate Professor of Anesthesia and Neurology
(Head, Section on Critical Care),
Bowman Gray School of Medicine;
Associate Chief of Professional Services,
North Carolina Baptist Hospital,
Winston-Salem, North Carolina
Critical Neurologic and Psychiatric Illness

HARRY S. RAFKIN, MD

Clinical Assistant Professor of Critical Care Medicine and Anesthesiology,
University of Pittsburgh School of Medicine;
Head of Critical Care Research and Physician Quality Assurance,
Department of Critical Care Medicine,
St. Francis Medical Center,
Pittsburgh, Pennsylvania
Assessing the Critically Ill Patient for Admission to the Intensive Care Unit

RAM E. RAJAGOPALAN, MB, BS

Fellow, Division of Critical Care Medicine, University of Pittsburgh
School of Medicine, Pittsburgh, Pennsylvania
Cardiovascular Disorders

ANTHONY R. RIELA, MD

Associate Professor of Neurology,
University of Texas Southwestern Medical School and
Children's Medical Center of Dallas,
Dallas, Texas
Critical Neurologic and Psychiatric Illness

DANIEL I. SESSLER, MD
Assistant Professor of Anesthesia,
School of Medicine,
University of California,
San Francisco, California
Temperature Disturbances

KEITH L. STEIN, MD
Associate Professor of Anesthesiology and Critical Care Medicine and Surgery,
University of Pittsburgh School of Medicine;
Associate Chief, Division of Critical Care Medicine,
and Director, Cardiothoracic Surgical Intensive Care Unit,
Presbyterian University Hospital,
Pittsburgh, Pennsylvania
Gastrointestinal Tract Function and Dysfunction in Critically Ill Patients;
Postoperative Intensive Care of Transplantation Patients

DAVID B. SWEDLOW, MD
Medical Vice President,
Nellcor Incorporated,
Hayward, California;
Staff Anesthesiologist,
Oakland Children's Hospital,
Oakland, California
Clinical and Technical Issues in Pulse Oximetry and Capnometry

ALAN S. TONNESEN, MD
Professor of Anesthesiology,
University of Texas Health Science Center;
Medical Director,
Shock Trauma Intensive Care Unit,
Hermann Hospital,
Houston, Texas
Initial Stabilization; Advanced Respiratory Life Support; Acute Renal Failure

ROBERT A. VESELIS, MD
Assistant Professor of Anesthesiology,
Cornell University Medical College;
Assistant Clinical Anesthesiologist,
Memorial Sloan-Kettering Cancer Center,
New York, New York
Psychologic Stress in the Intensive Care Unit

JOSEPH A. WAPENSKI, MD
Clinical Instructor and Chief,
Department of Nuclear Medicine,
St. Francis Medical Center,
Pittsburgh, Pennsylvania
Cardiovascular Disorders

LIN C. WEEKS, DrPH, RN,
Adjunct Assistant Professor,
University of Texas School of Nursing, Galveston and Houston;
Instructor in Medicine,
University of Texas Medical School;
Vice President for Nursing and
Chairman, Institutional Ethics Committee,
Hermann Hospital,
Houston, Texas
Legal and Ethical Issues in the Intensive Care Unit

Foreword

Critical Care Practice sponsored by the American Society of Critical Care Anesthesiologists, has been prepared primarily for anesthesiologists. Many undoubtedly will gain valuable information from this book, and hopefully, some will be motivated by it to become more involved in critical care medicine (CCM). This book offers a detailed knowledge base on a wide spectrum of topics, from life-support techniques via the pathophysiology of organ systems failure to special life-threatening diseases. Therefore, it will also be a valuable source of information for physicians from other disciplines who are embarking on work in CCM.

There is no uniform definition for CCM in the United States or abroad. The book's contents reflect the scope of critical care practice as extending beyond prolonged life-support of hospitalized intensive care unit (ICU) patients. This comes as no surprise, since one of the editor-authors is an alumnus and faculty member of the University of Pittsburgh CCM program. The Department of Anesthesiology of the University of Pittsburgh School of Medicine, which was initiated in 1961, "fathered" care, teaching and research programs in cardiopulmonary-cerebral resuscitation (CPCR), prehospital emergency medical services (EMS), respiratory therapy, and multidisciplinary intensive care. Thus, in this text CCM encompasses all three phases of CPCR (basic, advanced, and prolonged life-support) and their application to critically ill or injured patients throughout the life-support chain—from the prehospital scene (or anywhere inside the hospital where deterioration of vital organ systems begins) via transportation, through hospital emergency room, operating room, and ICU.

Before the 1950s the basic, advanced, and prolonged life-support methods available for use outside the operating room were largely unphysiologic and ineffective. Organized concentrations of patients in need of continuous monitoring and life-support were limited to a few specific medical problems. Examples were Cushing's and Dandy's neurosurgical recovery rooms and poliomyelitis wards stocked with iron lungs. Before and during World War II a few anesthesiologists in the United States and Great Britain created special recovery rooms where they could observe and provide life-support to still unconscious patients after anesthesia. I left surgery for anesthesia training in 1950, inspired by the belief that the development of modern surgery would depend on improved life-support. Other anesthesiologists at that time also recognized the importance of applying the life-support expertise gained in anesthesia to all of medicine and surgery.

In the early 1950s Scandinavian anesthesiologists were the first to apply the anesthesiologic skills of airway control and artificial ventilation on a large scale outside the operating room. They cared for patients paralyzed with poliomyelitis and patients in coma from barbiturate poisoning. Scandinavian cardiothoracic surgeons and anesthesiologists applied prolonged artificial ventilation to postoperative patients. The first physician-staffed ICU in the United States was initiated in 1958 by anesthesiologists of the Baltimore City Hospital. This was, however, a multidisciplinary medical-surgical ICU, where multiple-organ-systems support was provided jointly by resident and staff physicians of anesthesiology, medicine, and surgery and by specially trained nurses. In 1963 the first formal CCM physician fellowship training program was initiated at the University of Pittsburgh as a third year of anesthesiology residency training, which was supported in part by the National Institutes of Health. In the late 1960s it began to attract internists, surgeons, and pediatricians as well. The first two pediatric ICUs in the United States were also initiated by anesthesiologists in the 1960s.

Most of the early anesthesiologists who became intensivists did not abandon the operating room. Their skills and their willingness to provide continuous life-support to patients for long periods gained them the respect of their peers in other disciplines. In the late 1960s we anesthesiologists-intensivists discovered that the frustrations and obstacles we encountered in attempting to replace standard treatment by "rounds and prescription" with life-supporting treatment by "continual titration" were experienced also by some pioneering intensivists from medicine and surgery. This common understanding led in the early 1970s to the founding of the multidisciplinary Society of Critical Care Medicine (SCCM) and to the first guidelines for ICU organization and ICU physician training.

In the mid-1960s, under the aegis of then President Dr. John Bonica, the American Society of Anesthesiologists (ASA) established its first committee on acute medicine. This committee not only was to represent and promote the role of the anesthesiologist as intensivist but also was to lead the resuscitation-oriented organization of prehospital EMS throughout the community. The nation's first community councils on EMS, introduced in Pennsylvania, were spearheaded by anesthesiologists who were supported by some members of other disciplines. Previously, prehospital EMS either had been ignored or had been promoted by orthopedic surgeons who focused on fractures. Through the National Research Council (NRC), the American Medical Association (AMA), the American Heart Association (AHA), and other organizations, anesthesiologists helped to give EMS a multidisciplinary base.

Why in the 1980s did large numbers of U.S. anesthesiologists give up their involvement in prehospital and intrahospital CCM while European anesthesiologists remained active leaders in these fields? Numerous factors contributed to this trend. These probably include economics (earnings from anesthetic practice are higher than those from staffing of ICUs), frustration with the limits placed on their role in ICU patient care by internists and surgeons, new emphasis in academic anesthesiology on laboratory research rather than CCM, the fragmentation of all disciplines including anesthesiology, and a lack of commitment to EMS and CCM on the part of U.S. anesthesiology societies and boards. Abroad, socialized medicine made it easier for anesthesiologists to remain in EMS and CCM.

At present, the knowledge bases and techniques for resuscitation and multidisciplinary intensive care are established and are being continuously updated. Some of these anesthesiologists who had withdrawn into the operating room and who had become increasingly sophisticated in life-support of the anesthetized patient are returning to CCM. This is particularly true in the management of trauma cases and neurosurgical anesthesia and intensive care. Because of the mutual trust and respect gained during the collaboration of surgeons and anesthesiologists in the operating room, anesthesiologists have again become increasingly welcome in surgical hospital ICUs. The fact that few are eager or invited to work in medical ICUs is unfortunate for patients. Many internists-intensivists have not acquired life-support skills from rotation through operating room anesthesia or ambulance work. Anesthesiologists can and should provide more than airway control. As clinical physiologists, they should be experts in monitoring. As clinical pharmacologists, they should be experts in the care of drug overdose. Their anesthesia experience makes them particularly suited to teach and practice titrated life-support.

The founders of the SCCM had a multidisciplinary superspecialty in mind — the interaction of anesthesiologist, surgeon, internist (or pediatrician), and now also emergency physician, those with special interest and similar expertise in resuscitation and life-support — to jointly provide, guide, or supervise the "emergency and critical care medicine continuum" from scene through ICU. These specialists would share the fulltime emergency coverage of hospital ICUs, of resuscitation services in emergency departments and throughout the hospital, and for the guiding of prehospital resuscitation. In the subacute or long-term management of ICU patients their varied base specialty knowledge and expertise can contribute to the common purpose. The ideal of this multidisciplinary EMS-CCM continuum was fragmented by territorial, economic, and other disputes.

The forces that might rejoin this interdisciplinary continuum in the near future could be (1) the return of the anesthesiologist to acute medicine fulltime or part-time to act as coordinator, leader, or team member and (2) the joint pursuit of research in resuscitation medicine — in the laboratory, in patients, and in the community — by CCM physicians of various base disciplines and emergency physicians with additional CCM training. Thus, the science of emergency and critical care medicine, called resuscitology or reanimatology, could become a catalyst. To achieve this, emergency physicians in the United States who control the life-support services in the emergency department and outside the hospital, anesthesiologists, trauma surgeons, and intensivists of all base specialties, must work together not only in close cooperation but also with mutual respect, collegiality, and friendship where possible. This goal will undoubtedly be fostered through use of *Critical Care Practice*, edited by Drs. Hoyt, Tonnesen, and Allen.

PETER SAFAR MD

Preface

Anesthesiologists have played a major role in the development of critical care medicine from its earliest beginnings in treating life-threatening respiratory failure. To this day critical care has remained an important aspect of the practice of anesthesiology, with many anesthesiologists involved in various phases of the discipline. In recognition of its importance to the specialty, the American Board of Anesthesiology requires that candidates fulfill a minimum ICU rotation in the practice of critical care medicine under the direction of critical care–trained anesthesiologists.

Perhaps no anesthesia textbook has had the impact on the education of residents as has the *Introduction to Anesthesia* by the late Dr. Dripps and Drs. Eckenhoff and Vandam. The abiding usefulness of this book is due in part to its conciseness and readability. The text has gone through multiple editions, and its popularity remains undiminished.

One goal of our work has been to provide anesthesia residents fulfilling their critical care requirement with a text that is as readable and concise as the Dripps' book. This text is not meant to be a definitive reference; rather, it is an introduction to the essential knowledge of the subspecialty. A second goal is to provide a survey whereby the fellow starting critical care training can become oriented to the scope of its practice. We hope that this text can be digested during the first few months of fellowship training, to be followed by more in-depth reading.

Extremely ill patients are frequently admitted to the critical care unit with little advance notice and an incomplete history but with immediate, life-threatening problems. The organization of this book attempts to reflect this clinical reality. Thus, the most vital elements of maintaining major organ function are addressed in the first section. Following the discussion of stabilizing vital signs, more specific diagnoses and treatments are described in the next section. The third section handles specific aspects of critical care practice.

A major attraction of critical care to many intensivists is the enthusiastic involvement of physicians from many specialties who share their perspectives and ideas. This book, written largely by anesthesiologists, is an attempt to present our perspective. The practice styles of intensivists vary greatly. However, there is a basic core of information, presented in this book, with which every critical care practitioner should be familiar.

The practice of critical care involves resuscitation and titration of life support in its most basic form. This text is presented in a format that we hope will benefit all physicians, as full or part time intensivists, from whatever specialty, as they utilize the technologies of life support to save lives.

JOHN W. HOYT

ALAN S. TONNESEN

STEVEN J. ALLEN

Contents

SECTION II   ORGAN SYSTEM FAILURE

SECTION III   SPECIFIC CRITICAL CARE TOPICS

SECTION
I

CRITICAL
CARE
LIFE
SUPPORT

1

ASSESSING THE CRITICALLY ILL PATIENT FOR ADMISSION TO THE INTENSIVE CARE UNIT

HARRY S. RAFKIN, MD

Intensive care units (ICUs) were established so that the sickest individuals could receive the best care medicine could offer. Initially the sickest patients were always admitted to the ICU. In this way, critically ill patients were treated by medical personnel specially trained in intensive care medicine and were monitored by the most sophisticated equipment available.

Over the past 20 years, physicians, as well as the public, have refined their attitudes toward the ICU. Physicians realize that despite advances in medicine and technology, certain disease processes cannot be reversed under any circumstances. Furthermore, many individuals are unwilling to submit themselves or family members to prolonged hospitalization in the ICU, with its inherent discomfort, if the physician cannot state that the patient has a reasonable chance of survival. Thus both the physician and the layperson have grown to appreciate the limitations of medicine and the psychologic costs of prolonged but fruitless hospitalization.

During this same period, the costs of medicine have come under close scrutiny. ICUs account for more than 20% of hospital costs. Critical care units account for $20 billion to $40 billion of expenses annually in the United States. Total annual cost of health care in the United States is $400 billion, which represents 10% of the gross national product. Total annual hospital costs in the United States equal 4% of the gross national product. Since ICU costs equal approximately 25% of hospital costs, the cost of intensive care represents 1% of the gross national product.

The issues of cost and unnecessary treatment take on even more significance in light of the fact that 15% to 25% of people admitted to ICUs in the United States die. If certain subpopulations of ICU patients, such as stable postoperative patients, are eliminated, it is apparent that certain subgroups of patients have a remarkably high mortality rate.

Because of changing attitudes of physicians and society, as well as economic pressures, the issue of appropriate ICU admission policy has recently been debated in medical, economic, and ethical circles. Nonetheless, present policy in the United States is to admit virtually any critically ill patient to the ICU. This is because criteria for admission are essentially based on the need for monitoring, technologic support, or pharmacologic support. This is not true in many other countries, where one criterion for admission to the ICU is the potential benefit to the patient, as perceived by the physician. Hence, when septic shock develops in an elderly patient with chronically poor health, he may be refused admission to the ICU because his physician judges him unlikely to survive. Such practice is considered appropriate in these countries because both physicians and society recognize the need to limit health care expenses and to direct spending. The United States must adopt a similar policy. Physicians must somehow learn to identify patients with a reasonable chance of survival and not subject the others to the rigors of the ICU.

In addition to the problem of admitting irreversibly ill patients to the ICU, there is the

3

question of stable patients who are unnecessarily admitted to the ICU for monitoring. Physicians must learn to identify the patients admitted for prophylactic monitoring who have a high potential for complications that can best be treated in the ICU. For example, physicians need to determine which patients in the process of being evaluated for a myocardial infarction would benefit from ICU monitoring rather than telemetry on the medical floor and which patients admitted for postoperative monitoring would actually benefit from the ICU.

Although no perfectly accurate way exists to predict which patients can most benefit from the ICU, the physician can approach the situation systematically. This chapter attempts to demonstrate how this problem can be evaluated and managed.

The physician must learn to predict, at an early stage, when survival is possible and when death is inevitable. Despite attempts to approach this problem systematically, the difficulty of this endeavor must be recognized. The challenge is best summarized by Hippocrates' aphorism: "It is unwise to prophesy either death or recovery in acute disease."

INDICATIONS, INTERVENTIONS, AND OUTCOMES OF MEDICAL AND SURGICAL INTENSIVE CARE

The discussion begins with an evaluation of present indications for hospitalization in the ICU, the percentage of patients who require major therapeutic interventions, and the outcomes of these patients. ICU patients can be classified into two categories: patients admitted for prophylactic monitoring and patients admitted for active critical illness requiring immediate therapy. This chapter is particularly concerned with the percentage of patients admitted for prophylactic monitoring who actually require active interventions, as well as the survival rates for patients admitted to the ICU for active critical illness. The discussion addresses medical and surgical ICU populations separately.

Thibault looked at 2693 consecutive admissions to a single medical ICU during a 2-year period: 39% of patients were admitted because of chest pain or suspected myocardial infarction, 28% because of other cardiovascular disease, 11% because of respiratory problems, and 5% because of drug overdoses.

In this study population, myocardial infarction was confirmed in only 35% of patients admitted for a suspected myocardial infarction.

Nevertheless, myocardial infarction accounted for 20% of ICU discharge diagnoses. Thus, although myocardial infarction is a common diagnosis in the medical ICU, in this study more than half the patients admitted with this diagnosis did not have a myocardial infarction. An additional 15% of patients were discharged with the diagnosis of coronary insufficiency. Clearly, coronary vascular disease is a major cause of ICU admission, accounting for 35% of all discharge diagnoses in this study population. What is less clear is the percentage of these patients who actually required ICU care.

Thibault offered some insight into this question. Only 631 patients in his study (23%) were admitted to the ICU so that active interventions could be performed. Among the 2062 patients (77%) admitted for noninvasive monitoring, only 10% actually required a major procedure. Less than 10% of patients admitted because of precordial chest pain or suspected myocardial infarction actually required active intervention at the time of admission. These data suggest that a large proportion of patients admitted to the ICU are stable at admission and are admitted for prophylactic monitoring because of potential problems, which most often fail to develop. A significant number of these patients have an admission diagnosis of coronary artery disease.

Table 1–1 shows overall mortality for the 2693 patients included in Thibault's study. The overall mortality rate during hospitalization was 10%. The highest mortality rates occurred among patients with hepatic failure (71% mortality rate), respiratory failure (48%), and following a cardiopulmonary arrest (68%). These patients accounted for 80 (19%) of the 279 hospital deaths that occurred in patients included in this study. In contrast, a 5% death rate occurred among ICU patients with cardiovascular disease. It is apparent that mortality rates vary markedly according to diagnosis.

After hospital discharge Thibault followed 1230 patients during a 15-month period. The cumulative mortality rate during this period was 25%. Table 1–2 shows deaths during hospitalization and during the follow-up period. The mortality rate was highest in patients with congestive heart disease and chronic obstructive pulmonary disease. More people died during the follow-up period than during hospitalization (307 versus 279), and these deaths correlated directly with age. Patients older than 70 years had a mortality rate of 27%, whereas patients less than 50 years had a mortality rate of less than 7%.

TABLE 1–1. Mortality in ICU/CCU and in Hospital after 2693 Admissions to ICU/CCU during Two-Year Study Period

PRIMARY DISCHARGE DIAGNOSIS*	MORTALITY IN THE UNIT	MORTALITY IN THE HOSPITAL
	NUMBER OF PATIENTS†	
Acute myocardial infarction (527)	46 (9)	76 (14)
Coronary insufficiency (389)	0	9 (2)
Heart rhythm disturbance (284)	6 (2)	13 (5)
Precordial pain (192)	0	1 (1)
Congestive heart failure (191)	7 (4)	13 (7)
Drug overdose (159)	0	0
Gastrointestinal hemorrhage (100)	8 (8)	17 (17)
Chronic obstructive pulmonary disease (90)	4 (4)	8 (9)
Primary pneumonia (63)	10 (16)	15 (24)
Syncope (52)	0	0
Cardiopulmonary arrest (41)	21 (51)	28 (68)
Sepsis (39)	13 (33)	15 (38)
Renal failure (34)	7 (21)	9 (26)
Diabetic ketoacidosis (26)	0	0
Respiratory failure (25)	8 (32)	12 (48)
Delirium tremens (23)	0	0
Hepatic failure (14)	5 (36)	10 (71)
Other cardiovascular diagnoses (128)	3 (2)	9 (7)
Miscellaneous (316)	30 (10)	44 (14)
Total (2693)	168 (6)	279 (10)

*Figures in parentheses denote number of patients.
†Figures in parentheses denote percent of patients.
 Reprinted by permission of the New England Journal of Medicine from Thibault GE: N Engl J Med 1980;302(17):941.

TABLE 1–2. Mortality during Hospitalization and Total Mortality at Follow-up among 1230 Patients Admitted during First Year of Study

PRIMARY DISCHARGE DIAGNOSIS*	AGE (Y)†	HOSPITAL MORTALITY	TOTAL MORTALITY AT FOLLOW-UP‡	LOST TO FOLLOW-UP§
		NUMBER OF PATIENTS¶		
Acute myocardial infarction (258)	64 ± 0.8	34 (13)	71 (28)	3 (1)
Coronary insufficiency (190)	62 ± 0.9	4 (2)	26 (14)	8 (4)
Heart-rhythm disturbance (114)	64 ± 1.4	5 (4)	23 (15)	5 (4)
Precordial pain (90)	56 ± 1.4	0	6 (7)	9 (10)
Congestive heart failure (86)	70 ± 1.3	5 (6)	36 (42)	2 (2)
Drug overdose (79)	33 ± 1.5	0	3 (4)	23 (29)
Gastrointestinal hemorrhage (39)	54 ± 2.8	6 (15)	15 (39)	1 (3)
Chronic obstructive pulmonary disease (35)	64 ± 2.3	3 (9)	13 (37)	2 (6)
Primary pneumonia (41)	63 ± 2.9	12 (29)	21 (51)	4 (10)
Syncope (23)	69 ± 3.5	0	5 (22)	0
Cardiopulmonary arrest (19)	66 ± 4.2	12 (63)	13 (68)	1 (5)
Sepsis (15)	62 ± 4.4	5 (33)	6 (40)	2 (13)
Renal failure (19)	55 ± 3.7	5 (26)	9 (47)	0
Diabetic ketoacidosis (9)	55 ± 5.9	0	2 (22)	0
Respiratory failure (11)	66 ± 4.0	5 (45)	7 (64)	1 (9)
Delirium tremens (14)	45 ± 3.1	0	1 (7)	5 (36)
Hepatic failure (5)	50 ± 5.9	3 (60)	4 (80)	0
Other cardiovascular diagnoses (57)	62 ± 2.2	5 (9)	13 (23)	2 (3)
Miscellaneous (126)	57 ± 1.7	13 (10)	39 (31)	13 (10)
Total (1230)	60 ± 0.5	117 (10)	313 (25)	81 (7)

*Figures in parentheses denote number of patients.
†Mean ± S.E.M.
‡Mean interval between discharge and follow-up of survivors was 15 months (range, 5 to 25 months).
§Includes patients who did not give permission for posthospitalization follow-up.
¶Figures in parentheses denote percent of patients.
 Reprinted by permission of the New England Journal of Medicine from Thibault GE: N Engl J Med 1980;302(17):941.

TABLE 1–3.   Benefit from Overnight ICU Stay

OPERATIVE GROUP	TOTAL NUMBER OF PATIENTS	NUMBER OF PATIENTS BENEFITING	PATIENTS BENEFITING (%)
Carotid endarterectomy	48	33	69 (52–79)*
Abdominal vascular	40	16	10 (25–57)
Intracranial vascular	29	13	45 (7–60)
Peripheral vascular	60	16	27 (16–40)
Subtentorial craniotomy	18	3	17 (4–41)
Supratentorial craniotomy	55	7	13 (5–24)
Cervical laminectomy	13	0	0 (0–21)
All groups	263	88	33 (29–34)

*Numbers in parentheses are 95% confidence limits.
Reprinted with permission from the International Anesthesia Research Society from "Benefit of elective intensive care after certain operations," by R. Teplick, Anesthesia and Analgesia 62:572, 1983.

Several conclusions can be drawn from Thibault's study. The ICU is often used unnecessarily as an observation area for patients who are erroneously thought to have a potential for serious complications. Patients admitted for possible coronary artery disease represent a considerable proportion of patients admitted for prophylactic monitoring. Clearly, ICU admission practices could be made more efficient. In addition, this analysis indicates that a large proportion of ICU deaths result from respiratory failure, hepatic failure, renal failure, or cardiopulmonary arrest. The prognosis is clearly poor for patients with these complications.

The study appropriately points out that prognosis varies according to diagnosis. But even among patients with diagnoses associated with high death rates, a certain proportion survive. Some critically ill patients have a greater chance of survival than do others and in this sense have a greater chance to benefit from the ICU. Other patients are so ill at the time of admission that even intensive therapy cannot reverse their deterioration.

The study does not indicate how critically ill patients with a good chance can be differentiated prospectively from those with a poor chance. Although Thibault pointed out that ICU practices could be made more efficient by reducing the number of patients admitted for prophylactic monitoring, he did not suggest how this might be safely accomplished. These issues are explored later in this chapter.

Surgical patients in the ICU differ from medical patients. Postoperative patients are commonly placed in the ICU for 24-hour observation because certain surgical procedures carry a potential for complications that require immediate therapy. Although medical patients admitted to the ICU for prophylactic monitoring commonly derive no clear benefit, this may not be true for the surgical population.

Teplick performed a retrospective analysis of 263 patients who were placed in the ICU after a surgical procedure. The 57 different procedures represented were divided for analysis into seven groups: carotid endarterectomy, abdominal vascular surgery, intracranial vascular surgery, peripheral vascular surgery, subtentorial craniotomy, supratentorial craniotomy, and cervical laminectomy. The benefit of systematic 24-hour postoperative observation in the ICU was determined. Benefit was considered to have accrued if such problems as myocardial ischemia, hypotension, or hypertension developed, which could lead to serious consequences without rapid detection and treatment.

Table 1–3 shows the result of Teplick's study. Based on his criteria, 33% of the 263 patients studied benefited from 24-hour observation in the ICU. Patients who underwent vascular surgery derived clear benefit from the ICU. Specifically, 69% of patients undergoing carotid endarterectomies and 40% of patients undergoing abdominal vascular surgery benefited. Patients who underwent craniotomies also benefited significantly. Patients who underwent cervical laminectomies derived no benefit.

Hypotension and hypertension were the problems most commonly requiring immediate therapy. Acute hypotension occurred in 48%, 10%, 10%, and 11%, respectively, of patients who underwent carotid endarterectomy, abdominal vascular surgery, intracranial vascular surgery, and peripheral vascular surgery. Acute hypertension occurred in 10%, 18%, 15%, and 4%, respectively, of patients who underwent these same procedures. Among the patients undergoing carotid endarterectomy, hypotension lasted longer than hypertension and both fluids and vasopressors were required to restore hemodynamic stability. In other patients hypotension usually responded to fluids.

Teplick attempted to determine whether these problems occurred in the immediate postoperative period. He reasoned that any problem occurring within the first 4 hours after surgery could be treated in a recovery room, eliminating the need for admission to the ICU. However, he found that 34% of the problems requiring immediate treatment occurred after the initial 4-hour period. Thus a significant percentage of postoperative problems are not diagnosed during a routine or even a prolonged stay in a recovery room.

Teplick's findings suggest that systematic postoperative observation in the ICU is indicated for many surgical procedures, particularly abdominal, intracranial, and peripheral vascular surgery. Carotid endarterectomy, which is now performed less frequently than previously, clearly leads to problems that are best treated in the ICU. A significant percentage of postoperative problems occur after the immediate postoperative period and therefore cannot be detected in the recovery room. Hypotension and hypertension are the two most frequently encountered postoperative problems.

POPULATIONS AND SURVIVAL IN THE INTENSIVE CARE UNIT

The discussion now focuses on specific populations of patients commonly admitted to the medical ICU. As noted previously, ICU patients can be divided into two populations: those who are critically sick and require active therapy, and those who are relatively stable but require specific monitoring not found outside the ICU. The population of critically ill patients is discussed first.

As Thibault noted, certain diagnoses are associated with a high death rate. Some critically ill patients have virtually no chance of survival from the time they are admitted to the ICU. This discussion is aimed at identifying prognostic factors that might distinguish survivors from nonsurvivors, in other words, ways to identify prospectively those patients who might benefit from ICU care. The supposition is that patients who might benefit from the ICU should be admitted, whereas those who cannot benefit should not be admitted. The diseases considered here are respiratory failure, acute renal failure, infection and multiple system organ failure, coronary artery disease, acquired immunodeficiency syndrome complicated by respiratory failure resulting from

Pneumocystis carinii pneumonia, and nontraumatic coma.

Respiratory Failure

Mechanical ventilation has become more sophisticated over the past 20 years. Innovations such as positive end-expiratory pressure and pressure support have improved the ability to supply oxygen and ventilation to patients with severe respiratory failure. These innovations were expected to increase survival of patients with acute respiratory failure. Documenting increased survival is important because care of the ICU patient requiring mechanical ventilation is particularly expensive. Large amounts of resources are being directed toward a small percentage of the population near the end of their lives. In addition, prolonged dependence on mechanical ventilation is physically difficult for the patient and places an emotional burden on the family. This section examines the prognosis of patients with acute respiratory failure to determine whether modern technology has increased survival. Three types of respiratory failure are examined: adult respiratory distress syndrome (ARDS), chronic obstructive pulmonary disease (COPD), and pneumonia.

Adult Respiratory Distress Syndrome

Although understanding of the pathophysiologic mechanisms that contribute to ARDS has advanced, therapeutic progress has lagged behind. Mortality rates still exceed 60% in some reports. Several recent prospective studies have attempted to evaluate factors that might influence outcome.

Montgomery evaluated 207 patients with conditions that lead to ARDS, such as sepsis syndrome, gastric aspiration, and multiple fractures. ARDS developed in 47 patients (22.7%), and 36 (68%) of these died. Fourteen deaths occurred within the first 72 hours and in most cases were caused by the underlying disease, whereas 22 deaths occurred after 72 hours and were related to sepsis syndrome. The source of sepsis was most commonly the abdomen or the lung. This study reveals a remarkably high death rate produced by ARDS and shows virtually no improvement over mortality rates in earlier studies by Ashbaugh.

Bell confirmed the high mortality rate associated with ARDS and added to understanding of this process by assessing the influence of multisystem organ failure and infection in ARDS. This investigator looked at 84 patients with ARDS, including 37 survivors and 47 nonsurvivors on whom autopsies were performed. Extrapulmonary organ system failure occurred more frequently in nonsurvivors. The organ systems most commonly involved were the central nervous system, renal system, coagulation cascade, endocrine system, and gastrointestinal system. Infection was noted in 46 of 47 nonsurvivors but in only 23 of 37 survivors. Moreover, extrapulmonary organ failure was present in 64 of 69 infected patients but in only 7 of 15 noninfected patients. These data suggest that ARDS is more likely to result in death when severe infection and multisystem organ failure are present.

The studies show that the mortality rate from ARDS remains high. Death is more likely to result from infection producing sepsis syndrome and from multisystem organ failure than from respiratory failure itself. This is crucial to bear in mind. Most patients receive adequate oxygenation and ventilation with an FIO_2 level of 0.5 and positive end-expiratory pressure levels of 10 to 15 cm H_2O. These levels can be safely maintained until the underlying pathophysiologic process can be reversed. As Gillepsie has shown, the duration of mechanical ventilation is not related to survival.

Unfortunately, studies have failed to demonstrate other parameters that consistently correlate with survival in patients with ARDS. Fowler looked at clinical, cardiopulmonary, and demographic data in 88 patients at the outset of ARDS. The only factors he identified as significantly related to deaths were less than 10% band forms on the peripheral smear and acidemia secondary to metabolic acidosis. Although both these findings could certainly represent severe disease, neither would conclusively suggest at the time of admission that clinical deterioration was inevitable.

Other researchers have looked strictly at pulmonary parameters in attempting to identify potential survivors. Mancebo and Bell in separate studies looked at the influence of static compliance at the onset of symptoms. Neither found a significant correlation. Royston evaluated the permeability of the alveolar-capillary membrane by measuring the clearance of a radiolabeled low–molecular weight solute (^{99m}Tc-DTPA). Clearance of ^{99m}Tc-DTPA is increased in diseases, such as ARDS, that increase permeability of the pulmonary epithelium. However, Royston found that clearance of ^{99m}Tc-DTPA did not differentiate survivors from nonsurvivors. Nor did it differentiate between patients who were weaned from me-

chanical ventilation and those who were not. Thus at present it is not possible to look at pulmonary parameters at the onset of ARDS and determine who will survive.

CONCLUSION

In ARDS the physician is confronted with a syndrome that has a high mortality rate and few factors to predict survival. Clearly, ARDS without sepsis syndrome or multisystem organ failure should be treated aggressively. In patients in whom sepsis syndrome or multisystem organ failure develops, the mortality rate is considerably higher but not 100%. Furthermore, pulmonary function returns to normal in survivors of ARDS. Therefore it is reasonable to admit all patients with ARDS but without evidence of extrapulmonary failure to the ICU. If sepsis syndrome or multisystem organ failure develops and does not show signs of resolution within 72 hours, the physician should initiate discussion of withdrawing aggressive therapy.

Chronic Obstructive Pulmonary Disease

COPD is a particularly challenging disease because it is typified by progressive deterioration. Usually this deterioration is slow for many years and then accelerates over a relatively short period. The ICU physician sees the patient at a specific point in this continuum. In the early stages of COPD the prognosis is reasonably good, but it becomes progressively poorer. The physician needs to know the specific factors that influence the prognosis of COPD and which patients are most likely to survive and therefore benefit from the ICU.

One might hypothesize that pulmonary function tests should offer insight into this problem. Several authors have looked at the relationship between survival and pulmonary function as measured by forced expiratory volume in 1 second (FEV_1), forced vital capacity (FVC), and the FEV_1/FVC ratio. Unfortunately, some of these studies involved outpatients, some involved hospitalized patients, and the majority of patients did not require mechanical ventilation. Nevertheless, several of the studies suggest that patients with a more rapid decline of FEV_1 tend to have worse survival rates. This observation could be used at the time of ICU admission to identify patients who are in the terminal phase of COPD. A patient who received mechanical ventilation twice in the past 6 months, had clear signs of clinical deterioration during that time, and has a rapidly declining FEV_1 might no longer be a candidate for admission to the ICU.

There is one helpful study focusing on patients admitted to the ICU because of COPD. Kaelin retrospectively reviewed 35 patients requiring mechanical ventilation for COPD. Patients were divided into two groups: those surviving less than 6 months and those surviving more than 6 months. The author attempted unsuccessfully to identify predictors of 6-month survival available to the physician at the time of intubation. Three key parameters—results of pulmonary function tests, arterial blood gas concentrations at admission, and nutritional indexes (serum protein, albumin, and creatinine levels)—were similar in both groups. Only a multivariate analysis accounting for eight variables could identify with 78% accuracy the two groups of patients. On the basis of this analysis, however, 22% of survivors would still have been incorrectly classified as nonsurvivors. The single parameter that differed between the two subgroups was duration of mechanical ventilation, which was longer in patients surviving less than 6 months. This variable of course is not useful at the time of admission.

Further analysis of Kaelin's data provides useful information. Among patients surviving less than 6 months, the FVC at the time of admission was able to identify patients who died while receiving mechanical ventilation or within 10 days after extubation. An average FVC of 52% ± 9.3% predicted was noted for those who died during mechanical ventilation or within 10 days after extubation. For patients who survived up to 6 months following extubation, an average FVC of 71% ± 11.6% predicted was observed. This provides at least one criterion that can be used to identify patients receiving mechanical ventilation for COPD who have a poor chance of even short-term survival.

Finally, when patients do survive an exacerbation of COPD, the evolution of their disease is worth evaluating. Dardes studied 152 patients hospitalized for acute respiratory failure secondary to exacerbation of COPD. The author noted that 46 of 127 survivors were readmitted for additional episodes of respiratory failure. Of these patients, 16 were readmitted once, 17 twice, 4 three times, 1 five times, and 1 six times. Although the short-term prognosis of COPD is better than that of ARDS, the overall course is continued deterioration marked by frequent readmission.

CONCLUSION

The ICU physician is again faced with a lack of prognostic indicators available at the time a patient with COPD is admitted to the ICU. Among all the variables, FEV_1 appears to identify most reliably the patients with a potential for improvement. FVC may be useful in identifying patients without a reasonable chance at even short-term survival. Age has not been shown to correlate significantly with either survival or duration of mechanical ventilation. In survivors of earlier hospitalizations, the course is one of repeated exacerbations. Functional quality of life is an issue in survivors of COPD, whereas survivors of ARDS usually regain their baseline level of function. Therefore patients with exacerbations of COPD should be hospitalized in the ICU for most of the duration of their disease. However, during the terminal phase of COPD when FVC is rapidly declining and exacerbations are frequent, admission to the ICU may be inappropriate.

Pneumonia

The significance of pneumonia becomes obvious when it is recognized that (1) in critically ill patients, nosocomial pneumonia is the leading cause of death; (2) among hospitalized patients, nosocomial pneumonia has the highest mortality rate of all the nosocomial infections; and (3) although community-acquired pneumonia has a more favorable prognosis than nosocomial pneumonia, its mortality rate can exceed 50%. Woodhead retrospectively analyzed 50 patients admitted to the ICU with severe community-acquired pneumonia and found an overall mortality rate of 54%. The mortality rate from any type of pneumonia is high. This section discusses studies of both nosocomial and community-acquired pneumonia and attempts to identify factors that distinguish potential survivors from patients with only marginal chance for survival.

Community-acquired pneumonias, in particular pneumococcal pneumonias, have been the subject of several recent studies. In 1987 a prospective multicenter study to identify factors associated with poor prognosis was conducted in Great Britain. Using multivariate analysis, the authors found 10 factors to be associated with death. They believed the most useful to be age, confusion, leukocytosis, leukopenia, elevated blood urea nitrogen level, and diastolic hypertension. These findings have not yet been confirmed prospectively by other studies.

In addition to the preceding factors, bacteremia is associated with a poor prognosis in patients with pneumonia. Brewin evaluated 123 patients with pneumococcal pneumonia in whom the overall mortality rate was 8.9%. Only 7 (6.9%) of 109 nonbacteremic patients died, but 4 (28.6%) of 14 bacteremic patients died. Other authors have confirmed these findings and have identified other factors that suggest a poor prognosis in pneumococcal pneumonia. These include multilobar pneumonia, age of 60 years or greater, leukocyte count of 5000 cells/cu mm or less, and a preexisting chronic illness.

A high proportion of the total deaths occur within 24 hours of admission. For example, Austrian and Gold reported 19.5% and 31% mortality rates, respectively, for bacteremic pneumococcal pneumonia. Of these deaths, 36% and 27%, respectively, occurred within the first 24 hours. This suggests that factors ultimately responsible for the death of the patient are commonly present at the time of admission or shortly thereafter.

Nosocomial pneumonias are associated with an even higher mortality rate. Gram-negative pneumonias are the most common hospital-acquired pneumonias, which helps explain the high mortality rate. Stevens retrospectively evaluated 153 patients who were admitted to the ICU from other areas of the hospital for pneumonia or in whom pneumonia developed in the ICU. His analysis led him to define several subpopulations of patients. Patients with gram-positive pneumonia had a mortality rate of 5%, which is essentially the same as the mortality rate of patients without pneumonia (3.8%). When infections including both gram-positive and gram-negative pneumonias occurred, 22 (35%) of 63 patients died. Significantly, in a subgroup of 75 patients with *Pseudomonas* pneumonia, 53 (71%) died. Moreover, 33 of 53 patients taken from the original group of 153 died despite appropriate antibiotic therapy.

Given the high mortality rate associated with nosocomial pneumonia, Celis attempted to identify factors associated with a poor prognosis. He reported the following factors associated with a poor outcome: pneumonias resulting from one or more virulent organisms (such as *Pseudomonas,* other gram-negative bacilli, and *Staphylococcus aureus*), bilateral pneumonia, respiratory failure (PaO_2 less than 60 mm Hg or $PaCO_2$ greater than 50 mm Hg while breathing room air), age greater than 60 years, inappropriate antibiotic therapy, and an ultimately fatal underlying condition.

CONCLUSION

Several factors are associated with a poor prognosis in both community-acquired pneumonia and nosocomial pneumonia. The death rate varies from 15% to 30%, which, although considerable, is much less than the mortality rate of ARDS. The majority of patients with pneumonia should be admitted to the ICU. However, in some instances, particularly when the patient is elderly, the physician could reasonably argue against admission. In the case of community-acquired pneumonia, bacteremia, PaO_2 less than 60 mm Hg while breathing room air, and a severe underlying illness portend a poor prognosis. In the case of hospital-acquired pneumonia, bilateral involvement, PaO_2 of 50 mm Hg while breathing room air, and *Pseudomonas* or *Staphylococcus aureus* pneumonia are associated with a poor prognosis. Clinical research is being done on the manipulation of gastric pH to reduce the frequency of aspiration pneumonia in patients receiving mechanical ventilation. If this approach is successful, the incidence of nosocomial pneumonia in the ICU may decrease.

In summary, respiratory failure, especially resulting from ARDS and pneumonia, is a major cause of death in the ICU. Early predictors of survival in ARDS are unknown. Therefore, despite its high mortality rate, this disease should be treated initially in most instances. Exceptions are the presence of multisystem organ failure at admission, an underlying disease that is fatal in the relative short term, such as metastatic cancer, or a severely moribund baseline state, as an elderly, demented, nursing home patient might have. Patients with COPD usually overcome exacerbations, but despite a high rate of survival during the early phases of the illness, the natural history of this disease is a progressive deterioration. With each exacerbation the prognosis worsens. These patients must always be admitted to the ICU and treated aggressively until exacerbations become so frequent that aggressive therapy, in particular mechanical ventilation, no longer provides any real benefit. In this case the quality of life becomes so poor that mechanical ventilation is inappropriate. Factors associated with a high mortality rate from pneumonia are known. Although the mortality rate of pneumonia is significant, the majority of these patients improve. However, it seems reasonable to counsel against ICU admission for a patient who is older than 80 years, has bilateral gram-negative pneumonia, and is hypoxic while breathing room air.

Acute Renal Failure

The mortality rate for acute renal failure approaches 60%. However, the death rate varies according to the cause of renal failure. For example, dialysis has improved the prognosis of acute renal failure secondary to primary uncomplicated glomerulonephritis (mortality rate 24%) and secondary to an exacerbation of chronic renal failure (mortality rate 27%). On the other hand, the mortality rate in patients with acute renal failure secondary to acute tubular necrosis increased from 55% in the 1950s to 68% in the 1970s. This trend can be explained partly by the emergence of multisystem organ failure, often seen with acute tubular necrosis, as a significant cause of death.

Since the advent of dialysis, patients no longer die of renal failure per se. The most important cause of death in patients with renal failure is coexistent systemic illness and dysfunction of other organ systems. It is precisely because of these complications that many patients with acute renal failure are transferred to the ICU. This section explores the effects of organ system dysfunction on the prognosis of patients with acute renal failure. It concludes with recommendations concerning which patients should receive ICU care.

Infections are the most common complications in patients with acute renal failure. Studies suggest that infections are responsible for 30% to 72% of deaths in patients with renal failure. In a prospective evaluation of 276 patients with acute tubular necrosis, McMurray noted that infections were present in 74% of patients and were implicated in 54% of deaths. Gornik and Kjellstrand evaluated 50 patients with acute renal failure after surgery for aortic aneurysms and correlated decreased survival with either a temperature more than 100° Fahrenheit or a white blood cell count higher than 10,000/mm^3 2 weeks after the onset of renal failure. Thirty percent of these patients died of infection, and no patient with positive blood cultures while receiving antibiotics survived.

The infections most frequently associated with poor outcome are pulmonary. Reported rates of pneumonia or tracheobronchitis in patients with acute renal failure vary from 25%

to 50%, and overall, pulmonary infections have been reported to be responsible from 14% to 25% of deaths in these patients. In addition, gastrointestinal infections have been reported to worsen the prognosis of patients with acute renal failure. Peritonitis and intraabdominal abscess formation have been implicated in particular. Urinary tract infections, although common, do not affect the prognosis.

Thus severe infection, in particular sepsis, pulmonary infections, and gastrointestinal infections, worsens the prognosis of patients with acute renal failure. Certainly, denying ICU care to a patient with acute renal failure caused by sepsis is difficult. However, if this patient is elderly and shows no signs of improvement after several days of therapy, withdrawing aggressive therapy at that point might be appropriate. Several qualifications should be kept in mind when looking at these reports. Some of these studies were done more than 10 years ago. The patient populations include both ICU and non-ICU patients. Finally, these studies do not indicate whether the high rate of sepsis in these patients occurs because of iatrogenic factors or simply because the population is more critically ill and immunosuppressed. In light of advances in antibiotic therapy, the effect of infection on the outcome of patients with acute renal failure must be reevaluated. Moreover, ICU populations must be looked at specifically. Two recent studies failed to confirm that infection worsened the prognosis of patients with acute renal failure.

Certain noninfectious complications can also influence the prognosis of critically ill patients with acute renal failure. Bullock noted six factors that affect the death rate: age, urine flow at the time of discovery of renal failure, pulmonary complications, cardiovascular complications, jaundice, and hypercatabolism.

The effect of age on the prognosis of patients with acute renal failure is unclear. Several authors support the contention that age has a major influence on survival, whereas others show evidence to refute that finding. In support of a strong relationship between age and mortality rate, Bullock reported the following mortality rates in patients with acute renal failure: for ages 10 to 29, 60.7% mortality; for ages 30 to 59, 60.7%; for ages 60 to 79, 71.9%; and for ages 80 to 100, 78.8%. In a study by Kjellstrand, mortality rates were 25% for patients under age 10 and 70% for patients age 21 to 50. Consistent with these findings, McMurray reported that the mortality rate was 25% in patients under age 40 and increased steadily with advancing age. In contrast, Gornick, Hou, and Fisher did not find age to be a prognostic indicator in patients with acute renal failure.

Several studies have documented a high rate of cardiovascular complications in patients with acute renal failure. In Kumar's study myocardial infarctions accounted for 27% of deaths in patients with acute renal failure over the age of 70. Myocardial infarction was second only to infection as a cause of death in these patients. McMurray noted in his series that myocardial infarction occurred in 7% of patients. The average age of these patients was 64 years, in contrast to 51 years of age for patients without myocardial infarction. In the study by Bullock, 62.3% of patients with acute renal failure had cardiovascular complications, leading to an 81.9% mortality rate, or an increased risk of mortality of 3.37 as compared with patients without cardiovascular complications. Clearly, cardiovascular complications, particularly myocardial infarction, worsen the prognosis of patients with acute renal failure.

Pulmonary complications also increase the likelihood of death in patients with acute renal failure. In Bullock's study 54.1% of patients with acute renal failure also had pulmonary complications and the overall mortality rate of patients with dysfunction of these two organ systems was 87.2%. Bullock concluded that these patients had an increased risk of mortality of 8.22. Cameron studied 29 patients with acute renal failure requiring mechanical ventilation and observed a mortality rate of 76%. Pulmonary complications in a patient with acute renal failure portend a poor prognosis.

Terminal cirrhosis and fulminant hepatic failure have been shown to worsen the prognosis of patients with renal failure. Ring-Larsen studied the effect of liver disease on the prognosis of patients with renal failure. In that series the mortality rates were 88% in patients with cirrhosis and 71% in those without cirrhosis. Likewise, the mortality rates were 100% in patients with fulminant hepatic failure and 67% in those without hepatic failure. Bullock observed an 84.3% mortality rate in jaundiced individuals in his series of patients with acute renal failure. He concluded that patients with jaundice had a 4.06 greater risk of dying. Thus an easily recognizable clinical sign appears to correlate reliably with mortality.

Prospective data correlating the effects of hyperalimentation on the outcome of patients with renal failure are lacking. However, retrospective analysis suggests that hypercatabolic patients have worse prognoses than do patients receiving adequate caloric intake. Rainford looked at 352 patients with acute renal failure hospitalized over three decades. Survival increased from 48% to 58% to 71%, respectively, for the periods 1958 to 1964, 1965 to 1975, and 1976 to 1980. This correlated with increases in daily caloric intake recommended to critically ill patients over these periods from 1000 calories to 2000 calories to 3000 calories. Bartlett evaluated a series of 56 patients with acute renal failure following a surgical procedure. He noted a 37.5% survival rate in patients with a positive nitrogen balance but only a 9.4% survival rate in patients with a negative balance. These data suggest that survival in acute renal failure is improved by adequate nutrition. Conversely, it appears that acute renal failure in a severely malnourished patient is associated with a greater likelihood of death. However, the degree to which adequate hyperalimentation can reverse this situation is not clear. Much more prospective evaluation of this relationship must be done before reliable conclusions can be drawn. Nevertheless, it seems reasonable that a critically ill patient with acute renal failure, who has a poor baseline nutritional status, is at a higher risk of death than a comparable patient with a better nutritional status.

The type of renal failure has not been shown to influence prognosis. Toxic and ischemic renal failure alter survival similarly. Some authors contend that the degree of renal failure does influence outcome. In a series of 2262 patients with hospital-acquired renal insufficiency, Hou observed that the mortality rate for patients with a creatinine level of 3 mg/dl or higher was 64%, whereas it was only 15% in those with a creatinine level of less than 3 mg/dl. Several studies have shown that patients with nonoliguric renal failure have a better prognosis than those with oliguric renal failure.

CONCLUSION

A significant proportion of deaths among patients with acute renal failure result from infection or extrarenal organ system failure. The death rate increases with the extent of multisystem organ failure. McMurray's series indicates that when isolated renal failure is present, the survival rate is 90%, whereas when seven organ systems are dysfunctioning, the survival rate is as low as 25%.

Although more studies are needed in this area, patients with acute renal failure may not be reasonable candidates for admission to the

ICU if multisystem organ disease is present. Age has not been conclusively shown to be an independent risk factor for death in this group of patients and therefore should not be used independently to determine the appropriateness of either hemodialysis or admission to the ICU.

Infection and Multiple System Organ Failure

The preceding discussion makes it clear that infection and multiple system organ failure are major causes of mortality in critically ill patients. Sepsis and nosocomial pneumonia are, respectively, the first and second leading causes of death in the ICU. ARDS and multisystem organ failure often occur in association with nosocomial pneumonia and sepsis. Hence a sequence of events leads to irreversible deterioration and death.

As the data on infection are considered, the following points should be kept in mind. Most studies have documented a statistically significant association between death and sepsis. This is not the same as showing an independent causal relationship. Moreover, the definition of sepsis varies from one study to the next. Finally, authors may measure the incidence of infection differently. One method is to measure the total number of infections against the total number of patients discharged. The result, termed the "gross" infection rate, takes into account the possibility of multiple infections in an individual patient. A second method is to measure the number of infected patients against the total number of patients discharged. The result, termed the "true" infection rate, reflects the probability of a patient becoming infected during the hospital stay. Last, not all studies were performed on ICU patients. With these caveats, the various studies will be presented and conclusions will be suggested.

Sepsis is one of the most discouraging diseases to treat. The reported incidence in ICUs ranges from 0.2% to 19%. Unfortunately, most analyses of deaths caused by sepsis reflect overall hospital sepsis and not uniquely ICU sepsis. These studies suggest that the mortality rate ranges from 13% to 62%, with rates of approximately 40% reported most frequently. Kreger reviewed 612 episodes of gram-negative bacteremia spanning a 25-year period and observed an overall mortality rate of 35%. Closer inspection revealed that patients with rapidly fatal underlying diseases had a mortality rate of 40%, whereas those without an ultimately fatal disease had a 31% fatality rate. This observation underscores not only the degree of mortality produced by sepsis, but also the influence of host factors on the eventual outcome.

When sepsis produces shock, the prognosis is much poorer. Clinically apparent septic shock occurs in 10% to 16% of septic episodes. The mortality rate in septic shock varies from 60% to 90%. When hypotension occurs but clinical shock is not present, the mortality rate is approximately 44%. When sepsis is not complicated by either shock or hypotension, the mortality rate is only 9%. Septic shock or any type of hemodynamic instability produced by sepsis reduces the chance of survival.

Clearly, sepsis is a highly lethal disease, particularly when a gram-negative organism is involved. Nevertheless, not all patients with sepsis die. The state of health at the time of admission has been shown to influence the chance not only of becoming septic, but also of surviving sepsis. In addition, several studies have shown that polymicrobial sepsis produces a higher mortality rate than unimicrobial sepsis. Moreover, the development of septic shock markedly decreases the chances of survival. Most significantly, the development of multisystem organ failure radically alters the prognosis. Thus the physician can use several factors to identify patients at a higher risk of death from sepsis.

Associated with sepsis and the sepsis syndrome is multisystem organ failure (MSOF). Although the cause of MSOF is not precisely understood, it is apparent that severe infection initiates a process that compromises host defenses. This produces more invasive infection, altered peripheral metabolism, and hemodynamic instability. Some patients with MSOF can be stabilized with a combination of vasoactive drugs, mechanical ventilation, and hemodialysis, but in a vast number of cases, death ensues.

MSOF is defined as dysfunction of the cardiovascular, respiratory, renal, hemolytic, and neurologic systems. Knaus performed the most complete study of patients with this syndrome. He evaluated 5677 consecutive admissions to 19 ICUs in 13 hospitals. Organ systems were evaluated daily, and patients with MSOF were identified. The mortality rate increased linearly as the number of failing organ systems increased and as duration of organ system failure increased. For example, after 7 days of organ system failure, Knaus noted a 41% mortality rate for single-system failure, a 68% mortality rate for two-system failure, and a 100% mortality rate in the presence of three or more failing systems. One day of single-system failure produced a 22% mortality rate, and a single day of two- and three-system failure produced 52% and 80% mortality, respectively. Chang confirmed these results in a separate study.

Survival of patients with MSOF is related to its duration, the number of failing organ systems, and age. For example, in Knaus' study population, failure of three or more organ systems within the first 24 hours of admission resulted in more than a 90% mortality. But for the subpopulation of patients 65 years or older, the presence of only two failing organ systems limited chances for recovery. Of 188 patients 65 years or older with two-system failure, 61% did not survive. Therefore the patient with the greatest chance of surviving MSOF is less than 65 years of age, has not more than two failing organ systems, and receives appropriate treatment early in the course of MSOF.

CONCLUSION

Gram-negative sepsis is most commonly responsible for death from sepsis syndrome. The elderly individual is particularly at risk. Polymicrobial sepsis results in a higher mortality rate than unimicrobial sepsis. Underlying host factors appear to play a role in likelihood of fatality. When sepsis produces septic shock, the prognosis becomes much worse. The main risk in sepsis and septic shock is the development of MSOF. The risk of death from MSOF is related to the number of organ systems involved, the duration of organ system failure, and the patient's age. For patients less than 65 years of age, three or more dysfunctioning organ systems are often necessary to result in death, whereas in patients more than 65 years of age the presence of only two failed organ systems decreases the chance for recovery. Therefore, in many situations, not admitting patients greater than 80 years of age to the ICU is appropriate if respiratory failure and one other failing organ system are present. In many instances, however, MSOF develops after the patient is admitted to the ICU, instead of being the reason for admission. In this situation the physician must determine whether the patient has a reasonable chance of survival and could benefit from continued aggressive therapy.

Coronary Artery Disease

Some of the most significant advances in medicine have come in the treatment of coronary artery disease. Thrombolytic agents, per-

cutaneous transcutaneous balloon angioplasty, improved surgical techniques, heart transplantation and artificial hearts have all improved the prognosis of patients with coronary artery disease. All patients with manifestations of active coronary artery disease should of course be admitted to the hospital. However, only some patients with coronary artery disease require intensive care.

In most hospitals patients with coronary artery disease can be admitted to a coronary care unit (CCU) or ICU, where they will receive intensive care; to a cardiac step-down unit; or to a medical floor equipped for telemetry. The factor determining appropriate placement is the degree of hemodynamic instability at the time of initial evaluation, or the potential for it to occur shortly after admission. Therefore the physician needs indexes for estimating the potential for hemodynamic instability.

To determine the most appropriate placement for a patient with coronary artery disease, the physician must know the nature and duration of the chest pain, as well as electrocardiographic (EKG) changes. Goldman developed a logic tree, a sequence of questions to identify which patients with chest pain are at high risk of acute myocardial infarction and therefore should be admitted to the ICU. The decision tree for classification of acute chest pain is shown in Table 1–4. Goldman's system takes into account such factors as the nature and duration of the chest pain, accompanying signs, EKG changes, age, and previous history. This logic tree is based on a model derived from data collected on 428 patients in an emergency room. The model was validated on 357 other patients seen in an emergency room. In a subsequent study Goldman demonstrated that use of this system is safe and cost effective. Despite this, the system has not gained widespread use.

Second, the risk of hemodynamic instability associated with specific EKG changes should be noted. Brush reported on 469 patients who were admitted to the ICU from the emergency department for observation to rule out myocardial infarction. The goal of the study was to evaluate the EKG as a predictive tool for ventricular fibrillation, sustained ventricular tachycardia, or heart block. A positive EKG was defined as evidence of acute myocardial infarction, acute ischemia, left ventricular strain, ventricular tachycardia, or heart block. In patients with a positive EKG by these criteria, ventricular fibrillation, sustained ventricular tachycardia, or heart block developed in 14% of the cases, whereas these conditions occurred in

TABLE 1–4. Decision Tree for Classification of Acute Chest Pain

1. Does the emergency room ECG show ST elevation or a Q wave that may be new?	Yes = MI	No = Go to 2
2. Did the present pain or episodes of recurrent pain begin 42 or more hours ago?	Yes = Go to 4	No = Go to 3
3. Is the pain primarily in the chest but radiating into the shoulder, neck, or arms?	Yes = Go to 5	No = Go to 6
4. Does the emergency room ECG show ST or T changes of ischemia or strain that may be new?	Yes = MI	No = Not MI
5. Does chest pressure produce the pain?	Yes = Not MI	No = Go to 9
6. Is the present pain either similar to but worse than previously diagnosed angina, or is it the same pain as a previously diagnosed MI?	Yes = MI	No = Go to 7
7. Was the chest pain associated with diaphoresis?	Yes = Go to 8	No = Not MI
8. Is the patient 70 years old or older?	Yes = MI	No = Not MI
9. Is the patient 40 years old or older?	Yes = Go to 10	No = Not MI
10. Was this same pain previously diagnosed as angina?	Yes = Go to 12	No = Go to 11
11. Is the pain primarily in the chest but radiating to the left shoulder?	Yes = MI	No = Go to 13
12. Did the present pain or episode of recurrent pain begin 10 or more hours ago?	Yes = MI	No = Not MI
13. Is the patient 50 years of age or older?	Yes = MI	No = Not MI

MI = Myocardial infarction.
From Davis RE: Curr Probl Crit Care 1989;3(4): 641.

only 0.6% of patients with a normal EKG. In addition, 18% of patients with a positive EKG required pulmonary artery catheters, whereas only 4% of patients with a normal EKG did. Finally, 3% of patients with a positive EKG in the emergency department required the assistance of an intraaortic balloon pump, in contrast to only 0.6% of patients with a normal EKG. These data demonstrate the prognostic capabilities of the initial EKG. They suggest that patients with one of the findings mentioned deserve to be placed in an ICU. They also suggest that patients admitted for an evaluation of chest pain, but with a normal EKG, are at less risk for complications that require immediate treatment. If these patients' chest pain resolves and the EKG remains normal, they could safely be placed in an intermediate step-down unit.

The logic tree for chest pain evaluation and the EKG, if used together, could potentially identify patients at risk for a myocardial infarction or complications. Use of these systems could reduce unnecessary admissions to the ICU.

CONCLUSION

Patients with coronary artery disease and a high potential for complications that can lead to hemodynamic instability should be placed in the ICU. To identify patients at risk for serious complications, the physician must ascertain the nature and duration of the chest pain, as well as the nature of EKG changes. A detailed history

is necessary to characterize the chest pain. To standardize the questions that should be included in the medical history, Goldman devised a logic tree, which has proved useful in identifying patients with coronary disease. Brush demonstrated that the EKG can be used to identify patients with coronary disease who are at risk for serious complications that could best be diagnosed and treated in the ICU. Patients at low risk for complications can often safely be monitored outside the ICU, in an intermediate care setting or another telemetry area.

Acquired Immunodeficiency Syndrome and Respiratory Failure

The acquired immunodeficiency syndrome (AIDS) is a unique disease because it is still essentially fatal. However, recent medical advances coupled with earlier diagnosis have extended the duration of survival in many AIDS patients. In the past, most experts questioned the usefulness of placing these patients in the ICU because of the inevitable and often rapid death associated with AIDS. However, in light of increased survival times following diagnosis, this issue merits reevaluation. Therefore respiratory failure in AIDS patients is briefly discussed.

The most common cause of respiratory failure in patients with AIDS is *Pneumocystis carinii* pneumonia (PCP). The reported mortality rates of AIDS patients with acute respiratory failure from PCP have varied from 84% to 100%.

However, Friedman recently conducted a prospective study of 58 patients with AIDS who required positive-pressure ventilation for acute respiratory failure. In 33 of these patients PCP was a cause of acute respiratory failure. Twelve (36%) of these 33 patients survived. Moreover, the mean duration of survival after discharge from the hospital was 7.9 ± 1.8 months, which compares favorably with other reports. The reason for improved survival in this group of patients is unclear. Treatment was the same as in other studies, with trimethoprim-sulfamethoxazole and pentamidine as initial therapy. The authors suggested that increasing awareness of the symptoms of PCP may cause patients to seek professional help earlier. Friedman refuted some of the conclusions of earlier authors that "patients with AIDS who develop respiratory failure would benefit maximally by not undergoing mechanical ventilation or other invasive therapies." They concluded, in fact, that when acute respiratory failure develops in patients with AIDS and PCP, the potential benefits of intensive care and mechanical ventilation should be offered.

Conclusion

Admission to the ICU now appears appropriate for AIDS patients with acute respiratory failure secondary to PCP. Friedman's findings should prompt further study. If they are supported by other authors, the current philosophy regarding AIDS patients in the ICU will change dramatically.

Nontraumatic Coma

Most patients with nontraumatic coma are admitted to the ICU because they require close monitoring or mechanical ventilation. Since overall prognosis is poor in this group of patients, prognostic factors that could help physicians judge the usefulness of the ICU are needed. Unfortunately, few studies exist in this area.

Levy carried out a detailed prospective study of the prognosis of patients with various types of nontraumatic coma. For 12 months he followed 500 U.S. and British patients who were admitted to hospitals for nontraumatic coma. Serial neurologic evaluations were performed to evaluate clinical changes over time. Sixty-one percent of patients died without recovery from the initial coma, 12% never improved beyond a vegetative state, and 11% regained consciousness but remained dependent on others for daily activities. Only 81 (16%) led an independent life at some point during the first year.

Levy found no relationship between age and functional recovery. He observed the highest recovery rates in patients with hepatic coma or coma secondary to other metabolic causes. The lowest recovery rates were in patients with coma secondary to subarachnoid hemorrhages and cerebrovascular accidents. Early clinical signs of brainstem dysfunction correlated strongly with poor prognosis. Absence of at least two reflexes among corneal, vestibular, or oculomotor reflexes correlated with a poor prognosis in 119 of 120 patients. Early evidence of forebrain dysfunction correlated much less with outcome. Chances for recovery diminished as length of coma increased.

Levy's findings suggest that intensive care may not be useful for patients with nontraumatic coma. Nevertheless, the decision to forego life-sustaining therapy at an early stage in these patients is often difficult. Their disease is commonly limited to the central nervous system. Early in the clinical course the hope is that if the brain recovers, the patient will improve. Thus the tendency is to initiate intensive diagnostic and therapeutic measures.

The usefulness of aggressive therapy in nontraumatic coma is unproven. An earlier report by Levy and other investigators, based on the first 310 patients enrolled in the analysis just described, looked at outcome after 1 month in the U.S. and British populations separately. British patients underwent fewer diagnostic and therapeutic procedures and were less commonly given mechanical ventilation. Understandably, 71% of British patients died within 3 days, whereas only 46% of U.S. patients died within this period. Despite this, the 1-month recovery rate in the two countries was equal. This suggests that many patients in the United States with nontraumatic coma are receiving aggressive therapy that simply delays an inevitable death.

Conclusion

Based on Levy's study, it appears that patients with more than one sign of brainstem dysfunction have a poorer prognosis than other patients with nontraumatic coma. Many of these patients do not profit from prolonged periods of mechanical ventilation or monitoring in the ICU. On the other hand, long-term outcome varies in patients with forebrain dysfunction, and it is therefore difficult to determine which patients will benefit from the ICU. These patients should be admitted and observed in the ICU for longer periods. Therapy can ultimately be continued or withdrawn, based on clinical evolution. Finally, patients with coma of metabolic origin have the best prognosis and should always be placed in the ICU. More studies need to be done in the area of nontraumatic coma, and investigators must delineate criteria that will allow physicians to initiate intensive care in a setting that has reasonable potential for a successful outcome.

SEVERITY-OF-DISEASE SCORING SYSTEMS

The preceding discussion has identified the major syndromes and diseases most frequently encountered in the ICU. Mortality statistics have been reviewed, and specific variables that would allow prediction of the risk of death have been considered. This information may permit identification of patients who would benefit from placement in an ICU and of patients who would die despite placement in the ICU.

This issue has been settled to a limited degree. In many situations, however, even though mortality rates for a given disease are high, no specific prognostic indicators exist that allow a separation of the probable survivors from those who will die. Clearly, in many situations, it is difficult to identify at an early stage those individuals who will not survive.

Severity-of-disease scoring systems have recently been developed. These scoring systems use diagnostic, clinical, and laboratory criteria to assign scores that reflect severity of disease. In addition, the scoring systems assign an estimated risk of death to each patient and then compute an estimated risk of death for the entire ICU population. It should be emphasized that none of these scoring systems is intended to be an absolute indicator of risk of death for individual patients. However, the physician can use this information in conjunction with clinical evaluation and information about the mortality statistics of the disease in question to more objectively estimate a patient's prognosis.

Three prognostic scoring systems have been used and extensively evaluated: the Acute Physiology and Chronic Health Evaluation (APACHE) system, the Mortality Prediction Model (MPM), and the Therapeutic Intervention Scoring System (TISS).

Acute Physiology and Chronic Health Evaluation

The most widely employed scoring system is the APACHE system, which initially was published by Knaus and associates in 1981. Several publications have confirmed the reliability of this scoring system. The APACHE system is based on three components: type of disease or diagnosis, acute physiologic derangements, and long-term health. For each patient, APACHE computes an acute physiology score (APS), which reflects physiologic derangement, and an APACHE score, which incorporates all three components mentioned previously and reflects the overall status of the patient. The higher the scores, the sicker the patient. APACHE is intended to establish an estimate of the patient's severity of disease on the first day of hospitalization. Therefore APACHE data are collected after 24 hours of hospitalization and the most abnormal physiologic values are used to compute the APS. A predicted risk of death for individual patients, as well as for the entire population of patients entered into the program, is then computed. Table 1–5 presents an overview of the APACHE system.

APACHE classifies postoperative admissions and nonoperative admissions separately. The specific diagnostic categories used by APACHE are shown in Table 1–6. If none of these diagnostic categories permits adequate classification of a patient, the major organ system responsible for the patient's illness is used for classification (Table 1–6).

Long-term health is measured by the presence or absence of comorbidities. Positive comorbidity is defined as the presence of a severe preexisting illness or a severely immunocompromised state. A severe preexisting illness is defined as a history of severe chronic insufficiency of the gastrointestinal, cardiovascular, renal, or respiratory system. The existence of a severely immunocompromised state is defined by one of the following: (1) the administration of high-dose methylprednisone (greater than 0.3 mg/kg/d) or its equivalent for 6 months or longer, (2) active radiotherapy or chemotherapy within 1 year of admission, (3) a documented immunohumoral or cellular immune deficiency, or (4) radiotherapy or chemotherapy at any time in the past for Hodgkin's disease or non-Hodgkin's lymphoma.

TABLE 1–5. APACHE II Severity of Disease Classification System

PHYSIOLOGIC VARIABLE	HIGH ABNORMAL RANGE					LOW ABNORMAL RANGE			
	+4	+3	+2	+1	0	+1	+2	+3	+4
TEMPERATURE—rectal (°C)	≥41°	39°-40.9°		38.5°-38.9°	36°-38.4°	34°-35.9°	32°-33.9°	30°-31.9°	≤29.9°
MEAN ARTERIAL PRESSURE—mm Hg	≥160	130-159	110-129		70-109		50-69		≤49
HEART RATE (ventricular response)	≥180	140-179	110-139		70-109		55-69	40-54	≤39
RESPIRATORY RATE— (non-ventilated or ventilated)	≥50	35-49		25-34	12-24	10-11	6-9		≤5
OXYGENATION: A-aDO$_2$ or PaO$_2$ (mm Hg) a. FiO$_2$ ≥0.5 record A-aDO$_2$	≥500	350-499	200-349		<200				
b. FiO$_2$ ≥0.5 record only PaO$_2$				PO$_2$ >70	PO$_2$ 61-70		PO$_2$ 55-60	PO$_2$ <55	
ARTERIAL pH	≥7.7	7.6-7.69		7.5-7.59	7.33-7.49		7.25-7.32	7.15-7.24	<7.15
SERUM SODIUM (mMol/L)	≥180	160-179	155-159	150-154	130-149		120-129	111-119	≤110
SERUM POTASSIUM (mMol/L)	≥7	6-6.9		5.5-5.9	3.5-5.4	3-3.4	2.5-2.9		<2.5
SERUM CREATININE (mg/100 ml) (Double point score for **acute** renal failure)	≥3.5	2-3.4	1.5-1.9		0.6-1.4		<0.6		
HEMATOCRIT (%)	≥60		50-59.9	46-49.9	30-45.9		20-29.9		<20
WHITE BLOOD COUNT (total/mm3) (in 1,000s)	≥40		20-39.9	15-19.9	3-14.9		1-2.9		<1
GLASGOW COMA SCORE (GCS): Score = 15 minus actual GCS									
A Total ACUTE PHYSIOLOGY SCORE (APS): Sum of the 12 individual variable points									
Serum HCO$_3$ (venous-mMol/L) [Not preferred, use if no ABGs]	≥52	41-51.9		32-40.9	22-31.9		18-21.9	15-17.9	<15

B AGE POINTS
Assign points to age as follows:

AGE (ys)	Points
≤44	0
45-54	2
55-64	3
65-74	5
≥75	6

C CHRONIC HEALTH POINTS
If the patient has a history of severe organ system insufficiency or is immunocompromised assign points as follows:
a. for nonoperative or emergency postoperative patients—5 points
or
b. for elective postoperative patients—2 points

DEFINITIONS
Organ insufficiency or immunocompromised state must have been evident prior to this hospital admission and must conform to the following criteria:
LIVER: Biopsy proven cirrhosis and documented portal hypertension; episodes of past upper GI bleeding attributed to portal hypertension; or prior episodes of hepatic failure/encephalopathy/coma.

CARDIOVASCULAR: New York Heart Association Class IV.
RESPIRATORY: chronic restrictive, obstructive, or vascular disease resulting in severe exercise restriction, i.e., unable to climb stairs or perform household duties; or documented chronic hypoxia, hypercapnia, secondary polycythemia, severe pulmonary hypertension (>40mmHg), or respirator dependency.
RENAL: Receiving chronic dialysis.
IMMUNOCOMPROMISED: The patient has received therapy that suppresses resistance to infection, e.g., immuno-suppression, chemotherapy, radiation, long term or recent high dose steroids, or has a disease that is sufficiently advanced to suppress resistance to infection, e.g., leukemia, lymphoma, AIDS.

APACHE II SCORE
Sum of *A* + *B* + *C*
A, APS points _____
B, Age points _____
C, Chronic health points _____
Total APACHE II _____

From Knaus WA, Draper EA, Wagner DP, Zimmerman JE: Crit Care Med 1985;13:818-828.

TABLE 1–6. Factors in APACHE System Used to Predict Risk of Mortality in an Individual Patient

Diagnostic Categories

Postoperative Admissions

Cardiovascular
  Chronic cardiovascular disease
  Peripheral vascular disease
  Heart valve surgery
  Sepsis (any etiology)
  Hemorrhagic shock
  Post cardiac arrest
Trauma
  Multiple trauma
  Head trauma
Respiratory
  Thoracic surgery for neoplasm
  Post respiratory arrest
  Respiratory insufficiency after surgery
Gastrointestinal
  Gastrointestinal bleeding
  Gastrointestinal surgery for neoplasm
  Gastrointestinal perforation/obstruction
Renal
  Renal surgery for neoplasm
  Renal transplant surgery
Neurologic
  Craniotomy for ICH, SDH, SAH
  Craniotomy for neoplasm
  Laminectomy or spinal surgery

Nonoperative Admissions

Respiratory insufficiency
  Asthma, allergy
  Chronic obstructive pulmonary disease
  Pulmonary edema (noncardiac)
  Respiratory infection
  Respiratory neoplasm
  Post respiratory arrest
  Pulmonary embolus
  Aspiration, poisoning, toxic reaction
Cardiovascular insufficiency
  Hypertension
  Congestive heart failure
  Hemorrhagic shock, hypovolemia
  Coronary artery disease
  Sepsis (any etiology)
  Post cardiac arrest
  Dissecting thoracic, abdominal aneurysm
  Rhythm disturbance
Trauma
  Multiple trauma
  Head trauma
Neurologic failure
  Seizure disorder
  ICH, SDH, SAH
Other
  Self drug overdose
  Diabetic ketoacidosis
  Gastrointestinal bleeding

Organ Systems for Classifying Patients in Absence of an Appropriate Diagnostic Category

Neurologic
Cardiovascular
Respiratory
Gastrointestinal
Renal
Hematologic
Metabolic

12 Physiologic Variables

Temperature	Oxygenation	Serum creatinine
Mean arterial pressure	Arterial pH	Hematocrit
Heart rate	Serum sodium	White blood cell count
Respiratory rate	Serum potassium	Glasgow Coma Score

Equation to Predict Risk of Mortality

$$L_N (R/1 - R) = -3.517 + (\text{APACHE II} \times 0.146 + S + D)$$

where
  R = Risk of hospital death
  S = Additional risk imposed by emergency surgery
  D = Risk (+ or −) imposed by specific disease

ICH, Intracranial hemorrhage; *SDH*, subdural hemorrhage, *SAH*, subarachnoid hemorrhage.

Physiologic reserve is determined by measurement of variables thought to best correlate with overall stability or instability. These variables were chosen by a multidisciplinary panel of experts in critical care medicine. Relative weights are assigned to the variables, depending on their perceived influence on outcome.

The original APS system included 34 variables, and although its efficacy was validated, it proved cumbersome for data collectors. Therefore Knaus developed APACHE II in 1985. This version uses 12 physiologic variables, which are shown in Table 1–6, plus age to determine APS. APACHE II has been validated by applications to several patient populations.

All the information recorded is used to compute an APACHE score. APACHE scores are based on diagnosis, chronic health status, and the APS. Therefore they reflect the patient's overall status. A predicted risk of death for each patient and a predicted mortality rate for the entire population of patients are then computed.

APACHE uses the equation shown in Table 1–6 to predict the risk of death in an individual patient. This equation was derived through multivariate logistic regression analysis of APACHE II data. Thus predicted risk of death is based on the APACHE score, the diagnosis, and whether the patient undergoes emergency surgery. Under the APACHE system the predicted individual death rate is based on a decision criterion of 0.50. Any patient with an estimated risk of death greater than 0.50 is simply predicted to die, without being assigned a specific risk. Thus no patient can be assigned a probability of death of 1.0. In the original validation study of APACHE II, 5030 consecutive ICU admissions from 13 ICUs were evaluated. A direct relation between APACHE II scores and observed deaths was observed. The decision criterion of 0.50 was used to compare observed and predicted death rates. The positive predictive value of APACHE was 69.9%; that is, 69.9% of the patients who were predicted to die actually died.

The APACHE II system has been validated in several studies, including validation outside the institution where the system was devised. Others have been able to use the APACHE system with as much success as its creators. Proven reliability is therefore a considerable strength of the APACHE system. Because of this, APACHE is the most widely used ICU severity-of-disease scoring system.

Certain aspects of APACHE can be criticized. As noted previously, APACHE requires that one diagnosis be accorded each patient. This is often difficult with ICU patients, who frequently have more than one organ system involved.

A final potential problem with APACHE II is data collection. Although APACHE II is a streamlined version of the original system, data collection can be time consuming and ideally is the sole function of a single individual.

APACHE is a validated severity-of-disease scoring system. It provides a reliable measure of severity of disease and can therefore dependably confirm a physician's evaluation of a critically ill patient. It is also a reliable predictor of death for groups of ICU patients,

and although intended for groups of patients, it can provide useful information concerning an individual patient's risk of death. APACHE II can be used in conjunction with bedside patient analysis and general information concerning a patient's disease to evaluate the appropriateness of an admission to the ICU.

Mortality Prediction Model

The second most widely used and studied scoring system in the United States is the Mortality Prediction Model (MPM). This program was developed by Teres and associates, who used statistical analysis to select variables that correlated best with mortality. Data were collected on 755 consecutive admissions to a single ICU. The authors recorded a total of 137 variables that covered (1) demographics; (2) information on prior ICU admissions; (3) specific organ system failures; (4) measures of functional status; (5) cancer-related variables; (6) arterial blood gases; (7) renal, neurologic, and respiratory variables; and (8) some treatment variables such as concentration of inspired oxygen and units of blood transfused. A multiple linear regression model was then used to determine which of these variables strongly correlated with survival and death. Each variable was assigned a relative weight, depending on its degree of correlation with mortality. The initial analysis is based on admission data. In this way a risk of death that is totally independent of any treatment is established. Although MPM computes a risk of death at the time of admission, it does not establish a severity-of-disease score per se. MPM has been validated at 14 ICUs in the United States.

The MPM admission analysis includes 12 variables, which are shown in Table 1–7 along with the possible responses provided by the program.

MPM assigns every patient a risk of mortality ranging from 0.0 to 1.0. Admission MPM was found to conform to observed data by goodness-of-fit testing ($p = 0.53$). Through use of the traditional approach to model classification employing a 0.5 decision criterion, MPM correctly classified 87% of the patients at admission in the validation study. The general form of the MLR model used to denote probability of death is shown in Table 1–7.

MPM is based on statistical modeling. This system contrasts with the APACHE II model, which employs the subjective opinion of experts to identify and assign relative weights to variables that influence outcome.

TABLE 1–7. Factors in Mortality Prediction Model (MPM)

12 Variables and Possible Responses Used to Predict Risk of Mortality in an Individual Patient

Variables	*Responses*
Presence of coma or deep stupor	Yes or no
Type of admission	Elective or emergency
Cardiopulmonary compression prior to ICU admission	Yes or no
Cancer as part of the problem	Yes or no
History of chronic renal failure	Yes or no
Probable infection	Yes or no
Age	
Previous ICU admission within past 6 months	Yes or no
Heart rate at ICU admission	
Surgical service at ICU admission	Yes or no
Systolic blood pressure admission	
Square of systolic blood pressure	

14 Variables Used by MPM 24-hour Analysis

Presence of coma or deep stupor
Cancer as part of problem
Emergency admission
Prothrombin time greater than 3 s above laboratory standard
Probable shock during first 24 h
Urine output less than 150 ml in any 8-h period
Infection confirmed
Pao_2 less than 60 mm Hg
Fio_2 greater than 0.50
Creatinine greater than 2 mg/dl
Age
Hours of mechanical ventilation
Number of IV lines
Surgical service

11 Variables Used by MPM 48-hour Analysis

Presence of coma or deep stupor
Urine output less than 150 ml in any 8-h period of day 2
Presence of coma or stupor at admission
Emergency admission
Prothrombin time greater than 3 s above laboratory standard
Fio_2 greater than 0.50 during day 2
Cancer as part of problem
Infection confirmed at 48 h
Age
Total hours of mechanical ventilation in ICU
Total hours of continuous IV vasoactive drug therapy

General Form of Multiple Linear Regression Model

$$Pr\ (Y = \mid 1X_1, X_2,....X_k\ ) = \frac{e\ (B_0 + B_1X_1 + B_2X_2 +...+ B_kX_k)}{1 + e\ (B_0 + B_1X_1 + B_2X_2 +...+ B_kX_k)}$$

where $Pr\ (Y = \mid 1\ X_1, X_2,...,X_k$ denotes the probability that a patient with values of the condition and treatment variables equal to $X_1, X_2,...X_k$ will die (i.e., $Y = 1$).

In addition, MPM allows a prediction of death immediately after admission. The APACHE model, on the other hand, bases its score and predictions on data obtained over the initial 24 hours of hospitalization. Thus MPM allows the physician to obtain a risk of death virtually as the patient is brought into the ICU.

Finally, MPM provides for reevaluation of the patient's status at 24 and 48 hours. The variables used to score patients at these intervals have also been selected through statistical analysis. Significantly, these sets of variables differ in

some respects from the set of variables used at admission. In this way trends in patient status can be documented. A 72-hour model is being formulated. The MPM 24-hour analysis, which includes 14 variables, and the MPM 48-hour analysis, which includes 11 variables, are shown in Table 1–7.

In addition, an MPM "overtime" model (MPM OT) is being tested. This model evaluates trends in the probabilities of death computed by MPM (0), MPM (24), and MPM (48) and formulates an overall probability of survival

TABLE 1–8.   Description of ICU Active Treatment, ICU Monitoring, and Standard Care Tasks

Active Treatment — ICU	Standard Care — Floor Care
4 Point	*4 Point*
Cardiac arrest and/or countershock within past 48 h	Peritoneal dialysis
Controlled ventilation with or without PEEP	Platelet transfusion
Controlled ventilation with intermittent or continuous muscle relaxants	*3 Point*
Balloon tamponade of varices	Central IV hyperalimentation (includes renal, cardiac, hepatic failure fluid)
Continuous arterial infusion	Chest tubes
Atrial and/or ventricular pacing	Blind intratracheal suctioning
Hemodialysis in unstable patient	Multiple blood gas, bleeding, and/or STAT studies (>4/shift)
Induced hypothermia	Complex metabolic balance (frequent intake and output)
Pressure-activated blood infusion	Frequent infusions of blood products (>5 units/24 h)
G-suit	Bolus IV medication (nonscheduled)
IABA (intra-aortic balloon assist)	Hypothermia blanket
Emergency operative procedures (within past 24 h)	Acute digitalization — within 48 h
Lavage of acute GI bleeding	Emergency thora-, para-, or pericardio-centesis
Emergency endoscopy or bronchoscopy	Active anticoagulation (initial 48 h)
Vasoactive drug infusion (>1 drug)	Phlebotomy for volume overload
	Coverage with more than two antibiotics
3 Point	Complicated orthopedic traction
Intermittent mandatory ventilation (IMV) or assisted ventilation	*2 Point*
Continuous positive airway pressure (CPAP)	CVP (central venous pressure)
Concentrated K⁺ infusion via central catheter	Two peripheral IV catheters
Nasotracheal or orotracheal intubation	Spontaneous respiration via endotracheal tube or tracheostomy (T-piece or trach mask)
Complex metabolic balance (frequent intake and output)	GI feedings
Vasoactive drug infusion (1 drug)	Parenteral chemotherapy
Continuous antiarrhythmia infusions	Multiple dressing changes
Cardioversion for arrhythmia (not defibrillation)	Pitressin infusion
Active diuresis for fluid overload or cerebral edema	*1 Point*
Active Rx for metabolic alkalosis	One peripheral IV catheter
Active Rx for metabolic acidosis	Chronic anticoagulation
Rx of seizures or metabolic encephalopathy (within 48 h of onset)	Standard intake and output (q 24 h)
	STAT blood tests
2 Point	Intermittent scheduled IV medications
Hemodialysis–stable patient	Routine dressing changes
Fresh tracheostomy (less than 48 h)	Standard orthopedic traction
Replacement of excess fluid loss	Tracheostomy care
	Decubitus ulcer
Monitoring — ICU	Urinary catheter
4 Point	Supplemental oxygen (nasal or mask)
Pulmonary artery catheter	IV antibiotics (2 or less)
Intracranial pressure monitoring	Chest physiotherapy
	Extensive irrigations, packings or debridement of wounds, fistula or colostomy
3 Point	GI decompression
Pacemaker on standby	Peripheral hyperalimentation/Intralipid therapy
Arterial line	
Measurement of cardiac output by any method	
2 Point	
ECG monitoring	
Hourly neuro vital signs	

From Cullen DJ, Nemeskal AR: Therapeutic intervention scoring system (TISS). Probl Crit Care 1989; 3(4): 550–551.

at 48 hours based on these trends. The initial evaluation of MPM (OT) demonstrated that decreasing probabilities of survival based on MPM (0), MPM (24), and MPM (48) led to an MPM (OT) probability of death that was higher than the MPM (48) probability of death. Therefore this model accounts for the possibility that in patients with worsening trends over the first 48 hours of admission, the overall effect on prognosis may in fact be greater than data from any single 24-hour period might suggest. This model has been evaluated only on a single cohort of 948 patients in a single ICU, so its ultimate validity remains to be proved.

Nevertheless, it adds to severity-of-disease scoring systems a dynamic component that conceptually appears logical.

MPM is a validated severity-of-disease scoring system. It establishes a risk of death at admission, as well as at 24 and 48 hours. It is generally as accurate a predictor of patient outcome as APACHE. Furthermore, data collection is simpler with this scoring system.

Therapeutic Index Scoring System

The Therapeutic Index Scoring System (TISS) was developed in 1974 by Cullen and associates and is the oldest severity-of-disease scoring system. TISS is composed of 76 monitoring and therapeutic interventions. Each modality is assigned a weighted score, ranging from 1 to 4, depending on the intensity of intervention. Points are totaled, and a TISS score is obtained. Table 1–8 shows the components of TISS and the weighted score for each component. Patients can be stratified into one of four classes based on the number of TISS points. Table 1-9 indicates the mean number of points thought to best represent the various TISS classes.

TISS is based on the premise that, regardless of the diagnosis, the amount of therapy required reflects the degree of physiologic impairment. TISS scores are not used to predict outcome per se. However, trends in TISS scores over the first 3 days in the ICU correlate well with survival. If TISS scores do not improve by the third day, the likelihood of death increases.

TISS is now used most frequently in conjunction with the APACHE system. Each TISS modality is assigned to one of three categories: active therapy, ICU monitoring, or standard floor care. Any patient receiving two or more modalities assigned to active therapy is classified by APACHE as an active patient. Other patients are classified as monitor patients and are designated by APACHE as either high-risk or low-risk monitor patients. This aspect of APACHE is discussed in more detail later in this chapter.

In summary, TISS scores reflect quantity of therapy and monitoring. TISS and APACHE can therefore be used to evaluate concordance between severity of illness and quantity of therapy. In addition, TISS scores identify those patients requiring monitoring only. It will be seen in the next section how APACHE is able to differentiate high-risk monitor patients from low-risk monitor patients.

TABLE 1–9. Mean Number of TISS Points Thought to Best Represent Various TISS Classes

43 points	Class IV	Physiologically unstable
23 points	Class III	Relatively stable physiologically but requires intensive nursing care
11 points	Class II	Requires intensive monitoring to detect potential catastrophes, but no therapy
5 points	Class I	Does not require intensive therapy for any reason

CONCLUSION

Three severity-of-disease scoring systems are reviewed. APACHE II has been validated most extensively and is used most commonly. It is reliable and can be used with confidence. However, it is time consuming, and to be effective, it requires one designated person dedicated to collecting the data. Most validation of APACHE data has evaluated day 1 scores. APACHE can be used on subsequent days, and trends in APACHE scores can be noted. However, use of APACHE in this manner has not been looked at on a broad scale. MPM has been validated but on a smaller scale. This scoring system has the advantage of a simpler data collection process. MPM also allows rescoring the patient at 24 and 48 hours and uses different parameters from those used at admission to obtain these scores. This could be useful for viewing patients' evolution over the first 3 days in the ICU. TISS provides useful information concerning the amount of therapy given by physicians and nurses. It is used to stratify patients according to intensity of therapy required. This information is then incorporated into the APACHE system.

HOW TO DECIDE WHICH PATIENTS CAN BENEFIT FROM THE INTENSIVE CARE UNIT

Two types of patients should be admitted to the ICU: critically ill patients with a reasonable chance of survival and patients who may be stable at admission but have a significant chance of requiring active therapy.

When determining whether a critically ill patient might benefit from the ICU, the physician should first consider the mortality statistics for the disease in question. The mortality statistics for diseases and syndromes most frequently seen in the ICU are reviewed earlier in the chapter. The mortality rates are strikingly high in many cases. Prognostic indicators exist for some diseases, but unfortunately not all. Therefore at admission it can be difficult to determine which critically ill patients have the best chance of benefiting from the ICU. Likewise, if the patient has already been admitted to the ICU, the physician may be hesitant to recommend discontinuing aggressive therapy.

It is in these situations that severity-of-disease scoring systems can help in estimating a patient's physiologic instability at admission. The authors of these scoring systems do not recommend using their systems as absolute indicators of the survival or death of an individual patient. However, a severity-of-disease score and predicted mortality for the patient's disease can be used in conjunction with the physician's clinical evaluation of a given patient to estimate chance of survival. For example, two patients with the same admitting diagnosis and same acute physiology scores might have different APACHE scores and predicted death rates because one patient has a history of a tumor. This information could be added to the arsenal of information already obtained by the physician when a decision is made concerning the usefulness of aggressive therapy.

It can be equally difficult to identify, among patients admitted to the ICU for monitoring, those at risk for complications that might require active therapy. APACHE can be helpful in this setting also. As noted previously, APACHE uses TISS information to differentiate patients requiring active therapy from those requiring monitoring only. Through the use of the logistic regression equation, APACHE then classifies monitor-only patients as either high-risk monitor or low-risk monitor. This equation takes into account acute physiology score, surgical status, and major indication for ICU admission. High-risk monitor patients are those requiring only monitoring at admission but with a greater than 10% risk that complications requiring active therapy will develop shortly after admission. Low-risk monitor patients require only monitoring at admission and have less than a 10% risk of complications requiring active therapy. Low-risk monitor patients therefore would do just as well outside the ICU. If these patients could reliably be identified in advance, many unnecessary ICU admissions could be avoided.

Knaus evaluated the accuracy of APACHE as a tool for identifying low-risk monitor patients. In Knaus's initial study, 778 patients from one ICU admitted for monitoring were evaluated. Of these, 509 (65%) were predicted to have less than a 10% risk of requiring active treatment and were classified as low-risk monitor patients. Only 21 (4.1%) of the 509 ever received active therapy. Review of the charts of these 21 patients showed that none had life-threatening complications. A validation study of 1163 patients from 12 different hospitals followed; 849 (73%) were identified as low-risk patients. Only 37 (4.4%) of these low-risk patients required active therapy. Review of available discharge summaries and computerized data on 31 of the 37 patients indicated that none would have been adversely affected had they not been admitted to the ICU. These data suggest that APACHE can be reliably used to identify patients who fit the traditional criteria for admission to the ICU but who would be equally safe (and far more comfortable) outside the ICU.

The diagnoses of low-risk monitor patients are of interest. In Knaus's study population, 218 low-risk patients had undergone craniotomies. These patients accounted for 73% of the total ICU low-risk admissions. Only five of these patients required active treatment. The data also revealed that 85%, 34%, and 41% of patients, respectively, admitted after laminectomy, after peripheral vascular surgery, or for diabetic ketoacidosis were classified as low-risk monitor patients. Many patients with these diagnoses could be hospitalized outside the ICU without any additional risk.

In conclusion, the physician must first determine by clinical evaluation whether a patient is an appropriate candidate for the ICU. Critically ill patients should be admitted if they have a reasonable chance for survival. When this is difficult to determine, the physician can use a severity-of-disease scoring system such as APACHE or MPM. At present, severity-of-disease scoring systems are not intended to evaluate an individual patient's chance of survival, but the information they give can be used to reinforce a clinical evaluation. In addition, it is difficult to determine clinically whether patients admitted to the ICU for prophylactic monitoring are likely to require active therapy soon after admission. APACHE reliably identifies patients who have been thought to require ICU monitoring but can in fact be safely hospitalized outside the ICU. Such patients are frequently those who have undergone craniotomy, laminectomy, or peripheral vascular surgery or who have diabetic ketoacidosis. This last finding may surprise many and deserves to be further evaluated.

ETHICS OF LIMITING ADMISSIONS TO THE INTENSIVE CARE UNIT

The aims of avoiding futile admissions to the ICU are to alleviate unnecessary suffering by the patient and family and to ensure that resources are allocated for curable patients. To achieve these goals, physicians must "return death to disease" (in the words of Daniel Callahan), learn to allocate resources, and learn to say no to patients.

The early development of ICUs and the advancement of medical technology in the United States were initially accompanied by an attitude that all medical illness could be reversed. Moreover, every individual was deemed to have the right to this technology even if it had not been shown to reduce the person's illness. Callahan has written that this belief grew out of a "deep respect for individual life" (new technology should be used under any circumstances because it may prolong life) "and a strong tradition of medical progress" (medical technology can be helpful under any circumstances).

The sentiments of both physicians and patients are changing to a small degree. No longer is the ICU thought to be the panacea for all diseases. Families more often prefer that aggressive therapy be ended when a fruitful outcome appears unlikely. Yet the discussion between physician and family concerning the desirability of ICU care most often takes place after admission to the ICU. Furthermore, aggressive therapy is most often discontinued after admission to the ICU, not withheld from the outset. So although it is true that physicians and society have gained a respect for what Engelhardt termed the "unintended power of medicine to extend life under undesirable circumstances," people have not easily accepted the decline of health as part of the life cycle. Modern technology cannot reverse some medical conditions, and it is the responsibility of physicians to inform patients and their families of the limitations as well as the virtues of modern medicine.

In addition, a system for allocating resources is needed. The notion that resources for human health must be limited goes against common American sentiment. Yet we live in an era when this is true. Englehardt (1986) has written, "humans have the aspirations of deities, but never the resources." Certain societies have recognized this fact, but the United States perhaps has not. In such countries as Great Britain and New Zealand, access to critical care is limited. Age is an often used criterion. In the United States, where age is often perceived as a frontier to be tamed, the idea of denying older patients access to certain facets of the health care system arouses discomfort. Nevertheless, Callahan has enthusiastically endorsed this approach. Much of the data discussed in this chapter indicates that age as an independent factor does not correlate with survival. Regardless of the criteria ultimately used, in the future hospitals will have to adopt some type of formal mechanism for rationing expenditures on critical care or limiting the number of critical care patients.

Although most people in other countries accept the need to ration access to the health care system, many Americans are uneasy about this concept. Why is it so hard to say no in the United States? And what makes this approach so easy to accept in countries such as Great Britain? Daniels discussed this issue in detail. He pointed out that in Great Britain, where a centralized budget is formulated, decisions about introducing new technology or providing access to critical care or hemodialysis are made within the constraints of that budget. When resources are restricted for a particular group, it is clear which resources become available for other groups. In the United States, when physicians limit access to the ICU, they cannot guarantee that the money saved will remain unspent (if the goal is to reduce total expenditures) or be spent more usefully for some other patient (if the goal is to allocate resources in a more efficient manner).

In conclusion, physicians must go beyond their traditional role of curing. Their goal must be to do what is best for the patient. In certain situations, allowing a patient to die is best. In addition, access to the ICU must be limited to patients who have a reasonable chance for a successful outcome. Physicians and hospitals must adopt a policy that formally defines situations in which admission to the ICU is undesirable. To increase the acceptance of such a policy by physicians and society, there must be a formal mechanism guaranteeing that any financial savings will remain unspent or will be directed toward more fruitful areas.

SUMMARY

ICUs were created so that unstable patients or those with a high potential for instability could be appropriately monitored and treated. Despite improvements in medical therapy and technology, however, certain critically ill patients cannot be saved. The survival rates for diseases and syndromes often treated in the ICU are given in the chapter.

Formal policy must be established to define situations in which admission to an ICU is not necessarily in the patient's best interests. Mechanisms allowing the physician and family to end aggressive therapy in futile situations exist in many hospitals and should be used when chances for survival are minimal. Determination of inevitable death must be based foremost on clinical evaluation and consideration of the overall survival rates for the disease in question. In critical disease, however, reliable prognostic indicators do not always exist.

Severity-of-disease scoring systems can provide objective and illuminating information concerning the patient's physiologic stability and chances for survival. Although mortality predictions of these systems are not officially recommended for use in individual patient decisions, they can be used to clarify judgments based on clinical evaluation.

A significant percentage of patients are admitted to the ICU to be monitored for complications that never develop. Unfortunately, clinical evaluation often does not provide insight in determining which patients will ultimately have serious complications. However, the APACHE system provides a reliable and validated way of identifying patients in whom complications are unlikely to develop. For patients with coronary disease, specific systems have been established for identifying patients at risk for hemodynamic instability.

By limiting admission to the ICU, physicians can eliminate unnecessary suffering by patients and families and reduce unnecessary expenditures. A system must be established through which the money saved by not inappropriately admitting a patient to the ICU definitively decreases overall expenses or increases available funds elsewhere.

SUGGESTED READINGS

Ashbaugh DG: Acute respiratory distress in adults. Lancet 1967;2:319

Austrian R et al: Pneumococcal bacteremia with special reference to bacteremic pneumococcal pneumonia. Ann Intern Med 1964;60:759

Baek SM et al: Clinical determinants of survival in postoperative renal failure. Surg Gynecol Obstet 1975; 140:685

Bartlett RH et al: Continuous arteriovenous hemofiltration: Improved in survival in surgical acute renal failure. Surgery 1986;100:400

Baslov JT et al: A survey of 499 patients with acute renal failure influencing causes, treatment, complication, and mortality. Am J Med 1963;34:75

Bates D et al: A prospective study of non traumatic coma: Methods and results in 310 patients. Ann Neurol 1977;2:211

Bell RC et al: Multiple organ failure and infection in adult respiratory distress syndrome. Ann Intern Med 1983;99:393

Brewin A et al: High dose penicillin therapy and pneumococcal pneumonia. JAMA 1974;230:409

Britt MR et al: Severity of underlying disease as a predictor of nosocomial infection. JAMA 1978;239:1047

Brown RB et al: A comparison of infections in different ICUs within the same hospital. Crit Care Med 1985; 13:472

Brush JE et al: Use of the initial electrocardiogram to predict inhospital complications of acute myocardial infarction. N Engl J Med 1985;312:1137

Bryan CS et al: Analysis of 1186 episodes of gram negative bacteremias and fungemia in adults. II. Clinical observations with special reference to factors influencing prognosis. Rev Infect Dis 1983;5:521

Bullock ML et al: The assessment of risk factors in 412 patients with acute renal failure. Am J Kidney Dis 1985;5:97

Callahan D: Can we return death to disease? Hastings Rep (Suppl) Jan/Feb 1989:4

Cameron JS: Acute renal failure — the continuing challenge. Q J Med 1986;228:337

Celis R et al: Nosocomial pneumonia: A multivariate analysis of risk and prognosis. Chest 1988;93:318

Chang RWA et al: Predicting deaths among intensive care unit patients. Crit Care Med 1988;16:34

Cioffi WG et al: Probability of surviving acute renal failure. Ann Surg 1984;200:205

Cox SC et al: Acute respiratory failure: Mortality associated with underlying disease. Crit Care Med 1985;13:1005

Craven DE et al: Nosocomial infection and fatality in medical and surgical intensive care unit patients. Arch Intern Med 1988;148:1161

Daniels N (ed): Why saying no to patients in the United States is so hard: Cost containment, justice, and provider autonomy. N Engl J Med 1986;314:1980

Dardes N et al: Prognosis of COPD patients after an episode of acute respiratory failure. Eur J Respir Dis 1986;69(S146):377

Davis H et al: Prolonged mechanical assisted ventilation. JAMA 1980;243:43

Devillota ED et al: Septicemia in a medical intensive care unit: Clinical, biochemical, and microbiological data of 109 cases. Intensive Care Med 1983;9:109

Donowitz LG et al: High risk of hospital acquired infection in the ICU patient. Crit Care Med 1982;10:355

Douglas PS et al: DRG payment for long-term ventilator patients. Chest 1987;91:413

Dupont HL et al: Infections due to gram negative organisms: An analysis of 860 patients with bacteremia at the University of Minnesota Medical Center, 1958–1966. Medicine 1969;48:307

Elliot CG et al: Pulmonary function and exercise gas exchange in survivors of adult respiratory distress syndrome. Am Rev Respir Dis 1981;123:492

Engelhardt HT: Intensive care units, scarce resources, and conflicting principles of justice. JAMA 1986;255(9):1159

Farmer JC (ed): Problems in critical care, prognostic scoring systems in the ICU, vol 3, no 4. Philadelphia, 1989, JB Lippincott

Fisher RP et al: Early diagnosis in the treatment of acute renal failure. Surg Gynecol Obstet 1966;123:1019

Fowler AA et al: Adult respiratory distress syndrome: Prognosis after onset. Am J Respir Dis 1985;132:472

Friedman Y et al: Improved survival in patients with AIDS, *Pneumocystis* chronic pneumonia, and severe respiratory failure. Chest 1989;96:862

Gillepsie DJ et al: Clinical outcome of respiratory failure in patients requiring prolonged (>24 hours) mechanical ventilation. Chest 1986;90:364

Goldman L et al: A computer-derived protocol to aid in the diagnosis of emergency room patients with acute chest pain. N Engl J Med 1982;307:588

Gornick CC et al: Acute renal failure complicating aortic aneurysm surgery. Nephron 1983;85:145

Gross PA et al: Deaths from nosocomial infections: Experience in a university hospital and community hospital. Am J Med 1980;68:219

Hook EW et al: Failure of intensive care unit support to influence mortality from pneumococcal bacteremia. JAMA 1983;249:1055

Hou SH et al: Hospital acquired renal insufficiency: A prospective study. Am J Med 1983;143:209

Kaelin RM et al: Failure to predict six month survival of patients with COPD requiring mechanical ventilation by analysis of simple indices. Chest 1987;92:971

Kennedy AC et al: Factors affecting the prognosis in acute renal failure, a survey of 251 cases. Q J Med 1973;42:73

Kiley JE et al: Acute renal failure, eight cases of renal tubular acidosis. N Engl J Med 1960; 262:481

Kjellstrand CM et al: Recovery from acute renal failure. Trans Am Soc Artif Organs 1981;27:45

Knaus WA. Evaluation of outcome from intensive care: A preliminary multihospital comparison. Crit Care Med 1982;10:491

Knaus WA et al: APACHE II: A severity of disease classification system. Crit Care Med 1985;13(10):818

Knaus WA et al: Prognosis in acute organ system failure. Ann Surg 1985;202(6):685

Kreger BE et al: Gram-negative bacteremia. III. Reassessment of etiology, epidemiology, and ecology in 612 patients. Am J Med 1980;68:332

Kumar R et al: Acute renal failure in the elderly. Lancet 1973;1:90

Lemeshow SL et al: A method for predicting survival and mortality of ICU patients using objectively derived weights. Crit Care Med 1985;13(7):519

Levy DE: Prognosis in nontraumatic coma. Ann Intern Med 1981;94(3):293

Mackowiak PA et al: Polymicrobial sepsis: An analysis of 11894 cases using log linear models. Am J Med Sci 1980;280:73

Mancebo J et al: Value of static pulmonary compliance in predicting mortality in patients with acute respiratory failure. Intensive Care Med 1988;14:110

Menashe PI et al: Acquired renal insufficiency in critically ill patients. Crit Care Med 1988;16:1106

Montgomery AB et al: Causes of mortality in patients with the adult respiratory distress syndrome. Am Rev Respir Dis 1985;132:485

McMurray SD et al: Prevailing patterns and predictor variables in patients with acute tubular necrosis. Arch Intern Med 1978;138:950

Myers BD et al: Hemodynamically mediated acute renal failure. N Engl J Med 1986;314:94

Raffin TA: Intensive care unit survival of patients with systemic illness. Am Rev Respir Dis 1989;140:528

Rainford DJ: Nutritional management of acute renal failure. Acta Chir Scand 1981;507(Suppl 1):327

Ring-Larsen H et al: Renal failure in fulminant hepatic failure and terminal cirrhosis: A comparison between incidence, types, and prognosis. Gut 1981;22:585

Rosen MJ et al: Outcome of intensive care in patients with the acquired immunodeficiency syndrome. J Intensive Care 1986;1:55

Rotman HH et al: Longterm physiologic consequences of the adult respiratory distress syndrome. Chest 1977;72:190

Royston D et al: Failure of aerosolized 99 mTC-DTPA clearance to predict outcome in patients with adult respiratory distress syndrome. Thorax 1977;42:494

Schacter EN et al: Mechanically assisted ventilation in a community hospital. Arch Intern Med 1985;145:235

Spicher JE et al: Outcome function following prolonged mechanical ventilation. Arch Intern Med 1987;147:421

Stevens RM et al: Pneumonia in an intensive care unit. Arch Intern Med 1974;134:106

Swann RC et al: The clinical course of acute renal failure. Medicine 1953;32:215

Teplick R: Benefit of elective intensive care after certain operations. Anesth Analg 1983;62:572

Teres D et al: Validation of the mortality prediction model for ICU patients. Crit Care Med 1987;15(3):208

Thibault GE: Medical intensive care: Indications, interventions, and outcomes. N Engl J Med 1980;302(17):939

Thorp JM: A survey of infection in an intensive care unit. Anesthesia 1979;34:643

Wagner DP: Identification of low-risk monitor admissions to medical-surgical ICUs. Chest 1987;92(3):423

Woodhead MA et al: Aetiology and outcome of severe community-acquired pneumonia. J Infect 1985;10:204

Zimmerman JE: Patient selection for intensive care: A comparison of New Zealand and United States hospitals. Crit Care Med 1988;16(4):318

2

INITIAL STABILIZATION

ALAN S. TONNESEN, MD

The purposes of this chapter are to provide a conceptual framework for assessment of the patient at the time of admission to an intensive care unit (ICU), to describe the initial management steps that ensure the most rapid stabilization of the respiratory and circulatory systems possible, and to set the stage for further elaboration of the diagnosis and management of critical illness. The initial assessment is meant to detect life-threatening problems. This should be accompanied by immediate correction of identified abnormalities. A secondary, more complete assessment should follow initial assessment to detect less severe problems and to devise a plan that minimizes the chances of later complications. These principles should be reassessed if the patient's condition deteriorates while he or she is in the ICU.

INITIAL ASSESSMENT

An organized assessment of the patient on arrival in the ICU ensures that no immediately life-threatening problems are missed (Table 2–1). An initial, brief assessment should be performed, modeled on the ABCs of resuscitation (airway, breathe, circulate), and any indicated resuscitative measures should be instituted. This is followed by a more detailed history and physical examination and the planning of an approach to monitoring, diagnosing, and treating the identified problems. In the early phases of the ICU stay, specific diagnoses are often not yet made. Thus supportive care is initiated based on the current state of vital organ systems. The initial plans are modified as further information becomes available.

The first priority is to ensure adequate oxygen delivery to tissues (Fig. 2–1). The ABCs

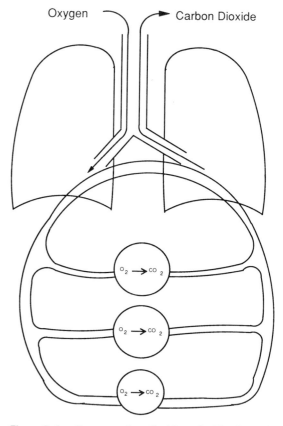

Figure 2–1. Oxygen–carbon dioxide cycle. The first priority in critical care is provision of oxygen and substrate to tissues and removal of carbon dioxide and other wastes. The steps in this cycle include oxygen ventilation, provision of hemoglobin to carry the oxygen, cardiac output to deliver it to tissues, conversion of oxygen to carbon dioxide with release of energy by tissues, transport of carbon dioxide to the lungs, and ventilation to remove carbon dioxide from the lungs. Adherence to this simple concept is the basis of all resuscitation and life support.

TABLE 2–1.   ICU Admission Assessment

ABCs of resuscitation
Resuscitation
Examination
Planning

of resuscitation involve delivering oxygen via a patent *a*irway with adequate ventilation (*b*reathing) to the lungs, transfer of oxygen to the blood, and delivery of sufficient oxygenated blood with adequate glucose to the tissues (*c*irculation).

Since hypoxia kills within minutes, it must be detected and treated immediately. Hypercarbia and acidosis in the absence of hypoxia are not desirable but rarely kill a patient if hypoxia is avoided. Inadequate ventilation causes hypoxia by inducing a global low ventilation/perfusion ($\dot{V}/\dot{Q}$) ratio. The hypoxia caused by a low $\dot{V}/\dot{Q}$ ratio is relatively easily reversed by elevation of the fraction of inspired oxygen (FIO_2) to 1.0. Thus every effort must be made to provide a high FIO_2 to alveoli even if ventilation, as assessed by arterial partial pressure of carbon dioxide ($PaCO_2$), is grossly inadequate.

AIRWAY

First, airway patency and adequacy of ventilation should be assessed. If the patient is apneic, some form of mechanical ventilation must begin. If spontaneous or mechanical ventilation is present, signs of airway obstruction should be sought. The signs of obstruction differ between spontaneously breathing and mechanically ventilated patients. Table 2–2 lists some

TABLE 2–2.   Signs of Airway Obstruction

	SPONTANEOUS VENTILATION	POSITIVE-PRESSURE VENTILATION
Retraction	Yes	No
Accessory muscle use:	Yes	No
Tracheal tug	Yes	
Mandible drop	Yes	
Airway pressure	Very negative	Very positive
Chest movement	Paradoxic	Diminished or absent
Breath sounds	Diminished Wheezes Stridor Snoring	Diminished Wheezes
Abdominal movement	Paradoxic Active expiration	Diminished or absent

signs that may be present during airway obstruction. When the patient is receiving mechanical ventilation but also has spontaneous respiratory efforts, the signs may be mixed.

Management of airway obstruction differs between intubated and nonintubated patients (Table 2–3). The manifestations of obstruction may be due to increased airway resistance in the external breathing circuit, upper airway, tracheal tube, or large or small airways. Similar manifestations may be due to poor compliance caused by pulmonary disease, chest wall or abdominal disease, or extrinsic pulmonary compression.

If the initial steps in opening the airway are unsuccessful, intubation is required. If the airway is made patent by these initial maneuvers, the next step depends on the adequacy of spontaneous ventilation and the risk of aspiration. If the patient is at risk of aspiration (for example, because of a full stomach or upper airway bleeding) and is obtunded sufficiently to

TABLE 2–3.   Management of Airway Obstruction

Nonintubated Patient

Removal of foreign material from upper airway
   Manual extraction
   Suction
Alignment of head, neck, and body
Extension of neck unless neck injury is suspected
Jaw thrust
Chin lift
Nasal airway
Oral airway
Tracheal intubation
   Oral
   Nasal
   Cricothyrotomy
      Needle
      Seldinger cricothyrotomy
      Surgical

Intubated Patient

Obstruction in external breathing circuit
   Disconnect tracheal tube from breathing circuit
   Ventilate with self-inflating bag
Obstruction in tracheal tube
   Pass suction catheter
   Suction via endotracheal tube
Obstruction caused by tube malposition
   Confirm presence of bilateral breath sounds
   Deflate cuff
   Confirm translaryngeal placement visually
   Reposition tube
Obstruction in patient's airways
   Rule out or treat bronchospasm
   Rule out or remove foreign material in airways
Low compliance
   Rule out pneumothorax
   Rule out or treat elevated intraabdominal pressure

tolerate an oral or nasal airway without coughing and gagging, intubation should be performed. A patient at minimal risk (for example, a patient who is expected to awaken after an elective operation) may be placed in a lateral decubitus position and monitored.

Airway Management

The health care worker must always remember the universal precautions, which help prevent the spread of communicable diseases from patients to caregivers. Protective gloves and goggles are indicated for virtually all airway manipulations.

Primary Management

The airway must be opened. This may be achieved with the chin lift or with jaw thrust maneuvers in conjunction with insertion of an oral or nasal airway. High concentrations of oxygen are provided with mouth-to-mouth, mouth-to-airway, or bag-to-mask positive-pressure ventilation. If the patient has suffered trauma, these maneuvers must be accompanied by neck stabilization until radiologic studies have excluded cervical spine injury. These essential emergency measures are followed by intubation of the trachea.

Secondary Management

Endotracheal intubation is the preferred method for providing ventilation and protection against aspiration of material from the upper airway. The esophageal obturator airway and its variants are useful when the intubator's skill is limited and occasionally when endotracheal intubation is exceptionally difficult. Needle cricothyroidotomy and surgical cricothyroidotomy are rarely required but can be performed rapidly by trained personnel.

ESOPHAGEAL AIRWAY INTUBATION

The esophageal airways are modified endotracheal tubes. The distal end of the endotracheal tube is plugged, and holes are present in the wall of the tube above the cuff level. A special connector replaces the standard connector to make the tube easier to connect to a face mask. The tube is advanced blindly into the esophagus, the cuff is inflated to prevent regurgitation, the specially modified mask is applied to seal the airway, and the lumen is ventilated by any source. Air passes down the lumen of the tube, out through the perforations in the pharynx, through the larynx, and into the lungs. The advantages of esophageal airways are the minimal skill required to insert the airway, the rapidity with which placement can be performed, and possibly a reduced risk of regurgitation. Disadvantages include possible tracheal intubation, which prevents ventilation; esophageal rupture; inadequate ventilation; and lack of protection from aspiration of upper airway secretions, blood, or regurgitated material. Individuals trained in other ways of ensuring a patent airway rarely insert an esophageal airway but may encounter patients with the device in place. If the patient requires continued airway protection or ventilation, endotracheal intubation should be performed.

ENDOTRACHEAL INTUBATION

Successful endotracheal intubation depends on the availability of equipment and trained personnel. Ideally it should be performed after the patient has been oxygenated and ventilated by other means. Table 2–4 lists the minimal equipment needed for intubation. Before any attempts at visualization, all equipment should be checked and placed where the intubator can easily reach it and where it will not be pushed out of reach if the patient moves during intubation.

MONITORING DURING INTUBATION

Hypoxia, arrhythmias, hypertension, and hypotension are problems commonly encountered during emergency intubations. Monitoring of oxygenation with a pulse oximeter and electrocardiographic monitoring should be continuous during intubation. Blood pressure can be measured continuously by means of an indwelling arterial catheter or intermittently at 30- to 60-second intervals with an automated noninvasive blood pressure device or by an assistant

TABLE 2–4. Endotracheal Intubation

Equipment
Suction source and tubing: rigid suction catheter (Yankauer)
Endotracheal tube
Syringe for cuff inflation
Stylet for shaping tube
Laryngoscopes
Straight blade
Curved blade
Spare bulbs, batteries
Alternative means of ventilation

with a cuff and pulse detector. A precordial stethoscope is useful for alerting the intubator to changes in the heart rate during the procedure.

SUCTION

The vacuum source should be connected to the collection reservoir and a rigid curved suction cannula (Yankauer suction cannula). The cannula should not require covering a hole or pressing a button to establish suction. Flexible suction catheters are not useful for clearing the airway during laryngoscopy because they cannot be easily and rapidly directed to fluid collections deep in the pharynx or larynx. The vacuum should be strong enough to empty a glass of water in 10 seconds. The suction cannula should be placed under the patient's right shoulder to allow the operator to reach it without looking away from the airway during laryngoscopy and to ensure that the tubing is long enough.

ENDOTRACHEAL TUBE

A cuffed endotracheal tube of the appropriate size (Table 2–5) should be prepared by lubrication of the distal end of the tube and the stylet (if orotracheal intubation is planned) with water-soluble lubricant. The stylet should be inserted until its tip is about 1 cm proximal to the end of the endotracheal tube. The cuff should have a large residual volume; that is, the cuff should hold 12 to 15 ml of air before any pressure is generated within it. Many patients require prolonged intubation, and use of a large cuff lessens the risk of tracheal malacia and stenosis. To detect a leak in the cuff or the one-way inflation valve, the operator should inflate the cuff until tense and remove the syringe from the inflation port. The cuff should then be completely deflated and the syringe left attached to the inflation port. Generally tubes

less than 5 mm internal diameter are cuffless to avoid reducing the cross-sectional area for ventilation. The prepared tube should be either left on the bed above the patient's right shoulder or held by a trained assistant.

LARYNGOSCOPE

The choice of laryngoscope blade depends largely on the operator's experience. The curved MacIntosh blade is better tolerated by a conscious patient, controls the tongue more effectively, and gives more working room in the oral cavity. The straight blade occasionally provides better visualization of the entire larynx. The percentage of cases in which the larynx can be visualized is thought to be somewhat higher with straight blades than curved blades, although data are not available to support this view. For adults the MacIntosh No. 3 (curved) and the Miller No. 2 or No. 3 (straight) blades suffice for all except the largest patients. Straight blades are preferred for neonates and children up to about 20 kg. The operator should check the batteries, blades, and bulbs by mounting each blade on the battery handle, holding the laryngoscope in the intubating position, stressing the blade from side to side and up and down, and applying pressure against the bulb. If any of these maneuvers result in flickering or loss of light, the problem should be remedied before intubation is attempted. Both blades should be checked; if, despite prechecking, the first blade fails, the second blade will be known to be functional. The bulb should shine brilliantly white; if it is yellow or obviously dim, fresh batteries should be inserted and the contact points between blade and handle checked for corrosion. If corrosion is present, a pencil eraser can be used to clean the contact surfaces without damaging them. After the blade is checked and after intubation, the light should be turned off to preserve the batteries.

NASOGASTRIC TUBE

If a nasogastric tube is already present, the tape should be removed to allow rapid removal if the tube obstructs the intubator's view. The advantages of removing a nasogastric tube before endotracheal intubation include possible reestablishment of competence of the gastroesophageal and posterior pharyngeal sphincters, better efficacy of the cricoid compression maneuver (Sellick's maneuver), and no chance that the tube will obscure the intubator's view or become entangled with the endotracheal tube.

TABLE 2–5. Appropriate Endotracheal Tube Sizes

PATIENT	INTERNAL DIAMETER (mm)
Adult male	8.0
Adult female	7.0
Full-term neonates	3.5
Child	Diameter of patient's small finger

If the nasogastric tube is left in situ, the intubator should remove it immediately if it impedes intubation. The disadvantages of removing a nasogastric tube before intubation include the removal of a potential route of gastric decompression, possible induction of epistaxis, and difficulty in reinserting the nasogastric tube. If a nasogastric tube is not in situ before intubation, placement depends on the presence of upper airway protective reflexes. If the patient is obtunded, paralyzed, or unconscious, the nasogastric tube should be placed after endotracheal intubation because the act of placement may induce epistaxis, regurgitation, or vomiting and subsequent aspiration.

NECK STABILIZATION

The neck must be stabilized before, during, and after intubation by any route if injury has not been excluded. Maneuvers to stabilize the cervical spine include (1) placement of sandbags or large bags of intravenous fluids on each side of the patient's head followed by taping around the head and spine board and (2) bimanual traction by a trained assistant to prevent both lateral flexion and anteroposterior flexion or extension.

ROUTE OF INTUBATION

Several factors should influence the decision regarding the intubation route (Table 2–6) and the use of muscle relaxants or anesthesia (Table 2–7).

Intubation while the patient is sedated or after muscle relaxants are administered is acceptable only when a fully trained anesthesiologist or someone who has performed hundreds of intubations and is intimately familiar with the pharmacology of muscle relaxants is present. Once intubation has been achieved, sedation and muscle relaxants may be used as needed. Patients should be intubated either without any drugs or while fully paralyzed with neuromuscular blocking agents. Attempted intubation of a sedated patient is likely to lead to hypoxia, regurgitation or vomiting, aspiration of blood or gastric contents, aggravation of other injuries, hypertension, tachycardia, or laryngospasm.

Intubation under anesthesia without muscle relaxants is performed only for upper airway obstruction, as in croup; in all other circumstances anesthesia should be accompanied by muscle relaxation. Although intubation with muscle relaxants but without anesthesia is uncomfortable and anxiety provoking, it is probably more comfortable than awake intubation without muscle relaxants and carries little risk of hypotension.

Any traumatized patient should be presumed to have a full stomach and thus to be at risk of aspirating gastric contents.

BLIND NASAL INTUBATION

Blind nasal intubation (Table 2–8) is performed only in spontaneously breathing patients. In emergency situations, nasal intubation with a laryngoscope is not indicated because it cannot be performed as rapidly as oral intubation with laryngoscopy. If the patient is awake and the stomach is known to be empty (almost never in emergency situations), sedation and topical anesthesia before nasal intubation should be considered. The first step is to clear

TABLE 2–6.   Factors Influencing Decision on Route of Urgent or Emergency Intubation

FACTOR	ROUTE			
	ORAL	NASAL	NEEDLE	SURGICAL
Spontaneous ventilation	◐	◐	○	◐
Apnea	●	○	◐	●
Airway obstruction	◐	◐	●	●
Upper airway bleeding	◐	○	●	●
Oral intubation anticipated to be difficult or indeterminate	○	●	●	●
Neck unstable or stability unknown	○	●	●	●
Hypoxia	●	○	●	◐
Intracranial hypertension likely	●	○	○	○
Evidence of basilar skull fracture	●	○	◐	◐

● Technique favored; ◐ technique acceptable; ○ technique relatively contraindicated

**TABLE 2–7.　Factors Influencing Decisions on Use of Drugs
for Urgent or Emergency Intubation***

FACTOR	AWAKE	ANESTHETIC AGENT	MUSCLE RELAXANT
Airway obstruction	●	◐	○
Upper airway bleeding	●	○	○
Anticipated difficulty in oral intubation or indeterminate	●	○	○
Status of neck unknown or unstable	◐	○	○
Hypoxia	○	◐	●
Cardiovascular status			
Coronary disease	○	●	◐
Severe hypertension	○	●	◐
Aneurysm (cerebral, aortic)	○	●	●
Hypotension	◐	○	◐
Hypovolemia	◐	○	◐
Intracranial hypertension likely	○	●	●

●, Technique preferred; ◐, factor not relevant; ○, relatively contraindicated. not relevant.
*The table presents my opinions regarding the desirability of each technique if that factor alone were present. When more than one factor is present, conflict in the decision-making process may develop. In these circumstances the clinician must subjectively weigh the relative risks of each technique and the possible untoward consequences of that technique.

the nasal passages of blood and mucus. Unless this is done, vasoconstrictors and anesthetics will not reach the mucosa and will have little or no effect, and the tube will be filled with mucus and blood during passage. In addition, secretions obscure breath sounds and are carried into the trachea. If time permits, a topical vasoconstrictor should be sprayed into each nostril and allowed to act for several minutes; Neo-Synephrine 0.25% (2.5 mg/ml) is usually available. After this three or four puffs of 2% to 4% lidocaine or benzocaine should be sprayed into the nostrils. Cocaine is very effective but is seldom available on short notice because of legal requirements. Painting the nasal passages with 2% lidocaine jelly on cotton-tipped applicators anesthetizes and lubricates them. The pharynx and larynx should not be anesthetized

TABLE 2–8.　Blind Nasal Intubation

Contraindications

Basilar skull fracture
Meningitis
Severe nasal or midface trauma
Apnea

Complications

Immediate
  Bleeding
  Submucosal dissection
Late
  Sinusitis
  Otitis media
  Nasal ulceration

because this would make the patient susceptible to aspiration even though wide awake.

The neck should be stabilized if a neck injury is suspected, and oxygen should be administered via a face mask and nasal cannula. The tube should be inserted parallel to the hard palate and advanced while breath sounds are audible through the tube lumen. Touching the larynx or epiglottis with the tube often elicits a cough. Rapid advancement during the inspiratory phase of the cough aids in placement. Specially designed endotracheal tubes with a deflectable tip allow the end of the tube to be flexed anteriorly if the tube does not pass into the larynx.

ORAL INTUBATION

Oral intubation is the preferred emergency route for apneic patients and those without neck injury (Table 2–9). If the surgical procedure dictates the need for nasal intubation, the tube can be changed from the oral to nasal route under controlled conditions in the operating room.

Laryngoscopy. After all the equipment required for laryngoscopy is assembled, the laryngoscope is grasped in the left hand, with the blade placed in the on and locked position. If cervical spine injury has not been excluded, the neck is stabilized. An assistant grasps the cricoid cartilage between the thumb and forefinger and presses firmly posteriorly to push the broad posterior wall of the cricoid cartilage against the posterior esophageal wall, which prevents

TABLE 2–9.   Oral Intubation

Contraindications

Oral abscess
Inability to undergo laryngoscopy
Impacted upper airway foreign body

Complications (Immediate)

Mandibular dislocation
Dental trauma
Neck trauma
Spinal cord damage
Oral (lip, tongue) lacerations

TABLE 2–10.   Indications for Fiberoptic Guided Intubation

Potential Upper Airway Injury

Burns
Smoke or chemical inhalation
Blunt or penetrating laryngeal trauma
Blunt or penetrating tracheal trauma

Inability to Undergo Conventional Laryngoscopy

Inadequate oral aperture
Upper airway distortion by tumor, hematoma, etc.
Neck immobilization

Need for Bronchoscopy

Aspiration of particulate material or blood
Suspicion of tracheobronchial rupture
Major atelectasis

Contraindications

Apnea
Severe hypoxia
Upper airway bleeding

regurgitation (Sellick's maneuver). The blade is inserted at the right corner of the mouth, with the tongue displaced to the left. The blade is advanced under direct vision until the epiglottis is visualized. If a curved blade is used, the tip of the blade is slipped between the superior surface of the epiglottis and the base of the tongue (vallecula). If a straight blade is used, the tip of the blade is placed under the inferior surface of the epiglottis. Force is then applied parallel to the long axis of the handle of the laryngoscope. This displaces the mandible and tongue anteriorly and caudad. The posterior commissure and arytenoid cartilages of the larynx are then usually seen lying in contact with the posterior pharyngeal wall. With further elevation of the laryngoscope, the true vocal cords are seen to form a triangle whose apex is anterior.

Intubation.   The tube is introduced from the right side of the mouth until the tip is seen to pass through the triangular opening between the vocal cords. The endotracheal tube is not passed down the laryngoscope as through a guiding tube. The tube is advanced until the cuff has passed about 2 cm beyond the cords. The cuff is immediately inflated to protect against aspiration. Insertion of a lighted wand into the tube permits localization of the tube tip by transilluminating the anterior neck to guide further attempts.

FIBEROPTIC GUIDED INTUBATION

Flexible fiberoptic laryngoscopes or broncho-scopes can be extremely useful for elective or urgent endotracheal intubation (Table 2–10), especially via the nose, but have little role in emergency intubation attempts. If the intuba-tion is not an emergency and difficulties are anticipated, the fiberoptic scope should be used as the primary technique. When blind intuba-tion or direct laryngoscopy is attempted before use of the fiberoptic scope, secretions are

invariably stimulated and bleeding is common. These make use of the fiberoptic scope difficult if not impossible.

When fiberoptic intubation is planned, an anticholinergic agent should be administered to block saliva production. The nasal passages should be cleared by nose blowing or suctioning. A topical vasoconstrictor should be applied to both nostrils to enlarge the nasal passage, decrease the incidence and severity of bleeding, and enhance the effect of topical anesthetics. A few minutes after the topical vasoconstrictor is applied, local anesthetic (such as 4% lidocaine) should be sprayed or nebulized into the nose. If aspiration is possible, no further anesthetic should be applied. The patient may be sedated with a rapidly acting narcotic and benzodiaz-epine if indicated. The bronchoscope is lubri-cated and passed through the endotracheal tube. The bronchoscope must be at least 0.5 mm smaller in external diameter than the internal diameter of the tube. Unless the tube's internal diameter is about 2.5 mm larger than the external diameter of the bronchoscope, ventila-tion is not possible and the scope must be removed immediately after intubation of the trachea. In general, the scope's tip should be positioned just proximal to the distal end of the tube. If the scope is passed beyond the tube and advanced into the trachea before the endotra-cheal tube is passed through the nose, the tube may be unable to negotiate the nasal passage, wasting the effort. The advantage of the latter approach is that bleeding may be less if the endotracheal tube is not passed through the

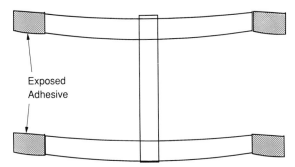

Figure 2–2. Adequate taping of an endotracheal tube requires that tape be applied to the tube in at least two planes. Two horizontal strips of tape are laid parallel, adhesive side up. Then a vertical connecting piece is applied at the midpoint of the horizontal pieces. The adhesive surfaces are covered except for the four ends of the horizontal tapes to prevent pulling on hair and beards.

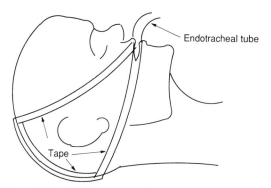

Figure 2–3. H-shaped tape described in Figure 2–2 is placed under the patient's occiput with the vertical strip in the posterior midline. One of the horizontal pieces is passed above the ear, and the other beneath. The exposed adhesive is then applied to the endotracheal tube. The lower tape prevents the tube from moving anteriorly; the upper tape prevents caudad movement.

nasal passage until after the bronchoscope is in the trachea. If the tube is passed into the nasopharynx before insertion of the scope into the tube, tube compression within the nose may prevent passage of the scope. The scope and tube are advanced together, with suctioning as necessary, until the tube passes over the soft palate into the oropharynx.

Fiberoptic guided intubation can also be performed orally. After application of topical anesthetic, a special oral airway, with a groove along the inferior surface to accommodate the fiberoptic bronchoscope, is positioned in the midline. The scope is passed through the groove.

At this point, whether the nasal or oral approach is used, the tongue and often the epiglottis can be seen. The tube is held in its position, and the bronchoscope is advanced through the glottis and into the trachea. The scope should be positioned about 3 cm above the carina and stabilized there while an assistant threads the tube over the scope into the trachea. The carina and the tip of the tube are then visualized with the scope to ensure appropriate positioning. The cuff is inflated, and the scope is withdrawn while the tube is held firmly in position. If hypoxia is a problem during intubation, oxygen may be insufflated down the bronchoscope channel. Jet ventilation with the Sanders jet attachment via the suction channel can also be used to remove carbon dioxide.

AFTER INTUBATION

Cricoid pressure should be maintained after intubation. The tube is grasped firmly with the hand resting on the patient's maxilla. Ventilation is begun with a self-inflating bag. The chest is auscultated in both axillae and the epi-gastrium to document equal breath sounds synchronous with ventilation and the absence of sounds in the epigastrium. The chest should move synchronously with ventilation, and no belching sounds should occur. If any of these conditions suggest improper placement, laryngoscopy should be repeated immediately. The intubator should note the distance markings on the endotracheal tube at the level of the incisors. The average depth of insertion is 23 cm in men and 21 cm in women. After confirmation of proper placement, cricoid pressure may be released. The intubator or a trusted assistant should never lose contact with the tube until it has been securely taped (Figs. 2–2 and 2–3). Many intubations have been lost when attention was momentarily distracted and the tube slipped from the larynx. After the tube is taped, signs of proper placement should again be confirmed. Chest radiography should be performed to confirm and document proper positioning.

Secure taping of the endotracheal tube is critical. The tape should encircle the neck and head and should tether the tube in two planes. One tape should encircle the lower part of the face, passing under the ear and occiput to prevent the tube's being pulled straight out. Another tape should be directed over the upper cheek, above the ear, and around the upper head to prevent the tube's being pulled caudad.

By meticulous attention to detail, the complications of endotracheal intubation can be minimized (Table 2–11).

ALTERNATIVE INTUBATION METHODS

Manually guided orotracheal intubation can be performed in unconscious patients. The

TABLE 2–11. Complications of Endotracheal Intubation

Immediate

Hypoxia
Esophageal intubation
Mainstem intubation
Hypertension
Vomiting
Laryngospasm
Laryngeal damage

Delayed

Oropharyngeal ulceration
Laryngeal ulceration

TABLE 2–12. Needle Cricothyrotomy

Equipment

12- or 14-gauge or larger needle with plastic external catheter
Empty syringe

Indications

Failure to intubate
Contraindications to other routes of intubation
Complete airway obstruction at or above larynx

Contraindications

Untrained personnel

Complications

Inadequate ventilation
Pneumomediastinum caused by malposition of catheter
Pneumothorax caused by lung overinflation
Tracheal and esophageal laceration
Hematoma

index and middle fingers of one gloved hand are placed over the tongue in the midline and pulled forward. An endotracheal tube with a stylet curved sharply anteriorly at the distal end is advanced into the larynx, with the fingers as a guide. The tube is then advanced off the stylet into the trachea. A number of alternative techniques for achieving endotracheal intubation have been described, but all require many minutes to perform. Thus they have limited applicability in an emergency. Several variations of a retrograde Seldinger-like technique have been reported. In this technique a catheter is introduced into the trachea via a cricothyroid membrane puncture in a cephalad direction. The wire is passed retrograde through the larynx and fished out via the mouth or nose. An endotracheal tube is then passed over the wire into the trachea. Unfortunately, the tube often passes into the esophagus, carrying the wire with it. Although this technique is occasionally successful, most clinicians do not find it useful or reliable.

CRICOTHYROTOMY

Needle or surgical cricothyrotomy is appropriate when endotracheal intubation is contraindicated or prolonged efforts have failed. Needle cricothyrotomy is a temporizing lifesaving measure that can be instituted quickly if the equipment is available and personnel are trained (Table 2–12). It provides adequate oxygenation in most cases and adequate ventilation in many. It does not protect against aspiration. A modification of needle cricothyrotomy has been described in which a guide wire is passed through the needle after the needle is positioned in the airway, followed by a dilator and small modified tracheostomy tube.

Needle   Cricothyrotomy. The cricothyroid membrane should be identified between the cricoid and thyroid cartilages. The skin is punctured with the needle, and gentle retraction is applied on the syringe handle (Fig. 2–4). The needle is advanced until the cricothyroid membrane is punctured as confirmed by free aspiration of air. The needle is aimed caudad, and the plastic catheter is advanced off the needle. The needle is removed, the catheter is advanced to its final position, and another check for free aspiration of air is made. The catheter is connected to a source of ventilation, which may be a jetting device or a self-inflating bag.

The jetting device consists of pressure tubing connected to a source of pressurized oxygen, a pressure regulator, and a manually operated valve, which is in turn connected to a male Luer-Lok fitting (Fig. 2–5). The latter attaches to the female Luer-Lok fitting on the plastic catheter. Adequate ventilation can be achieved for prolonged periods. When needle cricothyrotomy is used, exhalation must occur via the natural airway and the operator must ensure that the chest rises during inflation and falls with escape of air from the nose and mouth during exhalation. Ventilation cannot be provided for the patient with complete airway obstruction. The catheter also can be attached, via a 3 mm endotracheal tube connector, to a standard self-inflating bag-valve unit. Alternatively, an 8 mm endotracheal connector can be wedged into a 3 ml syringe, which is connected to the transtracheal catheter. When this device is used, ventilation is marginal because of the high resistance of the catheter and the rate of gas escape from the patient's lungs during exhalation via the catheter is low. Much of the gas is exhaled through the upper airway. With

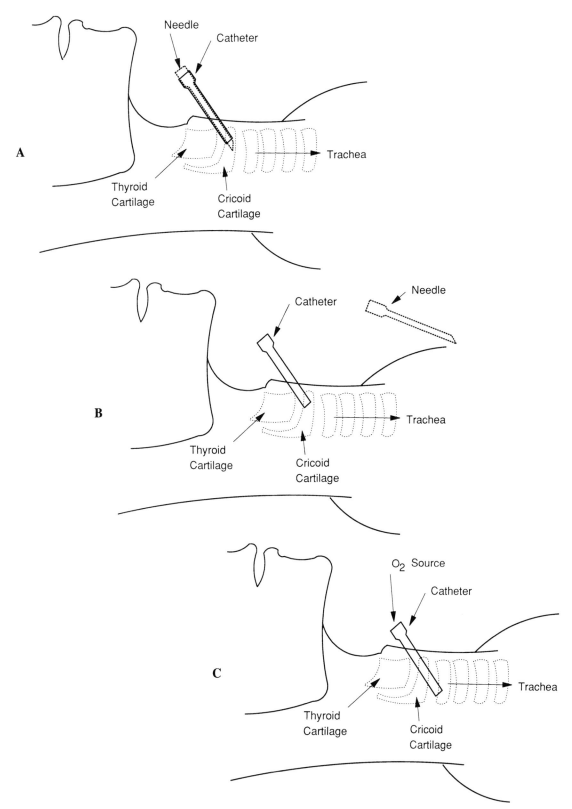

Figure 2–4. **A,** Catheter-needle assembly is positioned in the trachea. **B,** Needle is removed, leaving the tip of the plastic catheter in the tracheal lumen. **C,** Oxygen is injected via the catheter to sustain oxygen delivery.

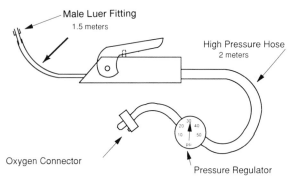

Figure 2–5. Jet attachment provides a high oxygen flow for ventilation via a needle cricothyrotomy or the suction channel of a fiberoptic bronchoscope.

either device the operator must guard against severe air trapping with lung overdistention because of restricted egress of air. Fortunately, hypoventilation with hypercarbia is a much less critical problem than hypoxia, and providing a high FIO_2 prevents hypoxia even when hypoventilation is severe.

Surgical Cricothyrotomy. Surgical cricothyrotomy can be performed rapidly, with little risk of significant bleeding (Table 2–13). The cricothyroid membrane is located, and the area is surgically prepared and anesthetized in the conscious patient. A skin incision is made horizontally and carried through the membrane (Fig. 2–6). After the wound is spread open, an endotracheal or tracheostomy tube is passed into the trachea. This airway can be left in place for hours to days before being replaced with a conventional tracheostomy.

TRACHEOSTOMY

Tracheostomy should almost always be performed as an elective procedure after the airway

TABLE 2–13. Surgical Cricothyrotomy

Equipment

Tracheostomy or endotracheal tube
Scalpel
Local anesthetic

Indications

Failure to intubate
Contraindications to other routes of intubation
Severe maxillofacial injury

Complications

Pneumomediastinum
Hemorrhage
Tracheal laceration
Esophageal laceration
Wound infection

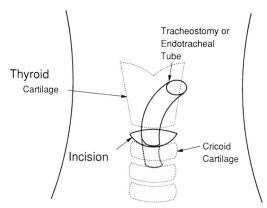

Figure 2–6. Surgical cricothyrotomy. See the text for a description of the technique. Placement of a tracheostomy tube by this method can be performed nearly as rapidly as endotracheal intubation.

is controlled by the simpler methods, such as endotracheal intubation or needle or surgical cricothyrotomy.

ASSESSMENT OF VENTILATION

After a patent airway has been established, the adequacy of ventilation should be assessed (Table 2–14). In the early moments after admission the assessment depends on clinical observation and application of noninvasive monitors. After initial stabilization, arterial blood gases should be measured and minute ventilation adjusted to maintain an arterial pH between 7.35 and 7.45.

TABLE 2–14. Initial Assessment of Ventilation

Observation

Respiratory rate
Chest expansion
Symmetry of chest expansion
Color

Auscultation

Symmetry
Air entry
Rales
Rhonchi
Wheezes

Measurements

Airway pressure
Tidal volume
Vital capacity
Negative inspiratory pressure
Pulse oximeter
Capnograph

BREATHING (VENTILATION)

Spontaneous Ventilation

After an open airway is established, some patients can maintain a normal minute ventilation and lung volumes spontaneously. This is generally not true if high doses of analgesics or sedatives are required, if weakness or respiration-induced pain is present, or if impedance to breathing (high resistance or low compliance) is high.

Positive-Pressure Ventilation

When spontaneous ventilation is judged inadequate, assisted or controlled positive-pressure ventilation is initiated. If the patient is not intubated, the airway is opened by maneuvers described previously.

Self-Inflating Bag

Ventilation is initially provided by a self-inflating bag supplied with 100% oxygen and a one-way valve. A variety of such bags are available, but all those capable of providing 100% oxygen have a reservoir attached to the inlet port of the bag. Without the reservoir, pure oxygen cannot be delivered because room air is entrained during the bag inflation cycle. Alternatively, any anesthetic breathing circuit may be used. These have the disadvantage of requiring a source of pressurized gas to inflate the bag; if the pressurized source is lost, no ventilation can be provided. Every occupied ICU bed should have an oxygen flowmeter mounted on a pressurized oxygen line, tubing to deliver oxygen to a bag or face mask, a self-inflating bag, and a tightfitting mask for positive-pressure ventilation. In emergencies the bag is attached to a face mask for ventilation. When oxygenation is reestablished, intubation should be performed while ventilation continues with the self-inflating bag.

Mechanical Ventilation

Mechanical ventilation should be started with a volume-preset ventilator. The initial tidal volume should be 12 to 15 ml/kg of ideal body weight, delivered 10 to 12 times/min, which provides total ventilation of about 150 ml/kg/min. This would hyperventilate some patients but would rarely hypoventilate patients. Sighs have shown no value during prolonged mechanical ventilation with these tidal volumes. Prolonged ventilation with smaller tidal volumes leads to progressive hypoxia.

Mode of Ventilation

Most patients can be managed initially with controlled, intermittent mandatory or assisted ventilation. The ventilation mode is chosen to ensure adequate ventilation during the stabilization phase in the ICU and then modified according to the patient's condition (see Chapter 3).

Fractional Concentration of Inspired Oxygen

The F_{IO_2} should be set at 1.0 unless adequate oxygenation has been documented with a lower F_{IO_2}. For nonintubated patients, supplemental oxygen can be provided through face masks with or without reservoir bags, by nasal cannula, or by a face shield or tent (see Chapter 3). The actual F_{IO_2} is variably lower than the concentration delivered to the device. The degree to which the F_{IO_2} is less than the delivered oxygen concentration depends on the patient's tidal volume, the inspiratory flow rate, the rate of oxygen delivery to the device, and the presence of anatomic or device dead space.

Positive End-Expiratory Pressure

Positive end-expiratory pressure (PEEP) should not be used initially in patients with acute or chronic airways obstructive diseases, such as asthma or emphysema, or in patients with low cardiac output, hypotension, or pneumothorax. Most other patients show better oxygenation if 3 to 5 cm H_2O PEEP is applied. This PEEP level should overcome the reduction in functional residual capacity caused by obesity, supine position, pain, narcotics, sedatives, and muscle relaxants. Although oxygenation is better during PEEP application, no long-term benefit has been attributed to the prophylactic administration of PEEP.

CIRCULATION

Assessment

The initial assessment of circulation is based on simple clinical observations (Table 2-15). Although the presence of blood pressure does

TABLE 2–15.   Initial Assessment of Circulation

Palpate central and peripheral pulses
  Heart rate and rhythm
Palpate peripheral skin temperature
Measure blood pressure
  Respiratory variation
Auscultate heart
Apply pulse oximeter
Assess venous distention
  Cardiac filling pressures
Apply EKG monitor

not ensure adequate perfusion, perfusion does not occur in the absence of a pressure gradient.

Pulses

Simple palpation of central and peripheral arterial pulses gives an impression of the systemic vascular resistance. If the patient is unresponsive and pulses are not present, cardiopulmonary resuscitation is begun. When central pulses are present and peripheral pulses weak, vascular resistance is likely to be high. Peripheral pulse volume is more closely related to pulse pressure (that is, systolic minus diastolic) than to absolute blood pressure. A narrow pulse pressure suggests vasoconstriction. While palpating the pulses, the physician should determine whether pulse volume varies noticeably in relation to ventilation. Large variation in the blood pressure correlates with relative hypovolemia, heart failure, or tamponade. Heart rate and rhythm should be noted as signs of compensatory tachycardia, and rhythm disturbance may be present.

Skin Temperature and Capillary Refill

When skin temperature decreases peripherally or capillary refill time is prolonged, vasoconstriction should be suspected.

Blood Pressure

Blood pressure should be determined. If an arterial catheter is in place, the blood pressure monitor should be the first monitor connected. Inspection of the tracing immediately reveals the absolute blood pressure, the presence of respiratory blood pressure variation, the width of the pulse tracing, and the regularity of rhythm and rate. Respiratory variation can also be detected by auscultation in which the examiner notes the pressure at which the first systolic sounds are heard and the pressure at which all heartbeats are heard. Excessive pressure variation with ventilation or a narrow pulse width suggests relative hypovolemia (see Chapter 4). Automated oscillometric blood pressure equipment may be applied if an arterial line is not in place. These monitors are reasonably accurate provided the patient is lying quietly and is not severely vasoconstricted. The systolic, diastolic, and mean pressures should be noted.

Cardiac Auscultation

The heart should be auscultated to determine intensity of heart sounds, rate, and rhythm. Muffled sounds are due either to a low amplitude of heart sounds or to interference with transmission to the stethoscope. Muffled sounds may imply poor contractility, hypovolemia, pulmonary overinflation, pneumothorax, or tamponade.

Pulse Oximetry

A pulse oximeter measures heart rate and oxyhemoglobin saturation. Because pulse oximeters function only when phasic changes in absorbance occur, they act as plethysmographs and suggest that reasonable peripheral perfusion is present when they display a saturation value (see Chapter 7).

Venous Pressure

The neck veins are assessed for distention. If central venous or pulmonary arterial catheters are present, the central venous pressure and wedge pressure are determined (see Chapter 4).

Electrocardiography

The EKG is much less important than the blood pressure tracing because it is unrelated to cardiac output or perfusion pressure unless an arrhythmia is present. When severe bradycardia or tachycardia or an irregular pulse is present, the EKG tracing should be inspected immediately for QRS and PR interval prolongations, obvious ST segment elevations or depressions, and marked T wave elevations or inversions. These findings on monitored EKG leads only suggest abnormalities because of the nonstandard placement of electrodes, as well as the electronic filtering required to obtain stable tracings (see Chapter 6). A standard 12-lead EKG is required for confirmation of morphologic abnormalities (see Chapter 4).

Management

The initial management of circulatory inadequacy is based on a four-step approach: (1) optimize cardiac rate, (2) optimize cardiac preload, (3) support cardiac contractility, and (4) optimize systemic vascular resistance (or cardiac afterload). During the early phase of stabilization, cerebral and myocardial perfusion pressures must be maintained to ensure flow to these critical organs. Fortunately, the circulation through the vasculature of heart and brain is relatively resistant to the effect of vasoconstrictor agents. Both require a perfusion pressure (mean arterial pressure minus venous pressure) of 50 to 60 mm Hg in normal individuals to sustain normal flow. Patients with hypertension and occlusive vascular disease may require higher perfusion pressures (see Chapter 4).

Heart Rate and Rhythm

Stroke volume is reasonably well maintained between 80 and 150 beats/min. Patients with heart disease may not tolerate rates between 120 and 150 beats/min. If the rate falls and the stroke volume fails to increase in a fully compensatory fashion, cardiac output must fall.

Anticholinergic or beta-adrenergic drugs or electrical pacing can improve cardiac output when bradycardia is present. Atropine (0.2 mg to a maximum of 1 mg) increases the rate in most supraventricular rhythms and may increase the number of transmitted impulses in the case of atrioventricular conduction block. Beta-adrenergic agonists such as isoproterenol (0.5 to 2 μg/min) or dopamine (5 to 15 $\mu g \cdot kg^{-1} \cdot min^{-1}$) increase the rate in both supraventricular and ventricular rhythms. Ventricular, esophageal, or transthoracic pacing is the only rapidly available option. If pacing is shown to be successful, atrial or sequential atrioventricular pacing should be considered later.

At high heart rates, impairment of ventricular filling causes stroke volume to fall more severely than the heart rate can compensate, with reduction in cardiac output. Tachyarrhythmias should be treated by finding and correcting precipitating factors (such as hypercarbia, theophylline or beta-adrenergic overdose, or hypokalemia), pharmacologic intervention, or electrical cardioversion.

Supraventricular tachycardias may be treated most rapidly with synchronized cardioversion. This should be the initial modality when hypotension is severe or symptomatic. Verapamil (1 to 5 mg boluses) or beta-adrenergic blockade (esmolol 0.2 to 0.5 mg/kg followed by a continuous infusion) is effective for most supraventricular arrhythmias. Both agents have the potential for worsening hypotension and decreasing myocardial contractility. If ventricular preexcitation is present, the agent of choice is a class I antiarrhythmic agent such as procainamide. Calcium channel blockade, beta-blockade, and digitalis may all actually increase conduction via the accessory pathways and worsen the rate. Digitalis is especially useful for control of atrial fibrillation, but its onset is relatively slow. When cardiac failure and acute atrial stretch are part of the pathogenesis of the arrhythmia, digitalis may also correct the underlying cause.

Ventricular tachycardia should generally be treated by administration of lidocaine and, if the patient is hypotensive, by synchronized cardioversion.

Preload

If the patient is hypotensive and shows no clear evidence of circulatory overload (neck vein distention, high central venous or wedge pressure, gallop rhythm), fluid 10 to 15 ml/kg should be infused rapidly while further assessment is performed. This should be continued until the circulatory status is adequate or the central venous pressure is greater than 15 mm Hg, wedge pressure is greater than 18 mm Hg, or other evidence of circulatory overload is present. If no filling pressures are available and the circulatory response to fluid loading is inadequate after 30 ml/kg has been administered, central filling pressures should be measured (see Chapter 4). Edema does not correlate well with blood volume or cardiac preload and should not be interpreted as a sign of circulatory overload.

Resuscitation Fluids

The choices of fluid for resuscitation include crystalloid, colloid, and red blood cells. Normally crystalloid solutions are the most readily available and are an appropriate first choice. Either saline solution or a balanced salt solution may be used. The latter prevents or minimizes later hyperchloremic acidosis. Colloids consist of concentrated albumin (25%), 5% albumin or plasma protein fraction, fresh-frozen plasma, dextran 70, and 6% hetastarch. If clotting factor deficiency is known to accompany hypovolemia, fresh-frozen plasma is the correct choice. Dextrans have fallen out of favor because they occasionally cause allergic reactions and interfere with the clotting process. Hetastarch is generally free of these problems, carries little or no risk of viral disease transmission, and is much less expensive than albumin or fresh-frozen plasma. Colloid and crystalloid solutions for resuscitation have been compared in emergency situations such as hypovolemic shock following trauma and in perioperative fluid loss. These studies generally show no difference in the incidence of pulmonary edema or death. Patients who receive colloid-containing solutions are generally resuscitated more quickly and with much less fluid than those receiving exclusively crystalloid solutions. When anemia or acute blood loss is known to be present, transfusion of red blood cells should begin. Type-specific blood and blood that has undergone typing and antibody screening carry a low risk of inducing an immediate or delayed hemolytic reaction. Thus a massively bleeding patient should receive blood before completion of the cross-matching procedure.

Inotropic Agents

If the patient shows clear evidence of circulatory overload in conjunction with hypotension and vasoconstriction, an agent with inotropic effect (such as dobutamine or dopamine) should be infused (see Chapter 4). Contractility is increased by alpha- and beta-adrenergic stimulation, ionized calcium, digitalis glycosides, and phosphodiesterase inhibitors such as amrinone. It is depressed by hypoxia, beta-adrenergic blockade, calcium channel blockers, and acidosis.

Vasoconstrictors

The primary circulatory priority is maintaining adequate perfusion pressure to the myocardial and cerebral vasculature so these vital organs will not sustain permanent ischemic damage. Identifying and correcting the underlying causes of the hypotension and weaning the patient from any vasoconstrictive agents as rapidly as possible are also critical. If hypotension, circulatory overload, and evidence of low peripheral resistance coexist, a mixed alpha- and beta-agonist (ephedrine, dopamine, epinephrine) infusion is appropriate (see Chapter 4). If hypotension is severe and the cause unclear, agents with alpha and beta activity are indicated.

INITIAL CENTRAL NERVOUS SYSTEM RESUSCITATION

The primary goal in central nervous system (CNS) resuscitation is an adequate flow of oxygenated blood with sufficient glucose. The determinants of cerebral oxygen delivery are arterial oxygen content and tension and cerebral blood flow. The latter depends on cerebral perfusion pressure (mean arterial pressure minus the greater of intracranial pressure or cerebral venous pressure) and cerebral vascular resistance. Maintenance of adequate blood pressure is critically important for cerebral resuscitation, especially if CNS injury is already present (see Chapter 5).

When intracranial hypertension is known or suspected to be present or when signs of herniation (pupillary dilation, hypertension with bradycardia, and ventilatory abnormalities) are present, initial supportive measures are provision of adequate oxygenated blood and mild hyperventilation. Mannitol should be used as an emergency measure when signs of herniation occur but should probably not be given for suspected intracranial hypertension. Steroids have few if any indications for treatment of intracranial hypertension except that caused by edema surrounding a tumor (see Chapter 5).

MANAGEMENT OF THE COMBATIVE PATIENT

The combative, agitated patient is a significant management problem because ability to diagnose and treat the underlying problems is impaired and treatment of the agitation may obscure its cause. The efficacy or safety of specific protocols or policies has not been well studied. First, the cause of the combative state is rarely obvious, and even when one obvious cause is present, frequently other factors are involved. Second, agitation precludes obtaining a clear history, which is often the most important diagnostic procedure, and impedes physical examination or performance of diagnostic or therapeutic procedures. Third, the combative patient may secondarily injure himself or herself. Fourth, these patients are a significant risk to personnel attempting to render care.

A few principles for managing the combative patient can be suggested, but their effectiveness and safety require verification. Empiric therapy (Table 2–16) includes establishment of an open airway, provision of oxygen and glucose, and

TABLE 2–16.   Emergency Management of Agitated Combative Patient

Empiric Emergency Therapy	*Intravenous Narcotics*

Empiric Emergency Therapy

Oxygen
Glucose
Restoration of adequate blood pressure
Reassurance, orientation
If history suggests sedative abuse, administer physostigmine
If phenothiazine toxic effects, administer diphenhydramine

Emergency Neurologic Examination

Pupils: size, shape, reactivity
Extraocular muscle function
Upper and lower extremity movement and symmetry
Glasgow Coma Scale score

Emergency History

Head trauma
Asphyxia
Medication, therapeutic and illicit
Preexisting abnormalities in mental status
Diabetes mellitus
Seizures

Emergency Blood Tests

Blood gases with carbon monoxide level
Glucose
Drug screen
    Alcohol blood level
    Urine and gastric contents
Hemoglobin
Blood urea nitrogen, creatinine
Liver function tests
Electrolytes and osmolality

Management of Agitated, Nonintubated Patient

Reassurance
Narcotics
    Small doses administered intravenously
Sedation
    Should follow analgesia
    Sedation in presence of pain causes agitation; titrate intravenously so that agitation is blunted
    Do not induce drowsiness
Monitoring
    Level of consciousness
    Rate and depth of ventilation
    Oxygenation with pulse oximeter
    Blood pressure

Intravenous Narcotics

Advantages

    Pain relief
    Sedation
    Reversibility
    Cardiovascular stability

Disadvantages

    Relatively slow onset
    Loss of validity of pain as a symptom
    Cardiovascular instability if hypovolemic
    Respiratory depression
        Hypoventilation
        Cough suppression
        Depression of protective airway reflexes

Pharmacologic Paralysis (Intubated Patients)

Advantages

    Rapid control
    Minimal cardiovascular effects
    Reversibility
    Improved ventilation/perfusion relations
    Decreased oxygen consumption
    Improved chest wall compliance

Disadvantages

    Loss of neurological examination
    Absence of cough
    Absence of sedation
    Absence of analgesia
    Inability for spontaneous ventilation
    Necessity for prior or simultaneous intubation
    Positional injuries
        Nerve compression
        Vascular compression
        Joint injury
        Eye abrasion, compression
        Genital compression
        Decubitus ulcers

---

restoration of blood pressure. Although necessarily limited, a rapid baseline neurologic examination should be performed (Table 2–16) and any available neuropsychiatric history (Table 2–16) should be obtained from the patient, family, friends, and bystanders. Blood, preferably arterial, should be obtained for detection of correctable abnormalities (Table 2–16).

Pain should be alleviated with small doses of intravenous narcotics and mechanical stabilization of the injured areas. Establishing communication via interpreters and providing reassurance can be effective. Simple maneuvers, such as emptying a distended bladder, are often surprisingly effective.

Drug therapy to suppress the combative or agitated state may be necessary to prevent further injury and permit more detailed assessment and therapy. Management frequently depends on the airway status (Table 2–16). Agents that can be reversed rapidly or have a short duration of action and that produce minimal respiratory or cardiovascular disturbance should be selected. Narcotics (Table 2–16) and muscle relaxants (Table 2–16) (for an intubated, ventilated patient) meet these criteria reasonably well. The doses and agents are determined by whether the patient's airway has been secured by intubation.

Muscle relaxants can be given to an intubated patient after mechanical ventilation has begun. Although neuromuscular blockade is useful for immediate control of an agitated patient, muscle relaxants should be viewed as temporizing agents while the underlying cause of agitation is sought and eliminated. When no treatable cause is found, analgesics and hypnotics should virtually always be given in high enough doses to eliminate or greatly reduce the need for muscle relaxants. For immediate control, succinylcholine is the most rapidly acting and has the shortest duration. However, it should not be given to patients at risk of acute hyperkalemia, such as patients with burns, sepsis, or central nervous system injuries. The newer nondepolarizing agents of intermediate duration such as vecuronium seem ideal and may be repeated as needed. Although the atracurium metabolic product laudanosine has not been a problem during intraoperative use, its lack of toxicity (seizures) if given for days in an ICU has not been proved. Longer-acting agents such as metocurine and pancuronium are less expensive and have tolerable incidences and severity of side effects for long-term use.

A sedative-hypnotic drug with rapid onset is required during the emergency control of a combative patient. Thiopental, etomidate, and midazolam are candidates, but each has specific limitations. Thiopental produces respiratory and cardiovascular depression. Etomidate suppresses adrenal function, which is undesirable in a patient under stress. Midazolam is less reliable for inducing unconsciousness and may also cause cardiovascular compromise and respiratory depression. Haloperidol is useful for long-term control of an agitated patient (see Chapter 21), but the onset of action is too slow for acute control.

The importance of securing an airway and providing adequate ventilation before administration of sedating and paralyzing drugs, and intense monitoring thereafter, cannot be overemphasized. This management method is equivalent to providing general anesthesia in an unprepared patient. Thus the physician is obligated to protect against complications of the therapy and to monitor vital organ systems. Once such drugs have been administered, the physician must assume that intracranial disease is present, institute the appropriate diagnostic tests, and presumptively treat the patient for such disease.

Although the list of potential causes of agitation is long (Table 2–17), it can be divided into those that limit oxygen and glucose delivery, metabolic abnormalities, central nervous system poisons, diseases or injuries, and psychiatric problems. Consideration of each of these categories minimizes the chances of missing a significant problem. Most of them are discussed elsewhere (see Chapters 5, 10, 17, and 21).

SECONDARY ASSESSMENT AND MANAGEMENT

The secondary assessment and initiation of therapy for diseases of lower priority should occur after the initial stabilization. An organized approach helps in covering all important areas quickly (Table 2–18). First the ABCs are quickly reviewed to ensure that no new problems have developed. Then the remainder of the patient's history and physical examination is assessed and a comprehensive plan of diagnosis, monitoring, and management is developed.

Drugs

Long-Term Medications

A complete list of medications the patient has been taking for an extended time should be obtained as soon as possible to prevent adverse drug interactions, overdosages, or the effects of inappropriate drug withdrawal. A history of allergy or other adverse reaction to any medications should be sought. Drugs that had been prescribed for valid indications before the acute illness should be continued or replaced with appropriate substitutes (see Chapter 4) whenever possible. The patient should be asked specifically about cardiovascular medications such as antiarrhythmic, antihypertensive, antianginal and diuretic agents. Informationabout drugs taken for pulmonary conditions such as asthma (see Chapter 8) should be sought. Steroid therapy for any condition has important implications regarding steroid replacement, as well as the potential complications of long-term steroid therapy (seeChapter 16).

Short-Term Medications

A complete list of agents administered in the hospital before arrival in the ICU is necessary for interpretation of the current physiologic

TABLE 2–17. Examples of Causes of Agitation or Combativeness

Substrate Insufficiency

Hypoxia
Hypoglycemia
Inadequate cerebral blood flow

Metabolic Abnormalities

Hypercarbia
Hyponatremia
Hypernatremia
Hyperglycemia
Hypophosphatemia
Calcium
Magnesium
Uremia
Hepatic failure

Drugs and Chemicals

Accidental administration
  Methanol
  Ethylene glycol
  Anticholinergics
  Organophosphates
Self-administered
  Alcohol
  Cocaine
  Amphetamines
  Sedatives
  Narcotics
  Hallucinogens
Prescribed
  Sedatives
  Phenothiazines
  Narcotics
  Butyrophenones

Drug Withdrawal Syndromes

Narcotics
Alcohol
Sedatives
Amphetamines

Central Nervous System (CNS) Disease

Postictal state
Fever
CNS infection
  Meningitis
  Encephalitis
  Abscess
Head injury
Subarachnoid hemorrhage
Intracerebral hemorrhage
Cerebral infarction
Elevated intracranial pressure

Psychiatric Problems

Sleep deprivation
Fear
Pain
Exacerbation of preexisting psychiatric illness
Inability to communicate
"ICU psychosis"
Hyperventilation syndrome

TABLE 2–18. Secondary Assessment and Management

Assessment (Alphabetically)

Airway
Breathing
Circulation
Drugs
Examination
Fluids
History
Plan of action

Physical Examination, Head to Toe

Head and neck
Brain and spinal cord
Chest
Abdomen
Extremities
Devices

Neurologic Examination

Level of consciousness
  Unstimulated
  Stimulated
Glasgow Coma Scale score
Muscle tone: right and left, upper and lower extremities
Sensory: touch, pain or temperature, proprioception
Pupils, right and left
  Size and shape
  Reaction to light
Eyes
  Position
  Motion: horizontal, vertical and diagonal, conjugate
Respiratory pattern
  Regularity
  Depth
  Rate
If depressed level of consciousness or signs of brainstem dysfunction
  Eyegrounds
    Optic disc clear
    Hemorrhages
  Plantar stimulation: toes up, down, no response
If comatose
  Corneal reflex
  Gag reflex
  Cough reflex
  Oculocephalic testing: horizontal and vertical
  Caloric testing: unilateral cold, bilateral cold and warm

state. Drugs used during anesthesia should be reviewed with the anesthesiologist, and the need to reverse the action of muscle relaxants and narcotics assessed.

Comprehensive Examination

During the initial evaluation a rapid physical examination is performed. In the secondary assessment the patient should be examined from head to toe (Table 2–18). The following are points of particular interest in a critically ill patient.

Head and Neck. The head and neck should be examined for signs of trauma in an injured patient. The eyes should be inspected for and protected from injury if the patient is not alert. The ears should be examined for later comparison if occult infection develops in patients with nasoenteral or endotracheal tubes. The teeth should be examined for signs of damage or looseness when an endotracheal tube is present.

Brain and Spinal Cord. The level of consciousness in the unstimulated and stimulated state should be described. The Glasgow Coma scoring should be repeated, and function of cranial nerves II to XII and the brainstem should be reevaluated in patients with known central nervous system disease and those who are not alert (Table 2–18). Completion of the baseline examination includes determination of muscle tone and voluntary or involuntary movement, as well as their symmetry, in upper and lower extremities. A gross check of sensory function should be performed. Babinski's reflex should be checked when the presence of brain or spinal cord disease, ischemia, or injury is possible. Any seizure activity should be described (see Chapter 5).

Chest. The chest wall, lungs, and heart should be more completely examined to supplement the findings of the initial screening examination. If the patient is intubated, the physician needs to know the reason for intubation and any difficulties encountered during intubation because the decision to extubate is influenced by this information. Relative cardiac position should be noted for evaluation of any later shifts induced by pneumothorax or atelectasis.

Abdomen. The abdomen should be assessed for distention, pain, and bowel sounds. If distention is present, assessment for tympany or dullness to indicate air or fluid, respectively, is performed. If the patient has abdominal pain, its location and response to direct and indirect stimulation should be determined.

Devices. The presence and position of all tubes and lines, ventilator settings, and monitors are noted. The presence of unexplained devices may be an important clue to abnormalities that were discovered or known before ICU admission, but not properly documented or communicated.

Extremities. Pulse symmetry, skin temperature, and presence of any deformities, wounds, dressings, pain, and traction devices are recorded.

Fluids

The current composition and rate of fluid administration should be ascertained in addition to the recent cumulative intake and output. The volume of urine, blood, and other drainage should be recorded and the container emptied or marked to make further losses easier to monitor after admission to the ICU. The net rate of glucose, sodium, and potassium administration should be calculated and adjusted if necessary. When multiple vascular lines are present, excessive administration may lead, rapidly or slowly, to complications. Even healthy individuals cannot metabolize more than 4 to 6 mg glucose/kg/min. This is roughly equivalent to 5% glucose 350 to 500 ml/h. Individuals in severe stress may tolerate even less.

PLAN OF ACTION

An initial plan of action should be formulated and ordered. This should include the items listed in Table 2–19. Each organ system should be evaluated to determine whether further diagnostic studies are needed. A plan for monitoring each system, disease, or symptom should be implemented. Monitoring should be designed to detect deterioration before it leads to significant damage. Appropriate therapy in addition to the initial resuscitative measures should be started. Prophylaxis against the common complications of ICU care and the known disease states should begin. Details of the appropriate monitoring, therapy, and prophylaxis for each of these are covered subsequently.

Activity. Every patient should be turned from side to side at least every 2 hours. If tubes,

TABLE 2–19.   Initial Plan Considerations

Activities
Cardiovascular
Respiratory
Renal
Hepatic
Metabolic
Nutrition
Musculoskeletal
Sepsis
Skin
Psychologic
Neurologic
Alimentary
Hematologic

intravenous lines, pain, or traction interferes with this, prescription of a special bed that mechanically turns the patient is indicated. Every patient should be encouraged to move out of bed unless specific contraindications exist.

Cardiovascular System. All patients should have EKG monitoring. Blood pressure monitoring frequency should be based on the current stability and the risk of sudden changes. Indications for invasive monitoring are considered in Chapter 4.

Respiratory System. The need for respiratory support is the most common indication for intensive care. Measures to mobilize secretions include providing adequate humidification of the inspired air, postural change at least every 2 hours (more frequently if unconscious, heavily sedated, or paralyzed by disease or drug), frequently inducing coughing, and suctioning when auscultation indicates the presence of secretions. The risk of laryngeal damage from endotracheal tubes should be minimized by ensuring that the tube is small enough to allow a significant leak when the cuff is deflated. The risk of tracheal damage is low if the cuff pressure is less than 20 mm Hg when the leak is occluded. Cuff pressure should be kept greater than 15 mm Hg to reduce the amount of upper airway material that slips past the cuff. All patients should be monitored for hypoxia. The best method is currently pulse oximetry. Although capnometry will be valuable, current equipment is poorly suited to ICU use because it frequently malfunctions owing to moisture (side stream) or secretions (in-line). Central mass spectrometers fail to monitor patients continuously, represent a single point failure node, and are more expensive than individual bedside oxygen and carbon dioxide monitors. Blood gases should be measured for clinical indications, such as when pulse oximetry reveals an abnormality, when respiratory distress is manifest, and after major ventilator changes, but not on a predesignated schedule.

Renal System. Urine output should be monitored at frequent intervals, and urine and plasma creatinine levels should be determined at least daily in any patient who has cardiovascular instability, evidence of sepsis, or a history of renal disease or is receiving nephrotoxic drugs.

Liver. General guidelines for monitoring liver function are difficult to formulate but include measurement of bilirubin, alkaline phosphatase, and transaminases. Measurement of bilirubin every 2 to 3 days seems reasonable, but enzymes need not be measured as frequently if the bilirubin level is normal. In critically ill patients, albumin and coagulation findings are frequently abnormal for reasons unrelated to liver dysfunction.

Metabolic System. Sodium, potassium, and glucose should be measured at least daily until levels are stable. Chloride need be measured only to clarify an acid-base abnormality identified in blood gas measurement.

Nutrition. Patients receiving nutritional support require extensive monitoring as outlined in Chapter 27.

Musculoskeletal System. Immobilization leads to muscle wasting, hypercalcemia, hypercalciuria, and contractures. If the patient cannot move voluntarily, the medical team must provide active and passive movement. This includes moving from bed to chair, bedside ambulation, weight lifting in bed, and passive range of motion. Considerable ingenuity may be required to maximize physical activity.

Sepsis. Temperature should be monitored every 1 to 4 hours or continuously. Total and differential white blood cell counts should be obtained daily and at the onset of new fever. Routine cultures are not indicated, but Gram stains of tracheal aspirates help in early identification of pneumonia and tracheobronchitis, which is highly lethal and the most common nosocomial infection in critically ill patients.

Skin. Routine turning to prevent pressure necrosis is an absolute requirement. The greater the hemodynamic instability, the more frequent the movement. Although a variety of special beds and mattresses are commercially available to help prevent decubitus ulcers, they give the staff false security and make the turning necessary for pulmonary toilet less likely to occur.

Psychologic Functioning. Alert patients require a variety of measures to enhance orientation and cooperation and allay anxiety (see Chapter 21).

Neurologic System. Routine informal assessment includes recording of level of consciousness, symmetry of movement, and evidence of agitation. More formal evaluation for patients with neurologic disease is discussed in Chapter 4.

Alimentary Tract. Gastric drainage should be considered for every critically ill patient until enteral nutrition has commenced. Drainage reduces the risk of aspiration and permits monitoring of the onset of motility, gastric pH, and blood. All critically ill patients should receive antibleeding prophylaxis with antacids, histamine blockers, or surface-active agents such as sucralfate. Enteral feedings should be started as soon as possible to sustain mucosal integrity. All stools should be recorded and tested for blood.

Blood. Coagulation tests should be performed on admission of critically ill patients. Those with abnormalities or at high risk of coagulopathy need to be tested until results are normal. Hemoglobin concentration is measured at least daily and when hemodynamic instability occurs.

HISTORY

The medical history should be completed with information from the patient, family, friends, other physicians, pharmacists, and old medical records. Particular attention should be paid to drugs, allergies, possible drug abuse, and history of usual illnesses.

SUGGESTED READINGS

Bruce DL, Applebaum EL: Tracheal intubation. Philadelphia, 1976, WB Saunders Co

Haddad LM, Winchester JF: Clinical management of poisoning and drug overdose. Philadelphia, 1983, WB Saunders Co

Oho K, Amemiya R: Practical fiberoptic bronchoscopy. New York, 1980, Igaku-Shoin

Plum F, Posner JB: The diagnosis of stupor and coma, ed 3. Philadelphia, 1982, FA Davis Co

Stehling LC: Fiberoptic intubation of the trachea. In 1988 Annual Refresher Course Lectures. Park Ridge, Ill, 1988, American Society of Anesthesiologists

3

ADVANCED RESPIRATORY LIFE SUPPORT

STEVEN J. ALLEN, MD, AND ALAN S. TONNESEN, MD

The primary life-sustaining functions of the respiratory system are to deliver oxygen to the pulmonary capillaries and carbon dioxide to the atmosphere. Transport of these two gases involves different physiologic processes. This chapter explains the various types of respiratory failure and their causes, describes techniques for assessment, and provides general guidelines for therapeutic intervention based on correction, when possible, of the disorder. Management of specific diseases is discussed later in the book.

Respiratory failure is broadly defined as the inability to maintain acceptable arterial values of oxygen, carbon dioxide, and pH. What determines "acceptable values" may vary from patient to patient depending on underlying conditions, as discussed in the weaning section of this chapter.

In a critically ill patient the first task is to ensure adequate gas exchange for survival. However, therapy itself may cause complications. For example, a patient may require a fraction of inspired oxygen (FIO_2) of 1.0 initially to prevent hypoxemia, but prolonged exposure to high concentrations of inspired oxygen results in pulmonary damage. Next, attention is turned to correcting the underlying problems, for example, treating pneumonia. Finally, ventilatory therapy is withdrawn as the patient's pulmonary function improves.

Chapter 2 outlines the initial steps taken to resuscitate and stabilize a critically ill patient. Once the patient is not in immediate danger of dying, attention focuses on understanding the cause of respiratory failure.

CLASSIFICATION

Respiratory failure may be due to a single factor or many. Full appreciation of a patient's respiratory failure requires a classification system that includes both clinical manifestations and underlying pathophysiologic processes (Table 3–1).

VENTILATORY FAILURE (ALVEOLAR HYPOVENTILATION)

Ventilatory failure, or alveolar hypoventilation, is the situation in which inadequate fresh gas is reaching the alveoli. This condition may be caused by primary weakness of the respiratory muscles, increased work of breathing, or impaired respiratory drive.

Respiratory muscle weakness may be due to a variety of causes such as muscle dysfunction (Duchenne's muscular dystrophy or starvation) or denervation (Guillain-Barré syndrome) or the effect of residual muscle relaxants.

Work of breathing may increase for a number of reasons, some of which are easily correctable. Bedside measurements quantitate certain components of work of breathing such as the degree

TABLE 3–1. Classification of Respiratory Failure

Ventilatory: insufficient bellows pump function
Oxygenation: ventilation/perfusion abnormalities
Airway defense: inability to protect airway

of increased airway resistance and decreased compliance. These tests involve measuring the airway pressure during mechanical ventilatory breaths. Tidal volume divided by peak inspiratory pressure (PIP), minus positive end-expiratory pressure (PEEP) if present, represents *dynamic compliance:*

$$\text{Dynamic compliance} = \frac{\text{Tidal volume}}{\text{PIP} - \text{PEEP}} \quad (1)$$

Dynamic compliance is a measure of the intrinsic compliance of the lungs and chest wall, as well as airway resistance. If the patient is held at end inspiration for a short time, the airway pressure decreases to a plateau (plateau pressure). Tidal volume divided by plateau pressure (minus PEEP if present) provides *static compliance:*

$$\text{Static compliance} = \frac{\text{Tidal volume}}{\text{Plateau pressure} - \text{PEEP}} \quad (2)$$

Static compliance is the true compliance of the lung-thorax unit. Normally 5 cm H_2O pressure results in a 500 ml breath; thus normal static compliance is 100 ml/cm H_2O. The difference between PIP and plateau pressure, then, provides an estimate of airway resistance. A more accurate measurement of airway resistance requires measuring the airflow with a pneumotachograph; airway resistance can then be calculated from the difference between PIP and plateau pressure divided by the airflow rate:

$$\text{Airway resistance} =$$
$$\frac{\text{Peak pressure} - \text{Plateau pressure}}{\text{Flow}} \quad (3)$$

RESPIRATORY DRIVE

Impaired respiratory drive implies dysfunction of the central control of ventilation. The most common culprit of this condition is narcotic overdose, which should respond to administration of narcotic antagonists. However, nonpharmacologic impairment in respiratory drive of a critically ill patient has only recently received much attention. Additional factors that suppress ventilatory drive are protein deprivation, hypothyroidism, and starvation.

Increased respiratory drive caused by acidosis and elevation of partial pressure of carbon dioxide in arterial blood ($Paco_2$) is due to stimulation of central chemoreceptors that produce a strong subjective response of dyspnea. These receptors adapt readily to chronic abnormalities of arterial pH and $Paco_2$. Thus the

baseline values of the patient's pH and $Paco_2$ should be used as a guide to realistic goals of ventilatory weaning. Normal persons manifest a breath-holding breakpoint when $Paco_2$ is in the high 40s to low 50s mm Hg. Sudden $Paco_2$ increases of more than 3 mm Hg cause intense stimulation of ventilation.

Hypoxic ventilatory drive differs from carbon dioxide/pH drive in that adaptation is slow and the primary receptors are located peripherally in the carotid and aortic bodies. Interestingly, a minimal subjective response (slight dyspnea) to hypoxia occurs even though hypoxia is a more potent and stable stimulus to ventilation. Hypoxic drive increases rapidly as the arterial partial pressure of oxygen (Pao_2) falls below 60 mm Hg, or the oxygen saturation (Sao_2) drops to less than 0.90. Most sedatives impair hypoxic ventilatory drive and carbon dioxide/pH drive.

Proprioception from lung and chest wall receptors provides a sense of ventilatory adequacy in many patients. The receptors are stimulated by small tidal volume, low functional residual capacity, and the lack of chest wall receptor stimulation, which may be lost in quadriplegia or during subarachnoid block anesthesia.

DEAD SPACE

Dead space is that portion of the respiratory system into which carbon dioxide does not diffuse. This includes the anatomic dead space, which consists of the respiratory tree proximal to the respiratory ducts, and the alveolar dead space, which consists of alveoli that are ventilated but not perfused ($\dot{V}/\dot{Q}$ = infinity). The difference between these two types of dead space is important in the interpretation of end-tidal capnometry. Increases in anatomic dead space may prolong the lag time (the time until the plateau of the capnogram is reached), but the gradient between the end-tidal carbon dioxide ($Petco_2$) and the $Paco_2$ should be unchanged. Conversely, an increase in alveolar dead space should not affect lag time but does increase the $Petco_2$-$Paco_2$ gradient. For clinical purposes *physiologic* dead space (anatomic plus alveolar dead space) is measured. The fraction of a tidal volume (V_T) that is dead space (V_{DS}) can be determined with $Paco_2$ and a *mixed* expired carbon dioxide ($Peco_2$) determination:

$$V_{DS}/V_T = \frac{Paco_2 - Peco_2}{Paco_2} \quad (4)$$

VDS/VT is normally 0.3 but may rise to 0.6 in severe pulmonary disease.

OXYGENATION FAILURE

Pao_2 represents the output of the lung. Thus Pao_2 is a function of the factors that serve as input into the lung such as inspired oxygen concentration, alveolar ventilation, mixed venous oxygen saturation, and ventilation/perfusion distributions within the lung. Normal individuals are not hypoxemic while breathing room air. Table 3–2 lists the relevant causes of hypoxemia. Decreased diffusion capacity is a cause of decreased oxygen but is usually of little clinical relevance for critically ill patients. These causes may interact with other pathologic processes to exacerbate hypoxemia.

The input factors play a major role in oxygenation because of the mechanism by which the blood carries oxygen. Oxygen is essentially insoluble in plasma. For every 1 mm Hg of oxygen partial pressure, only about 0.003 ml of oxygen is dissolved in each 100 ml of blood. Thus, a normal Pao_2 of about 100 mm Hg results in a whopping 0.3 ml of oxygen carried in each 100 ml of blood. Obviously, hyperbaric conditions would have to exist for adequate oxygen to be dissolved in plasma. On the other hand, each fully saturated gram of hemoglobin can carry 1.37 ml of oxygen. Concentration of arterial oxygen (Cao_2) in milliliters of oxygen per 100 ml of blood can be determined by the following equation:

$$Cao_2 = (0.003 \times Pao_2) + (Hgb \times Sao_2 \times 1.37) \quad (5)$$
$$\text{dissolved} \qquad\qquad \text{bound}$$

where Hgb is hemoglobin concentration in grams per deciliter of blood and Sao_2 is arterial oxygen saturation. Assuming a normal hemoglobin value of 14.7 g/dl and a normal Pao_2 and Sao_2, normal Cao_2 is about 20 ml of oxygen per deciliter of blood. Thus the important determinants of oxygen content are oxygen saturation and hemoglobin concentration. The hemoglobin–oxygen saturation dissociation curve

TABLE 3–2. Causes of Hypoxemia

Alveolar hypoventilation
Ventilation/perfusion abnormalities
Shunt
Impaired diffusion
Low Pao_2
   High altitude
   Hypoxic delivered gas
   Hypercarbia

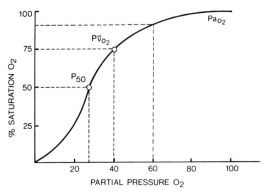

Figure 3-1. Hemoglobin dissociation curve. This curve represents the relationship between hemoglobin saturation and partial pressure of oxygen if pH, temperature, and concentration of 2,3 = diphosphoglycerate are all normal. Three points are noted along the curve: Pao_2 = 60 mm Hg when Sao_2 = 90%, showing that higher Pao_2 adds little to hemoglobin saturation; normal mixed venous oxygen partial pressure ($P\bar{v}o_2$) = 40 mm Hg when $S\bar{v}o_2$ = 75%; partial pressure at which 50% of the hemoglobin is saturated (P_{50}) = 27 mm Hg.

is presented in Figure 3–1. Under normal values of pH, temperature, and 2,3-diphosphoglycerate (2,3-DPG), partial pressure of oxygen (Po_2) levels of 60, 40, and 27 mm Hg are associated with 90%, 75%, and 50% oxygen saturation, respectively. Inspection of the curve shows that elevating the Pao_2 above 60 mm Hg improves Cao_2 relatively little. On the other hand, hemoglobin concentration is directly related to the oxygen content. The Po_2 that results in 50% oxygen saturation is called the P_{50} and serves as an indication of the shift of the hemoglobin dissociation curve. Decreases in pH or increases in temperature or 2,3-DPG shift the curve to the right. Alkalosis, hypothermia, or a decrease in 2,3-DPG shifts the hemoglobin dissociation curve to the left.

The oxygen content of the blood returning to the lungs ($C\bar{v}o_2$) can be calculated in a similar fashion by substituting $P\bar{v}o_2$ and $S\bar{v}o_2$ in equation 5. Assuming a normal $S\bar{v}o_2$ of 75%, normal $C\bar{v}o_2$ is about 15 ml of oxygen per deciliter of blood.

ALVEOLAR AIR EQUATION

The partial pressure of oxygen in the alveoli (Pao_2) is different from the partial pressure of oxygen in the atmosphere because the amounts of various components of gas in the alveoli differ from those in the atmosphere. The sum of all partial gas pressures in the alveoli must equal the atmospheric pressure, which at sea level is 760 mm Hg. The partial pressure of inspired oxygen (PIO$_2$) is calculated by the following equation:

$$PIO_2 = (PB - PH_2O) \times FIO_2 \qquad (6)$$

where PB is barometric pressure and PH$_2$O is the partial pressure of water. This equation corrects for the fact that alveolar gas is fully saturated with water (PB = 47 mm Hg at 37° C). Correcting for the presence of carbon dioxide in the alveolar gas gives the simplified alveolar air equation:

$$PAO_2 = PIO_2 - \frac{PacO_2}{R} \qquad (7)$$

where R is equal to the respiratory quotient typically assumed to be 0.8 and PACO$_2$ is assumed to be equal to PacO$_2$ for purposes of this calculation. This equation has two important characteristics. First, increasing FIO$_2$ results in a direct increase in PAO$_2$. Second, changes in PacO$_2$ affects PAO$_2$. Alveolar hypoventilation, which increases in PACO$_2$, decreases PAO$_2$. Conversely, hyperventilation increases PAO$_2$. This latter observation explains the respiratory changes occurring in response to hypoxia at high altitude. It is also used in severe respiratory failure to improve the PaO$_2$ when arterial desaturation is relentless. However, the elevation in PAO$_2$ is relatively small after alveolar ventilation is normalized, that is, when PacO$_2$ is less than 40 mm Hg (Fig. 3–2) and cannot exceed PIO$_2$. The difference between PAO$_2$ and PaO$_2$, the (A-a)DO$_2$, under normal conditions is small.

As a disease process produces hypoxemia, the (A-a)DO$_2$ widens. Some clinicians use (A-a)DO$_2$ gradient as an index of the severity of oxygen failure. Its main drawbacks are that changing FIO$_2$ has a major effect on the calculated value and that it fails to account for the influence of C$\bar{v}$O$_2$ on arterial oxygen.

VENTILATION/PERFUSION

Under normal conditions, pulmonary blood flow is about 5 L/min and alveolar ventilation is about 5 L/min. Thus the $\dot{V}/\dot{Q}$ ratio for the entire lung is 1. This match is not represented in every individual lung unit; $\dot{V}/\dot{Q}$ values vary throughout the lung, although most fall very near 1. The extremes of $\dot{V}/\dot{Q}$ ratios are zero and infinity. The latter, as described previously, is dead space and has relatively little direct effect on oxygenation. A $\dot{V}/\dot{Q}$ of zero means that some fraction of cardiac output is passing from the right side of

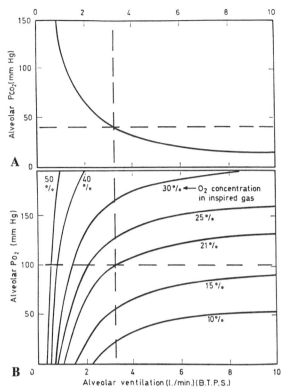

Figure 3-2. Alveolar gas tensions of carbon dioxide (**A**) and oxygen (**B**) at different levels of alveolar ventilation. The bottom graph also depicts the effect of increased FIO$_2$ on alveolar oxygen level. The vertical broken lines in both graphs mark normal alveolar ventilation of 3.2 L/min. The horizontal broken lines mark normal alveolar PCO$_2$ of 40 mm Hg and alveolar PO$_2$ of 100 mm Hg, respectively. (From Nunn JF: Applied respiratory physiology. Stoneham, Mass, 1969, Butterworths, p. 154.)

the heart to the left without perfusing a ventilated alveolus. This is also referred to as intrapulmonary shunt. $\dot{V}/\dot{Q}$ units below 1 but above zero represent less than ideal ventilation for a given amount of perfusion. In these units delivery of oxygen may be inadequate to fully saturate the blood perfusing the units. The level of arterial oxygenation depends on the fraction of pulmonary blood that is not fully saturated during its passage through the lungs. A mathematical explanation of this fact is found in the derivation of the so-called shunt equation. A model of pulmonary blood distribution is shown in Figure 3–3. The total amount of oxygen per minute entering the left atrium may be calculated by multiplying the cardiac output ($\dot{Q}$t) by the CaO$_2$. This is also equal (Equation 8) to the sum of the amount of oxygen leaving the unventilated ($\dot{Q}$s × C$\bar{v}$O$_2$) and ventilated portions [($\dot{Q}$t − $\dot{Q}$s) × CcO$_2$] of the pulmonary circuit.

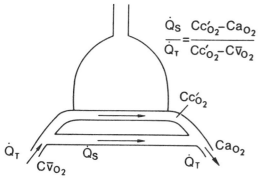

Figure 3-3. Two-compartment model for determining pulmonary shunt flow. The oxygen carried in the arterial blood is the sum of the oxygen carried in blood perfusing ventilated alveoli and that of shunted blood. (From West JB: Respiratory physiology, ed 3. © 1985, The Williams & Wilkins Co., Baltimore.)

$$\dot{Q}t \times Ca_{O_2} = (\dot{Q}s \times C\bar{v}_{O_2}) + (\dot{Q}t - \dot{Q}s) \times Cc_{O_2} \quad (8)$$

where $\dot{Q}s$ is the amount of blood flow through the shunted regions of the lung and Cc_{O_2} is the content of the pulmonary blood after it has left a ventilated alveolus. Rearranging the equation,

$$\dot{Q}s/\dot{Q}t = \frac{Cc_{O_2} - Ca_{O_2}}{Cc_{O_2} - C\bar{v}_{O_2}} \quad (9)$$

Cc_{O_2} cannot be measured directly. It is calculated with the alveolar air equation in the assumption that the hemoglobin is fully saturated. If the patient is breathing an F_{IO_2} of 1.0, the hemoglobin of the blood that passes any alveoli with any ventilation is assumed to be fully saturated. If the patient is not breathing 100% oxygen, this calculation more correctly provides the degree of venous admixture, $\dot{Q}va/\dot{Q}t$, than just true shunt. The term "venous admixture" includes true shunt and the effect of low $\dot{V}/\dot{Q}$ units. The presence of dyshemoglobinemias (carboxyhemoglobinemia and methemoglobinemia) reduces the maximal possible saturation. Thus the percentages of dyshemoglobinemias should be subtracted from 100% to obtain a more accurate Cc_{O_2} value. The amount of shunt present has important implications for the treatment of hypoxemia. Figure 3–4 displays the effect of increased F_{IO_2} on the Pa_{O_2} at increasing levels of $\dot{Q}s/\dot{Q}t$. As can be seen, the higher the shunt, the less effect of increasing F_{IO_2} on Pa_{O_2}.

In the normal state, very little shunt can be measured. Even in patients with evidence of collapsed or poorly ventilated lung, $\dot{Q}s/\dot{Q}t$ usually remains low. Hypoxic pulmonary vaso-

constriction is a protective mechanism that ameliorates the effect of areas of low ventilation. Quite simply, a low P_{O_2} in a lung unit results in constriction of the part of the pulmonary vasculature supplying that lung unit. The effect of this reflex is to minimize the impact of poorly ventilated units on Pa_{O_2}. Thus interference with this reflex, either by disease or by direct pulmonary vasodilators, may decrease Pa_{O_2}.

As the $\dot{V}/\dot{Q}$ ratio falls, the blood perfusing the alveoli removes oxygen more rapidly than it is replaced. If the F_{IO_2} is less than 1.0, the concentration of oxygen in the alveoli decreases and nitrogen level rises, reducing Pa_{O_2}. If Pa_{O_2} decreases below 150 mm Hg, hemoglobin saturation may become less than 1.0. Thus some reduced hemoglobin reaches the arterial circulation. Any excess dissolved oxygen from normal lung units combines with the reduced hemoglobin, reducing Pa_{O_2}. If 0.5 g of reduced hemoglobin reaches the left atrium, it can potentially combine with 0.695 ml of oxygen per deciliter of blood (0.5×1.37). Thus Pa_{O_2} could be reduced by more than 200 mm Hg ($200 \times 0.003 = 0.6$ ml/dl). Raising the F_{IO_2} to 1.0 overcomes the effect of low $\dot{V}/\dot{Q}$ units but not shunt. When the $F_{IO_2} = 1.0$, oxygen removal does not concentrate any remaining nitrogen in the alveoli. Thus the Pa_{O_2} remains constant at a level determined by the Pa_{CO_2} and P_{H_2O}.

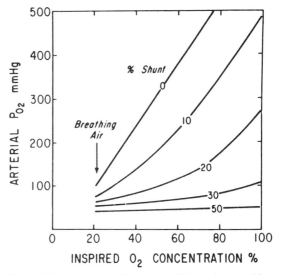

Figure 3-4. Response of the arterial P_{O_2} to increased inspired oxygen concentrations in a lung with various amounts of shunt. In the presence of a greater than 30% shunt, increases of inspired oxygen even to 100% only marginally improve Pa_{O_2}. (From West JB: Pulmonary pathophysiology, ed 3. © 1987, The Williams & Wilkins Co., Baltimore.)

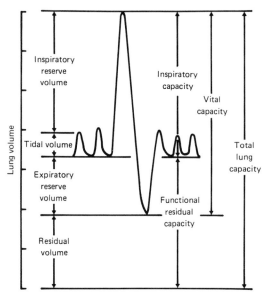

Figure 3-5. Lung volumes.

Arterial oxygenation may also depend on the saturation of the mixed venous blood if any shunt or venous admixture exists. Mixed venous blood that passes through shunt regions mixes with oxygenated blood in the pulmonary veins. Decreases in mixed venous oxygen saturation decrease the overall partial pressure of oxygen in arterial blood. From another perspective, the effect of any degree of shunt on the Pao_2 is directly related to the mixed venous oxygen saturation. Low mixed venous oxygen saturation reflects an imbalance in which the oxygen consumption/oxygen delivery ratio is increased. This is most often due to low cardiac output. Thus, hypoxemia may develop with relatively little pulmonary disease but poor cardiac function. This information is important in the care of patients with cardiac disease, especially postoperatively. By this mechanism, respiratory failure may develop because of the inability to increase cardiac output in response to ventilatory work, stress, or pain. Increased oxygen consumption and arterial hypoxemia are also causes of respiratory failure. However, cardiac output normally increases in these latter two situations, which tends to increase mixed venous oxygen saturation toward normal.

A complete review of the basic concepts of pulmonary function and an understanding of the common pathophysiologic problems in the critically ill requires discussion of lung volumes. Figure 3–5 demonstrates the four basic components of the total lung capacity. Inspiratory reserve volume (IRV), tidal volume (V_T), and expiratory reserve volume (ERV) may be measured with a spirometer at the bedside of a cooperative patient. Determination of residual volume (RV) requires an indirect method. Functional residual capacity (FRC) is the sum of ERV and RV. FRC represents the amount of gas left in the lungs at the end of a tidal breath. The unique aspect of FRC is that it represents the point in the respiratory cycle when the respiratory muscles are at rest. Thus FRC is determined by factors independent of the respiratory muscles. FRC is the lung volume that results from the interaction between the chest wall tending to expand outward and the lungs tending to collapse. Under normal conditions FRC is about 35% of total lung capacity. Clearly, any event that affects the balance of these factors may change FRC. Most clinical events, such as pneumonia, pulmonary edema, general anesthesia, and abdominal or thoracic surgery, that affect the pulmonary system result in a relative increase in the stiffness of the lungs and therefore a decrease in FRC. Decreased FRC has two important clinical implications: increased work of breathing and hypoxemia.

DECREASED FUNCTIONAL RESIDUAL CAPACITY AND WORK OF BREATHING

Figure 3–6 displays the pressure volume curve for the lungs. The lungs behave much like a child's balloon. When they are collapsed, a relatively large amount of pressure is required to move any air into them (low compliance). Once a critical volume has been reached, however, volume increases dramatically, even with small additional changes in pressure (high compliance). This continues until the lungs have reached the limits of inflation, when compliance again decreases. Clearly the most efficient region for ventilation is in the steep part of the curve. This also happens to be where a normal FRC value lies. However, a decrease in FRC moves the starting place for ventilation down along the curve. A great enough decrease may reduce lung compliance; that is, a given tidal volume requires a greater decrease in pleural pressure. This has the same effect as adding an inspiratory resistive load to the patient. The stereotypic response to this increased work of breathing is tachypnea and decreased tidal volume. Thus the first sign of decreased FRC may be an increase in the respiratory rate. Successful efforts to return the FRC to normal should resolve the tachypnea.

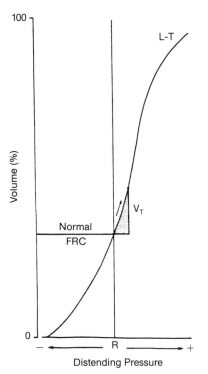

Figure 3-6. Pressure-volume curve of the pulmonary system. At normal FRC, lung compliance is high and relatively small pressure changes produce a normal tidal volume.

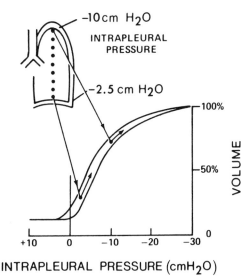

Figure 3-7. Effect of hydrostatic gradient on lung inflation in different parts of the lung. The pleural pressure is less negative in the dependent than in the nondependent aspect of the lung. Although the alveoli in the dependent region are smaller, they operate on a more compliant part of the lung inflation curve and thus expand more than alveoli in the nondependent region. (From West JB: Ventilation/blood flow and gas exchange, ed 3. Oxford, England, 1977, Blackwell, p. 28.)

DECREASED FUNCTIONAL RESIDUAL CAPACITY AND HYPOXEMIA

The concept of *closing volume* is needed to understand how decreased FRC leads to hypoxemia. Figure 3–7 demonstrates the hydrostatic differences in pleural pressure in an erect patient. The erect position is used for illustration; the discussion concerns the difference between dependent and nondependent lung regions. Pleural pressure is more negative at the apexes than at the bases. This is at least partly due to the weight of the lung pulling away from the apex and pressing down at the base. Because the pressure inside the alveoli is similar throughout the lung (0 at end expiration), the transpulmonary pressure gradient (pleural pressure − alveolar pressure), which represents the distending pressure of the alveoli, is more negative in the nondependent regions than at the base. This results in a greater volume of gas in the nondependent alveoli than in dependent areas. However, because the nondependent alveoli are at the less steep portion of their function curve (Fig. 3–7), they undergo less volume change during ventilation. The alveoli in the bases receive greater ventilation,

which is beneficial because the distribution of pulmonary blood flow is preferentially to the bases, optimizing matching of ventilation to perfusion.

At some point during expiration in a lung with decreased volumes, the transpulmonary pressure is insufficient to hold the airway open. Surface-active forces prevent the alveoli from collapsing. The major impact of an increase in pleural pressure is the tendency of small airways to collapse during expiration. A secondary consideration of pleural pressure increase is that the dependent alveoli are in a less steep portion of the pressure volume curve, so that ventilation is not as great for a given change in pleural pressure. Ventilation to alveoli distal to these closed airways is decreased, leading to decreased $\dot{V}/\dot{Q}$ units and eventual hypoxemia. The lung volume above residual volume at which dependent small airways begin to close is called closing volume (CV). In healthy individuals in their twenties, CV occurs at 10% of vital capacity and therefore well below tidal breathing. However, decreases in FRC may be sufficient for tidal breathing to begin to include CV. Furthermore, age is associated with a progressive rise in CV so that, at age 44, CV occurs within tidal breathing in the supine position. When CV exceeds FRC, some lung units remain collapsed during part of the tidal volume change. This reduces ventilation and thus the $\dot{V}/\dot{Q}$ ratio. Thus one principle of hypoxemia management is to restore FRC above CV.

INTERPRETATION OF ARTERIAL BLOOD GAS VALUES

Arterial Oxygen Partial Pressure. The factors that determine Pao_2 are discussed earlier in this chapter. A young person breathing room air normally has a Pao_2 of about 100 mm Hg (Table 3–3). A value less than 100 mm Hg but greater than 80 mm Hg is no physiologic threat to homeostasis, but it does imply that gas exchange is impaired. Pao_2 less than 80 mm Hg but greater than 60 mm Hg is considered hypoxemia because Pao_2 values in this range are definitely not found in normal individuals under the age of 60 years. However, oxygen delivery depends on oxygen saturation, and as long as the Pao_2 is greater than 60 mm Hg, oxygen loading of hemoglobin is not significantly impaired. Pao_2 less than 60 mm Hg does require intervention. Clinically, few critically ill patients are allowed to breathe room air (which is 20.9% oxygen). Thus, comparison of Pao_2 values obtained while subjects are breathing higher Fio_2 is desirable to track the pathologic process and monitor the effect of therapy. The best technique for routinely performing this task is use of the shunt equation described previously. However, this requires placement of a pulmonary artery catheter, which is impractical with many patients. A number of indexes have been proposed for estimating gas exchange efficiency without knowing the mixed venous gas values. $(A\text{-}a)Do_2$ gradient is calculated by subtracting the Pao_2 from the calculated Pao_2. In normal subjects breathing room air, $(A\text{-}a)Do_2$ is about 10 mm Hg. However, this index varies with the Fio_2. Pao_2/Pao_2 ratio is more stable in response to changes in Fio_2 but requires solving the alveolar air equation. Pao_2/Fio_2 is the easiest to calculate but is not sensitive to changes in $Paco_2$. Finally,

an "estimated" shunt equation has been proposed in which the $Cao_2/C\bar{v}o_2$ difference is assumed to be 3.5.

$$\frac{\dot{Q}s}{\dot{Q}t} = \frac{Cco_2 - Cao_2}{C(a\text{-}v)o_2 + (Cco_2 - Cao_2)} \tag{10}$$

None of these shortcut methods allows for the effect of changes in mixed venous oxygen saturation. Thus they give imprecise estimates of shunt and $\dot{V}A/\dot{Q}$. Hypoxemia is best monitored by use of the shunt equation as described previously.

Arterial Carbon Dioxide Partial Pressure. Carbon dioxide is transported in the blood mostly (65%) in the form of bicarbonate ion inside the red blood cell. This form results from the availability of carbonic anhydrase, which catalyzes the reaction

$$CO_2 + H_2O \rightarrow H^+ + {}^-HCO_3 \tag{11}$$

Because inspired gas contains essentially no carbon dioxide, $Paco_2$ is a function of carbon dioxide production ($\dot{V}co_2$) and alveolar ventilation ($\dot{V}A$),

$$Paco_2 = \frac{\dot{V}co_2}{\dot{V}A} \times K \tag{12}$$

where K is a constant. Examination of this equation reveals an exponential slope of $Paco_2$ to alveolar ventilation. Thus at a markedly elevated $\dot{V}A$, large changes in $\dot{V}A$ are associated with small changes in $Paco_2$. Conversely, when $\dot{V}A$ is below normal, relatively small changes in $\dot{V}A$ result in large changes in $Paco_2$. A rising $Paco_2$ represents a relative decrease in alveolar ventilation. This may be due to an absolute decrease in total minute ventilation, an increase in dead space, or an increase in carbon dioxide production. $Paco_2$ elevations sufficient to decrease pH below 7.35 require investigation.

Acid-Base Disturbances. The pH is determined by the ratio of bicarbonate concentration to $Paco_2$ in the Henderson-Hasselbalch equation,

$$pH = pKa + \log(HCO_3/0.03\ Paco_2) \tag{13}$$

where pKa is the dissociation constant. Thus, pH changes only when a ratio of bicarbonate and $Paco_2$ is altered. Because of the relation between HCO_3 and $Paco_2$, it might seem that increases in $Paco_2$ would result in equivalent changes in HCO_3 so that pH does not change. This is not the case, since HCO_3 changes relatively little in response to manipulations of $Paco_2$.

TABLE 3–3. Normal Arterial Blood Gas Values

	MEAN	RANGE
pH	7.4	7.3–7.5
$Paco_2$ (mm Hg)	40	30–50
Pao_2	97	60–105 (decreases with age)

RESPIRATORY ACIDOSIS. An increase in $Paco_2$ decreases the pH. A pH less than 7.30 associated with a $Paco_2$ greater than 50 mm Hg is defined as respiratory acidosis. This situation represents insufficient alveolar ventilation or ventilatory failure. Clinical conditions in which this may be found are narcotic overdose, residual muscle relaxants, neuromuscular disease, and respiratory muscle fatigue. In a normal patient an acute increase in $Paco_2$ causes a decrease in pH of 0.005 unit (and an increase in HCO_3 of 0.1 mmol/L)/mmHg $Paco_2$ change ($Paco_2$ change from 40 to 60 mm Hg changes pH from 7.4 to 7.3 and HCO_3 from 24 to 26 mmol/L.) If $Paco_2$ is elevated for several days, renal compensatory mechanisms increase the amount of HCO_3 reabsorbed in the distal nephron and thus its concentration in the extracellular fluid. Increasing the HCO_3 concentration in the extracellular fluid causes the pH to return toward normal. In this situation HCO_3 is elevated 3 to 4 mmol/L for each 10 mm Hg increase in $Paco_2$. The relationship of $Paco_2$ to $\dot{V}a$ benefits patients with abnormally low alveolar ventilation and concomitant hypercarbia because small increases in alveolar ventilation may correct respiratory acidosis.

RESPIRATORY ALKALOSIS. A decrease in $Paco_2$ increases pH. A pH greater than 7.50 associated with a $Paco_2$ less than 30 is defined as respiratory alkalosis. Normally a rapid decrease in $Paco_2$ causes an increase in pH of 0.01 unit (and a decrease in HCO_3 of 0.2 mmol/L) for each millimeter of mercury of $Paco_2$ change. For example, a rapid decrease in $Paco_2$ from 40 to 30 mm Hg should increase pH from 7.4 to 7.5 and decrease HCO_3 from 24 to 22 mmol/L. Respiratory alkalosis may have a number of causes, the most common of which is mechanical ventilation. This may be intentional to cause cerebral vasoconstriction and reduce intracranial pressure, or it may be due to improper choices of ventilator settings. Respiratory alkalosis may also be present as part of the systemic response to hypoxemia. Severe metabolic acidosis may stimulate ventilatory drive sufficiently to produce hypocarbia and mask the pH change. Finally, some central nervous system disorders produce abnormal ventilatory stimulation and may result in respiratory alkalosis. Renal compensation consists of loss of bicarbonate, which reduces HCO_3 in the extracellular fluid and decreases pH. In this situation, HCO_3 is decreased 5 to 6 mmol/L for each 10 mm Hg decrease in $Paco_2$. Once again, the degree of alkalemia provides information concerning the chronicity of the hypocarbia.

METABOLIC ACIDOSIS. Much of the metabolic activity of the body produces acids that must be buffered initially and excreted eventually to maintain the narrow range of pH acceptable for intracellular function. The major acid in the blood is carbonic acid, which dissociates to form water and carbon dioxide. Thus the major acid load is buffered in the blood but excreted through the lungs. Because of its ability to be excreted through the lungs, carbonic acid is termed a volatile acid. However, other acids produced as part of metabolic activity must be excreted through the kidneys. These are called fixed acids. In diabetic ketoacidosis the accumulation of ketone bodies may result in metabolic acidosis. More ominous is the development of metabolic acidosis caused by ischemia. When cells are deprived of adequate oxygen delivery, cellular metabolism switches from aerobic to anaerobic. Rather than being metabolized to carbon dioxide and water, which requires oxygen, pyruvate is converted to lactate. Accumulation of lactic acid not only may produce acidosis but heralds severe cellular distress. A pH less than 7.3 with a $Paco_2$ less than 50 mm Hg is defined as metabolic acidosis. As fixed acids accumulate in the blood, HCO_3 concentration decreases, causing a lesser ratio of $HCO_3/Paco_2$ with a resultant decrease in pH. A rapid decrease in pH stimulates the peripheral chemoreceptors, which increase ventilatory drive, decreasing $Paco_2$ and thereby providing respiratory compensation for the metabolic acidosis (see "Control of Breathing"). Over a longer time course, renal compensation of metabolic acidosis lowers urinary excretion of bicarbonate. Normally the $Paco_2 = 1.5\ HCO_3 + 8(\pm2)$ in compensated metabolic acidosis.

METABOLIC ALKALOSIS. A pH greater than 7.5 and a $Paco_2$ greater than 30 mm Hg are defined as metabolic alkalosis. Metabolic alkalosis is often a puzzling clinical situation of unclear cause. The simplest presentations of metabolic alkalosis involve a loss of organic acid through vomiting or gastric suction. The loss of hydrogen cations decreases the plasma bicarbonate concentration with little change in $Paco_2$, resulting in an increase in pH. Metabolic alkalosis may also be caused by administration of alkali in the form of sodium bicarbonate or occur in response to hypokalemia, hypochloremia, and chronic hypovolemia. Hypokalemia reflects profound intracellular loss of potassium. Hydrogen ions move intracellularly to maintain osmolality, resulting in plasma alkalosis and intracellular acidosis. Once diagnosed, the metabolic alkalosis is corrected by potassium repletion. Hypochloremia produces metabolic alkalosis by increasing renal excretion of hydrogen and potassium. Correction requires suitable amounts of volume and potassium. Chronic hypovolemia also causes metabolic alkalosis by a renal compensatory mechanism. In volume-contracted states the kidneys conserve bicarbonate and pH rises. Treatment centers on volume replacement. Respiratory compensation for metabolic alkalosis consists of mild hypoventilation, which rarely corrects the pH to near normal. Normally $Paco_2 = 0.7 \; HCO_3 + 20 \; (\pm 2)$ in compensated metabolic alkalosis.

Bicarbonate concentration may be elevated because of electrolyte disturbances or iatrogenic bicarbonate administration. Elevations may also develop as a response to chronic respiratory acidosis as occurs in patients with chronic obstructive pulmonary disease. Regardless of its cause, an elevated bicarbonate concentration may cause apnea or apparent weaning failure. If $Paco_2$ is lowered to normal, the pH is increased and the ventilatory drive depressed. Either the patient's $Paco_2$ should be allowed to rise to the baseline value if chronic hypercarbia is present, or 0.1 N hydrochloric acid should be infused at 10 ml/h (with a close eye on the serum potassium level and arterial pH).

MIXED ACID-BASE PROBLEMS. At initial examination patients may have a combination of metabolic and respiratory acid-base disturbances. In many cases it is difficult to determine which abnormalities were primary and which were compensatory, if any. Careful attention to maintaining adequate oxygen delivery and carbon dioxide removal should be the first priorities, followed by electrolyte concentration correction.

Intraarterial Sensors. The moment-to-moment management of critically ill patients is greatly improved with the introduction of intraarterial sensors such as optodes. These devices may be placed through an existing arterial line for continuous monitoring of Pao_2, $Paco_2$, and pH. Previous technology required adjusting ventilatory parameters, waiting 15 to 30 minutes, collecting an arterial sample, taking or sending the sample to the blood gas machine, and waiting for the results. With continuous blood gas analysis the clinician can titrate therapy at the bedside with immediate feedback. Furthermore, continuous monitoring with the device provides a better picture of blood gases than intermittent arterial blood gas analysis.

DIAGNOSTIC TECHNIQUES
Chest Roentgenography

Portable chest roentgenography is the most common radiographic examination performed in critically ill patients. The proper position of therapeutic and monitoring tubes and lines should be confirmed radiographically. An immediate roentgenogram should also be ordered whenever respiratory difficulties do not respond quickly to treatment. The portable chest roentgenogram is used in the diagnosis of a wide variety of pulmonary diseases in critically ill patients. However, the technique has limitations. Portable roentgenography images are not of the same quality as those produced in the radiology department. Comparing chest roentgenograms of a single patient may be difficult. Because of variation in exposure techniques, not only may patient position vary from one examination to the next, but the technician may choose different milliampere and kilovolt settings. One solution to this problem is to have the position and x-ray machine settings standardized for each patient and printed on a card that is then attached to the end of the bed. Another problem with portable chest roentgenograms is the anteroposterior direction of exposure, which magnifies the anterior structures such as the heart. Finally, even the best chest roentgenogram is still only a two-dimensional image. The position of structures within the chest at times challenges even the most experienced radiologist. The processes most likely to be missed on a portable anteroposterior roentgenogram of a supine patient are posterior layering hemothoraces or pleural effusions and pneumothoraces confined to the anterior pleural space (which is the least dependent part in a supine patient). Small and loculated empyemas are also easily missed.

Chest Computed Tomography

The limitations of routine chest radiography have led to increased computed tomography (CT) of the chest in critically ill patients. Few studies have detailed the role of this modality. However, patients whose pulmonary structural abnormalities require more exact definition are the most likely to benefit. In our institution we have been surprised at the extent of disease revealed by CT, which even retrospective review of the chest failed to demonstrate.

Thoracentesis

Thoracentesis is the removal of fluid or air from the pleural cavity, generally with a needle-introduced catheter. Thoracentesis may be performed for diagnosis, as of an empyema, or therapy, as for a small pneumothorax or large pleural effusion. The insertion site is determined by whether fluid or air is to be aspirated. An anterior, nondependent site is chosen for removal of air, and a posterior, dependent site is used for fluid removal. Regardless, an intercostal space below the seventh rib should almost never be used because of the risk of entering the abdominal cavity. After the skin is anesthetized, a thoracentesis catheter and needle are carefully advanced over the top of the rib just until fluid (or air) is aspirated. The catheter is then slipped off the end of the needle. As the needle is withdrawn, the end of the catheter is immediately occluded with a finger to prevent iatrogenic pneumothorax. The catheter may then be connected to either a syringe or an evacuation bottle or bag, depending on how much fluid is to be removed. At the conclusion of the procedure the catheter is removed without allowing air to enter and the puncture wound is dressed.

Pulmonary Arteriography

The pulmonary arteriogram is most commonly used to detect the presence of emboli in the pulmonary circulation (see "Pulmonary Thromboembolism," Chapter 8). Angiographic findings diagnostic of embolism include "pruning" of the pulmonary arterial tree (caused by occlusion of small branches) or filling defects of larger vessels. Modified pulmonary arteriography may be performed at the bedside to evaluate the effect of adult respiratory distress syndrome (ARDS) on the pulmonary circulation. A pulmonary artery balloon catheter is floated into wedge position, and radiopaque dye is injected while a portable chest roentgenogram is taken. Investigators have reported progressive occlusion of pulmonary arterioles as ARDS progresses. Some evidence suggests that prevention or reversal of the arterial occlusion increases survival from ARDS.

Pulmonary Perfusion and Ventilation Scanning

In the critically ill, pulmonary perfusion and ventilation scanning is most commonly performed when pulmonary embolism is suspected.

The perfusion scan is obtained with a gamma camera after albumin labeled with technetium-99m is injected. The radioisotope is trapped in perfused capillaries and thus provides information on pulmonary blood flow distribution. An optimally performed normal perfusion scan essentially excludes pulmonary embolism. However, a number of factors may interfere with the ability to obtain an optimal scan and to determine whether the scan is indeed normal. Trained and experienced technicians and radiologists are needed to obtain the several different views required to avoid missing a nonperfused area. Interpretation is often hampered if the patient has underlying pulmonary disease. Although the perfusion scan identifies areas of nonperfusion, several processes other than embolism may produce the same perfusion scan. Emphysema, pneumonia, atelectasis, and pneumothorax may directly reduce blood flow in affected portions of the lung. Diseases that reduce ventilation of part of the lung are associated with a reflex-driven decrease in blood flow to the poorly ventilated areas. Thus careful examination of an excellent chest roentgenogram is important. Since many critically ill patients do not have a normal chest roentgenogram, interpretation is made more difficult. Ventilation scanning is an additional test that may help. The patient breathes in a gaseous radioisotope such as xenon-133, and the wash-in rate is observed in lung areas that appeared suspect on the perfusion scan. Pulmonary embolism is more likely to be present in areas of absent perfusion and near normal ventilation. The ventilation scan is performed first for technical reasons.

Pulmonary Function Tests

Several bedside tests, some more routine than others, are performed in intensive care units to assess various aspects of ventilatory function. These tests are used to determine whether mechanical ventilation may be discontinued (or should be reinstituted) and to characterize increased ventilatory work. Unfortunately, no test or even group of tests is without false positives and false negatives. Thus pulmonary function tests may be used only as rough guidelines in clinical management.

Negative Inspiratory Force

Negative inspiratory force (NIF), also called negative inspiratory pressure (NIP) or maximum inspiratory force and pressure (MIF and MIP, respectively), is determined by having the patient perform an inspiratory maneuver while airflow is zero. Normal NIF is about 100 cm H_2O in men and somewhat less in women. An NIF greater than 25 cm H_2O is commonly accepted as predicting successful weaning from mechanical ventilation. NIF is primarily a measure of inspiratory muscle strength. However, it does not take into account pulmonary compliance, which may be low enough to prevent weaning. Also, NIF is highly dependent on the measurement technique. Like other muscles, the diaphragm exhibits greater contractility when its starting position is stretched. Thus NIF is least near total lung capacity and greatest at residual volume. Furthermore, NIF depends greatly on patient effort. Studies have shown that NIF varies with the length of time airflow is zero. NIF measurements should be standardized within a given unit so that values are comparable. One such technique uses one-way valves allowing only exhalation, which causes the patient eventually to reach residual volume. After oxygenation the test is conducted for 20 seconds to ensure a maximal response.

Vital Capacity

Vital capacity (VC) is also used primarily to determine the need for mechanical ventilation. The patient performs a maximal inspiratory maneuver without restriction of airflow and then exhales through a spirometer. Normal VC is 75 ml/kg ideal body weight. VC of 15 ml/kg is believed necessary for adequate spontaneous ventilation. VC is a measure of the balance between inspiratory muscle strength and impedance to breathing (pulmonary compliance). Results depend on the patient's ability to follow directions. Use of VC with NIF may reduce the number of false positives concerning successful ventilator weaning predicted by NIF alone. However, the use of NIF and VC still does not always predict who may be successfully removed from mechanical ventilation.

Forced Expiratory Volume in 1 Second and Forced Vital Capacity

Forced expiratory volume in 1 second (FEV_1) and FVC are measured by having the patient forcibly exhale from total lung capacity through a spirometer that plots volume versus time. A ratio of the volume exhaled during the first second (FEV_1) to the total FVC is calculated. The FEV_1/FVC ratio is normally greater than 70%. A lower ratio implies obstruction of airflow.

Peak Expiratory Flow

Peak expiratory flow (PEF) is also a test of airflow resistance and may be measured more easily at the bedside with disposable devices. Normal PEF is about 600 L/min. Bronchospasm is typically associated with values less than 350 L/min.

Tidal Volume

Tidal volume (V_T) is measured with a spirometer, typically before determination of VC or NIF. V_T in normal individuals is 6 to 7 ml/kg. V_T is not a reliable predictor of successful weaning and is more dependent on the underlying pulmonary disease than some other tests. Restrictive disease results in a decreased V_T, whereas obstructive changes often have the opposite effect.

Pressure Volume Loop

The pressure volume loop is generated by plotting the airflow against the airway pressure during a complete respiratory cycle. Flow volume loops give a graphic presentation of the magnitude of resistive versus viscoid work of breathing (Fig. 3–8).

FIBEROPTIC BRONCHOSCOPY

Fiberoptic bronchoscopy (FOB) is useful in a wide variety of clinical settings in and out of the hospital. The problems of the critically ill patient offer unique indications and techniques for FOB. For safety and efficacy, FOB should be performed by an experienced endoscopist.

The indications for FOB may be divided into diagnostic and therapeutic categories. To begin at the top, FOB may be used to evaluate and monitor upper airway obstruction such as stridor, inhalation injury, and vocal cord dysfunction. Patients with a large bronchopleural fistula may be evaluated for bronchial disruption. The presence of a persistent lobar collapse on chest roentgenogram can be a diagnostic problem. FOB may elucidate the reason for atelectasis. Although less common, hemoptysis in a critically ill patient occasionally necessitates FOB examination to determine the source. Finally, pneumonia is a common complication in critically ill patients and often the cause is unclear.

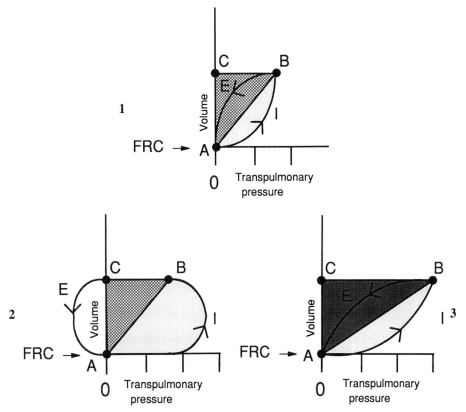

Figure 3-8. Pressure-volume loops. The various components of work of breathing (WOB) are graphically demonstrated for each of three situations: **1,** normal airway resistance and compliance; **2,** increased airway resistance; and **3,** decreased compliance. In each graph the slope of line *AB* is the lung-thorax compliance, area *AIBA* is inspiratory resistive WOB, area *ABCA* is elactic WOB, and area *AIBCA* is total WOB. *1,* Increase in transpulmonary pressure during *I* results in an increase in lung volume, followed by expiration and a return to FRC. *2,* Effect of increased airway resistance, such as bronchospasm, on spontaneous breathing. Although the slope of *AB* is unchanged because compliance is not altered, the increased airway resistance requires generation of higher transpulmonary pressures. The elastic WOB is unchanged, but the inspiratory and expiratory *(CEAC)* resistive components are much greater. *3,* Effect of decreased compliance, such as adult respiratory distress syndrome, on spontaneous breathing. The slope of *AB* is markedly decreased, which requires a much greater transpulmonary pressure to produce a normal tidal volume. Elastic WOB is markedly increased.

FOB techniques increase the chance of identifying the offending organism and directing antibiotic therapy.

Therapeutic indications for FOB follow from some of the diagnostic uses. If atelectasis is determined to be due to a mucus plug or foreign body, the bronchoscope may be used to clear the bronchus. FOB has also been advocated in the placement of double-lumen tubes. However, the most common therapeutic indication for FOB in critically ill patients involves securing an artificial airway. FOB has been invaluable in safely establishing airway control in a number of critical care situations, including those posing anatomic problems, such as cervical spine and facial trauma, and potentially life-threatening endotracheal tube changes in a patient requiring high levels of PEEP.

Contraindications to FOB are few but noteworthy. Since manipulation of a patient's airway

by an unskilled endoscopist invites disaster, absence of an experienced clinician is a contraindication. Inability to oxygenate the patient adequately during the procedure is also a contraindication. In some patients respiratory failure is severe enough to result in hypoxemia whenever FOB is attempted. The presence of coagulopathy is a relative contraindication. The bronchial mucosa is often friable in the critically ill, especially those with inflammatory changes. The benefits of FOB must be weighed against the risk of persistent bronchial bleeding in patients with thrombocytopenia, uremia, and other conditions associated with a prolonged bleeding time.

The most significant physiologic alteration occurring with FOB is a decrease in the Pao_2. This decrease has been reported to be 20 to 30 mm Hg in normal patients. The decrease may worsen with duration of bronchoscopy and is probably due to exacerbation of $\dot{V}/\dot{Q}$ mismatch. The decrease in Pao_2 does not usually resolve at the end of the procedure but may continue for several hours. Techniques such as bronchoalveolar lavage may also decrease Pao_2.

A brief review of tracheobronchial anatomy is presented to remind the reader of the asymmetric arrangement of pulmonary lobes and segments. The anatomy is presented as it appears to the endoscopist (Fig. 3–9). The trachea begins at the vocal cords and extends to the carina where it bifurcates into the left and right main bronchi. The carina normally looks like a knife pointed directly at the endoscopist. Following the right main bronchus, the right upper bronchus branches off near the level of the carina at about 180 degrees from the carina (from the lateral wall). The right upper bronchus is short and divides into the apical, anterior, and posterior bronchi. Below the right upper bronchus the right main bronchus becomes the intermediate bronchus. The right middle bronchus originates on the anterior aspect of the intermediate bronchus and gives rise to the lateral and medial bronchi. The right lower bronchus divides into five segmental bronchi including the superior branch, often arising from the posterior wall directly opposite the middle bronchus; the medial basal bronchus, originating medially; and the anterior basal, posterior basal, and lateral basal bronchi, which are variably distributed. When viewed from the carina the left main bronchus divides into the upper and lower bronchus. The secondary carina runs from anterolateral to posterior medial. The upper bronchus then divides into the upper and the lingular bronchi. The lingular, which is somewhat equivalent to the right middle bronchus, immediately divides into superior and inferior bronchi. The left upper lobe bronchus trifurcates into the apical, anterior, and posterior bronchi. The left lower bronchus gives rise to the superior bronchus from the posterior wall near the origin of the left upper bronchus in an analogous fashion to the right side. The left lower bronchus continues into the lower lobe and gives rise to the anterior basal, posterior basal, and lateral basal bronchi. Tracheobronchial tree anatomy varies greatly, and segmental bronchi distribution, especially in the lower lobes, may not conform to Figure 3–9.

The bronchial wall mucosa is normally tan. Erythematous mucosa suggests bronchitis or trauma. Normal mucosa appears to be stretched over the cartilage rings and to have a fine blood vessel network. Divisions in the healthy tracheobronchial tree appear sharp and knifelike.

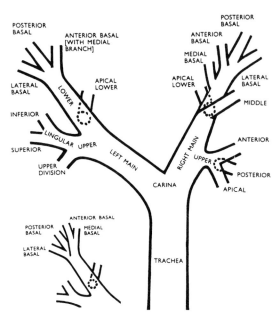

Figure 3-9. Tracheobronchial anatomy. The first posterior branch of the lower bronchus on each side is labeled "apical lower" in the diagram, but these bronchi are more commonly called "superior" in the United States. (From Stradling P: Diagnostic bronchoscopy, ed 5. New York, 1986, Churchill Livingstone, p. 41.)

Boggy, redundant mucosa suggests infection or inhalation injury. Secretions are not evident in the normal tracheobronchial tree because healthy individuals clear their secretions effectively.

TECHNIQUE

Appropriate attention to preparation cannot be overemphasized. Requirements include a stationary patient, a clean and properly functioning bronchoscope, and the equipment normally needed to intubate a patient with a laryngoscope. The patient is prepared with an explanation of the procedure and intravenous administration of an antisialogogue such as atropine 0.4 mg or glycopyrrolate 0.2 mg. Unless comatose, the patient should be given a sedative, such as a benzodiazepine or a narcotic or both, at dosages appropriate for the cardiovascular stability. Before, during, and after the procedure, someone must monitor the pulse oximeter, electrocardiogram, and blood pressure. The patient's risk for aspiration of gastric contents should be considered and reduced if deemed high.

The nonintubated patient may be examined by either the nasal or the oral route. The nasal route is greatly preferable because the bronchoscope is easily positioned in the supraglottic region and is not damaged by the patient's teeth. The nares are prepared in a fashion similar to that used for nasal intubation (see Chapter 2). Oral FOB is made easier with a hollow bite block to protect the scope. Oral airways designed to guide the bronchoscope into position are available commercially. After the vocal cords are identified, their shape and movement are evaluated, and 2 to 4 ml 2% lidocaine is injected via the bronchoscope, the endoscopist advances the bronchoscope through the cords during an inspiration. This usually causes vigorous coughing.

Intubated patients may be examined while receiving mechanical ventilation. Commercially available adapters allow passage of the bronchoscope into the endotracheal tube without an airleak even when PEEP is being administered. Although the presence of an endotracheal tube makes passage of the bronchoscope easier, certain physical factors should be considered before FOB. The bronchoscope partially occludes the lumen of any endotracheal tube and increases the resistance to airflow. Poiseuille's law states that flow is proportional to the radius to the fourth power. Thus even small decreases in the lumen available for gas flow require large increases in inspiratory pressure to maintain airflow rate. Expiration is also retarded by the presence of the bronchoscope and may be manifested by auto-PEEP (unwanted residual positive pressure at end expiration) and decreased P_{ETCO_2}. Current bronchoscopes are generally 5 mm in diameter. The smallest endotracheal tube that should be used is one with a 7 mm internal diameter. However, a larger tube may be desirable if ventilation is significantly impaired. If the patient is receiving intermittent mandatory ventilation or pressure support, the level of ventilatory support should be increased. One option is to reintubate the patient with a larger endotracheal tube. Another is to use a helium-oxygen mixture for ventilation. The substitution of helium for nitrogen in the inspired mixture reduces the density of the gas and increases airflow. A final option is to pass the bronchoscope alongside the endotracheal tube.

Once the bronchoscope is placed within the trachea, the instillation of local anesthetics may be desired. To prevent toxic effects, 2% lidocaine in 3 to 5 ml aliquots may be instilled, up to a total of 400 mg (20 ml).

Specific Techniques. The removal of mucus plugs often requires little other than suctioning. Extraction of tenacious sputum may be made easier by saline lavage. However, the bronchoscope itself may become plugged. In this case the bronchoscope must be removed entirely and irrigated, and the procedure resumed.

Foreign body removal may provide some of the more challenging encounters with critically ill patients. Traditionally, rigid bronchoscopy has been the technique of choice, but a number of reports support the selective use of FOB in foreign body removal. Several techniques are available to aid extraction. A biopsy forceps is usually effective in capturing the foreign body. The bronchoscope, forceps, and foreign body are then removed together. Wire baskets are useful when the foreign body can be encircled but not grabbed or when crushing the foreign body is a concern. Finally, a thin balloon catheter may be passed alongside the foreign body, the balloon inflated, and the foreign body removed with retraction of the catheter.

Bronchoalveolar lavage is performed in critically ill patients to obtain material for diagnostic study (if malignancy, infection, or an interstitial process is suspected) and to treat pulmonary alveolar proteinosis. After the bronchoscope is wedged into the appropriate bronchus, 100 to 200 ml of warmed saline solution is instilled and suctioned in 20 ml aliquots.

Techniques for Diagnosis of Pulmonary Infection. Despite the high incidence of pneumonia in critically ill patients, identification of the causative organism is often difficult. The main confounding factor is the presence of organisms in the airway above the glottis, which contaminate sputum specimens. Bronchial washings consist of instilling three to five 10 ml aliquots of saline solution. Since the bronchoscope itself is contaminated by passage through the oropharynx or nasopharynx, the washings may be contaminated. Similarly, bronchial brushings may be contaminated by the bronchoscope. To reduce upper airway contamination, protected brush catheters have been developed. Such a catheter consists of a brush enclosed within two sheaths, the outer of which is sealed with paraffin. After the catheter is passed through the bronchoscope and into the chosen bronchus, the inner sheath is pushed to dislodge the plug and the brush is advanced to sample the bronchi. The brush is then retracted into the catheter to prevent contamination and sent for culture study. Some contamination still occurs with this technique. Transbronchial biopsy with a cup forceps is performed to obtain lung parenchymal tissue. Transbronchial biopsy carries a greater risk of pneumothorax and hemorrhage than do other FOB techniques and thus is relatively contraindicated in patients who have coagulopathy or are receiving high levels of PEEP.

Inductive Plethysmography

The mechanics of breathing involves the complex interaction of a number of chest and abdominal muscles. Efficient breathing is normally associated with synchronous activity of all these muscles. In disease states and especially in patients who cannot be weaned from mechanical ventilation, these muscle groups act out of phase, resulting in clinically evident respiratory paradox ("rocking chest"). Inductive plethysmography is a technique for noninvasively quantifying the degree of respiratory paradox, as well as a number of parameters that describe ventilatory drive. Although not routinely used, it offers a sensitive and noninvasive technique for providing insights into abnormal ventilation.

SUPPORT OF OXYGENATION

Positive airway pressure is applied to expand lung volumes decreased by pathologic processes. This maneuver can be explained by a consideration of the lower curve in Figure 3–10. This curve portrays the pressure-volume relationship in a patient with acute respiratory dysfunction. The problem is that at end-expiration, with an airway pressure of zero, lung volume decreases to an abnormally low level. Providing large tidal volumes does not correct the condition. If positive pressure is applied during expiration, however, the lungs do not deflate as much. This is the concept behind positive end-expiratory pressure (PEEP). With PEEP, the two problems of decreased FRC outlined previously should be improved or at least made no worse. Collapsed alveoli should have been opened, ventilation/perfusion mismatching reduced, and the PaO_2 and calculated shunt improved. Also, pulmonary compliance should improve or at least not decrease. A decrease in pulmonary compliance suggests that the upper end of the lung inflation curve has been reached and further increases in positive airway pressure are relatively contraindicated. Because of developments in equipment (CPAP mask), positive airway pressure may be applied to patients without intubation.

The two techniques for increasing arterial oxygenation (SaO_2, PaO_2) when no mechanically correctable problem (pneumothorax, atelectasis, mainstem intubation) is present are increased FIO_2 and PEEP. Their indications and applications differ markedly.

Fraction of Inspired Oxygen. Oxygen is a drug; enough is good, too much may be bad. Oxygen is used to rapidly raise or prevent life-

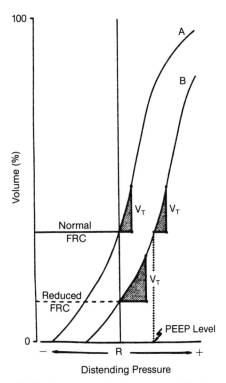

Figure 3-10. Pressure volume curves of the lung and thorax. Curve *A* represents a normal relationship and is identical to the curve in Figure 3-6. Curve *B* represents the changes associated with decreased functional reserve capacity (FRC). Lung inflation during inspiration occurs in a less steep (decreased compliance) part of the curve. Thus a greater transpulmonary pressure is required to produce a similar tidal volume. However, restoring FRC to normal with positive end-expiratory pressure should increase compliance.

threatening low levels of arterial oxygenation. However, the administration of oxygen does not reverse the pathologic process that has led to hypoxemia. Furthermore, high FIO_2 may add pulmonary damage to the underlying disease. The pulmonary manifestations of excessive oxygen include loss of alveolar epithelial type I cells, decreased bronchial ciliary transport, and tracheal inflammation. Oxygen administration may depress hypoxemic ventilatory drive in patients with chronic hypercarbia, greatly exacerbating respiratory acidosis. Finally, administration of FIO_2 greater than 70% may exacerbate the development of intrapulmonary shunt through absorption atelectasis in low $\dot{V}/\dot{Q}$ units. Thus only the amount of oxygen needed to prevent hypoxemia should be administered.

Equipment. Oxygen may be delivered with a number of devices. The choice should be based on whether the patient is intubated, the FIO_2 desired, whether hypercarbia is present, and the patient's comfort.

Source and Flow of Inspiratory Gas. A major factor in the choice of oxygen delivery devices is the patient's inspiratory flow rate and tidal volume. A patient who has a spontaneous tidal volume of 350 ml inhaled over 1 to 1.5 seconds has a mean inspiratory flow rate of 14 to 21 L/min and a peak value two to three times this mean. Thus an oxygen delivery device with a lower flow rate (most deliver up to 15 L of oxygen per minute) connected to a nasal cannula or open face mask is associated with entrainment of room air. If an FIO_2 of 1.0 is not desired, this characteristic is used to provide the patient with an FIO_2 that depends on the rate of oxygen flow, as well as the patient's tidal volume and respiratory rate. Because the latter two parameters vary from patient to patient and even in the same patient, the exact FIO_2 being delivered is often difficult to determine. For example, hypoventilation results in a higher effective FIO_2. If an FIO_2 of 1.0 is desired, a reservoir of gas and one-way valves may be attached to the face mask, producing a nonrebreathing system.

More consistent FIO_2 may be delivered with high-flow devices. These devices generate a high flow that is used to prevent entrainment of room air by the patient. These devices themselves entrain room air by a Venturi effect (and thus are called Venturi masks) in controlled quantities to provide accurate FIO_2 mixtures. They are most useful when a low FIO_2 is required. An example is a patient with chronic hypercarbia who is dependent on his hypoxic ventilatory drive. Venturi masks may be used to deliver FIO_2s of 0.24 and 0.28, which may be sufficient to alleviate systemic effects of hypoxia but not depress alveolar ventilation. Hypoxemia caused by low $\dot{V}/\dot{Q}$ units typically responds well to even small increments of FIO_2, although that caused by a shunt does not.

Continuous Positive Airway Pressure (CPAP) Mask. As discussed previously, hypoxemia may be caused by decreases in FRC. Positive airway pressure is a technique for reexpanding FRC. The ability to deliver positive airway pressure with a mask may obviate the need for intubation in some patients with respiratory failure. Patient selection is important to the success of mask CPAP. Inclusion criteria are presented in Table 3–4. Requisite equipment includes a clear CPAP mask with a soft seal, high–gas flow generator capable of entraining room air, oxygen analyzer, pulse oximeter, CPAP valve with threshold resistor characteristics, head strap, and manometer to monitor level of CPAP. Inappropriate application of

TABLE 3–4. Patient Criteria for Continuous Positive Airway Pressure Mask

Awake and alert
Unrestrained
No aerophagia
No ileus
No recent upper gastrointestinal surgery

CPAP mask has led to unfavorable experience with the device. However, with a few key principles kept in mind, CPAP mask may be used to improve gas exchange and tachypnea as well as avoid intubation. The mask makes a relatively airtight seal with the aid of the head strap. The head strap should be adjusted only tight enough to minimize air leak. A small leak is preferable to discomfort from mask compression. Air flow is adjusted to the 60 to 90 L/min range. The CPAP valve is set to 5 cm H_2O, and the physician at the bedside monitors the patient's response. CPAP is increased at 2.5 to 5 cm H_2O increments until either SaO_2 has improved to greater than 88% on FIO_2 less than 0.4 or 15 cm H_2O is reached. One complication of decreased FRC is decreased pulmonary compliance with resultant tachypnea. Application of CPAP should decrease the respiratory rate if the therapy is effective. Because of this the patient should feel less dyspneic with the mask on. Patients should be observed for the development of gastric distention, at which point the CPAP mask is removed promptly. Some clinicians always insert a nasogastric tube if a CPAP mask is to be used, but this is not a universal practice.

SUPPORT OF VENTILATION

Intubation is performed when certain indications are present (Table 3–5). Mechanical ventilation is applied to the intubated patient to prevent or treat respiratory acidosis. However, some patients with respiratory acidosis may not require mechanical ventilation. The underlying process in these patients may be quickly reversible as in the case of narcotic overdose or

TABLE 3–5. Indications for Intubation

Inability to protect airway
Ventilatory failure
Need to apply PEEP
Inability to handle secretions
Salvageable patient
Need to provide hyperventilation

residual muscle relaxant. If adequate reversal does not occur within a few minutes, intubation should be considered. Chronic respiratory acidosis presents a special problem. These patients have marginal alveolar ventilation. A number of respiratory stimulants have been administered in this situation to improve ventilatory function. These are covered in the section on weaning but are not considered to be consistently reliable means of supporting ventilation.

Mechanical ventilation may be required in certain therapeutic interventions such as administration of muscle relaxants. Mechanical ventilation may also be applied to induce respiratory alkalosis in patients with intracranial hypertension.

Once alveolar ventilation is deemed to require mechanical support, a number of considerations determine appropriate ventilator settings. Tidal volume is set to 10 to 15 ml/kg, although normal spontaneous tidal volume is 5 ml/kg. Less efficient distribution of positive-pressure breaths requires larger mechanical volumes. Furthermore, normal individuals exhibit sighs (intermittent large tidal volumes) at varying intervals, which most likely prevent atelectasis and resulting hypoxemia. The use of mechanical breaths of this volume has been shown to inhibit the development of hypoxemia better than with smaller tidal volumes. Alternatively, smaller tidal volumes may be used with programmed intermittent mechanical sighing to prevent atelectasis.

Ventilator tubing and humidifiers are compliant. This means that some of the tidal volume delivered by the ventilator does not go to the patient but rather expands the tubing. The higher the inflation pressure, the greater the loss of mechanical tidal volume in the ventilatory circuit. Although the exact number varies, for each liter of ventilator circuit, 1.5 to 3 ml/cm H_2O peak inspiratory pressure is lost from each tidal volume. Thus, in the presence of increased peak airway pressure as occurs with severe respiratory failure, the tidal volume set on the ventilator has to be greater than that desired for delivery to the patient. For accuracy, the tidal volume returned from the patient's lungs should be measured at the endotracheal tube with a spirometer.

Frequency. After an appropriate tidal volume has been selected, frequency is adjusted to provide minute ventilation (respiratory rate × tidal volume) of about 100 to 150 ml/kg/min. Carbon dioxide and pH are monitored, usually by arterial blood gas analysis, and the respiratory rate is adjusted to correct pH.

Inspiratory/Expiratory Ratio. Sufficient time should be allowed for complete passive exhalation to occur. Therefore inspiratory/expiratory (I/E) ratios should be adjusted to less than or equal to 1:1. A higher I/E ratio may result in auto-PEEP with subsequent patient deterioration. I/E ratio may be reversed in special circumstances (see "Inverse Ratio Ventilation") for the treatment of severe respiratory failure.

Inspiratory Flow Rate. As pointed out previously, patient inspiratory flow rate demand is frequently in the range of 60 to 100 L/min. Thus inspiratory flow rates must be at least this high to prevent dyspnea. In some ventilators inspiratory flow rate is a function of the I/E ratio. The ventilators choose an inspiratory flow rate that delivers the selected tidal volume over a time period determined by the I/E ratio.

MODES OF VENTILATION

Many modes are available for the delivery of positive-pressure ventilation. Although each has its proponents, little consensus has developed as to choice of modes. The mode selected is less important than the particular ventilator. Commercially available ventilators have different mechanisms for providing various modes of mechanical ventilation. A patient's response to assist-control, intermittent mandatory ventilation, or CPAP on one machine may be quite different from these same modes on another. More important issues are the added work of breathing a particular ventilator imposes on a patient because of the performance of the demand valve (if present), the inspiratory flow rate, and the flow-resistive properties of the exhalation valve.

Control. The simplest, and perhaps the least controversial, form of mechanical positive-pressure ventilation is the control mode. The ventilator delivers all the breaths; the patient not only does not, but cannot, initiate any breaths. No provision is made for allowing the patient to breathe spontaneously with this mode. The control mode is appropriate only for patients who have no spontaneous respiratory movement and offers no advantages over the use of other modes.

Assist-Control. With assist-control ventilation the patient receives breaths of preselected tidal volume equal to control mode. However, if the patient performs an inspiratory maneuver, thus decreasing the airway pressure in the ventilator circuit, the machine delivers another mechanical breath of the same preset volume. The rate may be set high enough to suppress patient respiratory activity or low enough to encourage inspiratory effort. The appeal of this mode is that the patient's work of breathing should be minimized. However, a number of mechanical difficulties have plagued this mode. Although unintubated individuals do not generate negative airway pressure even to achieve high inspiratory flow rates, a negative airway pressure is required with assist-control mode to open the demand valve. If the sensitivity is not set low enough, considerable additional work may be imposed on the patient. Furthermore, after the demand valve is opened, additional work of breathing may arise from inadequate inspiratory flow rates.

Intermittent Mandatory Ventilation. Intermittent mandatory ventilation (IMV) was developed to minimize the number of positive-pressure breaths delivered to patients and to provide a circuit that imposed little or no additional work of breathing. When the number of positive-pressure breaths is reduced, less barotrauma and cardiovascular depression are thought to occur than with the assist-control mode. Furthermore, the concept of IMV allows the use of continuous flow circuits. Rather than having the patient open a demand valve, fresh gas is delivered past the end of the endotracheal tube continuously so that when a spontaneous breath is initiated, the patient merely diverts the gas flow into the lungs. However, IMV is also associated with mechanical problems. If the exhalation valve has flow-resistive characteristics, that is, airway pressure rises when flow increases, additional work of breathing may be imposed. Some ventilators offer synchronized IMV (SIMV) in which a demand valve circuit is substituted for the continuous flow circuit. SIMV modes are subject to the same problems outlined in the discussion of the assist-control mode.

Pressure Support. The issue of increased work of breathing caused by resistance to airflow imposed by the endotracheal tube, as well as ventilator characteristics, has generated interest in pressure support. Although the exact control mechanism varies among ventilators, the resultant airway pressure is similar to that associated with pressure-limited ventilators. When the patient opens the demand valve, the ventilator injects gas into the circuit until the airway pressure rises to the preselected pressure support level. The ventilator then constantly monitors the airway pressure and adjusts the inspiratory flow to maintain the pressure sup-

port level until end inspiration, at which time the patient is allowed to breathe out passively. The end of inspiration is usually detected by monitoring inspiratory flow. The inspiratory support mode is terminated when flow rate decreases to 25% of its peak value. The effect of pressure support is to boost spontaneous tidal volume by increasing transpulmonary pressure at a given level of inspiratory effort. The appeal of this form of partial assist ventilation lies in its perceived ability to adjust to the patient's needs on a breath by breath basis. The level of pressure support required to offset work imposed by standard endotracheal tubes and ventilators ranges from 4 to 8 cm H_2O depending on the size of the endotracheal tube. However, there is lack of consensus about the optimal level of pressure support. Clearly, if the pressure support level is set high enough, the ventilator performs essentially all of the work of breathing. Conversely, if the level of pressure support is set too low, the purpose of the mode is defeated.

High-Frequency Ventilation. Despite enormous interest, high-frequency ventilation has not replaced more conventional forms of mechanical ventilation. Although a number of forms of high-frequency ventilation have been shown to support gas exchange as well as conventional ventilation does, it has rarely been shown to be superior in adults. In the United States most work has been with high-frequency jet ventilation (HFJV). HFJV has been instituted in a number of situations, including bronchopleural fistula, thoracic surgery, and raised intracranial pressure, with mixed results. HFJV use in bronchopleural fistula does not always improve gas exchange and typically increases the measured leak of gas out of the chest tube. A randomized trial of HFJV versus conventional ventilation in ARDS failed to demonstrate significant differences in outcome, cardiovascular depression, and barotrauma.

Airway Pressure Release Ventilation. Not yet commercially available, airway pressure release ventilation (APRV) was developed to reduce the greatly increased airway pressures associated with acute respiratory failure. The level of airway pressure to maintain PaO_2 is selected as in conventional ventilation analogous to selection of PEEP levels. However, to remove carbon dioxide, the patient is allowed to deflate for 1.5 seconds from the CPAP level and then CPAP is reapplied rapidly. Peak airway pressure in this mode of ventilation is only as high as the CPAP. The circuit is designed to allow spontaneous breathing by a continuous flow technique. The

TABLE 3–6.   Independent Lung Ventilation

Indications

Unilateral aspiration
Unilateral lung contusion
Unilateral adult respiratory distress syndrome (one lung
   worse than the other)
Bronchopleural fistula

Proposed Techniques

Continuous positive airway pressure (CPAP)–CPAP
CPAP–High-frequency ventilation (HFV)
Conventional ventilation (CV)–CPAP
CV–HFV
CV–CV with breaths given together (synchronized)
CV–CV with alternating breaths

place of APRV has yet to be determined by clinical studies.

Inverse Ratio Ventilation.   Inverse ratio ventilation (IRV), also known as pressure control, is similar to APRV. IRV was used initially in neonates to ventilate with low peak inspiratory pressure. With IRV the patient is held in end inspiration, at the preselected pressure control level, for a time determined by the I/E ratio. Often an I/E of 4:1 is chosen, producing short periods of deflation from the pressure control level followed by rapid reinstitution of airway pressure. The major difference between IRV and APRV is that the former does not allow spontaneous ventilation. As with APRV, insufficient clinical data exist to determine the ultimate place of IRV.

Independent Lung Ventilation.   Occasionally patients have respiratory failure primarily affecting one lung. Using PEEP in these patients overdistends the alveoli in the more normal lung and compresses the pulmonary vasculature. If pulmonary vascular resistance in the "good lung" is increased sufficiently, pulmonary blood may be shunted away from the good lung to the more diseased lung, resulting in a paradoxic worsening of blood gas concentrations. One method for managing such a condition is to keep the patient in the lateral position (with the good lung down), shifting blood flow away from the injured lung and into the normal lung. However, maintaining a critically ill patient in one position precludes the performance of many necessary nursing activities. Another option is to place a double-lumen tube and selectively provide PEEP to the more diseased lung, while using lower airway pressures in the good lung. Indications for independent lung ventilation (ILV) are listed in Table 3–6.

DOUBLE-LUMEN TUBES TECHNIQUE.   Despite the benefits that double-lumen tubes may offer selected critically ill patients, safe placement and maintenance require appropriate equipment, physicians experienced with the technique, and nurses and respiratory therapists familiar with the use of the device. The suggested readings for this chapter offer a more detailed discussion of techniques and management.

For most situations a disposable, clear plastic, left-sided double-lumen tube is chosen. The reasons include larger internal diameter of the individual lumens and avoidance of occlusion of the right upper bronchus. The operator views the larynx and places the tube through the vocal cords with the tip directed anteriorly. After the tip passes the larynx, the tube is turned counterclockwise one-quarter turn to align the curve of the bronchial lumen with the branching off of the left main bronchus. The tube is advanced until a slight resistance is felt. The tracheal cuff is inflated, and bilateral ventilation is confirmed by auscultation. Then 1 to 2 ml of air is placed in the bronchial cuff. Appropriate tube placement can be verified by a series of tube clamping and ventilation, descriptions of which may be found in the suggested readings. However, direct visualization with a fiberoptic bronchoscope is strongly recommended as a more convincing assessment. A fiberoptic bronchoscope is passed through the tracheal lumen of the tube to visualize the carina and the endobronchial tip of the tube disappearing down the left main bronchus. The tube is in optimal position when the bronchial cuff sits just inside the left main bronchus when inflated. The bronchial cuff should not be overinflated because the cuff may compromise the bronchial tube lumen or herniate and obstruct the right mainstem bronchus.

The tube should be securely taped in place or secured by wire to the teeth and an immediate portable chest roentgenogram obtained. Only 1 to 2 cm movement of the tube may obstruct airflow.

MANAGEMENT.   Several techniques can maximize ventilatory support with ILV (Table 3–6). However, two conventional ventilators are typically used, and the issues of major concern are distribution of the tidal volumes and amount of PEEP to be used on each lung. Definitive guidelines supported by clinical evidence do not exist for either of these issues. Based on experimental evidence, most clinicians deliver equal tidal volumes to both lungs. Although the more diseased lung should receive more PEEP, the choice of the level is less clear.

COMPLICATIONS. Practical considerations involving the use of double-lumen tubes in the intensive care unit should be kept in mind. Inability to suction adequately through the lumens is often cited as a reason to discontinue the use of these tubes. The tube may be dislodged with little movement. Bronchial rupture because of inappropriate tube size has also been reported.

MONITORS OF VENTILATOR FUNCTION

The institution of ventilator therapy is often a lifesaving maneuver. However, no system of mechanical ventilation is without hazards. Ventilator monitors are used to provide early warnings of critical events, occurrences that would lead to significant negative outcomes if not recognized and treated. However, monitors themselves may fail to warn because of equipment failure (rare) or human error (common); for example, alarms may be set to inaudible levels, ignored, or not activated.

The most common critical event associated with mechanical ventilation is disconnection somewhere in the patient-ventilator circuit. All ventilators should have an alarm that identifies this critical event, which may lead to hypoxemia, hypercarbia, cardiovascular depression, and neurologic devastation. Three techniques are available for monitoring for disconnection. Breath to breath determination of the exhaled tidal volume allows an alarm to be set off if disconnection occurs. This type of alarm is most commonly an intrinsic component of the ventilator, requiring a pneumotachograph. Another technique is to monitor airway pressure in the circuit. The third technique involves monitoring exhaled carbon dioxide concentration. Alarms also detect excessive peak inspiratory pressure, absence of positive pressure, and absence of pressure variation (apnea).

MUSCLE RELAXANTS

Muscle relaxants are frequently used in the management of pulmonary disease. Because improved pulmonary function after administration of these agents is not well documented, specific guidelines have not been widely accepted.

Muscle relaxants are sometimes administered to patients who appear to be fighting the ventilator. Although this may be an appropriate intervention, the clinician should first determine

TABLE 3–7. Causes of Fighting the Ventilator

Hypermetabolism
Hypoxia
Hypercarbia
Acidosis
Inadequate tidal volume
Pain related to breathing
Excessive inspiratory temperature
Tube impinging on carina
Anxiety
Pain
Bladder distention
Copious secretions or foreign body
Inspiratory or expiratory obstruction or leaks in ventilator circuit
Delirium

whether the ventilator settings are adequate to meet the patient's cardiopulmonary needs. A wide variety of causes of fighting the ventilator exist (Table 3–7), and the specific reason should be identified and treated if appropriate.

In some patients with severe pulmonary disease, ventilator therapy increases peak inspiratory pressure to more than 50 cm H_2O, placing the patient at risk for barotrauma. Some clinicians administer muscle relaxants in the hope that paralyzing the chest wall will decrease the peak inspiratory pressure. This desired benefit is not obtainable in all such patients who receive muscle relaxants.

After prolonged surgery and massive transfusion the core temperature frequently decreases to about 33° C. Once these patients begin to rewarm in the critical care unit, they shiver. The disadvantages of shivering include significantly increased oxygen consumption and carbon dioxide production, which place additional demands on cardiopulmonary function. Some clinicians administer muscle relaxants to abolish shivering if the metabolic demand of the increased muscle activity appears to be exceeding the patient's ability to compensate. The administration of muscle relaxants may increase the time needed to rewarm the patient. Muscle relaxants may also be used to prevent shivering when the temperature of a febrile patient is being lowered.

Disadvantages of administering muscle relaxants to critically ill patients include unimpaired awareness, the need for positive-pressure ventilation, and complete absence of cough or spontaneous movement, leading to position-related injury. Modern muscle relaxants such as metocurine, pancuronium, atracurium, vecuronium, and succinylcholine do not blunt awareness. Therefore critical care physicians must always guard against instituting chemical paralysis in an unsedated patient. Once a patient is paralyzed, all ventilatory function must be assumed by positive-pressure ventilation. In some patients with marginal intravascular volume the conversion from a net negative intrathoracic pressure to a net positive intrathoracic pressure decreases venous return sufficiently to cause hypotension. The hypotension generally responds to intravascular volume enhancement. However, awareness of this complication and vigilance after chemical paralysis are essential.

COMPLICATIONS OF MECHANICAL VENTILATION

Positive-pressure ventilation has long been associated with two major problems, barotrauma and cardiovascular depression. The culprit in both cases is the unphysiologic positive intrathoracic pressure associated with mechanical ventilation.

Barotrauma. Barotrauma occurs when gas escapes from the respiratory tree. The exact mechanism is not clear, but many clinicians believe that barotrauma begins when increased transpulmonary pressure ruptures the respiratory ducts and alveoli. This is most likely to occur in relatively normal parts of the lung because compliance in these areas is high and overdistention more likely. The incidence of pneumothorax correlates with elevated peak inspiratory pressure and the frequency of positive-pressure breaths. However, some clinicians believe that mean airway pressure is to blame for barotrauma. The pathophysiology of barotrauma is discussed in Chapter 18. Barotrauma becomes of physiologic importance when air enters the pleural space (pneumothorax). Bronchopleural fistula occurs when the air leak into the pleural space is continuous. Tension pneumothorax arises when the site of the air leak into the pleural space acts as a unidirectional valve. Pressure in the pleural space may rise enough to cause cardiovascular embarrassment. The signs of tension pneumothorax are absent or transmitted breath sounds on the affected side, overinflation of one hemithorax, tympany to percussion, shift of the trachea or cardiac impulse, respiratory distress, tachycardia, distended neck veins, hypoxia, and hypotension. Radiographic signs include inverted diaphragm, massive pneumothorax, and shift of the mediastinal structures to the contralateral side. In patients with underlying severe pulmonary disease such as ARDS, the lungs may be incapable of collapsing much or adhesions may cause loculation. Thus tension pneumothorax may be present when a relatively small pneumothorax appears on the chest roentgenogram. The important physiologic alteration is the increased intrapleural pressure, not the size of the pneumothorax. Pneumothorax also occurs in 1% to 2% of patients who have had a central line placed. Pulmonary abscesses or pulmonary lacerations from blunt or penetrating trauma may destroy sufficient lung parenchyma to result in pneumothorax.

Tension pneumothorax requires immediate intervention. The most expeditious technique is to place a 14- or 16-gauge intravenous cannula in the affected hemithorax. The catheter should be placed appropriately (in the third or fourth intercostal space at the anterior axillary line) to avoid causing additional complications. The catheter should be passed just over the top of the rib so as not to lacerate components of the intercostal neurovascular bundle. As soon as the needle enters the pleural space, the catheter is advanced and the needle withdrawn. A syringe and stopcock are attached to the catheter, and the pneumothorax is evacuated with care to avoid allowing air to leak back into the chest. The pneumothorax may then be decompressed while preparations are made for a more stable tube thoracostomy.

Indications for tube thoracostomy placement include pneumothorax and collections of pleural fluid, especially blood. Although air may be evacuated with a small tube, the presence of fluid (particularly blood) requires the placement of a large-bore (36 to 40 French) tube. Tube thoracostomy may be established with either a chest tube or a catheter attached to a one-way valve (Heimlich valve). Before the chest tube is placed, the skin over the upper and lateral chest on the affected side is cleansed with a antiseptic solution and draped in a sterile fashion. The site of insertion of a chest tube for pneumothorax has been debated. Traditionally the second intercostal space is used with the chest tube placed in the midclavicular line and directed into the apex. Three problems are associated with this approach: tubes in the apex may cause Horner's syndrome on the ipsilateral side, air collects in the least dependent regions, and an unsightly scar is likely to occur. In a supine patient the midchest area is the least dependent region. A chest tube with its tip in the apex may be unable to completely evacuate an anterior pneumothorax, which may not be apparent on the postplacement chest roentgenogram. Many clinicians choose to place a chest tube for pneumothorax in the fourth or fifth intercostal space at the middle to anterior axillary line and direct the tube superiorly and medially. The problem that may arise with this approach, especially on the right side, is that the tube slips into a lobar fissure, limiting its ability to reexpand the lung. The tube should not be placed through breast tissue.

After the site has been selected, the skin is anesthetized with a local anesthetic and a skin incision is made. The pleural space is entered bluntly with a large hemostat. An obvious rush of air out of the chest should accompany this maneuver if tension pneumothorax is present. The insertion track should be explored with a finger to ensure pleural placement and the absence of adhesions between the lung and parietal pleura. The end of a chest tube can be grasped with a large curved hemostat and directed into the pleural space in the desired direction. If the patient is breathing spontaneously, the tube should be clamped before insertion to prevent further collapse. After placement in the pleural space the chest tube is connected to an underwater seal device or one-way valve and the skin is loosely approximated. Massive subcutaneous emphysema has been reported when the skin was closed tightly around the chest tube.

For placement of a catheter with a Heimlich valve, the site is selected, prepared, and anesthetized as described previously. A 1 cm skin incision is made, and the catheter is passed into the pleural space and guided into position. The valve is attached to the catheter, and low suction is applied to the valve outlet.

Chest tube drainage devices have three functions: providing a one-way path of egress for air, collecting and measuring fluid or bloody drainage, and providing a mechanism for application of negative pressure. The amount of negative pressure is regulated by the depth of the opening of the atmospheric vent tube beneath the surface of the water in the vacuum-regulated chamber. Air leaks are seen as bubbles passing from the patient side to the vacuum side of the one-way seal chamber. Generally, persistent air leaks are treated expectantly. Immediate major risks of placing tube thoracostomies are bleeding from an intercostal vessel and laceration of the lung parenchyma. Later major risks include empyema and tube malfunction with development of tension pneumothorax.

A tube thoracostomy placed for pneumothorax can be removed when no air leak has been demonstrated for 8 to 12 hours and fluid drainage is less than 100 ml in 24 hours. This may occur within 24 hours or may take 2 weeks or longer. If the patient requires positive-pressure ventilation, suction is discontinued for 6 to 12 hours, leaving the tube connected to an underwater seal. If pneumothorax does not recur and fluid drainage is acceptable, the tube is removed.

Tube removal is performed by ensuring that pleural pressure is positive by applying a positive-pressure breath or having the patient perform a Valsalva maneuver. The tube is rapidly withdrawn, and an occlusive pad is immediately applied to prevent aspiration of air. Removal of tubes that have been in place for several days may tear the lung surface and cause bleeding or recurrence of air leak, although both are rare. Thus a chest roentgenogram should be obtained after tube removal.

Cardiovascular Complications. For more than 40 years, positive-pressure ventilation has been associated with cardiovascular depression, and the exact mechanisms have yet to be fully elucidated. Increasing airway pressure has been associated with a decrease in blood pressure but more commonly with a fall in cardiac output. Several mechanisms have been proposed, including compression of the great veins in the thorax, shift of the cardiac septum, right ventricular dysfunction caused by elevated pulmonary vascular resistance, and direct myocardial depression. Most likely positive airway pressure induces cardiovascular changes by increasing pleural pressure. Thus the less compliant the lung, the less severe the cardiovascular manifestations. Conversely, emphysematous patients with their abnormally high pulmonary compliance may demonstrate exquisite sensitivity to even small increases in airway pressure. Airway pressure elevations in these patients should be minimized by using tidal volumes of 8 ml/kg and little if any PEEP.

Positive airway pressure expands the lungs. The amount of lung expansion for a given amount of positive pressure is determined by compliance of the lung, diaphragm, and chest wall. The stiffer the ventilatory apparatus, the greater the airway pressure (and therefore intrathoracic pressure) required to deliver a given tidal volume. One possible mechanism of positive airway pressure–induced cardiovascular depression is as follows. Intrathoracic pressure compresses the great veins, increasing venous pressure. The latter decreases the gradient between extrathoracic and central venous pressure and the venous return to the heart.

This reduces cardiac filling. The pericardial pressure is increased, which may lead to decreased cardiac chamber pressure gradient. This also leads to decreased filling. Finally, the pulmonary vasculature is compressed, leading to increased pulmonary vascular resistance. Thus right ventricular function is impaired by the combination of decreased preload and increased afterload. Left ventricular function may also be impaired by the increased pericardial pressure, decreasing left ventricular filling. Furthermore, some studies have indicated that the interventricular septum is shifted into the left ventricle, decreasing left ventricular compliance.

Positive airway pressure may decrease cardiac output sufficiently to activate compensatory reflexes. These include stimulation or release of the sympathetic nervous system, antidiuretic hormone, renin-angiotensin-aldosterone, and atrial natriuretic factor, which act in concert to increase venous tone, peripheral vascular resistance, and extracellular fluid volume. This should result in restoration of venous return, cardiac filling volumes, cardiac output, and blood pressure.

Intravascular volume is a major determinant of the severity of cardiovascular depression associated with positive airway pressure. Hemodynamic changes that occur with routine ventilatory settings invariably respond well to volume enhancement. However, it is possible to reach levels of positive airway pressure that require inotropic agents to maintain cardiac output. The question often arises as to the reliability of pulmonary artery and pulmonary artery occlusion pressures when a patient is receiving elevated airway pressure in a form such as PEEP. Studies have been performed in which patients receiving high PEEP underwent simultaneous measurement of pulmonary artery occlusion pressure and direct left ventricular end-diastolic pressure (LVEDP) or left atrial pressure. Pulmonary artery occlusion pressure was found to correlate remarkably well with LVEDP regardless of PEEP level. The information really needed is the distending pressure of the vessels; this is determined by the pressure inside the vessel, which can be measured accurately, and the pressure outside the vessel (pleural pressure), which cannot. Pleural pressure rises with positive airway pressure but is not predictable because it depends on pulmonary compliance. Therefore, PEEP application elevates pulmonary vascular pressures, left ventricular filling pressures, and pleural pressures, but whether their relationship and thus the distending pressures are changed cannot be determined.

AIRWAY INFECTION DEFENSE MECHANISMS

Pulmonary infection is probably the most common nosocomial infection in critically ill patients. Infection results when the balance between potentially pathogenic organisms and pulmonary defense mechanisms shifts in favor of the organisms. Many factors permit an increased burden of pathogens to reach the lower airway in a critically ill patient, including depressed level of consciousness, weakness from associated illness or drugs, increased volumes of contaminated oropharyngeal secretions, presence of foreign bodies such as endotracheal tubes, performance of suctioning, and contamination of ventilator circuits. Furthermore, antibiotics and inhalation of high oxygen concentrations may change the upper airway flora, favoring growth of enteric gram-negative organisms. The patient's defense systems may be bypassed mechanically or suppressed by drugs or disease. The physiology of the normal defense mechanisms and the impacts of disease and therapy are presented in this section.

The lung is in direct continuity with the ambient atmosphere, but a variety of mechanisms protect it from noxious gases and particles, including pathogenic organisms. Defense mechanisms include filtration, impaction, sedimentation, sneezing, swallowing, coughing, laryngospasm, the mucociliary apparatus, pulmonary macrophages, and immune responses.

The nose filters particles larger than 100 μm, and those less than 10 μm remain in the air. The stimulation of sneeze, cough, and laryngospasm reflexes impedes the passage of mechanical and chemical irritants. However, aging depresses the sensitivity of these reflexes.

Chemical or mechanical stimulation can initiate the cough reflex anywhere between the larynx and the carina, the two most sensitive areas. Afferent impulses travel via the vagus nerve to the medulla, which integrates a sharp inspiration followed by glottic closure, contraction of the expiratory musculature with an increase in intrathoracic pressure to between 50 and 100 cm H_2O. The glottis suddenly opens, resulting in explosive exhalation. When airflow velocity exceeds 25 m/s, excess secretions are separated from the walls of the trachea or main bronchi and carried cephalad. Cough is effective only in removing secretions by rapid airflow from the trachea and mainstem bronchi. In addition, cough removes secretions only when excess secretions or foreign bodies are present. Cough may also move secretions from smaller airways by direct compression or "milking," although this mechanism has not been well studied. The cough reflex is suppressed by aging, ipratropium, diphenhydramine, sedatives, and narcotics and may be eliminated by topical application of local anesthetic drugs.

The protective effect of mucus derives from its ability to dilute deleterious material, thereby reducing the concentration, and to inhibit adhesion of bacteria and viruses to epithelial cells. Mucus also acts as a solvent that allows antibacterial substances, such as lysozymes, lactoferrin, and immunoglobulins, to come into contact with their targets. Mucus is secreted by goblet cells, submucosal glands, and Clara cells. Cholinergic agonists stimulate mucus secretion, whereas antagonists such as atropine block secretion. Adrenergic drugs may cause mucus secretion, but adrenergic nerve stimulation does not. Mechanical stimulation of the upper airway causes secretion in the trachea. This effect is blocked by combined vagal and sympathetic block. Other mediators that induce mucus secretion include histamine, leukotrienes, and prostaglandin E_2. Dust and dry air cause secretion by local irritation. Nicotine increases secretion by ganglionic stimulation.

Adding topical water decreases the viscosity of mucus, but the administration of 100% humidity has no effect. The latter might be expected because the humidity in the airways is already close to 100%. No other drugs have been found effective in stimulating production of mucus. However, hypertonic saline solution improves cough clearance of mucus.

Mucociliary Escalator. The cilia in the nose beat downward toward the pharynx, while those in the lower airway beat cephalad at a rate of 1000 to 1500 strokes each minute.

DEPRESSED CILIARY ACTIVITY. Ciliary beating is impaired by increased inspired oxygen concentrations, inhalation of dry air, cigarette smoke (2 to 3 months of abstinence is required for recovery), sleep, cough, advancing age, anesthetics, alcohol, viral infection, *Mycoplasma* infection, and congenital ciliary abnormalities. Beta-adrenergic receptor blockade, atropine, aspirin, bronchitis, bronchiectasis, asthma, and tracheostomy also impair clearance. Adequate humidity is required for optimal function because dry air dehydrates mucus and increases its viscosity, which depresses clearance. FIO_2 greater than 0.25 depresses mucociliary clearance significantly in as little as 20 minutes.

ENHANCED CILIARY ACTIVITY. Physical stimulation of the mucosa and beta-adrenergic agonists increase mucus clearance. The latter may act indirectly by stimulating mucus secretion, which is known to stimulate ciliary activity. Cholinergic agents also may act indirectly by stimulating mucus secretion. Methylxanthines and systemic steroids, but not aerosolized steroids, stimulate ciliary activity. Vigorous exercise, but not ordinary exercise such as walking, stimulates clearance of the tracheobronchial tree.

The mucociliary escalator moves particles deposited in the tracheobronchial tree at a velocity of 0.5 to 1.0 mm/min in small airways, with a clearance half-time of several hours. The velocity is more rapid (5 to 20 mm/min) in the trachea and main bronchi, with a clearance half-time of about 30 minutes.

Pulmonary Macrophages. Cellular defense mechanisms remove particles deposited distal to the ciliated epithelium. The pulmonary macrophages perform a variety of defensive functions, including foreign particle recognition, phagocytosis, release of chemotaxins, and presentation of antigen to lymphocytes for initiation of the immune response. Pulmonary macrophages are effective in removing gram-positive but not gram-negative bacteria. Particles are removed with a clearance half-time of many days, in contrast to the mucociliary system, which clears material within hours. The chemotactic mediators released by the macrophages attract polymorphonuclear cells and are effective against *Klebsiella, Pseudomonas,* and other gram-negative organisms.

Immunoglobulins. Immunoglobulins A and G (IgA and IgG) account for 13% and 3.5% of protein content, respectively, in nasal secretions. Immunoglobulin activity is induced by exposure to specific antigens but is short lived. Saliva contains IgA but little IgG. However, the ratio of IgG to IgA in mucus increases the more distal in the tracheobronchial tree secretions are sampled. IgG is found in about the same concentration in plasma, suggesting that it is not actively secreted into the airways. IgA found in the airways is predominantly in the secretory form and thus is probably actively secreted.

CHEST PHYSICAL THERAPY

Chest physical therapy consists of maneuvers to enhance ventilation and clear pulmonary secretions. An understanding of this frequently ordered but rarely appreciated therapy is crucial to optimal critical care practice. Appropriate goals of chest physical therapy are presented in Table 3–8.

Improvement of Ventilation. As discussed previously, decreased lung volumes are common in critically ill patients. Chest physical therapy attempts to return lung volumes toward normal by a variety of inspiratory maneuvers. These include self-initiated deep breathing, incentive spirometry, CPAP, and, in patients with respiratory muscle weakness, intermittent positive-pressure breathing. All these techniques tend to increase lung volumes, and those involving spontaneous effort may improve respiratory muscle strength. Furthermore, cough is more effective when initiated at higher lung volumes. Inspiratory maneuvers should be performed at least every 6 hours and the patients encouraged to initiate such maneuvers on their own. The performance of 10 deep breaths per hour has been shown to decrease postoperative pulmonary complications. Maneuvers such as using blow bottles and expiring to residual volume may adversely affect oxygenation and ventilation and should not be encouraged.

Secretion Clearance. Secretion clearance may be impaired in critically ill patients for a number of reasons such as increased production, impaired mucociliary escalator, muscle weakness, decreased cough reflex, and splinting caused by pain. Chest physical therapy techniques help mobilize secretions from the periphery to the trachea where they may be expectorated or suctioned. Chest physical therapy is as effective as bronchoscopy in providing pulmonary toilet. However, these positive effects can be demonstrated only in patients with excessive secretions and intact ventilatory and cough mechanisms. Chest physiotherapy does not hasten resolution of pneumonia, nor is it effective prophylaxis against postoperative pulmonary complications in patients without pre-existing lung disease.

Postural Drainage. Positioning of the patient has a number of beneficial effects. The patient can be placed so that gravity helps drain secretions from each of the lobes. Extreme degrees of position are not necessary. Positioning can be provided to the vast majority of patients, although patients who are immobilized, are paralyzed by disease or drugs, or have or are suspected of having intracranial hypertension may pose certain limitation to positioning. Besides lobar drainage, positioning allows a diseased lung and a good lung to be placed nondepen-

TABLE 3–8. Goals of Chest Physical Therapy

Prevent accumulation of secretions
Improve mobilization and drainage of secretions
Promote relaxation to improve breathing patterns
Promote development of respiratory strength and endurance
Improve cardiopulmonary exercise tolerance

dent and dependent, respectively. This may speed the resolution of atelectasis and improve gas exchange by allowing greater aeration of the diseased (uppermost) lung and increased perfusion to the good (dependent) lung.

Manual Techniques. A skilled chest physical therapist can perform a number of manual techniques to mobilize secretions. Appropriate training is necessary to deliver effective therapy without causing harm. Few absolute contraindications to manual techniques exist (tension pneumothorax is one). An experienced therapist should be consulted as to their advisability in patients with relative contraindications such as intracranial hypertension and rib fractures. Often a modified approach can be developed to at least ameliorate secretion retention.

PERCUSSION. Percussion is delivered with a cupped hand repetitively striking the nondependent chest to clear secretions. Skilled delivery of percussion is the mainstay of manual techniques and should not cause patient discomfort. Pneumatically driven mechanical percussion devices are commercially available.

VIBRATION. A therapist applies vibration during expiration by rapidly making small compressions of the rib cage.

SHAKING. Shaking is used to dislodge extremely tenacious secretions. Like vibration it is delivered during expiration, but with greater force. Another name is rib springing.

WEANING FROM MECHANICAL VENTILATION

The difficulty of weaning patients from mechanical ventilatory support is roughly proportional to the duration of support, the degree of respiratory dysfunction, and the severity of underlying illness. Success in weaning depends more on the patient's overall medical and pulmonary condition than on the weaning technique. The intubated patient receiving mechanical ventilation is exposed to a number of factors that may increase the work of breathing. These include factors that increase the resistance of airflow through the ventilator circuit and endo-tracheal tube, such as a narrow endotracheal tube, kinking of the circuit or endotracheal tube, secretions or water in the tube or circuit, inappropriate sensitivity of the mechanical ven-tilator, and inadequate inspiratory flow rates. Work of breathing may be increased by intrinsic pulmonary diseases that decrease pulmonary compliance or increase airway resistance. In-creased airway resistance requires active effort to reduce lung volume. If a patient is not readily weaned from ventilatory support, the intensivist should examine the patient and the ventilatory apparatus for these and other conditions that if corrected might improve the balance between respiratory workload and work capacity.

Respiratory Workload. The respiratory work-load depends on the required minute ventilation and the compliance and resistance of the respiratory system. Minute ventilation require-ments are determined by carbon dioxide pro-duction, dead space, and respiratory drive. Before any serious attempt to wean a difficult patient, the rate of carbon dioxide production should be minimized by control of sepsis, fever, shivering, agitation, anxiety, beta-adrenergic stimulation, and carbohydrate overload, all of which increase metabolic rate. Carbohydrate administration in excess of the patient's needs causes fat production, which generates 8 to 9 moles of carbon dioxide for each mole of oxygen consumed. This is of concern in patients with a fixed, low maximal minute alveolar ventilation. These patients may require careful titration of calorie intake (measured by indirect calorime-try), as well as reduction in the respiratory quotient to 0.7 to 0.8 by supplying 40% to 60% of the total calories in the form of fat.

Increases in dead space require augmentation of minute ventilation, which is the sum of alveolar and dead space ventilation. Unfortu-nately, dead space can rarely be reduced by any specific therapy in patients with acute or chronic respiratory failure. Normal V_{DS}/V_T is 0.3; when it exceeds 0.65, successful weaning is unlikely because the increased respiratory work needed to produce the alveolar ventilation necessary for carbon dioxide elimination may produce more carbon dioxide than is eliminated.

Respiratory drive is a critical factor in suc-cessful weaning. Either impaired or exaggerated drive may impede weaning. Depressed drive results in hypoventilation, hypercarbia, and hypoxemia. Exaggerated drive may cause failure because the resultant higher minute ventilation and work of breathing lead to fatigue and eventually hypoventilation.

When hypoventilation is the problem, the first task is to decide whether drive is impaired or the patient is unable to perform the work needed to eliminate carbon dioxide. Suppressed drive is most commonly due to narcotics and sedative drugs. The latter may allow hypoventilation to occur primarily by suppressing carbon dioxide/pH drive and virtually eliminating hypoxic ven-tilatory drive. Drive is also suppressed by hy-pothyroidism, starvation, and sleep deprivation. Amino acid infusions and ammonia stimulate drive. The methylxanthines stimulate carbon di-oxide drive, and doxapram stimulates hypoxic drive. Acidosis, hypercarbia, or hypoxemia should stimulate ventilation if ventilatory drive is intact. If ventilation is unable to meet needs, signs of respiratory muscle fatigue (tachypnea, dyspnea, accessory muscle activation) and sympathetic stimulation result. The patient with suppressed drive does not manifest these signs of failure despite hypoxia, hypercarbia, or acidosis.

Exaggerated drive causes signs of ventilatory failure despite an adequate arterial pH, $Paco_2$, and oxygenation. These patients may need judicious pharmacologic drive suppression to facilitate weaning.

Psychologic factors may impede weaning of the patient after prolonged mechanical ventila-tion. These patients have learned to associate disconnection from the ventilator with feelings of suffocation. The patient should be reassured that weaning, although difficult, is a sign of progress and requires hard work. Sedation may occasionally help as long as it does not suppress ventilatory drive. The butyrophenones, halo-peridol and droperidol, cause minimal if any suppression of ventilatory drive. Use of weaning techniques that do not require disconnection from the ventilator, such as pressure support or IMV, and that can decrease mechanical ventila-tion very slowly is often better than T-piece trial weaning.

Compliance. Poor compliance of the res-piratory system represents a major imped-ance to spontaneous ventilation in acute respiratory failure but is usually normal or higher than normal in emphysema. Lung compliance also depends on lung volume be-cause pulmonary compliance decreases at very low or very high lung volumes. Thus lung vol-ume (that is, FRC) should be optimized as part of the weaning process. PEEP should be ad-justed to produce a maximal compliance as determined by measuring inspiratory plateau pressure and tidal volume at a series of PEEP values.

Overinflation may result from increased airway resistance. Thus reducing airway resistance helps optimize lung volume. Compliance may be reduced by pulmonary edema, infiltration of inflammatory or neoplastic cells, fibrosis, sarcoid, and amyloid. Extrinsic compression of the lung by pneumothorax, hemothorax, or hydrothorax should be treated, especially if they appear to be causing significant compressive atelectasis.

Chest wall compliance should be considered to include the diaphragm, ribs, and intercostal musculature. It may be reduced by obesity, body wall edema, tense subcutaneous emphysema, circumferential burn eschar or scar, extrinsic compression by tightfitting braces, casts, or dressings, and abdominal distention.

Resistance. Resistance to airflow may be found either in the mechanical breathing circuit or within the bronchopulmonary system. The mechanical circuit resistance may be increased if the endotracheal tube has kinks, is compressed, or is too small. Nasal endotracheal tubes are especially prone to compression by the nasal turbinates and to kinking as the endotracheal tube makes the nasopharyngeal bend. Cuff overinflation may cause tube compression or cuff herniation, although these have become rare with newer plastic tubes. The tube tip may impinge on the tracheal wall, causing impedance during both exhalation and inhalation or a flap valve effect, which leads to severe overinflation because of expiratory obstruction. The widespread use of endotracheal tubes that have an extra hole in the side wall near the tube tip has significantly reduced these complications. Increases in tracheobronchial resistance can result from extrinsic compression by tumors or cardiomegaly, edema of the mucosa, intraluminal material (sputum or foreign bodies), stenosis caused by scar or neoplasm, or bronchospasm. These factors should be identified and eliminated or reduced.

The resistance of the inspiratory limb of the mechanical circuit may be increased by kinks or by pools of water from condensation of humidified gas. Inspiratory flow limitation may be imposed by demand valves that produce a flow proportional to the negative pressure produced by the patient and by those with a response time too slow to meet patient needs. Flow-by systems, which use a continuous flow of gas through the inspiratory circuit, are generally associated with lower work of breathing than demand valves, but they require a reservoir for optimal performance. A condition for flow-by systems is that the flow rate and reservoir bag must be able to deliver whatever inspiratory flow rate the patient demands.

Work Capacity. The various impedances to breathing just discussed must be overcome by the ventilatory bellows function of the chest wall, as well as the intercostal, accessory, and diaphragmatic musculature. The structural integrity of the chest wall can be impaired by multiple fractured ribs, costochondral separations (such as flail chest), or other chest wall defects. By themselves these are rarely limiting factors, but they impair the efficiency of the inspiratory and expiratory musculature.

The diaphragm is the primary inspiratory muscle. The function of the inspiratory muscles depends on preload (the amount of stretch at the beginning of inspiration), afterload (the resistance, compliance, and requirement for minute ventilation), and contractility. Diaphragmatic preload is determined by elevation into the typical rounded end-expiratory shape. When the diaphragm is flat, as in asthma and emphysema, little stretch is imparted and the muscle does not contract optimally. Quadriplegics have flaccid abdominal musculature, allowing gravity to cause the diaphragm to descend and flatten when the patient is upright. They may breathe more easily supine or with an abdominal binder.

Diaphragmatic contractility is determined by the neural system's ability to deliver an adequate stimulus for contraction. Thus the central drive mechanisms must be intact to send the appropriate synchronized volley down the intact phrenic nerves and across the neuromuscular junction. The electrical impulse must cause sufficient influx of calcium to couple excitation with contraction. Oxygen and substrate must be available to supply the required energy. Finally, the contractile tissue mass must be sufficient. Deficits at any link in this chain impede weaning ability.

The diaphragm's metabolic environment requires good delivery of oxygen and substrate. This may be impeded by low cardiac output or insufficient arterial oxygen concentrations. Optimal contractility requires adequate phosphate levels (greater than 1 mmol/L). Certain drugs, including methylxanthines and beta agonists, can stimulate diaphragmatic contractility or make it less susceptible to fatigue. Neuromuscular junction blockade may result from disease (myasthenia gravis) or drugs (aminoglycosides, curare-like drugs). The mass of contractile tissue depends on adequate exercise, rest, and caloric and protein balance. Strengthening exercises may help wean a debilitated patient or one with greatly increased impedance to breathing.

Excessive respiratory muscle afterload (resistance, compliance, minute ventilation, or rate) may lead to fatigue. Fatigue is difficult to quantitate at the bedside. Clinical signs include nasal flaring, tachypnea, recruitment of accessory muscles of ventilation, and possibly chest wall–abdominal dyssynchrony. However, these are imperfect correlates of fatigue.

Weaning Criteria. No single factor or combination of factors has been shown to predict accurately the success or duration of the weaning process in all cases. Factors that should be considered before weaning and factors generally associated with weaning failure are given in Table 3–9.

Weaning Techniques. Several weaning techniques are available, but none has clearly been documented as superior in rapidity, cost, or complications. Judging when to wean is probably more important than how to wean. No technique succeeds when the impedances to breathing exceed the capacity to produce ventilation, but any method works when capacity greatly exceeds the load.

The basal conditions outlined previously should be corrected or optimized before or during the weaning process. It is important to monitor for and to prevent severe respiratory muscle fatigue, dangerous drops in oxygen tension, saturation, or pH, and cardiovascular deterioration during the weaning process. Thus any weaning technique chosen should be titrated to maintain the respiratory rate below 30 breaths per minute; ventilatory accessory muscle use should be avoided; no new or increased arrhythmias should occur; signs of sympathetic stimulation should be minimal or absent, that is, heart rate and blood pressure within 15% of baseline; arterial pH should remain above 7.35 or not decrease by more than 0.05 unit; $Paco_2$ should be stable; $Petco_2$ should increase not more than 5 mm Hg; Pao_2 should be greater than 60 mm Hg; and saturation measured by pulse oximeter should remain above 0.90 and not decrease more than 5%.

Intermittent Mandatory Ventilation. The IMV should be set to the lowest rate at which the patient sustains the goals just described. The rate can be decreased every 30 minutes to 12 hours, depending on the rate of improvement in the patient's condition.

T Tube. The vital capacity should be greater than 10 ml/kg of ideal body weight before T tube trials are started. If the vital capacity is less than this, IMV or pressure support may be a less

TABLE 3–9. Weaning from Mechanical Ventilation

Extubation Criteria and Considerations

Overall salvageability of patient
Oxygenation (PEEP $\leq$ 5 cm H_2O)
Patency of airway
Protective reflexes
  Cough
  Gag
  Swallow
Cardiovascular function
  Stability
  Adequacy of O_2 delivery
  Filling pressures
Secretions
  Quantity
  Viscosity
  Adhesiveness
Premorbid status
Chest radiograph
Ventilation
  $Paco_2$, arterial pH
  Minute ventilation
    $\leq$ 10 L/min
    Voluntarily double minute ventilation
  Vital capacity
    > 10 ml/kg ideal body weight to wean
    > 15 ml/kg ideal body weight to extubate
  Negative inspiratory force
    > -25 cm H_2O
    Greater than peak positive pressure to produce tidal volume
Recent trends

Criteria of Weaning Failure

Signs of sympathetic stimulation
  Tachycardia
  Hypertension
  Arrythmias
  Sweating
  Anxiety
Tachypnea
Signs of accessory muscle use
  Tracheal tug
  Jaw drop
Nasal flaring
Arterial pH decreasing (increasing metabolic or respiratory acidosis)
Oxygenation decreasing

stressful method for weaning. The Fio_2 is usually increased by 5% to 10% above that maintained during mechanical ventilation. The duration of the T tube trial is determined by the patient's ability to meet the weaning goals. This may be as little as 15 minutes at the onset of the weaning process. If the patient cannot tolerate at least 15 minutes, another weaning technique should be considered. Lung inflation techniques (such as manual hyperinflations or intermittent CPAP) should be used every 2 to 3 hours to prevent progressive atelectasis in patients recovering from ARDS. The T tube trials can be stressful, with hypertension, arrhythmias, and hypoxia occurring within 3 minutes of onset of weaning. Continuous observation by trained personnel is mandatory throughout the trial period.

PRESSURE SUPPORT. The initial pressure support level for weaning is chosen to sustain a tidal volume of at least 6 ml/kg of ideal body weight. If the patient meets the weaning goals and sustains a tidal volume of 6 to 7 ml/kg for 2 to 4 hours, the support level is decreased. Lung inflation techniques (such as IMV breaths or PEEP) are usually required for patients recovering from ARDS.

FATIGUE-REST. Some clinicians advocate a program of fatigue alternating with rest to improve ventilatory function, whereas others believe that inducing fatigue is harmful. The rationale for exercising the respiratory muscles to the point of fatigue, followed by rest, has been extrapolated from skeletal muscle training in athletes. In such training a muscle achieves maximal strength when it is fatigued by exercise, followed by complete rest. This regimen does not result in more rapid weaning than any other technique. We use the following guidelines for rest. The patient is returned to fully controlled ventilation for 15 to 20 minutes every 2 to 4 hours if no fatigue was evidenced at the completion of the exercise period. If the patient showed mild fatigue (increase in respiratory rate, early recruitment of accessory muscle activity, more than a 30% fall in vital capacity from the beginning to the end of the exercise period), 2 to 4 hours of rest is prescribed. Complete rest for 24 hours is prescribed if the patient shows severe fatigue (carbon dioxide elevation and acidosis, hypoxia, respiratory rate greater than 40 breaths per minute or an increase of more than 15 breaths per minute, arrhythmias, postweaning vital capacity less than 5 ml/kg or negative inspiratory force less negative than -10 cm H_2O, or severe accessory muscle activity).

Close monitoring is required because the goal is to induce respiratory muscle fatigue. The patient must be observed every 5 minutes for the criteria listed earlier. At the end of the initial trial, arterial blood gases, vital capacity, and negative inspiratory force are measured. Subsequently the arterial blood gas measurement is optional if the pulse oximeter and PETCO$_2$ values are stable and the patient is not severely fatigued.

The rest-fatigue regimen can be done with any of the weaning techniques. The T tube trial is carried out in the usual fashion except that it is terminated when signs of fatigue are noted.

Pressure support can be used to exercise patients who need PEEP for oxygenation or who cannot tolerate at least 15 minutes on the T tube. The pressure support level is simply decreased by 10% to 20% until the patient manifests signs of fatigue within 15 to 30 minutes. The duration on this exercise level is increased until the patient tolerates 2 to 4 hours before fatigue develops, at which time the support level is again decreased by 10% to 20%. When fatigue develops, the pressure support level is increased, IMV breaths are added, or a controlled mode of ventilation is chosen. The level of mechanical support should cause the patient to cease respiratory efforts.

IMV is used to exercise the patient by decreasing the rate by about 20%. If no signs of fatigue develop in 15 to 30 minutes, the rate is decreased again. When the patient requires 2 to 4 hours of the exercise IMV rate to induce fatigue, the rate is decreased further. When fatigue occurs, guidelines for rest are followed by increasing the IMV rate to a level that causes the patient to cease spontaneous respiratory activity.

Inspiratory resistive training can be used to increase the respiratory system reserve in patients who have chronic elevations in their impendance to ventilation. A 5 to 6 cm segment of endotracheal tube with an inner diameter 1 to 1.5 mm smaller than the patient's current tube is placed in series with the endotracheal tube. Exercise, followed by complete rest with a ventilator, is carried out as described previously. The size of the interposed segment of tube is decreased when the patient tolerates 2 to 4 hours of breathing.

TUBE COMPLICATIONS

A number of complications may arise from the placement and maintenance of artificial airways. Many of these have been minimized because of improved tube design and acquired knowledge, but problems remain.

Laryngeal injuries may be divided into those caused by pressure necrosis and those caused by tube movement. Abrasions or lacerations are due to the trauma of insertion. Compression of the mucosa may produce ischemia, which allows ulcers to involve deeper structures in the larynx. Cartilaginous destruction and tracheomalacia may result in uncontrollable air leak and increase the risk for tracheoesophageal fistula. Furthermore, inflammatory response to the structural damage eventually may lead to scarring and life-threatening airway stenosis. Tracheal injury may be minimized by using high-volume, low-pressure cuffs, inflating cuffs to less than 20 mm Hg, and choosing endotracheal tubes not large enough to dilate the larynx and not small enough that cuffs have to be overdistended to create a seal. Movement of the endotracheal tube abrades laryngeal and tracheal mucosa and should be minimized by support of the ventilator circuit. However, flexion and extension of the neck cause the endotracheal tube to move a mean of 3.8 cm.

Mechanical factors may lead to complications of artificial airways. Tubes are commonly made from materials that soften at body temperature. This property allows the tube to conform better to the patient's airway and reduce trauma but also increases the risks of kinking and compression. Other complications include unobserved disconnection or extubation, herniation of the cuff over the end of the endotracheal tube creating obstruction, obstruction by secretions, and sinusitis with the nasotracheal route. We believe the endotracheal tube should never be amputated because (1) it may be impossible to advance the tube into proper position, necessitating a change of the tube, (2) the protruding tube buffers the forces applied by the ventilator circuit, and (3) the staff may not be able to glance at the length of tube protruding from the patient and know whether the tube has been moved.

TRACHEOSTOMY

Clear indications for tracheostomy include immediate need to establish an airway when intubation is not possible and protection of the airway after oromaxillofacial surgery or when a disease process obstructs the upper airway. The need for or timing of tracheostomy in a patient requiring long-term ventilatory support is not clear. Long-term translaryngeal intubation is associated with complications of laryngeal stenosis and inadvertent extubation. Advantages of tracheostomy include better tolerance by the patient, easier speech and oral feeding, improved efficacy of suctioning, and more secure access to the airway. However, the performance of tracheostomy after prolonged translaryngeal intubation may exacerbate laryngeal stenosis. Furthermore, the risks of tracheostomy include tracheal injury with subsequent tracheal stenosis, bleeding, infection, and pneumothorax. A recent consensus conference highlighted the need to tailor the timing of tracheostomy to the patient. The following were suggested as general guidelines. Tracheostomy is not needed if an artificial airway would be required for less than 10 days. If intubation would last more than 21 days, tracheostomy should be performed as early in the hospital course as possible to reduce laryngeal injury. However, we defer tracheostomy indefinitely if we anticipate that PEEP will exceed 12 to 15 cm H_2O or peak inspiratory pressure will exceed 50 cm H_2O.

WORK OF BREATHING

Classically, the physical concept of work consists of moving a mass over a distance. In contrast, ventilatory work is determined by the pressure required to generate a given lung volume, such as tidal volume. However, work done does not always reflect effort exerted. Interestingly, if force is applied to the lung and no air is moved, effort may be great but no work is performed. The pressure component is the transpulmonary pressure, which is the difference between the pleural pressure (commonly estimated by esophageal balloon techniques) and the alveolar pressure. Transpulmonary pressure is the pressure that determines alveolar volume for any given pulmonary compliance. Because of the mechanical characteristics of the lung, the work performed on the lung may be divided into that used to overcome the tissue-resistive elements (lung stiffness) and that used to overcome the viscous elements, largely composed of airflow resistance (Fig. 3–8). To minimize the work of breathing, patients with low total pulmonary compliance choose rapid, shallow tidal breaths. In contrast, asthmatic patients have increased airflow resistance. These patients often change breathing pattern to a slower respiratory rate and larger tidal volume, again to minimize the effect of airflow resistance on work of breathing.

SUGGESTED READINGS

Basic Pulmonary Physiology and Pathophysiology

West JB: Respiratory physiology — the essentials, ed 3. Baltimore, 1985, Williams & Wilkins

West JB: Pulmonary pathophysiology — the essentials, ed 3. Baltimore, 1987, Williams & Wilkins

Arterial Blood Gases

Shapiro BA, Harrison RA, Walton JR: Clinical application of blood gases, ed 3. Chicago, 1982, Year Book, chapters 8-11

Diagnostic Techniques

Stradling P: Diagnostic bronchoscopy. New York, 1986, Churchill Livingstone, chapters 3, 5, and 9

Tobin MJ: Respiratory monitoring in the intensive care unit. Am Rev Respir Dis 1988;138:1625-1642

Support of Oxygenation and Ventilation

Banner MJ, Smith RA: Mechanical ventilation. In Civetta J, Taylor RW, Kirby RR, eds: Critical care. New York, 1988, JB Lippincott, pp. 1161-1181

Downs JB: Airway pressure support. In Civetta J, Taylor RW, Kirby RR, eds: Critical care. New York, 1988, JB Lippincott, pp. 1151-1159

Shapiro BA: General principles of airway pressure therapy. In Shoemaker WC, Ayres S, Grenvik A, et al, eds: Textbook of critical care, Philadelphia, 1989, WB Saunders, pp. 505-515

Ventilator Modes

Kirby RR: Continuous positive airway pressure: to breathe or not to breathe. Anesthesiology 1985;63:578-580

Slutsky AS: Nonconventional methods of ventilation. Am Rev Respir Dis 1988;138:175-183

Stock MC. Mechanical ventilation: old vs new (Refresher Lecture No. 522). In American Society of Anesthesiologists Refresher Course Lectures. Philadelphia, 1989, The Society.

Tharratt RS, Allen RP, Albertson TE: Pressure controlled inverse ratio ventilation in severe adult respiratory failure. Chest 1988;94:755-762

Muscle Relaxants

Lumb, PD: Sedatives and muscle relaxants in the intensive care unit. In Fuhrman BP, Shoemaker WC, eds: Critical care state of the art, vol 10. Fullerton, Calif, 1989, Society of Critical Care Medicine, pp. 145-171

Complications of Mechanical Ventilation

Broaddus V, Berthiaume Y, Biondi JW, Matthay MA: Hemodynamic management of the adult respiratory distress syndrome. Intensive Care Med 1987; 2:190-213

Haake R, Schlichtig R, Ulstad DR, Henschen RR: Barotrauma: pathophysiology, risk factors and prevention. Chest 1987;91:608-613

Powner DJ: Pulmonary barotrauma in the intensive care unit. J Intensive Care Med 1988;3:224-232

Regel G, Sturm JA, Neumann C, et al: Occlusion of bronchopleural fistula after lung injury—a new treatment by bronchoscopy. J Trauma 1989;29:223-226

Airway Infection and Defense

Reynolds H: Pulmonary host defenses—state of the art. Chest 1989;95:223S-230S

Richardson PS, Peatfield AC: The control of airway mucus secretion. Eur J Respir Dis 1987;71(suppl 153):43-51

Chest Physical Therapy

Frownfelter DJ: Chest physical therapy and airway care. In Barnes TA, ed: Respiratory care practice. Chicago, 1988, Year Book, pp. 181-200

Mackenzie CF: Chest physiotherapy in the intensive care unit, ed 2. Baltimore, 1989, Williams & Wilkins, chapters 1, 3, 4, and 5

Weaning

Benotti P, Bistrian B: Metabolic and nutritional aspects of weaning from mechanical ventilation. Crit Care Med 1989;17:181-185

Sassoon C: Weaning from mechanical ventilation: how to predict the problem patient. J Crit Illness 1988;3: 29-38

Tube Complications and Tracheostomy

Bishop MJ: Mechanisms of laryngotracheal injury following prolonged tracheal intubation. Chest 1989;96:185-186

Consensus conference on artificial airways in patients receiving mechanical ventilation. Chest 1989;96:178-180.

Heffner JE: Medical indications for tracheotomy. Chest 1989;96:186-190

4

ADVANCED CARDIOVASCULAR LIFE SUPPORT

JOHN W. HOYT, MD

The primary physiologic role of the cardiovascular system is to deliver oxygenated blood and nutrients to the cells, tissues, and organs. Without a constant oxygen supply, many cells, such as those in the brain and heart, cannot continue their metabolic activities and are at risk of cellular death.

Three cardiovascular elements are required for tissue perfusion: cardiac output or flow, an intravascular volume of oxygenated hemoglobin and cellular nutrients, and peripheral resistance to create a pressure for perfusion. If any one of these three requirements is substantially reduced or missing, the system fails.

A significant goal of critical care medicine is to provide an environment in which a patient with shock or inadequate tissue perfusion can be examined, diagnosed, and treated expeditiously to reduce the organ damage caused by a failing cardiovascular system. For that to occur, skilled critical care physicians, nurses, respiratory therapists, and technologists must be available to assess the critically ill patient and act on physiologic abnormalities. As mentioned in Chapter 3, this team must immediately look at heart rate and rhythm, blood pressure, oxygen saturation of hemoglobin in arterial blood (SaO_2), level of consciousness, urine output, pulses, skin warmth, and color. The team must quickly act on the first impressions received in this clinical assessment to stabilize the critically ill patient. Second-level assessment can begin after attention has been paid to the ABCs: airway, breathing, and circulation.

PRELIMINARY CARDIOVASCULAR ASSESSMENT

For admission assessment of a patient with a failing cardiovascular system, the ICU bedside should be equipped with a monitor for electrocardiography, noninvasive blood pressure monitoring, and pulse oximetry (Fig. 4-1). This basic equipment permits the automated collection of

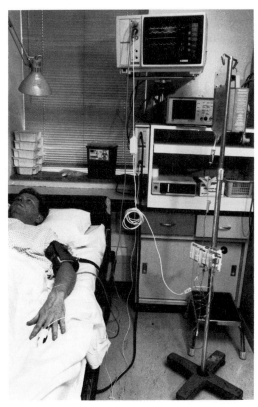

Figure 4–1 The preliminary cardiac assessment of a critically ill patient requires a bedside monitor with electrocardiogram, noninvasive blood pressure, and pulse oximetry. New computer-based monitors have been able to incorporate preliminary assessment devices, as well as more invasive equipment such as monitors of intravascular pressure and cardiac output. This has greatly reduced the monitoring clutter at the bedside. Collected data can be expressed in both tabular and graphic fashion for easy review and interpretation.

vital sign data and allows the critical care team to assess other areas of concern, such as level of consciousness, pulses, skin color, and warmth. If shock is suspected, a Foley catheter should be inserted immediately to monitor hourly urine output. Because of peripheral vasoconstriction, pulse oximetry is often unsuccessful in patients with shock. With appropriate resuscitation of the cardiovascular system, the pulse oximeter will begin to work, signaling restoration of peripheral perfusion.

The initial stabilization of circulation is directed toward heart rate and blood pressure. Bradycardia can be treated with atropine, isoproterenol, or a pacemaker depending on the cause of the problem. Blood pressure is restored by an initial bolus of crystalloid, 10 to 20 ml/kg, given over 1 hour and by the use of the inotropic and vasoconstrictor agent dopamine. Doses greater than 10 μg/kg/min cause significant beta and alpha stimulation, increasing cardiac output and systemic vascular resistance.

At one time, critical care treatment ended when blood pressure was stabilized. In the late 1960s and early 1970s, blood pressure was the center of attention in attempts to restore tissue perfusion. Alpha-agonist drugs such as norepinephrine and phenylephrine were commonly used to maintain blood pressure.

Blood pressure is an essential requirement for tissue perfusion, but by itself it is an inadequate physiologic variable for restoring proper perfusion. Blood pressure is a product of cardiac output and system vascular resistance. It is possible to have a normal blood pressure with a low cardiac output and a high systemic vascular resistance, or to have a normal blood pressure with a high cardiac output and a low systemic vascular resistance. In both situations tissue perfusion may be inadequate.

Therefore, during stabilization of the circulation, it is appropriate to focus on blood pressure, but subsequent evaluations must look at other findings such as level of consciousness, urine output, and skin warmth and color as the clinician moves from initial concerns about heart rate and blood pressure to concerns about cardiac output, intravascular volume, systemic vascular resistance, and most important, tissue perfusion.

ADVANCED CARDIOVASCULAR ASSESSMENT

If the patient has not responded rapidly to fluid and dopamine therapy, he or she is a candidate for advanced cardiovascular assessment with arterial, central venous, and pulmonary artery catheters. Many patients require only an arterial catheter or arterial and central venous catheters, but a definitive evaluation of peripheral perfusion should include hemodynamic monitoring with a pulmonary artery catheter.

Blood pressure monitoring in the ICU has advanced significantly from the mercury or aneroid manometer (Riva-Rocci) technique in which every hour the bedside nurse inflated and deflated an arm cuff, listened for Korotkoff sounds, and recorded systolic and diastolic measurements. Automated blood pressure cuffs are now routine in the ICU. By an oscillotonometer technique, the automated cuff determines systolic, diastolic, and mean blood pressure every few minutes, saving significant nursing time. Despite the technologic advances in noninvasive blood pressure monitoring, arterial catheters are still essential in the ICU for monitoring systemic blood pressure in a patient with shock of cardiovascular origin.

Arterial Catheters

The bedside display of an arterial waveform provides significant information beyond the convenience of beat-to-beat systolic, diastolic, and mean blood pressure. Analysis of the arterial waveform is most valuable in the early assessment of the cardiovascular system. Many patients with poor peripheral perfusion but a "normal" blood pressure have little area under the pressure waveform. They may have a tall, spiked arterial wave with little width, indicating the possibility of inadequate cardiac output. Other patients have a significant beat-to-beat variation in arterial waveform. A hypovolemic patient receiving mechanical ventilation has a substantially reduced arterial waveform after each cycle of the ventilator. The positive airway pressure increases intrathoracic pressure and significantly limits venous return. Stroke volumes after the cycle of the ventilator are reduced. Significant beat-to-beat arterial waveform variation can also be seen in patients with marked bronchospasm who are struggling with spontaneous respiration.

Fifteen years of the safe use of arterial catheters in the critical care environment has resulted in liberal indications for the use of these catheters. In many critical care centers, 90% to 95% of patients have arterial catheters at some time during their ICU stay for evaluation of beat-to-beat blood pressure or for the frequent drawing of blood for arterial blood gas and other blood analyses. Any hypotensive patient who is receiving inotropic or vasoconstrictor therapy by continuous intravenous infusion should have an arterial catheter. Any ICU patient receiving vasodilator therapy by continuous infusion should also have an arterial catheter. Any patient receiving mechanical ventilation or positive end-expiratory pressure therapy should have an arterial catheter for frequent and convenient blood gas analysis (Table 4-1).

Relative contraindications for arterial catheters include severe vascular disease, anticoagulant therapy, and thrombolytic therapy (Table 4-1). Whether these are contraindications depends on the severity of the patient's illness. A critically ill patient needing continuous resuscitation must have an arterial catheter to help guide therapy.

When placement of an arterial catheter is elective, the Allen test has been recommended for evaluating blood supply to the hand before insertion of a radial artery catheter. This test involves draining the raised hand of blood and compressing both the radial and ulnar arteries. When the patient opens the hand, the ulnar artery is released and the thenar eminence is observed for return of flow. A flash of red should occur in the palm within 5 seconds while the radial artery is compressed if the patient has good palmar arch flow from the ulnar artery.

The Allen test should be reserved for hemodynamically stable patients about to undergo major surgery and anesthesia. In the critical care setting many candidates for arterial catheters have inadequate peripheral perfusion because of shock and the Allen test is uninterpretable. However, arterial catheters have been used extensively in the critical care environment with rare incidence of extremity ischemia.

Four techniques are used for insertion of an arterial catheter. First is surgical cutdown, which is still used in small infants but otherwise is mostly of historical significance and has been replaced by various percutaneous techniques. Second is the percutaneous, over-the-needle technique using a standard intravenous catheter. Third is the percutaneous, over-the-needle technique using a built-in guidewire that rests in a protective sheath so that the wire can be advanced through the needle without hand contact (Fig. 4-2). Last is the true Seldinger technique in which use of a locating needle is followed by a wire and then a catheter. The percutaneous, over-the-needle technique with a protected guidewire has become universally popular because of its ease of use. This catheter allows the clinician to sterilely insert an arterial catheter without wearing gloves to preserve the tactile sensation of the pulse. Unfortunately, the

TABLE 4–1. Arterial Catheters

Indications

Beat-to-beat blood pressure monitoring
Frequent sampling of blood for analysis
Continuous infusion of vasoactive drugs
Shock with or without hypotension
Hypertensive crisis
Mechanical ventilation
Refractory hypoxia

Relative Contraindications

Peripheral vascular disease
Coagulopathy
Thrombolytic therapy
Inadequate collateral circulation

Complications

Bleeding
Peripheral ischemia
Proximal embolization to the central nervous system
Infection
Arterial aneurysm
Arterial or venous fistula
Vessel thrombosis
Arterial spasm
Pain
Distal embolization

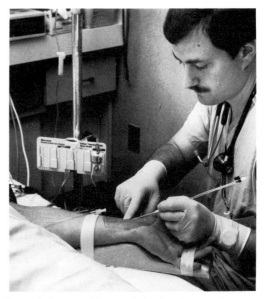

Figure 4–2 Arterial cannulation has been made convenient, safe, and easy by the use of a protected guidewire. After the artery is entered percutaneously by following the pulse, a flash of blood is seen in the needle hub chamber. A flexible-tip wire is advanced into the vessel through a protected plastic shield. The arterial catheter is then threaded off the wire and secured in place with suture.

growing incidence of acquired immunodeficiency syndrome makes the insertion of arterial catheters without protective gloves unwise for the clinician. Even with the best ungloved technique, some blood is lost during the procedure and the clinician's hands are certain to be contaminated.

The usual first choice for arterial catheterization is a 20-gauge 1½-inch catheter in the radial artery. On many occasions an 18-gauge catheter can be used in the radial artery, but this carries a higher risk of thrombotic occlusion of the vessel. Occlusion may have no clinical significance in the presence of good collateral flow, since most vessels recanalize within 8 weeks after removal of the catheter. A 20-gauge catheter can also be inserted into the dorsalis pedis artery. The double blood supply to the foot makes a dorsalis pedis catheter quite safe. Blood pressure determinations from this catheter are slightly higher than from a radial catheter. In general, the farther from the heart in a major artery, the more peaked the wave and the higher the systolic determination.

The second most common site for an arterial catheter is the femoral artery. The 1½-inch, 20-gauge catheter used in the radial artery is not a good choice for the femoral artery because it is likely to be dislodged. A 6-inch, 20- or 18-gauge catheter inserted by the Seldinger technique should be considered. Femoral artery catheters have proved quite safe with no higher incidence of infection than other sites if the groin area is shaved and cleansed with a bactericidal solution.

An axillary arterial catheter can be used when other possibilities have been exhausted. A 6-inch catheter is recommended. A 20-gauge catheter in the axillary artery permits better flow to the arm around the catheter.

In all circumstances the arterial catheter should be inserted under sterile conditions with local anesthetic. The site should be shaved if appropriate and cleaned with povidone-iodine solution. Local anesthetic such as 1% lidocaine should be infiltrated in the skin for the patient's comfort and to minimize arterial spasm during insertion. The site should be draped with sterile towels, and the clinician should wear sterile surgical gloves. Once the artery has been cannulated, the catheter should be connected to a saline-filled, high-pressure tubing that leads to a transducer. The tubing can be of variable length depending on whether the transducer is positioned on the patient or at the bedside on a transducer holder. Tubing should not be longer than 4 feet for accurate transmission of pressure.

The catheter should be secured in place with a 2-0 or 3-0 suture.

A continuous flush system (3 ml/h) with heparinized saline (1000 U heparin in 500 ml normal saline) from a pressurized intravenous fluid bag maintains the vessel's patency. The flush system is connected to a transducer that converts the pressure energy of the arterial pulse into an electrical signal that can be displayed on the bedside monitor as an arterial waveform. In the past, reusable transducers were routinely used in the ICU. During the last 5 years, however, disposable transducers have largely replaced reusable transducers because of their convenience, low cost, and safety. Nosocomial epidemics of bloodstream infection associated with reusable transducers, which were previously common, have essentially been eliminated by the use of disposable transducers. The Centers for Disease Control recommends that the transducer, tubing, and flush device be discarded after 48 hours' use.

Once the arterial catheter has been inserted, a dry sterile dressing is applied and changed daily. Blood samples can be drawn from a stopcock in the line, but blood should be prevented from accumulating in any part of the line because of the risk of infectious disease. All ports should be protected by caps.

The incidence of hospital-acquired infections from arterial catheters is lower than with other vascular lines such as pulmonary artery catheters. Therefore no time limit on the use of an arterial catheter is generally accepted. Rather, the nurse inspects the site daily and determines the time when the catheter is removed. If a fever of unknown origin or unexplained bacteremia develops, the catheter should be removed. Should the catheter become nonfunctional because of bending or clotting, it can be changed over a wire if the insertion site looks good. A 0.021-inch wire is used to change a 20-gauge catheter, and a 0.028-inch wire is used for an 18-gauge catheter. It is not wise to "rewire" an arterial catheter when the risk of infectious disease is significant.

Since the evolution of the continuous flush heparinized saline system, sterile technique, and disposable transducer, complications from arterial catheters have been minimal. An arterial catheter may be one of the safest monitors in the ICU when the amount of information obtained is weighed against the risk to the patient. Bleeding at the insertion site is the most common complication. Other possible complications include peripheral ischemia, peripheral embolization of clots, proximal embolization of clots during flushing, infection, arterial aneurysm, and arteriovenous fistula. These rare events are reversible if the catheter is removed when problems are first detected (Table 4-1).

Central Venous Catheter

The second part of advanced cardiovascular life support and monitoring is the insertion of a central venous catheter. In the past, this catheter was known as a central venous pressure (CVP) catheter, emphasizing the technique of monitoring right-sided filling pressures. In a previously healthy patient without significant cardiopulmonary disease, such as a trauma patient, a central venous catheter can be valuable in determining intravascular volume by recording filling pressures in the right side of the heart. Unfortunately, most critically ill patients have some cardiac or respiratory problem that may invalidate a CVP catheter as a useful monitor of intravascular volume. As a result, the primary indication for inserting a central venous catheter is for the administration of drugs and fluids (Table 4-2).

Three techniques are used for central venous access. First is surgical cutdown, which is rarely indicated today. Antecubital cutdowns were once used frequently but were replaced by the second approach, the through-the-needle technique. In this method a 14-gauge needle was used to puncture the subclavian vein and then as a conduit for a 16-gauge catheter. This technique has also largely been discarded because of advances in the Seldinger technique.

TABLE 4–2. Central Venous Catheters

Indications

Rapid fluid administration
Pharmacologic therapy
Monitoring right-sided preload
Parenteral nutrition
Venous access

Relative Contraindications

Coagulopathy
Thrombolytic therapy
Infection or tissue problem at proposed site
Risk of pneumothorax
Severe peripheral vascular disease at proposed site

Complications

Bleeding
Pneumothorax or hemothorax
Infection
Phlebitis and thrombosis
Air embolus
Hydrothorax
Catheter shearing, kinking, knotting

Seldinger, a radiologist, developed the prevalent approach to inserting a central venous catheter. A small (18-gauge) needle is used to puncture the vein, followed by a 0.035-inch wire through the needle, a vein dilator, and then a central venous catheter threaded off the wire (Fig. 4-3). This approach became popular in the ICU because of the need to insert large sheaths for placing pulmonary artery catheters. Since that time the Seldinger concept has been applied to central venous, arterial, dialysis, intra-aortic balloon, pericardial, and thoracentesis catheters.

Single-, double-, and triple-lumen catheters can be inserted by the Seldinger technique. The technology that created multiple-lumen pulmonary artery catheters has been applied to central venous catheters for administering fluids and drugs when certain infusions cannot be mixed because of incompatibility. The usual catheter in the ICU is a 20 or 30 cm, triple-lumen CVP that is threaded to the superior vena cava by one of several routes. For long-term use a very soft, flexible catheter can be surgically inserted and tunneled under the skin away from the site of venipuncture to reduce infections. An ICU physician who is not a surgeon can insert such a catheter by a modified Seldinger technique in which a peel-away sheath is used.

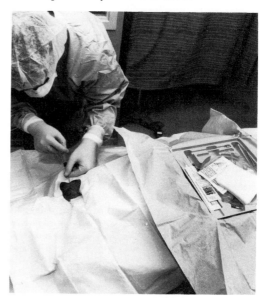

Figure 4–3 The Seldinger technique is now the standard technique for placing a central venous catheter. Sterile disposable kits provide the clinician with all supplies for placing a triple-lumen central venous catheter: sterile prep solution and drapes, local anesthetic, needles and syringes, wire, triple-lumen catheter, vein dilator, suture, and knife blade. Because of the increased risk of nosocomial infections for central venous and pulmonary artery catheters, the clinician should wear a hat, mask, sterile gown, and gloves.

Central venous catheters are divided into two types depending on the reason for insertion. First is the short but large-gauge catheter used for rapid fluid resuscitation. To minimize resistance to flow, the catheter diameter should be as large as possible (8½ French) and as short as possible, since resistance to flow is related to radius to the fourth power and length. Commonly ICU physicians insert a pulmonary artery catheter sidearm introducer to accomplish rapid fluid administration. Any patient with significant hypovolemia admitted to the ICU for rapid fluid administration should have such a catheter inserted at the time of admission.

The second type, the triple- or double-lumen central venous catheter, does not work well for rapid fluid administration but is better for giving drugs, hyperalimentation, and lesser amounts of fluid. The triple-lumen catheter has two 18-gauge ports and one 16-gauge port. Through either the 18- or 16-gauge lumen, 1000 ml of colloid can be given in 60 minutes with a volumetric infusion pump. This represents a significant fluid challenge when trying to improve cardiac function or urine output. Faster rates must be given through a sidearm pulmonary artery catheter introducer. The role of the single-lumen central vein catheter seems to be decreasing in the ICU because it is less versatile than a triple-lumen catheter. The most common sites of insertion for central venous catheters are the internal jugular, subclavian, and femoral veins. The external jugular and antecubital veins are also possibilities but are used less frequently. Usually the right internal jugular vein is used because of concerns about damaging the thoracic duct when puncturing the left internal jugular vein. The internal jugular vein is entered by insertion of the needle at the top of the triangle created by the sternal and clavicular heads of the sternocleidomastoid muscle. The top of the triangle is usually located at the level of cricoid cartilage. The vein lies behind the belly of the clavicular head of the muscle. The needle is inserted at a 30-degree angle to the skin and aimed at the nipple on the same side of the body. The vein is 2 to 5 cm under the skin.

Either the right or left subclavian vein can be used for a central venous catheter. If an 8½ French sidearm introducer is being inserted for large-volume fluid replacement, it should be inserted through the left subclavian vein because of the sharp angle the right subclavian vein takes as it enters the superior vena cava. This angle frequently leads to kinking and reduced lumen size of the thin-walled pulmonary artery catheter introducer. To enter the subclavian vein the needle should be inserted about two-thirds the distance of the clavicle from the midline. At this point the clavicle is usually easy to palpate and most prominent in its curve over the upper chest. The needle should be inserted onto the surface of the clavicle, "walked" under the inferior edge of the bone, and then aimed at the supraclavicular notch. The vein is 2 to 5 cm under the skin.

The right and left femoral veins are also accessible to venous cannulation. The femoral vein lies medial to the femoral artery and is easily entered. If the clinician palpates the femoral artery, the vein can be entered by inserting the needle 1 to 2 cm medial to the center of the femoral pulse. The needle should be inserted at a 30-degree angle to the skin and should enter the vessel at a 2 to 5 cm depth depending on the size of the patient.

The right and left external jugular veins are accessible for venous catheters but are a second choice to the previous sites because of the difficulty of rounding the corner into the central jugular vein even with a J wire. The antecubital vein is also a second choice because of the need for a long catheter and the problems rounding the corner at the axilla to enter the veins in the chest.

For all insertions of central venous catheters the site should be cleansed with povidone-iodine solution and draped with sterile towels. The critical care physician should wear a hat, mask, gown, and gloves to guarantee a sterile insertion, since in many situations the catheter is used for hyperalimentation, which has a high potential for hospital-acquired infection. Local anesthetic should be generously infiltrated in the skin. After the catheter has been threaded 15 to 20 cm into the superior vena cava if inserted from the subclavian or internal jugular approach, it should be sutured in place. If inserted from the femoral vein, the catheter should be inserted a full 30 cm and sutured in place.

After insertion, all lumens should be checked for free flow of blood and flushed with heparinized saline or connected to infusion products or high-pressure tubing from a central venous transducer. If hyperalimentation is to be used, one of the ports should be flushed and left unused to preserve it for the total parenteral nutrition solution. The remaining lumens can be used for drug or fluid infusions. Manifold-type, multichannel infusion pumps permit the mixing of compatible drugs into a single delivery port. The manifold pump might be connected to one of the 18-gauge ports, leaving the other

18-gauge lumen for fluid therapy or monitoring of right-sided filling pressures.

After a sterile dressing has been applied, the catheter's position should be verified by chest roentgenogram. When the catheter is inserted by the internal jugular or subclavian route, the tip should be in the superior vena cava or at the junction of the superior vena cava (SVC) and right atrium. Central venous catheters inserted from the left subclavian approach should be noted on roentgenogram to have rounded the curve into the SVC rather than aiming at the right wall of the SVC. Numerous reports have described SVC perforation by left subclavian vein catheters when not properly positioned. The tip of the catheter should be kept away from the right atrium to avoid perforating the atrium or crossing the tricuspid valve and causing ventricular irritation.

The catheter site dressing should be changed daily and the skin inspected. The tubing should be changed every 48 hours. Most parenteral nutrition catheters are left in place indefinitely unless the patient shows signs of infection. The heavily used ICU triple-lumen catheter probably should not be left in place indefinitely but should be changed every 5 days. If the site is clean and the patient has no sign of infection, the catheter can be changed over a wire. Culture studies of the tip of the old catheter should be performed. If more than 15 colonies are found, the new catheter inserted over a wire should be removed and a fresh venipuncture should be carried out.

Several new devices are designed to limit infection that might begin at the skin site. One of these is a silver-impregnated collagen ring that slides over the catheter and is placed just under the skin to inhibit bacterial growth at the puncture site. Early results indicate that this may be helpful. Other approaches have included coating the catheter with surfactant and binding antibiotics to limit bacterial colonization. These protective techniques need further evaluation.

Complications from central venous catheters include pneumothorax, bleeding, infection, venous thrombosis, and air embolus (Table 4-2). Pneumothorax occurs with the highest frequency in subclavian vein insertions. Internal jugular vein punctures also cause pneumothorax but less frequently. If pneumothorax occurs, particularly in an intubated patient receiving mechanical ventilation, a tension pneumothorax can cause cardiac compromise. Air should be removed immediately by insertion of a chest tube. If only air is present, a chest tube can be inserted in the midclavicular line between the second and third ribs. This can be done most efficiently with a percutaneous, small-bore tube connected to an underwater seal with 10 to 20 cm of negative pressure.

Bleeding can occur at the insertion site, particularly if the clinician enters the carotid artery instead of the vein. A tear in the subclavian artery can lead to a hemothorax. Patients with a coagulopathy are at greater risk of bleeding. The femoral vein site is easily compressed and is the site of choice when a significant coagulopathy exists.

A central venous catheter can become infected in two ways. If the skin site is infected, bacteria pass down the catheter and enter the bloodstream. This is an exogenous catheter infection with secondary spread to the bloodstream. The central venous catheter can also be seeded with bacteria present in the bloodstream from another infected site such as the lung or bladder. This is an endogenous secondary colonization of the catheter when bacteria proliferate on the fibrin coating of the catheter.

Venous thrombosis can occur with a central venous catheter, leading to complete occlusion of the vein. Thrombosis can be sterile or infected. Significant arm edema may accumulate if a subclavian vein is occluded.

Air embolus can occur during central venous catheter insertion or after the catheter is in place. If a patient is breathing spontaneously during insertion, a negative intrathoracic pressure lowers venous pressure and allows air to enter a disconnected needle. Likewise, an accidental intravenous line disconnection can permit air embolus with devastating cardiac complications.

Central venous catheters are a routine part of ICU patient care. They are associated with few complications when properly inserted and maintained. Relative contraindications to the use of central venous catheters include coagulopathy, use of heparin or thrombolytic agents, or the presence of large bullae in the upper lobes of the lung if the subclavian approach is contemplated. The femoral vein catheter has the lowest incidence of complications, since there is no risk of pneumothorax and bleeding can be well controlled at the site. The incidence of infection is no higher than with other catheters.

Advanced Hemodynamic Assessment

Most patients admitted to the ICU, regardless of their medical and surgical problems, have their circulation adequately improved by the measures listed thus far in the chapter. Further collection of information from auscultation of the heart and lungs, history and physical examination, and radiologic examination yields enough information for the clinician to make a cardiac diagnosis and begin corrective measures. For example, a patient with chronic congestive heart failure who has pulmonary edema at admission is easily stabilized with oxygen, morphine, nitroglycerin, and a diuretic. Likewise, a patient with a first myocardial infarction who has some arrhythmias but maintains appropriate peripheral perfusion is easily managed without further invasive assessment of the cardiovascular system. When preliminary diagnostic and therapeutic measures fail to provide a clear diagnosis and restore peripheral perfusion, a pulmonary artery catheter should be inserted for further hemodynamic study.

Considerable controversy exists about the value of the pulmonary artery catheter in improving the condition and survival of critically ill patients. No controlled study has ever been designed and carried out to show that pulmonary artery catheters reduce mortality rates. However, evidence from other studies shows the limitations of physical diagnosis in the ICU and the inability even of senior clinicians to predict pulmonary capillary wedge pressure (PCWP) and cardiac index in patients with complicated diseases who failed to respond to first-pass stabilization techniques. Hemodynamic monitoring enables clinicians to make a clearer diagnosis and plan more effective therapy.

Pulmonary Artery Catheters

Pulmonary artery catheters should be inserted for three reasons. First is for an intravascular volume and preload assessment based on PCWP. The pulmonary artery catheter can frequently provide helpful information in determining whether the origin of pulmonary edema is cardiogenic or noncardiogenic. Second is for a cardiac output analysis or assessment of peripheral perfusion. When the adequacy of peripheral perfusion is in question (for example, because of low urine output, metabolic acidosis, or peripheral vasoconstriction), a pulmonary artery catheter can be used to monitor thermodilution cardiac output and sample mixed venous blood for measurement of oxygen saturation (Svo_2). The third indication for inserting a pulmonary artery catheter is afterload analysis, the systemic vascular resistance index (SVRI) (Table 4-3). Once the pulmonary artery catheter is in place, decisions can be made about the use of fluid, inotropes, and vasodilators.

The two techniques for insertion of pulmonary artery catheters are cutdown and percutaneous by the Seldinger technique. The latter has overwhelming popularity in the ICU and has led to the development of many insertion kits with sidearm introducers for percutaneous placement of pulmonary artery catheters.

Many types of pulmonary artery catheters are available. The standard is a 7½ French catheter that has a pulmonary artery port for measuring pulmonary artery pressures and PCWP, a balloon port for inflating the 1.5 ml balloon on the tip of the catheter, a thermistor wire for thermodilution cardiac output, a central venous port 30 cm from the tip for measuring central venous pressure, and a venous infusion port (also 30 cm from the tip) for administering drugs or fluids. Other choices include an oximetry

TABLE 4–3. Pulmonary Artery Catheters

Indications

Monitoring left-sided preload
Complicated hypovolemic shock
Fluid challenge protocol
Monitoring cardiac output
Svo_2 assessment
Cardiogenic shock
Inotropic therapy
Insertion of pacer wire
Monitoring right ventricular ejection fraction
Afterload monitoring and therapy
Construction of hemodynamic profile
Differentiation of cardiogenic from noncardiogenic pulmonary edema
Diagnosis of mitral regurgitation or ventricular septal rupture in myocardial infarction
Determination of pulmonary artery hypertension
Diagnosis of pericardial tamponade

Relative Contraindications

Coagulopathy
Thrombolytic therapy
Risk of pneumothorax
Infection or tissue problem at proposed site
Severe peripheral vascular disease at proposed site
Ventricular dysrhythmias
Pulmonary hypertension

Complications

Dysrhythmias
Bleeding
Pulmonary embolus or infarct
Pulmonary artery rupture
Infection
Catheter coiling and knotting
Endocarditis and valve damage
Air embolus or balloon rupture
Right ventricular perforation and cardiac tamponade
Inaccurate information

catheter, which has two fiberoptic bundles for reflection spectrophotometry of blood in the pulmonary artery to determine mixed venous oxygen saturation; a pacing catheter, which has a port 20 cm from the catheter tip to permit insertion of a pacer wire into the right ventricle without fluoroscopic guidance; and a right ventricular ejection fraction catheter, which has sensitive thermistors for measuring washout of the temperature indicator from the right ventricle.

The internal jugular and subclavian veins are the most common sites for inserting pulmonary artery catheters. The right internal jugular vein provides a nearly straight path to the right atrium and right ventricle and is the usual first choice. The technique for entering the right internal jugular vein is the same as that described for central venous catheters. The left internal jugular vein is less often used because of the risk of damaging the thoracic duct.

The subclavian vein is the second most common site. The left subclavian vein is preferred because of the smooth anatomic curve from this vein into the right atrium. In the right subclavian vein the pulmonary artery catheter and introducer have to make a sharp angle to enter the superior vena cava. This can kink the catheter and compromise function of one of the ports or the thermistor.

Other choices for insertion are the femoral, antecubital, and external jugular veins. All of these choices are more difficult because of anatomic obstructions in the venous pathway to the heart. The femoral vein is the most frequently used of these alternative sites.

Sterile technique is particularly important during insertion of a pulmonary artery catheter because of the high nosocomial infection rate associated with hemodynamic monitoring. The clinician inserting the catheter should always wear gown, hat, mask, and gloves. The site should be cleansed with povidone-iodine or other bactericidal solution, and the work area should be widely draped. Generous amounts of local anesthetic (5 to 10 ml 1% lidocaine) should be injected into the right side of the neck at the juncture of the sternal and clavicular heads of the sternocleidomastoid muscle or into the midclavicular area of the left clavicle, including infiltration of the periosteum.

The Seldinger technique should be used to insert an 8½ French introducer sheath into the vein. The pulmonary artery catheter should be prepared for insertion by injection of 1.5 ml of air into the balloon to evaluate its inflation,

size, and shape. All ports should be flushed and checked for patency. The thermistor should be connected to the bedside thermodilution cardiac output monitor to check for function. Finally, a protective sleeve should be placed over the pulmonary artery catheter and moved past the 60 cm mark. The bedside transducers should be filled with saline solution, calibrated, and leveled. A bedside monitor and strip chart recorder should be prepared to provide a pressure trace during insertion.

The pulmonary artery catheter is threaded through the hemostasis valve on the end of the introducer sheath and advanced to the 20 cm mark. When insertion is by the right internal jugular or left subclavian route, this distance places the catheter tip in the superior vena cava. The clinician should check for a clear trace on the bedside monitor and look for air bubbles in the bedside transducer and tubing. Blood can be aspirated at this point to evaluate the free flow of fluid in the catheter and to remove any hidden bubbles that might dampen the tracing and make interpretation of the waveforms seen during insertion more difficult.

The clinician inflates the balloon on the catheter tip with 1.5 ml of air and locks the balloon port in the closed position. As the catheter is advanced, the bedside monitor is observed for typical right ventricular, pulmonary artery, and pulmonary capillary wedge traces. The catheter tip usually enters the right ventricle when 30 to 35 cm of catheter has been advanced through the introducer. The occurrence of premature ventricular contractions on the electrocardiogram heralds passage through the ventricle and across the pulmonary valve into the pulmonary artery. Usually 35 to 40 cm of catheter is required to enter the pulmonary artery. The wedge position is reached at 50 to 55 cm of catheter. The inflated balloon on the catheter tip pulls the catheter along with the flow of blood from right atrium to right ventricle to pulmonary artery. Once a wedge trace is obtained, the balloon should be deflated; a pulmonary artery trace then appears on the bedside monitor.

One reason for the popularity of the pulmonary artery catheter is the ability to insert the catheter by pressure waveform analysis instead of fluoroscopic guidance. Rarely the catheter coils in the right atrium or right ventricle in the presence of tricuspid valve disease or right ventricular enlargement from pulmonary valve disease or pulmonary artery hypertension. Then roentgenography is essential. Insertion of more than 40 cm of catheter without the advent of a right ventricular trace or more than 50 cm without the appearance of a pulmonary artery trace is evidence of catheter coiling. Knotting of the catheter is one complication of coiling.

Once the clinician has established a position for the pulmonary artery catheter that permits easy wedging with 1 to 1.5 ml of air, the catheter should be secured and the protective sterile sleeve pulled over the catheter and connected to the sidearm introducer. The distal end of the sleeve should be secured to the catheter to prevent slipping of the sleeve and contamination of the catheter. Often during catheter use the tip must be advanced or pulled back to maintain a proper wedge position, and this can be accomplished only with a sterile catheter.

A dry sterile dressing should be applied to the insertion site, and the catheter position evaluated with a portable chest roentgenogram. Normally the catheter passes into the right pulmonary artery and is 2 to 3 cm past the midline curling toward the right lower lobe. If this position provides a sharp and clear pulmonary artery trace on the bedside monitor and the catheter tip can be wedged by injection of 1.5 ml of air, the catheter is in good position. In a patient with pulmonary artery hypertension, significantly more catheter may be inserted to obtain a wedge trace and the risk of pulmonary artery perforation is higher. Regular monitoring of the bedside pulmonary artery trace by the nurse ensures proper position of the catheter and reduces the risk of occlusion of a branch of the pulmonary artery with subsequent pulmonary infarct.

Both the pulmonary artery port and the central venous port can be connected to bedside transducers to display pulmonary artery and central venous pressures. Instead of continuous display of central venous pressure, the clinician may want intermittent measurement for developing a hemodynamic profile or recording hourly vital signs. The pulmonary artery and central venous ports can be connected by a high-pressure tubing bridge that permits intermittent central venous measurement and saves the use of one transducer. Continuous infusion medications should not be administered through the central venous port, since the rapid injection of 10 ml of cardiac output fluid gives a bolus of drug that resides in the central venous port at the time of injection. In the case of nitroprusside, that volume of drug can lead to a clinically significant drop in blood pressure. Fluid and drugs can be infused through both the sidearm introducer port and the venous infusion port, leaving the central venous port free for measuring thermodilution cardiac output. If more fluid or drug infusion sites are needed, insertion of a triple-lumen central venous catheter should be considered.

Probably the most common complication of pulmonary artery catheters is the occurrence of ventricular dysrhythmias at the time of insertion (Table 4-3). This is normally brief and of no clinical significance, but occasionally ventricular tachycardia or fibrillation can occur in a patient with an irritable ventricle. Treating such a patient with lidocaine (1 to 1.5 mg/kg bolus) before catheter insertion can reduce the frequency of arrhythmias. When the catheter is in place in the pulmonary artery and the catheter tip is not touching the ventricle wall, the occurrence of arrhythmias is uncommon. Occasionally, supraventricular arrhythmias such as paroxysmal atrial tachycardia occur with insertion of a pulmonary artery catheter. This can usually be managed with verapamil 2.5 to 5 mg as an intravenous bolus.

Another complication is bleeding at the site of insertion of the introducer sheath, particularly if the carotid or subclavian artery is punctured. If patients have fewer than 50,000 platelets/cu mm or other coagulation disorders, correction of the coagulopathy should be considered before insertion of a pulmonary artery catheter. In an emergency situation when hemodynamic information is essential to the patient's survival, platelets and fresh-frozen plasma can be given just before catheter insertion.

A pulmonary infarct can occur when a catheter migrates from the pulmonary artery into a small vessel, leading to occlusion and cessation of blood flow. Vigilant observation of the pulmonary artery trace on the bedside monitor usually prevents this problem. If the pulmonary artery trace is lost and a wedge trace appears when the balloon is deflated, the catheter should be pulled back. When pulmonary artery catheters were first used, there was a problem with accumulation of clot on the catheter tip and pulmonary vessel occlusion when the clot embolized. The continuous infusion of the pulmonary artery catheter with 3 to 6 ml/h of heparinized saline (500 U heparin/250 ml normal saline) has essentially eliminated this complication.

Two significant complications of pulmonary artery catheters are (1) rupture of the pulmonary artery with hemorrhage into the lung and (2) infection. Rupture of the pulmonary artery usually occurs in patients with pulmonary artery hypertension, which causes difficult wedging of the catheter and necessitates frequent repositioning. Eventually the balloon ruptures a small vessel, leading to exsanguination into the lung and a quick death from hypoxia. This complication is rare. Infection is more common, especially after 5 days of pulmonary artery monitoring. This has led to the recommendation that the catheter be changed every 5 days and inserted via a fresh venipuncture if hemodynamic information is still needed. If the catheter cannot be replaced, it should be removed from the introducer. The introducer can be removed over a wire and the tips of both catheters cultured. A new introducer can be threaded over the wire. If the cultures of the old catheters are positive, the new catheters should be removed and another pulmonary artery catheter inserted from a fresh venipuncture. If the cultures are negative, the risk of infection can be considered minimal for the next 3 or 4 days.

Determination of an accurate PCWP requires considerable clinical experience. Negative airway pressures associated with spontaneous respiration and positive airway pressures associated with mechanical ventilation are transferred across the lung to the pulmonary vasculature. By convention PCWP is read at end exhalation to minimize the effect of changes in airway pressure. This requires a bedside strip chart recorder for accurate determination of PCWP. The usual clinical procedure is to start the recorder and obtain several respiratory cycles of the pulmonary artery trace. The balloon on the tip of the pulmonary artery catheter should then be inflated to obtain a PCWP. Several respiratory cycles of PCWP trace should be obtained, after which the balloon is deflated.

PCWP should never be obtained from the digital readout of the bedside monitor, which is designed to look for the lowest point on the pulmonary artery waveform as diastole and highest point on the waveform as systole. Both pulmonary artery pressure and PCWP determinations are inaccurate with this approach because of respiratory variations.

Some of the newer ICU equipment has a freeze frame on the bedside monitor and a movable cursor that allows the bedside clinician to make the same determination on the monitor as has been described for the strip chart recorder. Some pressure modules are programmed to read out respiratory variation, but this requires significant validation for clinical applicability. Clinicians often have difficulty determining end exhalation and accurate pulmonary artery pressures. Also, a bedside monitor cannot make independent interpretations, particularly in a patient with marked respiratory failure and tachypnea.

Cardiac output is measured with the pulmonary artery catheter by injection of 10 ml of thermal indicator through the central venous port and measuring the change in temperature over time as blood and indicator pass the thermistor on the catheter tip. A bedside cardiac output monitor determines the area under the temperature curve, and with body and injectate temperature and volume of indicator the monitor solves an equation for thermodilution cardiac output. Normally 10 ml of room temperature or iced 5% dextrose and water (D5W) injected in less than 4 seconds provides a good curve. To minimize technical errors, the clinician should measure injectate temperature at the entrance to the central venous port with a second thermistor probe. Injectate can be delivered from a bag of D5W passing through a coil in an ice bucket. Injection should be synchronized with the ventilator, and at least three injections should be performed to look for repeatability of the measurement. An average of three close values gives an accuracy of 10% of the indocyanine green or direct Fick technique.

Hemodynamic Profile

The original pulmonary artery catheter, introduced in 1970 by Swan and Ganz, was developed to measure PCWP with the belief that this measurement would more accurately reflect left ventricular end-diastolic volume (LVEDV) than had been accomplished with central venous or right atrial pressure. It was hoped that PCWP would be the same as left atrial pressure and as left ventricular end-diastolic pressure (LVEDP). For the most part this latter relationship has held, but the ability to use LVEDP or PCWP to predict LVEDV or preload or intravascular volume has not been possible in many patients. Clinicians are realizing that the pressure/volume relationship of the left ventricle varies with changes in compliance initiated by cardiac ischemia.

The pulmonary artery catheter in the critical care unit is a data collection system for constructing a hemodynamic profile of cardiac performance (Table 4-4). The hemodynamic analysis has four components: preload, output, afterload, and heart rate.

PRELOAD

Preload is the volume of blood in the ventricle at end diastole (LVEDV). Starling noted that with increased stretch on the cardiac muscle, tension increased when the muscle contracted.

TABLE 4–4. Hemodynamic Definitions and Formulas

Definitions

BSA = Body surface area
CI = Cardiac index
CO = Cardiac output
CVP = Central venous pressure
HR = Heart rate
LVSWI = Left ventricular stroke work index
MAP = Mean arterial pressure
MPAP = Mean pulmonary artery pressure
PCWP = Pulmonary capillary wedge pressure
PVRI = Pulmonary vascular resistance index
SI = Stroke index
SVRI = Systemic vascular resistance index

Hemodynamic Formulas

$$SI = \frac{CI}{HR}$$
$$SI = 40 \pm 10 \text{ ml/m}^2 \text{ BSA}$$

$$CI = \frac{CO}{BSA}$$
$$CI = 3.0 \pm 0.5 \text{ L/min/m}^2 \text{ BSA}$$

$$LVSWI = SI \times MAP \times 0.0136$$
$$LVSWI = 60 \pm 20 \text{ g m/m}^2 \text{ BSA/beat}$$

$$SVRI = \frac{MAP - CVP}{CI} \times 80$$
$$SVRI = 2000 \pm 500 \text{ dyne s cm}^{-5}/\text{m}^2 \text{ BSA}$$

$$PVRI = \frac{MPAP - PCWP}{CI} \times 80$$
$$PVRI = 400 \pm 100 \text{ dyne s cm}^{-5}/\text{m}^2 \text{ BSA}$$

In an intact heart, LVEDV creates stretch on the cardiac muscle. Increasing LVEDV increases stretch, resulting in improved stroke volume and cardiac output. At a cellular and subcellular level, diastolic volume stretches the sarcomere of the cardiac muscle myofibril, improving contractility. This relationship has a limit, after which excessive stretch on the sarcomere causes ventricular failure. The relationship between LVEDV and cardiac output or contractility is used in the ICU to augment cardiac output by fluid challenge.

Unfortunately, LVEDV is not easily monitored in the ICU, so clinicians rely on LVEDP, which can be determined more easily and accurately. Because LVEDP cannot be monitored directly in the ICU, the clinician bases the measurement on the relationship between LVEDP and left atrial pressure and PCWP. With some uncommon but clinically significant exceptions, PCWP monitoring accurately reflects LVEDP.

The problem of interpretation occurs when LVEDP turns out to be a poor monitor of LVEDV. In the healthy patient without myocardial disease, the relationship between LVEDP and LVEDV permits an accurate interpretation of preload and a helpful indication of intravascular volume. In the event of ventricular dysfunction, particularly caused by episodes of ischemia, the reliable relationship between LVEDP and LVEDV fails. With intermittent ischemic events, patients can move from one ventricular pressure/volume curve to another in a matter of minutes. For example, at one moment a LVEDV of 150 ml creates a PCWP of 8 mm Hg or an LVEDP of 8 mm Hg while the left ventricle is well perfused and contracting properly. With the onset of ischemia, LVEDV may stay at 150 ml but LVEDP increases to 30 mm Hg because of decreased ventricular compliance. This can cause functional mitral insufficiency with V waves on the PCWP tracing. Intervention with an agent such as nitroglycerin to improve compliance can reverse this process and return PCWP to 8 mm Hg. Such an ischemic episode with elevated PCWP, left untreated, would result in congestive heart failure and pulmonary edema despite a normal vascular volume.

Clearly, PCWP in a critically ill patient is a helpful but potentially misleading measurement of preload and intravascular volume. Several things can be said about the previous clinical example. PCWP accurately reflected the impending congestive heart failure and pulmonary edema, since it is hydrostatic pressure that leads to pulmonary edema. PCWP did not reflect vascular volume, since the patient in a nonischemic state had a normal PCWP and was normovolemic. PCWP did not indicate preload because LVEDV never changed in this example and was always the best indicator of preload despite an elevated PCWP and pulmonary edema.

These criticisms of PCWP should not decrease the clinical value of a pulmonary artery catheter as a monitor in the ICU, but data concerning vascular volume, preload, and hydrostatic pressure should be interpreted with caution.

CARDIAC OUTPUT

The second important determinant of cardiac function is contractility or inotropic state, which in the ICU is monitored as cardiac output determined by a thermodilution technique. Like PCWP and preload, thermodilution cardiac output is a distant variable of inotropy when compared with the more sophisticated measurements that can be made in the cardiology laboratory. Routine and repeatable measurements of ejection fraction, pressure change/time change (dP/dT), and fiber length shortening would be helpful in assessing cardiac function in the ICU but are not routinely available. Therefore thermodilution cardiac output is measured and compared with a standard of normal. The effectiveness of a patient's cardiac output can be interpreted by looking at oxygen transport as a marker of peripheral perfusion. Monitoring mixed venous oxygen partial pressure ($P\bar{v}O_2$) and $S\bar{v}O_2$, arterial/venous oxygen content differences, and oxygen extraction ratio can help in interpreting the normality of a particular thermodilution cardiac output measurement.

One helpful way of interpreting the inotropic state is to examine the relationship between cardiac output and PCWP. If a patient continuously requires an elevated PCWP to have a borderline cardiac output, this is an indicator of a depressed ventricle that may benefit from inotropic therapy. Inotropic state can also be examined by plotting the left ventricular stroke work index (LVSWI) against cardiac output to create a Sarnoff ventricular function curve. Just as ICU physicians interpret a PaO_2 obtained in arterial blood gas analysis by looking at fraction of inspired oxygen (FIO_2) and positive end-expiratory pressure (PEEP), they interpret the significance of any particular cardiac output in the light of preload and inotropic support.

Contractility is manipulated in the ICU by use of a beta$_1$ agonist drug to activate the beta receptor on the surface of the myocardial cell. Activation of the beta receptor increases intracellular cyclic adenosine monophosphate (AMP), which participates in a chain reaction with calcium to increase the strength of contraction of the actin and myosin fibers in the sarcomere. The result of this stimulation is monitored as changes in thermal dilution cardiac output, not as changes in blood pressure. Blood pressure is a complex result of cardiac output and systemic vascular resistance and in a critically ill patient is a poor indicator of peripheral perfusion.

In addition to the use of beta-agonist drugs to improve cardiac output, the clinician can use a phosphodiesterase inhibitor agent such as amrinone, which prevents the breakdown of cyclic AMP and increases contractility. There is some evidence of synergism between beta-agonist drugs and phosphodiesterase inhibitors when used in combination to augment inotropic state. Traditionally critical care physicians have used both a beta agonist and a phosphodiesterase inhibitor (albuterol and aminophylline) to manage severe bronchospasm in the ICU. Now the same is possible for inotropic support.

Cardiac glycosides seem to have a minimal role in managing inotropic failure in the ICU. Digoxin is used regularly for rate and rhythm control but has a minimal effect on improving contractility. Long-term management of cardiac compromise in an outpatient, who cannot be given traditional intravenous inotropic agents, should be done with unloading agents such as hydralazine or captopril, which reduce afterload and ease ventricular emptying.

SYSTEMIC VASCULAR RESISTANCE

A third important determinant of cardiac function and peripheral perfusion is afterload, or the resistance to ejection. This is calculated from mean arterial pressure, central venous pressure, and cardiac output and is expressed as systemic vascular resistance (SVR). SVR is interpreted as the degree of vascular tone created by arteriolar smooth muscle vasoconstriction. Afterload has other causes, such as valvular resistance to ejection created by aortic stenosis, but using afterload and SVR as a measure of vasoconstriction and acting on that determination to improve cardiac output or blood pressure has proved clinically useful.

Monitoring patients in shock in the ICU over the past 10 to 15 years has demonstrated a single reaction to loss of peripheral perfusion for both hypovolemic and cardiogenic shock. In hypovolemia the release of catecholamines leads to marked vasoconstriction, reducing vascular volume and maintaining blood pressure to perfuse the vital tissue beds of the brain and heart. This reaction works well and is easily reversed when vascular volume is restored. With a loss of contractility and cardiac output as occurs in cardiogenic shock, an identical reaction occurs in response to loss of peripheral perfusion. Once again the release of catecholamines leads to vasoconstriction and elevated SVR. The dysfunctional myocardium of cardiogenic shock tolerates this increased afterload poorly, and ejection fraction and cardiac output are further reduced with the onset of left ventricular failure and pulmonary edema. The reduction in afterload by vasodilators increases cardiac output. Likewise, patients with chronic congestive heart failure do well with long-term afterload reduction as a primary approach to the management of their ventricular failure.

Afterload is a beneficial component of the cardiovascular system because it creates pressure within the vascular space to move oxygenated blood to all organs against the effects of gravity. In hypovolemia, afterload is an important part of cardiovascular physiology to distribute flow to various organs despite the loss of intravascular volume. However, afterload is a disadvantage to the failing myocardium because it further reduces ejection fraction, stroke volume, and cardiac output.

HEART RATE

Heart rate is the final determinant of cardiac output. Acceptable heart rates in adults in an ICU are usually between 50 and 100 beats/min as long as stroke volume is reasonably well preserved. Sustained heart rates much below 50 beats/min may lead to hypoperfusion. Common causes of bradycardia include various types of heart block, which responds to atropine, isoproterenol, or a transvenous pacemaker depending on the cause of the problem.

In the shock state oxygen delivery is significantly reduced. If left unreversed, this problem leads to severe cellular dysfunction and ultimately cellular death. In the same manner that cardiovascular system function can be analyzed by looking at the components of preload, output, afterload, and heart rate, shock can be roughly categorized as preload failure, output failure, afterload failure, and heart rate failure.

PRELOAD FAILURE

Preload failure is a clinically significant decrease in intravascular volume either by external losses as in hemorrhage from trauma or by internal losses as in third space fluid movement during extensive intraabdominal surgery. Loss of intravascular volume leads to a decrease in LVEDV, which reduces the stretch on the sarcomere of cardiac muscle and therefore reduces contractility and cardiac output. At fluid losses of 20% to 30% of intravascular volume, vasoconstriction and increased afterload compensate for the LVEDV decrease by reduced flow to specific organ beds such as muscle, skin, and bowel. Flow to the heart and brain is preserved with much less compensatory vasoconstriction. These changes are caused by the release of catecholamines as the body perceives a decrease in peripheral perfusion. Monitoring of PCWP and cardiac output during such a bleeding process reveals a less than expected drop in preload and output because of these compensatory mechanisms. At losses greater than 30% of intravascular volume, compensatory mechanisms progressively fail and hypotension begins with poor organ perfusion and the onset of metabolic acidosis.

This scenario of shock occurs every day in ICUs across the United States. Trauma, with its significant blood loss and hypovolemic shock, has led to the development of a national network of emergency medical services (EMS) and trauma centers to transport injured patients rapidly so the preload failure process can be quickly reversed. These trauma centers have demonstrated that hemorrhagic shock, if corrected early, is treatable and has minimal long-term sequelae. Transport time is important because vasoconstriction causes many organs to be dangerously hypoperfused in hypovolemic patients: thus the term "golden hour" for time of transport and resuscitation after trauma.

Initial resuscitation of these patients should be with crystalloid (normal saline or lactated Ringer's solution) to restore vascular volume. Blood should follow as quickly as possible to restore oxygen transport. Colloid solutions such as 6% hydroxyethyl starch and 5% albumin, which remain in the circulation longer, are also appropriate for replenishing vascular volume. Once LVEDV has been restored, cardiac output and organ perfusion return to normal with minimal long term-problems if vascular volume is restored before the onset of organ damage from poor perfusion (Table 4-5).

Preload failure is not restricted to hypovolemia; excessive amounts of preload like wise have a negative impact on the cardiovascular system. There are two categories of increased preload. First is fluid overload with a markedly increased intravascular volume and LVEDV. Second is the appearance of fluid overload with high PCWP but a normal or reduced LVEDV. Both entities lead to congestive heart failure and pulmonary edema, but their acute management is quite different.

TABLE 4–5. Preload Failure

Preload			
CVP	2.0	4.0	6.0
PCWP	2.0	4.0	6.0
Output			
BSA	1.7	1.7	1.7
HR	110.0	100.0	95.0
CO	3.0	4.0	4.6
CI	1.8	2.3	2.7
SI	16.0	23.0	28.0
LVSWI	16.0	22.0	30.0
Afterload			
MAP	70.0	72.0	75.0
SVRI	3022.0	2365.0	2044.0
MPAP	12.0	16.0	18.0
PVRI	444.0	417.0	355.0
Therapy			
		1000 ml colloid	1000 ml colloid

Differentiating these two types of preload failure is difficult.

True preload failure with elevated LVEDV caused by fluid overload is much less common in the ICU because the kidney compensates for errors in intravenous fluid administration. With renal failure, nonoliguric or oliguric, the kidney is no longer able to manage wide swings in intravascular volume. Therefore a patient with renal failure is the most likely candidate for true preload failure with pulmonary edema. Administration of large volumes of blood, colloid, or hypertonic saline can precipitate preload failure in patients with normal renal function. Appropriate clinical responses to excessive preload include administration of intravenous diuretics, such as furosemide, and emergency dialysis or ultrafiltration for patients with renal insufficiency.

Two important problems occur with high LVEDV preload failure. The first is congestive heart failure and pulmonary edema, which lead to hypoxia and respiratory failure. Hypoxia can be managed by endotracheal intubation, increased FIO_2, and PEEP. The second problem is myocardial ischemia caused by a large, dilated, tense ventricle, which increases myocardial oxygen consumption. The three chief determinants of myocardial oxygen consumption are heart rate, systolic blood pressure, and tension of the left ventricle. Excessive levels of LVEDV in preload failure can lead to functional mitral insufficiency with V waves on the PCWP trace and the risk of ischemia or infarction when myocardial oxygen demand exceeds myocardial oxygen supply.

The second and more common type of preload failure occurs with an elevated PCWP but normal to decreased intravascular volume and LVEDV. This type of preload failure is caused by changes in left ventricular compliance, usually initiated by ischemia. When the ventricle becomes ischemic, compliance changes and PCWP rises without a change in LVEDV. Intravascular volume remains normal. The elevated PCWP creates adequate hydrostatic pressure in the pulmonary capillaries to increase the flow of fluid into the interstitial space of the lung. Eventually the lymphatics can no longer clear fluid from the lung and the alveoli fill with fluid, leading to congestive heart failure and pulmonary edema. Appropriate treatment in this situation is not the reduction of LVEDV and intravascular volume with diuretics but rather the adjustment of left ventricular compliance with preload-reducing agents such as nitroglycerin and nifedipine. Both agents directly reduce tenseness in myocardial muscle and lower PCWP.

The use of diuretics in this second type of preload failure is controversial. Furosemide is helpful because it reduces PCWP by being a pulmonary capillary vasodilator. However, furosemide is harmful because it leads to active diuresis and lowers an already normal LVEDV. An appropriate compromise might be one low dose of diuretic for the pulmonary capillary vasodilating effect with more appropriate agents such as nitrates.

Differentiating between normal LVEDV preload failure and elevated LVEDV preload failure is difficult as noted previously. In both situations PCWP is elevated and the patient shows signs of congestive heart failure and pulmonary edema. In the first situation there is no evidence of excessive intravenous fluid administration to justify a high intravascular volume and no evidence of renal insufficiency to explain an inability to handle fluids. Since physiologic parameters such as LVEDV and ejection fraction cannot be routinely measured in the ICU, data must be gathered indirectly from many areas to build a case for normal LVEDV preload failure. If all information, such as fluid balance, daily weight, and clinical chemistry determinations, points to a normal intravascular volume, preload reduction by manipulation of ventricular compliance should be attempted first. In the situation of high LVEDV preload failure, when direct and indirect data point to excessive fluid administration and retention, diuresis should be started.

OUTPUT FAILURE

The second type of shock is output failure caused by a decrease in organ perfusion from primary pump failure. Failure can occur in the rate at which the pump delivers a stroke volume (heart rate) or in the amount of stroke volume. Rate failure bradycardia is caused by an abnormality of the heart pacemaker or a failure to conduct the pacing signal as in heart block. In both situations the clinical correction includes atropine, isoproterenol, and pacing. In an adult patient 0.6 to 1 mg of atropine given intravenously usually corrects, although temporarily, a supraventricular bradycardia. If there is heart block with a slow ventricular rate, the ventricle responds to isoproterenol to improve heart rate temporarily until more definitive diagnostic and therapeutic measures can be taken. If both pharmacologic measures fail, a demand transthoracic pacemaker should be used until a transvenous pacemaker can be floated into the ventricle or a permanent pacemaker can be surgically implanted. The new transthoracic demand pacemaker has been helpful in managing the patient with intermittent bradycardia episodes as seen in sick sinus syndrome. Large pads are placed on the anterior and posterior chest. The pacer senses heart rate and is programmed to deliver a variable-milliampere discharge if a long sinus arrest or low heart rate is detected.

A number of different pacemaker wires exist for use in the ICU. One of the easiest ways to place the wire is the pulmonary artery catheter with a pacing port 20 cm from the catheter tip. This port lies in the right ventricle and can be used as a channel for the insertion of a pacer wire. About 3 to 6 cm of wire is required in the right ventricle to achieve capture of heart rate. This pacer wire can be used in the control or demand mode. Many ICUs routinely use pacing pulmonary artery catheters so that a pacing wire can be inserted quickly whenever bradycardia develops.

A second type of pacing wire is balloon tipped so that, like the pulmonary artery catheter, it will pass into the right ventricle by following the natural flow of blood through the chambers of the heart. Insertion of this catheter requires some cardiac function to advance the balloon on the tip of the pacer wire through the circulation.

Finally, standard pacing catheters are available and in the elective situation should be inserted with fluoroscopic guidance to achieve the appropriate position in the right ventricle. This type of pacing catheter can be inserted from a right internal jugular or left subclavian vein puncture during a cardiac arrest or emergency bradycardia if the clinician advances the catheter with the pacer activated and looks for capture on the electrocardiogram.

The second type of output failure is a primary cardiac muscle problem as occurs in myocardial infarction, cardiac contusion, myocarditis, or myocardiopathy. Inotropic status is reduced with poor muscle contraction. Ejection fraction, cardiac output, and peripheral perfusion are also reduced (Table 4-6).

The physiologic reaction to primary pump failure is almost identical to that of preload failure with hypovolemia. The body perceives the drop in cardiac output and peripheral perfusion as hypovolemia and elaborates catecholamines, leading to vasoconstriction and an afterload elevation to maintain blood pressure. Nonessential organs, such as skin, kidney, and viscera, lose flow and are at risk of cellular hypoxia as

TABLE 4-6. Output Failure

Preload			
CVP	14.0	12.0	12.0
PCWP	19.0	16.0	14.0
Output			
BSA	1.7	1.7	1.7
HR	120.0	115.0	110.0
CO	3.2	4.5	5.2
CI	1.9	2.6	3.1
SI	16.0	23.0	28.0
LVSWI	17.0	22.0	25.0
Afterload			
MAP	78.0	70.0	65.0
SVRI	2694.0	1784.0	1367.0
MPAP	26.0	24.0	23.0
PVRI	294.0	246.0	232.0
Therapy			
		Dobutamine 5 μg/kg/min	Dobutamine 10 μg/kg/min

the heart and brain receive the majority of flow. This sharp increase in afterload causes further cardiac failure, since the weakened myocardium cannot eject against a high afterload. Peripheral perfusion declines more and venous return backs up to the left side of the heart, giving the perception of preload failure with high PCWP, congestive heart failure, and pulmonary edema. Depending on the degree of cardiac function, this downward slide of cardiac function may stop and plateau, creating various clinical pictures of failure.

In acute myocardial infarction, categories of cardiac failure are predictive of the chances of death. Normal PCWP and cardiac output are associated with the best survival. A decreased cardiac output or increased PCWP worsens the prognosis. When both reduced cardiac output and increased PCWP are present, the worst prognosis exists. Early intervention in the last three classes of myocardial infarction patients permits the salvage of myocardial muscle and reduces the risk of death.

Correction of output failure is directed at improving inotropic state and reducing afterload to ease ejection of stroke volume. Either of these techniques can be employed as a first-line approach with good results. Dobutamine and amrinone are excellent inotropic agents for the failing myocardium. Beginning with a peripheral vasodilator, such as nifedipine or nitroprusside, significantly improves cardiac output and peripheral perfusion. The choice of inotropic agent or vasodilator is based on analysis of the hemodynamic profile derived from the thermodilution pulmonary artery catheter. If the greatest decrease in function is in cardiac output and vasoconstriction is only mild, beginning with an inotropic agent may be better. If increased afterload with a high SVR is the predominant cardiovascular abnormality, starting with a vasodilator may be preferable.

Before pharmacologic manipulation of the cardiovascular system is used to treat any form of output failure, adequate LVEDV must be guaranteed. If PCWP is less than 18 mm Hg, fluid challenge should be attempted first. Boluses of crystalloid, 500 to 1000 ml given over 30 to 60 minutes, or colloid, 250 to 500 ml given over 30 to 60 minutes, challenge the ventricle to improve contractility and cardiac output. As LVEDV increases, the force of contraction increases, which improves cardiac output and peripheral perfusion (Fig. 4-4).

During a fluid challenge protocol, frequent monitoring of PCWP is essential. A compliant ventricle absorbs significant increases in LVEDV without changes in LVEDP or PCWP. When maximum stretch on the ventricle in diastole has been achieved, the PCWP increases rapidly, signalling the knee of the pressure volume curve (Fig. 4-5). Fluid administration should be stopped at this point, and a full hemodynamic evaluation of the cardiovascular system should be performed, including cardiac output, LVSWI, and SVRI.

If fluid therapy fails to achieve adequate inotropic results with improved cardiac output and peripheral perfusion, pharmacologic manipulation of the cardiovascular system should be added to the cardiac support. The use of inotropic agents may further decrease preload in output failure, creating opportunities for further fluid resuscitation.

Dopamine was the most popular inotrope in the ICU during the late 1970s and early 1980s. It replaced norepinephrine and epinephrine, which were difficult to use beneficially in the management of cardiogenic shock. Dopamine has a dose-dependent response with significant alpha-agonist properties at high doses. Therefore, like epinephrine, it is difficult to use for the correction of pump failure. At low doses of up to 3 μg/kg/min, dopamine activates the dopaminergic receptor in the renal vasculature to increase renal blood flow and improve urine output. At higher doses of 3 to 10 μg/kg/min, dopamine has strong beta-agonist properties to improve contractility. At doses greater than 10 μg/kg/min, dopamine becomes an alpha-agonist drug with a major vasoconstrictive response.

Two pharmacologic responses to dopamine make it unsatisfactory for use in cardiogenic shock. First is the alpha-agonist property, which begins in the middle dose ranges and increases vasoconstriction and afterload in patients who already have problems with elevated afterload. Second, dopamine's chronotropic effect increases heart rate and myocardial oxygen consumption. The vasoconstriction property worsens ejection fraction and lowers stroke volume, although cardiac output will initially increase because of the beta-agonist properties. The chronotropic property decreases diastolic time by increasing heart rate and can reduce myocardial oxygen supply and blood flow to the coronary arteries. Overall, in cardiogenic shock, dopamine is expected to increase blood pressure, systemic vascular resistance, cardiac output, heart rate, and myocardial oxygen consumption and to increase or maintain PCWP at the same level. The only valuable aspect of this

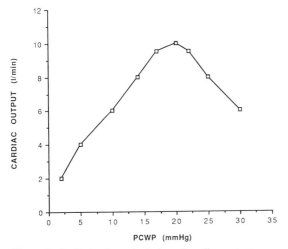

Figure 4–4 Preload manipulation of cardiac output.

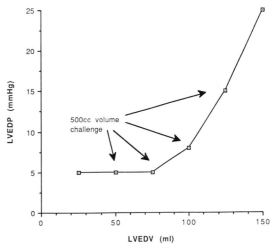

Figure 4–5 Left ventricular pressure/volume relationship.

pharmacologic profile in cardiogenic shock is the increase in cardiac output. The concomitant use of nitroprusside with dopamine in cardiogenic shock can counteract many of the negative effects by reducing afterload.

Dobutamine is clearly superior to dopamine in the management of cardiogenic shock. As a beta$_1$- and beta$_2$-agonist drug, dobutamine increases cardiac output, minimally changes blood pressure and heart rate, and reduces SVR and PCWP. The results are improved peripheral perfusion, without an increase in myocardial oxygen consumption, and decreased preload to lessen the risk of congestive heart failure and pulmonary edema (Table 4-6). At higher doses dobutamine has some alpha-agonist properties, which are largely counteracted by the beta$_2$-agonist vasodilating properties. Usual doses of dobutamine vary from 0 to 20 μg/kg/min with a rather flat dose-response curve above 15 μg/kg/min.

Dobutamine is a synthetic catecholamine that is metabolized much like natural catecholamines. This means that the onset of action is rapid when the drug is started and a loading dose is not needed. Dobutamine has a short half-life and is gone from the circulation in minutes after the infusion is discontinued. One problem with the long-term use of dobutamine for the support of cardiogenic shock is tachyphylaxis. This necessitates progressively larger doses to achieve the same clinical improvement.

In cardiogenic shock dobutamine is often an effective single agent because it increases contractility and cardiac output, reduces preload, and reduces afterload. Unlike dopamine, nitroprusside is not usually required for further afterload reduction. The addition of a continuous intravenous infusion of nitroglycerin can often be helpful for further preload reduction, improvement in ventricular compliance, and reduction in coronary vascular resistance.

If adequate correction of cardiac output and peripheral perfusion is not achieved with dobutamine alone, amrinone, a phosphodiesterase inhibitor with inotropic and vasodilating properties, should be added to the dobutamine. Amrinone increases cardiac output; reduces PCWP, SVR, and blood pressure; and maintains heart rate and myocardial oxygen consumption at approximately the same level. The vasodilating properties of amrinone are significantly greater than those of dobutamine, and often the concomitant rise in cardiac output is not enough to maintain blood pressure at a pre-infusion level, particularly in the hypovolemic

patient. Amrinone has been shown to be synergistic with dobutamine and is a natural agent to be used with a beta$_1$-agonist drug.

Since amrinone is not a catecholamine, it is not metabolized in the same manner as dobutamine. Amrinone is degraded largely in the liver. It has a 4- to 5-hour half-life and a long onset of action if a loading dose is not used. With a loading dose of 0.75 mg/kg the onset of action and peak effect occur minutes after the drug is administered. The clinically effective dose ranges up to 20 μg/kg/min. Increases in infusion rate of 5 μg/kg/min or greater should be preceded with another loading dose of 0.75 mg/kg to ensure the rapid onset of action of the new dose. The only significant complication or side effect of the drug is thrombocytopenia. This generally occurs slowly over days and is reversible when the infusion is stopped. Tachyphylaxis, as occurs with dobutamine, has not been reported with amrinone, making it a better long-term drug for the management of poor cardiac function.

Amrinone can replace dobutamine as a first-line drug in correcting poor cardiac function when vasoconstriction is the predominant dysfunction. Amrinone is approximately twice as effective as a vasodilator and is appropriate as a first-line agent to reduce SVR. Hypovolemia and vasoconstriction are difficult to manage with amrinone as a first-line agent, since hypotension occurs quickly after administration of the loading dose. Hypotension should be managed by volume loading and not by the use of vasoconstrictive agents, which are counterproductive to forward blood flow in cardiogenic shock.

In some ICU patients with reduced peripheral perfusion and predominant vasoconstriction, afterload reduction instead of inotropic therapy can be considered as the initial approach. These patients generally have acceptable left ventricular function, but excessive peripheral vasoconstriction sharply reduces cardiac output and ejection fraction. An example is a patient after coronary artery bypass (CABG). The post-CABG patient usually has acceptable ventricular function if this is a first bypass procedure, but because of hypothermia in the operating room the patient is vasoconstricted in the ICU. Nitroprusside has been used effectively in this situation. Sublingual nifedipine or intravenous hydralazine or enalaprilat might be considered appropriate agents to reduce afterload. Nitroglycerin has some afterload-reducing properties, but only in large doses. One problem with using any of the pure afterload reducers in this situation is a reflex tachycardia and potential for compromising diastolic filling of the coronary arteries if heart rate is much greater than 110 beats/min. The effective vasodilating properties of the inotropic agents dobutamine and amrinone make them more reasonable agents for restoring cardiac function, since they cause little increase in heart rate.

In both approaches to restoring left ventricular function, increasing inotropy and decreasing afterload, the first-line ICU monitors of arterial and central venous catheters are inadequate. It is possible to monitor the effects of dopamine by observing the trend of blood pressure with an arterial catheter and assessing other aspects of peripheral perfusion indirectly by looking at urine output and skin color and warmth. Doing the same with dobutamine and amrinone is difficult, if not impossible. Since both of these agents usually maintain heart rate and blood pressure at approximately preinfusion levels, the only direct quantifiable monitor of patient response to the drugs is the measurement of thermal dilution cardiac output from a pulmonary artery catheter and the calculation of SVR. Hemodynamic monitoring with a pulmonary artery catheter seems essential when the inotropic agents dobutamine and amrinone are used.

If hemodynamic monitoring and inotropic/afterload therapy have not adequately corrected peripheral perfusion, the patient should be considered for mechanical afterload reduction. The use of the intraaortic counterpulsation balloon (IACB) in the past was limited to desperate situations such as inability to separate from cardiopulmonary bypass and terminal cardiogenic shock. The indications have expanded to refractory angina before cardiac catheterization and severe left main artery disease before surgery. Now IACB is being used more frequently as an important part of the inotropic/afterload armamentarium for correction of left ventricular dysfunction.

There are probably at least two reasons for increased use of the IACB. First is improved technology with better bedside equipment and better balloons. The Seldinger technique has made it possible to insert a 30 ml balloon percutaneously and avoid any use of a cutdown. Therefore both cardiologists and critical care physicians can use IACB as an emergency technique in the management of cardiac dysfunction. Second is Braunwald's evolving concept of the stunned but reversibly injured myocardium. Various cardiac muscle insults

that lead to ischemia can cause 7 to 14 days of inadequate left ventricular function. The damaged heart remains responsive to inotropic agents and afterload reduction, which limit the ischemia and buy time for recovery. In the situation of the stunned myocardium, agents that do not increase heart rate or myocardial oxygen consumption must be used so the heart can recover from the ischemic insult. Inotropic-afterload agents such as dobutamine and amrinone, preload reducers such as nitroglycerin, and mechanical afterload reducers such as IACB all fall into that category. Just as there are deficiencies and excesses of preload that lead to cardiac compromise, there are also deficiencies (cardiogenic shock) and excesses of cardiac muscle performance. The deficient myocardium is discussed in the preceding paragraphs. The review of inotropic problems is completed by an examination of increased contractility. Clinical examples include hyperthyroidism, delirium tremens, and pheochromocytoma, all of which are associated with high cardiac output, tachycardia, and hypertension. The hypercontractile state alone should not lead to shock unless myocardial oxygen demands exceed myocardial oxygen supply and ischemia ensues. Beta blockers are useful in controlling excessive cardiac performance and preventing ischemic episodes. Long-acting cardioselective blockers such as metoprolol or atenolol may be used and are probably preferable to the older nonselective propranolol. The ideal emergency beta blocker in the ICU may be esmolol, which has a 9-minute half-life and must be given as a continuous intravenous infusion. This agent allows the critical care physician to test patient response to beta blockers without any long-term effects if the drug is poorly tolerated. After an initial loading dose, esmolol is usually effective at doses of 100 to 200 μg/kg/min.

AFTERLOAD FAILURE

The third and final essential determinant of cardiac function and peripheral perfusion is afterload. Both excessive and inadequate afterload can lead to inadequacies of peripheral perfusion.

Excessive afterload occurs in a number of clinical situations, some of which are discussed previously in the chapter. As noted in the preceding discussion of preload and contractility, sudden decreases in preload (hypovolemic shock) and sudden decreases in cardiac output (cardiogenic shock) are associated with the release of catecholamines and increased afterload in an attempt to maintain blood pressure to perfuse vital organs such as the brain and heart. The management of this entity has been well reviewed and is not covered here in more detail. Instead this discussion concerns excesses of afterload or vasoconstriction with normal intravascular volume and normal cardiac function. This is known in the ICU as hypertensive crisis and may lead to a shock state if myocardial ischemia compromises cardiac function. The routine management of a hypertensive crisis in the ICU does not normally require a pulmonary artery catheter but should include an arterial catheter for accurate beat-to-beat pressure measurements. Selection of therapy depends on the assessment of heart rate. If hypertension alone is present and heart rate is 70 beats/min or less, an agent with vasodilating properties alone is appropriate. If hypertension is accompanied by tachycardia, both vasodilating and beta-blocking properties may be necessary.

The antihypertensive agents for emergency intravenous therapy in the ICU include nitroprusside, hydralazine, and diazoxide. Nitroprusside is a potent vasodilator with a rapid onset of action and short half-life. It must be given as a continuous infusion starting at 0.1 µg/kg/min and increasing doses to 6 to 7 µg/kg/min to achieve control of blood pressure. Nitroprusside has an excellent track record for treating hypertension in the ICU and should be the first-line agent for dangerously high blood pressure when heart rate is near normal. The major side effect of the drug is the accumulation of cyanide as a result of the nitroprusside metabolism. This can be monitored by looking for metabolic acidosis, since cyanide poisons the electron transport systems and leads to anerobic metabolism with the accumulation of lactate. If metabolic acidosis is detected, nitroprusside should be stopped and the acidosis will normally correct. The cyanide toxic effect can be treated with hydroxycobalamin, which forms cyanocobalamin to remove the cyanide from the circulation.

In less serious situations intermittent bolus injections of hydralazine, 5 to 10 mg, can be given to treat hypertension. Hydralazine is a direct smooth muscle vasodilator with rapid onset and a 4-hour half-life. Unlike nitroprusside, it has no serious side effects in the acute situation. Both agents are well known for causing reflex tachycardia.

Diazoxide, a drug related to chlorothiazide, is another emergency antihypertensive agent that can be used in the ICU. This agent must be given rapidly to cause an antihypertensive effect, since it is heavily protein bound and is quickly inactivated if given slowly. Given as a 300 mg bolus in less than 10 seconds, diazoxide rapidly lowers blood pressure. Overdosage can be a problem because the drug has a long half-life. At present diazoxide is not a popular antihypertensive in the ICU.

Two other agents are useful in the ICU for the management of excessive afterload leading to severe hypertension. First is oral nifedipine, which has become popular in emergency rooms and ICUs. Nifedipine is a liquid in a capsule. The tip of the capsule can be perforated with a needle and the contents poured into the mouth of the hypertensive patient. An initial dose of 10 mg significantly lowers blood pressure in 10 to 15 minutes. The drug's half-life is about 4 hours. Since nifedipine is a direct vasodilator, reflex tachycardia is associated with the decrease in blood pressure.

The second drug is trimethaphan camsylate, a ganglionic blocker and potent antihypertensive agent. Trimethaphan must be given by continuous intravenous infusion. It has a rapid onset and short half-life, disappearing from the circulation quickly when the infusion is stopped. No reflex tachycardia occurs. The major difficulty with this agent for extended use in the ICU is tachyphylaxis. Trimethaphan is not a first-line agent at present but has been used in the past to cause hypotension in the operating room and to manage the hypertension associated with dissection of the thoracic aorta when increases in heart rate and contractility, as occur with hydralazine, were contraindicated.

Nifedipine, intermittent boluses of intravenous hydralazine, and a continuous intravenous infusion of nitroprusside seem to be the mainstay of acute antihypertensive therapy when the heart rate is normal (70 beats/min) or below. A new agent for use in the ICU is the converting enzyme inhibitor enalaprilat, which is available for intravenous administration. Recommended starting dose is 1.25 mg every 6 hours. This agent's effectiveness in hypertensive crises remains to be evaluated.

Hypertension is often associated with some elevation in heart rate or frank tachycardia (more than 100 beats/min). In that situation, when the use of a vasodilator would lead to reflex tachycardia, using both a beta blocker and a vasodilator would more effectively control afterload and reduce the ischemic effect of tachycardia on the myocardium.

In the past, a combination of hydralazine or nitroprusside and intermittent intravenous boluses of propranolol was used. In the last several years a new drug, labetalol, has been successful in the management of hypertensive crises.

Labetalol is both an alpha and a beta blocker with a rapid onset of action when given in bolus intravenous doses of 5 to 10 mg. It has a 4-hour half-life. Blood pressure and heart rate can be slowly reduced to a desired level with increasing bolus doses up to 20 mg at a time. A continuous infusion of 2 mg/min also lowers blood pressure gradually over 60 to 90 minutes. When blood pressure has reached a desirable level, the continuous infusion can be decreased to 0.5 to 1 mg/min to maintain the pressure until afterload is controlled or an oral antihypertensive agent can be started.

Given intravenously, labetalol is said to have one part alpha and seven parts beta effects. Nevertheless, an equal, proportional lowering of heart rate and blood pressure occurs when labetalol is given intravenously. If labetalol is administered to a patient with a normal or low heart rate, an unfavorable bradycardia often results. This can be managed with combined doses of hydralazine and labetalol to lower blood pressure more than heart rate. The beta-blocking properties of labetalol prevent the reflex tachycardia that often occurs with hydralazine alone. Labetalol maintains good ventricular function even when given to patients with reduced ventricular function.

In addition to excesses of afterload, inadequacies of afterload can be caused by several clinical entities and can lead to hypotension because of the loss of SVR. Sepsis, anaphylactic shock, and neurogenic shock associated with spinal cord trauma produce peripheral vascular collapse and hypotension (Table 4-7). In response to the drop in afterload, heart rate and cardiac output increase in an attempt to maintain blood pressure. Afterload failure in the ICU is most commonly associated with septic shock. Down-regulation of the alpha receptor produces wide-open vasodilation. A cardiac index greater than 4 L/min/m^2 and a systemic vascular resistance index less than 1000 dyne s cm^{-5} meets the hemodynamic definition for septic shock. The reversal of this process calls for fluid resuscitation to fill up the dilated intravascular space and the restoration of vasoconstriction by the use of alpha-agonist drugs. In anaphylaxis natural body products cause the vasodilatation. In neurogenic shock a

TABLE 4–7. Afterload Failure

		Preload	
CVP	2.0	6.0	8.0
PCWP	2.0	6.0	10.0
		Output	
BSA	1.7	1.7	1.7
HR	110.0	105.0	115.0
CO	9.0	9.5	8.5
CI	5.3	5.6	5.0
SI	48.0	53.0	43.0
LVSWI	36.0	47.0	
		Afterload	
MAP	55.0	65.0	75.0
SVRI	800.0	842.0	1072.0
MPAP	12.0	15.0	20.0
PVRI	151.0	128.0	160.0
		Therapy	
		1000 ml colloid	norepinephrine 0.1 μg/kg/min

loss of sympathetic tone occurs similar to that occurring with high spinal anesthesia. In all three entities the problem is loss of afterload and not cardiac function.

The critical care physician must restore enough vascular tone to preserve blood pressure for the purpose of perfusing organs. As in hypovolemic and cardiogenic shock, renal perfusion is often compromised, leading to a drop in urine output and possible kidney damage. Restoration of blood pressure by the use of alpha-agonist drugs such as high-dose dopamine (greater than 10 μg/kg/min), phenylephrine, and norepinephrine often restores organ perfusion and urine output. The first-line therapy in afterload failure is fluid administration to increase vascular volume in the vasodilated patient. If that fails to restore blood pressure, alpha-agonist agents should be used to restore mean blood pressure to 60 to 70 mm Hg and SVRI to 1500 dyne s cm^{-5}.

The management of afterload failure in sepsis is a complex matter requiring more than blood pressure monitoring. Hemodynamic monitoring with pulmonary artery catheter is essential for accurate restoration of afterload without excessive vasoconstriction and an inappropriate fall in cardiac output. In the septic patient afterload manipulation with an alpha-agonist drug is a temporizing measure until antibiotic therapy and possible drainage of pus can correct the basis of the septic process. When the infection is controlled, normal vasoconstriction returns and the patient can be weaned from the alpha drugs.

OXYGEN TRANSPORT

In all of this discussion of monitoring and therapy for the cardiovascular system, one important target should be kept in sight, the transport of oxygen to the tissues for metabolic needs and cellular survival. It is appropriate to end this chapter with a brief look at how oxygen is transported to the various organs of the body and how monitoring of the oxygen transport system is helpful in understanding the function of the cardiovascular system.

Oxygen is brought to the cardiovascular system by the lungs and crosses the pulmonary alveolar-capillary barrier to enter the bloodstream. It is carried in two forms in the circulation. First, oxygen is dissolved in plasma and measured with a Clark electrode in a blood gas analyzer as partial pressure (PaO_2). Second, oxygen is carried attached to the hemoglobin molecule, and its presence is detected by looking for the color change from blue with deoxyhemoglobin to bright red with oxyhemoglobin. This is measured by using transmission spectrophotometry with a CO-oximeter and is recorded as percent saturation of hemoglobin (SaO_2). The oxygen content in the blood (CaO_2) is obtained from the sum of the dissolved and the bound oxygen. Normally each 100 ml of blood with 15 g of hemoglobin that is 95% saturated carries 20 ml of oxygen. Each liter of cardiac output contains 200 ml of oxygen. A 5 L cardiac output transports 1000 ml of oxygen to the peripheral tissues per minute (Table 4-8).

Within the hemoglobin molecule, oxygen is carried in the heme crevice with four oxygen molecules per molecule of hemoglobin. Other molecules such as carbon monoxide can compete for the heme crevice with oxygen. Carbon monoxide binds with 200 times the affinity to the hemoglobin molecule and can be displaced over time only with high concentrations or pressures of oxygen. Carbon monoxide also turns the hemoglobin molecule from blue to red so that the clinical diagnosis of carboxyhemoglobin is not immediately apparent. A CO-oximeter can differentiate between oxyhemoglobin and carboxyhemoglobin using a multiple wavelength spectrophotometric technique. A standard blood gas measurement with a calculated saturation does not reveal the presence of carbon monoxide, since the Clark electrode is measuring oxygen in the plasma. The iron in the heme molecule can become oxidized and unable to carry oxygen, leading to methemoglobin. This creates chocolate brown blood and is clinically apparent. Once again, a CO-oximeter can report

TABLE 4–8. Oxygen Transport Definitions and Formulas

Definitions

CaO_2 = Arterial content of oxygen
$C\bar{v}O_2$ = Mixed venous content of oxygen
DO_2 = Oxygen transport
Hgb = Hemoglobin
PaO_2 = Arterial partial pressure of oxygen
$P\bar{v}O_2$ = Mixed venous partial pressure of oxygen
SaO_2 = Arterial hemoglobin oxygen saturation
$S\bar{v}O_2$ = Mixed venous hemoglobin oxygen saturation

Formulas

$$CaO_2 = (PaO_2 \times 0.0031) + (Hgb \times 1.34 \times SaO_2)$$
$$= 20 \pm 2 \text{ ml } O_2/\text{dl blood}$$
$$C\bar{v}O_2 = (P\bar{v}O_2 \times 0.0031) + (Hgb \times 1.34 \times S\bar{v}O_2)$$
$$= 16 \pm 2 \text{ ml } O_2/\text{dl blood}$$
$$DO_2 = CO \times CaO_2 \times 10$$
$$= 1000 \pm 100 \text{ ml/}O_2/\text{min}$$

percentage of methemoglobin. Finally, sulfur can irreversibly bind to the heme molecule and prevent the transport of oxygen.

The affinity of oxygen for the hemoglobin molecule is regulated by several factors. First, the presence of increased hydrogen ions in the blood decreases the affinity and raises partial pressure of oxygen at 50% saturation of hemoglobin (P_{50}), which is a measure of affinity. P_{50} of adult hemoglobin is 27 mm Hg. With acidosis (Bohr effect) the P_{50} increases and affinity decreases, making oxygen more available to be released from the hemoglobin molecule and enter the tissues. Likewise, increases in 2,3-diphosphoglycerate (DPG), a molecule that fits into the hemoglobin structure at the amino acid N-termini, decrease affinity and increase P_{50}. Both anemia and high altitude are capable of increasing 2,3-DPG. Hypophosphatemia decreases 2,3-DPG and increases affinity, making oxygen less available. In the ICU this information becomes helpful when the critical care physician knows that increased temperature, acidosis, and hypercarbia all make oxygen more available for cellular metabolism.

In the past, oxygen transport was monitored by comparison of arterial blood gases to mixed venous blood gases drawn from the tip of the pulmonary artery catheter. The clinician could calculate arterial and mixed venous oxygen contents and determine the difference. If 20 ml of oxygen per 100 ml of blood is normal for the arterial side of the circulation, 16 ml of oxygen per 100 ml of blood is normal for the venous side and the arterial/venous oxygen content difference is 4 ml. This is an oxygen extraction ratio of 20%. The cardiovascular system normally transports 1000 ml of oxygen to the peripheral tissues per minute. An oxygen consumption of 250 ml/min allows 750 ml of oxygen to return to the venous side of the circulation. Normal $P\bar{v}O_2$ is 40, and normal $S\bar{v}O_2$ is 70.

The four primary determinants of the oxygen transport system are hemoglobin level, pulmonary loading of oxygen, cardiac output, and oxygen consumption. If an uncompensated decrease in hemoglobin, PaO_2, or cardiac output occurs while oxygen consumption stays the same, $S\bar{v}O_2$ falls. Likewise, if oxygen consumption increases while the other three factors remain the same, $P\bar{v}O_2$ and $S\bar{v}O_2$ must fall. The continuous monitoring of $S\bar{v}O_2$ by a technique of reflection spectrophotometry with use of a fiberoptic pulmonary artery catheter allows the critical care physician a unique opportunity for continuous tracking of oxygen transport. Adding pulse oximetry to the fiberoptic pulmonary artery catheter, dual oximetry, provides even more valuable information on oxygen transport. With this combination both the arterial and venous components of the circulation can be continuously monitored for the quality of oxygen loading and unloading.

Probably dual oximetry as a real-time monitor of oxygen transport will be increasingly popular in the ICU, since the circulation's primary task is the movement of oxygen to peripheral tissues to support metabolism.

SUGGESTED READINGS

Adams JM, Speer ME, Rudolph AJ: Bacterial colonization of radial artery catheters. Pediatrics 1980;65:94-97

Band JD, Maki DG: Infections caused by arterial catheters used for hemodynamic monitoring. Am J Med 1979; 67:735-741

Bedford RF: Radial arterial function following percutaneous cannulation with 18- and 20-gauge catheters. Anesthesiology 1977;47:37-39

Buchbinder N, Ganz W: Hemodynamic monitoring. Anesthesiology 1976;45(2):146-155

Carroll GC: Blood pressure monitoring. Crit Care Clin 1988;4(3):411-434

Cerra FB: The systemic septic response: multiple systems organ failure. Crit Care Clin 1985;1(3):591-608

Chatterjee K: Myocardial infarction shock. Crit Care Clin 1985;1(3):563-590

Daily EK, Tilkian AG: Cardiovascular procedures. St Louis, 1986, CV Mosby, pp. 3-82

Forrester JS, Diamond G, Chatterjee K, et al: Medical therapy of acute myocardial infarction by application of hemodynamic subsets. N Engl J Med 1976;295(25): 1404-1413

Forrester JS, Diamond G, McHugh TJ, et al: Filling pressures in the right and left sides of the heart in acute myocardial infarction. N Engl J Med 1971;285:190-193

Forrester JS, Ganz W, Diamond G, et al: Thermodilution cardiac output determination with a single flow directed catheter. Am Heart J 1972;83(3):306-311

Gardner RM, Schwartz R, Wong HC, et al: Percutaneous indwelling radial-artery catheters for monitoring cardiovascular function. N Engl J Med 1974;290:1227-1231

Harmon E: Arterial cannulation. Probl Crit Care 1988; 2(2):286-295

Kapadia CB, Heard SO, Yeston NS: Delayed recognition of vascular complications caused by central venous catheters. J Clin Monitor 1988;4:267-271

Kaufman JL, Rodriguez JL, McFadden JA, et al: Clinical experience with the multiple lumen central venous catheter. JPEN 1986;10(5):487-489

King EG, Chin WDN: Shock: an overview of pathophysiology and general treatment goals. Crit Care Clin 1985; 1(3):547-562

Lowenstein E, Little JW, Lo HH: Prevention of cerebral embolization from flushing radial-artery cannulas. N Engl J Med 1971;285(25):1414-1415

Marshall JP, Chadwick SJ, Meyers DS: Catheter perforation of the right ventricle. N Engl J Med 1974;290(16):890-891

Matthay MA, Chatterjee K: Bedside catheterization of the pulmonary artery: risks compared with benefits. Ann Intern Med 1988;109:826-834.

McGee WT, Mallory DL: Cannulation of the internal and external jugular veins. Probl Crit Care 1988;2(2):217-241

Michaelson ED, Walsh RE: Osler's node — a complication of prolonged arterial cannulation. N Engl J Med 1970;283(9):472-474

Novak RA, Venus B: Clavicular approaches for central vein cannulation. Probl Crit Care 1988;2(2):242-265

Rose SG, Pitsch RJ, Karrer W, et al: Subclavian catheter infections. JPEN 1988;12(5):511-512

Scott WL: Complications associated with central venous catheters. Chest 1988;94(6):1221-1224

Shabot MM, Shoemaker WC, State D: Rapid bedside computation of cardiorespiratory variables with a programmable calculator. Crit Care Med 1977;5(2):105-111

Shanji FM, Todd TRJ: Hypovolemic shock. Crit Care Clin 1985;1(3):609-630

Sprung CL, Jacobs LJ, Caralis PV, et al: Ventricular arrhythmias during Swan-Ganz catheterization of the critically ill. Chest 1981;79:413-415

Sprung CL, Drescher M, Schein RMH: Clinical investigation of the cardiovascular system in the critically ill: invasive techniques. Crit Care Clin 1985;1(3):533-546

Thys DM: Cardiac output. Anesthesiol Clin North Am 1988;6(4):803-824

Tribbet D, Brenner M: Peripheral and femoral vein cannulation. Probl Crit Care 1988;2(2):266-285

Vender JS: Invasive cardiac monitoring. Crit Care Clin 1988;4(3):455-478

Vender JS: Pulmonary artery catheter monitoring. Anesthesiol Clin North Am 1988;6(4):743-765

Weisel RD, Berger RL, Hechtman HB: Measurement of cardiac output by thermodilution. N Engl J Med 1975;292(13):682-684

Wyatt R, Glaves I, Cooper DJ: Proximal skin necrosis after radial-artery cannulation. Lancet 1974;8

5

ADVANCED NEUROLOGIC LIFE SUPPORT

STEVEN J. ALLEN, MD

Expeditious assessment and appropriate treatment of the patient with altered central nervous system (CNS) states are crucial for optimal outcome. The reason for this lies in the rapidity with which life-threatening neurologic deterioration may occur, as well as the inability of neurons to hypertrophy or regenerate. Thus prevention of further neuronal loss becomes a major goal in the treatment of critically ill patients. The first priority in a patient with evidence of neurologic impairment, as with any critically ill patient, is to secure the airway and ensure adequate ventilation and circulation as described in previous chapters.

PATHOPHYSIOLOGY OF STUPOR AND COMA

Not all cerebral lesions decrease the level of consciousness. A number of discrete lesions, such as frontal lobe contusion or medullary infarction, may cause neurologic deficits without coma. From an anatomic standpoint, coma occurs only when a process affects (1) both cerebral hemispheres, (2) the arousal centers in the diencephalon and upper brainstem, or (3) both by metabolic interference. Pathologic states associated with coma can be divided into three categories (Table 5-1): supratentorial and subtentorial lesions that disrupt function of the upper brainstem arousal centers or both cerebral hemispheres, metabolic processes diffusely affecting the brain, and psychiatric disorders. Mechanisms, diagnosis, and treatment of the more common causes of coma are discussed in Chapter 10.

ASSESSMENT

Level of consciousness consists of two components, arousal and awareness. Level of *arousal* refers to the patient's ability to awaken, that is, open his or her eyes. The intensity of the stimulus required to cause eye opening is a measure of the arousal level. *Awareness* is the patient's ability to interact meaningfully with the environment. Level of awareness is a measure of the content of consciousness. Normal awareness includes orientation to person, place, and time. An important distinction should be made between arousal and awareness. For example, regardless of the severity of injury, patients with a cerebral insult begin to have spontaneous eye opening after 2 to 3 weeks. They may be fully arousable but have no response to any stimulus other than pain. This state does not fit the classic definition of coma, since patients appear to be awake. The term "persistent vegetative state" has gained popularity to describe patients who are arousable but are not aware.

Neurologic dysfunction is best assessed initially by a history and an appropriate neurologic examination (Table 5-2). History is important because it often reveals the cause of the neurologic dysfunction. A careful history may indicate whether the neurologic dysfunction is due to an acute episode or was presaged by

TABLE 5–1. Pathologic Causes of Coma

Supratentorial and subtentorial lesions
Metabolic processes
Psychiatric disorders

104

TABLE 5–2. Initial Assessment for Neurologic Dysfunction

History (often elucidates cause)
   Past medical history
   Drugs (psychoactive, hypoglycemics, etc.)
Physical examination: Head to toe
Neurologic examination
   Level of consciousness: Glasgow Coma Scale score
   Focal examination
       Cranial nerves
       Motor examination
       Reflexes
       Sensory examination

symptoms. For example, a patient in coma after an accident may have only minor physical evidence of head trauma. Although head injury is a possibility, so are subarachnoid hemorrhage, intracerebral hematoma, and arrhythmia, each of which is managed differently. Past medical problems, such as diabetes, recent injury, access to drugs (including hypoglycemic agents), and psychiatric history, should be elicited. All too often the reason for an altered state of consciousness is inapparent. After initial stabilization a careful head-to-toe examination should be performed to look for signs of trauma, needle puncture sites, and the smell of alcohol or acetone on the breath.

Despite the recent proliferation of CNS monitors, none is as valuable as the performance of serial examinations by a conscientious observer. The initial examination after stabilization of a critically ill patient is more detailed than subsequent ones so that subtle findings are not overlooked. It should be performed as soon after admission as possible. The results serve as a baseline with which subsequent neurologic findings can be compared. Often the decision to intervene is made because of neurologic deterioration or failure to improve. The neurologic examination may be divided into two categories, level of consciousness and focal.

Decreased Level of Consciousness

The objective description of altered responsiveness has been hampered by the subjective nature of such words as "stuporous," "semicomatose," and "lethargic." Head-injured patients form a large population of critically ill patients in whom decreased level of consciousness is a major presenting sign. It was for these patients that a simple, reliable, reproducible scale, the Glasgow Coma Scale (GCS), was designed and validated in a multinational study. The GCS has become widely accepted and can be used to assess altered responsiveness in patients with coma of other etiology. GCS is obtained by scoring the response of three aspects (motor, eye opening, and verbal response) of the clinical examination (Table 5-3). The awake and oriented patient receives the highest score in each section (total 15), whereas the mute, flaccid, unarousable patient receives a 1 in each category (total 3). The sum can be used to describe the severity of altered responsiveness, with a score of less than 8 considered coma. However, more information is conveyed when the individual category scores are reported. The first part of the GCS involves the type of stimulus required to cause eye opening. Spontaneous eye opening implies that the brainstem arousal centers are intact. If the patient appears to be asleep, the examiner speaks to the patient. If this fails to result in eye opening, a standardized stimulus, such as nailbed pressure, is used to stimulate the arousal centers. Verbal response is assessed by conversation and observation of the patient. The utterance of any formed speech is a sign of high-level cerebral function. Patients who are intubated or have aphasia may not be accurately categorized with this approach and should be assessed on the basis of their motor response. To assess motor response, the clinician observes the movement of the extremities in response to command or stimulus. A patient

TABLE 5–3. Glasgow Coma Scale

EYE OPENING		MOTOR		VERBAL	
Spontaneous	4	Follows command	6	Oriented	5
Voice	3	Localizes	5	Confused	4
Pain	2	Flexion/withdrawal	4	Words	3
None	1	Flexion	3	Moans	2
		Extensor	2	None	1
		Flaccid	1		
	Range 3-15		Coma < 8		

who follows commands receives a 6 in this category. The command should require some understanding on the patient's part. If a patient squeezes the examiner's hand, this may reflect only reflex activity. More accurate assessment may be obtained by asking the patient to protrude his or her tongue (especially a quadriplegic patient) or to hold up two fingers. A patient who does not follow commands but reaches toward the noxious stimulus is said to be localizing. The GCS makes a distinction in the response to pain that is nonlocalizing but also nonposturing (flexion-withdrawal). With this level of motor response the patient may appear to thrash the arm but not reach for the stimulus. However, if the response is supination of the forearm and flexion at the elbow, the patient is exhibiting flexion. Pronation and extension of the upper extremities form the extensor response. The use of anatomic terms such as decortication and decerebration should be avoided because their interpretation may not be clear and their use implies specific anatomic sites of injury that may not be correct. The GCS does not take the place of a neurologic examination but rather attempts to assess the level of consciousness. A patient who extends on one side but localizes on the other is given a motor score of 5. Although the unilateral extensor response implies a focal problem, the ability to localize conveys a better assessment of the functional state of the rest of the brain.

Focal neurologic examination

Major goals of the focal neurologic examination in the ICU are to document the level of function and localize the structural site of the lesion. Although a textbook neurologic examination is not practical in critically ill patients, an examination that explicitly details cranial nerve, motor, and sensory function on admission is still helpful. Examining an uncooperative patient does have limitations, but careful observation often provides insight into the degree of neurologic function. Appropriately focused serial examinations are unsurpassed as a monitor of neurologic function. New cranial nerve deficits or changing sensory and motor levels should initiate an evaluation to determine the cause. Two important distinctions to be made when any focal neurologic deficit is identified are whether the deficit is of long standing and whether it is due to a central (brain or spinal cord) or peripheral process.

Eye examination

The pupillary light reflex consists of an afferent pathway via the cranial nerve II (optic) and an afferent pathway via cranial nerve III (oculomotor) and the ciliary ganglion (Fig. 5-1). Normal pupillary reaction to light is brisk, and the normal difference in size between the two pupils may be as much as 1 mm. Unreactiveness of the pupils may be due to factors other than brain damage, such as drugs, ocular trauma, seizures, or hypoxia. If these causes are excluded, unilateral pupillary dilatation suggests an intracranial process on the ipsilateral side that is compressing the cranial nerve III pathway. The presence of an elliptic (football-shaped) pupil has been reported in patients with brainstem compression despite a low intracranial pressure. The pupillary reflex is relatively resistant to metabolic processes, so the presence of an intact pupillary response may help differentiate these processes from a structural lesion. Some drugs, such as systemic narcotics and antiglaucoma drugs, constrict pupils, whereas topically applied anticholinergics (for example, atropine) and sympathomimetics (epinephrine) and intravenous ganglionic blockers (trimethaphan) dilate pupils, which interferes with the usefulness of this examination.

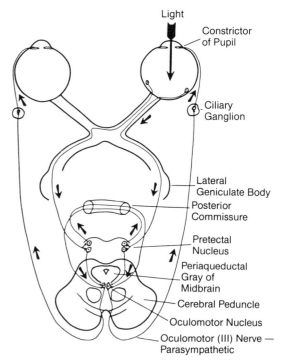

Figure 5–1. Pathways for the pupillary light reflex. (From Garoutte B: Survey of functional neuroanatomy, ed 2. Greenbrae, Calif., Jones Medical, p 107. With permission.)

In comatose patients the eyelids are closed by the resting tone in the orbicularis oculi muscles. If the eyelids are manually elevated and released, the lids should gradually close. A hysterical patient cannot reproduce this movement. Spontaneous blinking implies that the arousal centers are intact. Unilateral blinking implies that the facial nerve is damaged.

Normally in an awake person the eyes move conjugately and do not have spontaneous roving movement. In patients who are comatose but whose oculomotor pathways are unaffected, the eyes are conjugate or slightly dysconjugate and either are directed forward or display slow roving movements. The eyes do not appear to fix on any object and generally move side to side. Normal awake persons involuntarily fix on objects and cannot mimic these roving movements. The direction of the eyes toward one side or the other is called gazing. The cerebral cortex (frontal eyefield) associated with gazing to the right is located in the left frontal lobe. The right frontal eyefield directs the eyes to gaze conjugately to the left. Comatose patients who have damage to one frontal eyefield or are postictal may have conjugate gaze toward the side of the damage or seizure focus. If a comatose patient has damage to the midbrain where the oculomotor nuclei are located, the eyes are fixed and directed straight ahead. The patient does not respond to oculocephalic or oculovestibular testing (see the following). Ocular bobbing is a term used to describe the phenomenon of sudden downward gaze of both eyes with a slow rise followed by another sudden but shorter downward movement, resembling bobbing. This response generally is seen when the eyelids are opened in a patient with caudal pontine lesions, although it also has been reported in metabolic coma.

The corneal reflex is a protective response to a noxious stimulus applied to the cornea. A normal corneal reflex consists of attempted eyelid closure and an upward and outward deviation of the pupil (Bell's phenomenon), which indicates normal lower brainstem integrity.

When the possibility of a cervical fracture has been ruled out, the oculocephalic reflex (doll's eye) maneuver may be performed. The eyelids are held open and the head is suddenly rotated to one side and held in that position, followed by a rotation to the other side. In comatose patients with intact pathways the eyes move conjugately in the direction opposite to the rotation. If an eye fails to move medially or laterally, dysfunction of cranial nerves III or VI is implied. The doll's eye reflex is not seen in an awake patient unless the subject fixes the gaze on a target during the test.

Combined function of cranial nerves III, VI, and VIII is demonstrated by oculovestibular testing. The ear canal is determined to be clear of debris and the tympanum noted to be intact. With the head elevated 30 degrees above horizontal, the ear canal is slowly irrigated with up to 120 ml of ice water. In the awake patient the eyes stay generally in the midline but a nystagmus develops with the slow phase toward the irrigated ear. The nystagmus is regular and lasts 2 or 3 minutes. The presence of coma results in loss of the fast component with preservation of the tonic movement of the eyes toward the irrigated ear (Fig. 5-2). In metabolic coma the oculovestibular and oculocephalic responses may be very brisk even when signs of brainstem compression such as flexor or extensor posturing have developed. However, as coma deepens, regardless of the cause, the responses are lost. Among the many factors that may prevent oculovestibular response are ear wax, ototoxic agents, barbiturates and other anesthetic agents, phenytoin, muscle relaxants, and diseases of the vestibular system. Third and sixth cranial nerve palsies decrease the degree of movement with caloric stimulation. Thus a negative oculovestibular response must be interpreted with care. Testing both ears decreases the incidence of false-negative results.

Motor signs

The examination of motor function must be tailored to the patient's degree of arousal and cooperation. If a patient is agitated and uncooperative, simply observing the movement and strength of a particular extremity may provide a reasonably complete picture of any motor deficits. Motor examination of the comatose patient generally requires that a stimulus be applied to an extremity to elicit movement. The examiner must be careful in the choice of stimulus so that repeat, as well as initial, testing does not result in tissue trauma. For this reason many clinicians recommend nailbed pressure with a hard object such as a pencil. The examiner classifies the motor response of each extremity as (1) no movement, (2) extension, (3) flexion, (4) flexion-withdrawal, (5) localization, or (6) follows command. The test is performed as part of the GCS as discussed previously. A

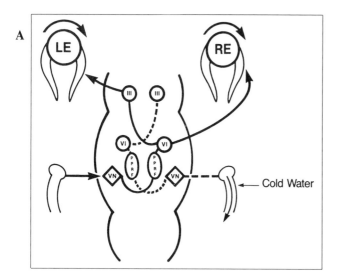

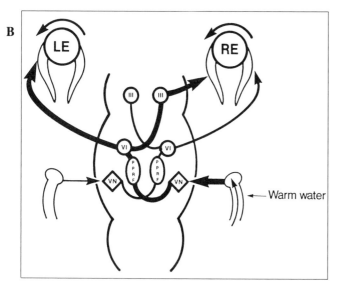

Figure 5–2. *A,* Cold water in the right ear causes shift of endolymph away from the ampulla, decreasing the ipsilateral vestibular tone and allowing the contralateral vestibular tone to dominate. The result is a slow movement toward the cold water and a fast, compensatory movement away. *B,* Warm water in the right ear causes shift of endolymph toward the ampulla, thereby increasing the ipsilateral vestibular tone and resulting slow movement of eyes toward the contralateral side with fast, compensatory movement toward the warm water. (LE = left eye. RE = right eye. III and VI = cranial nerves. VN = vestibular nuclei. PPRF = paramedial pontine reticular formation.) (From Bajandas FL, Kline LB: Neuro ophthalmology review manual, ed 2. Thorofore, NJ, 1987, Slack. With permission.)

number of different intracranial processes may cause abnormalities on the motor examination. Supratentorial lesions that do not compress the brainstem can produce motor weakness, flaccidity, or spasticity. Early brainstem compression may be accompanied by loss of localization that may progress to withdrawal. As brainstem compression worsens, the withdrawal response is replaced by abnormal flexion in the upper extremities and extension in the lower extremities. Extension of the upper extremities reflects an extremely severe injury and may proceed to flaccidity. Evidence of neurologic deterioration in the motor examination should trigger immediate evaluation for the presence of a surgically correctable lesion such as an epidural or intracerebral hematoma or hydrocephalus.

Neurologic examination in spinal cord injury

A careful examination of individual muscle function assists in the determination of underlying spinal cord injury. Table 5-4 provides a list of commonly tested muscles with their predominant spinal nerve innervation. Motor testing remains a somewhat subjective practice. However, a common grading system is provided in Table 5-5.

Sensory testing

Knowledge of the distribution of the spinal sensory innervation is necessary for accurate determination of the functional level of spinal cord injury. The spinal nerve innervations of extremity muscles and sensory dermatomes are displayed in Figure 5-3. The lower cervical and upper thoracic spinal nerves are often not represented on the trunk (Fig. 5-3, *A* and *B*). Thus sensory testing of the arms is necessary to determine the correct sensory level.

Reflex testing

The stretch reflexes of the extremities, which are normally part of the neurologic examination, are called tendon reflexes. Tendon reflexes are elicited by sharply striking the appropriate tendon (not muscle) and palpating the resultant muscle contraction. These reflexes include the biceps (C5-6), triceps jerk (C7), knee jerk (L2-4), and ankle jerk (S1-2). Absence or decrease of a normal response may be due to impairment of the afferent sensory nerve, impairment of the lower motor neuron supplying the muscle, or a myopathy that has affected the muscle itself. Acute CNS injury may also result in the loss of reflex activity, even if the process does not directly impinge on the reflex circuit (spinal shock). All tendon reflexes may be increased in response in situations of agitation, tension, or metabolic derangements. Some CNS lesions, such as those affecting the pyramidal tracts, disinhibit the tendon reflexes, markedly increasing reflex activity. One example of this disinhibition is ankle clonus. For this response to occur, the patient's foot and leg must be relaxed. The examiner briskly dorsiflexes the foot. A normal response is a reflex plantar flexion and relaxation after one or two beats. However, pyramidal tract injury is associated with clonus, a sustained repetitive cycle of plantar flexion and relaxation.

To elicit superficial reflexes, the examiner

TABLE 5–5. Motor Strength Scale

Full strength: full resistance	5
Weakness: resistance but less than normal	4
Cannot develop resistance but can overcome gravity	3
Can move only in a horizontal plane	2
Flicker	1
Flaccid	0

lightly strokes the skin in certain areas and observes whether an appropriate muscle contraction occurs. The abdominal reflexes are tested by stroking of the abdomen across dermatomes in each of the four quadrants. A normal response is movement of the umbilicus in the direction of the stimulus. The anal reflex is tested by stroking of the perianal skin. If S4 and S5 are intact, the external sphincter contracts.

The examiner elicits the plantar response by stroking the lateral aspect of the sole of the foot from back to front. The normal response is flexion of the toes. The abnormal response, called the extensor or Babinski response, consists of dorsiflexion of the great toe and fanning out of the other toes. Presence of an abnormal plantar response is considered pathognomonic for a pyramidal tract lesion somewhere between the contralateral motor cortex and the ipsilateral lateral corticospinal column of the spinal cord. The extensor response is part of a disinhibited primitive withdrawal reflex. In some cases elicitation of the plantar response results not only in an extensor response, but also in flexion of the hip and knee and possibly bowel and bladder evacuation (mass reflex).

IMMEDIATE STABILIZATION IN THE COMATOSE PATIENT

The priority in stabilizing a patient with an altered CNS state is to support and protect cerebral oxygen delivery. Expeditious therapy to protect the brain from further injury takes precedence over a detailed history and physical examination. The brain is capable of storing only a few minutes' supply of energy substrates. Oxygen deprivation from hypoxia or decreased perfusion quickly causes irreversible injury. Thus, before any CNS problem is addressed, basic respiratory and circulatory life support as described in the preceding chapters must be instituted. Decreased consciousness and other neurologic deficits often resolve or improve remarkably when the patient has been resuscitated.

TABLE 5–4. Spinal Nerve Innervation

MUSCLE	SPINAL ROOTS
Trapezius	C4
Shoulder external rotators	C5
Shoulder internal rotators	C5
Shoulder abductors	C5
Biceps	C5,6
Triceps	C7
Wrist extensors	C6,7
Wrist flexors	C7,8
Finger extensors	C8
Grasp	C8, T1
Hip flexors	L1,2
Hip extensors	L5, S1
Knee flexors	S1
Knee extensors	L3,4
Dorsiflexion	L4
Plantar flexion	S1,2

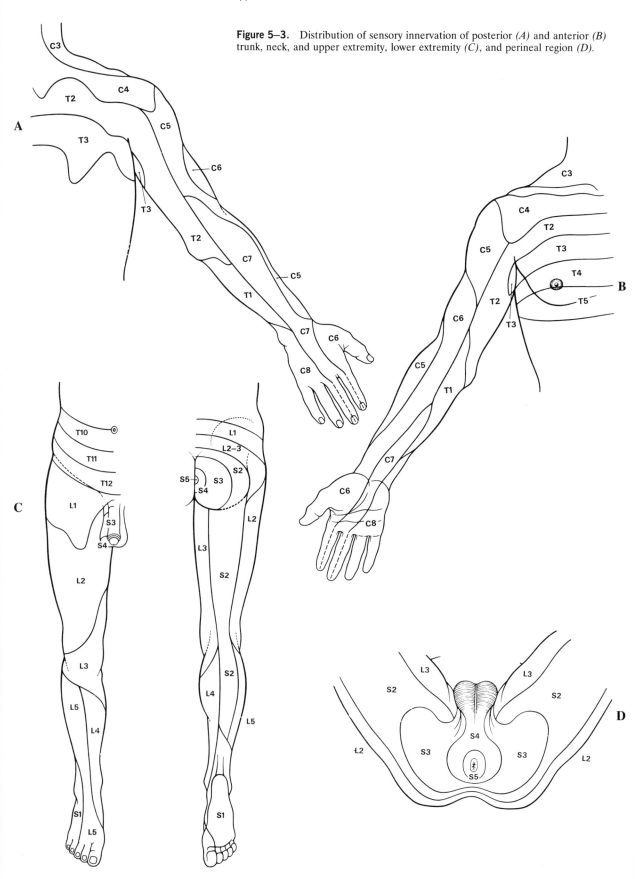

Figure 5–3. Distribution of sensory innervation of posterior *(A)* and anterior *(B)* trunk, neck, and upper extremity, lower extremity *(C)*, and perineal region *(D)*.

After hypoxemia and hypotension have been addressed, patients with coma of unclear origin may require treatment before a complete diagnostic workup can be performed. A series of treatments is recommended in the following paragraphs to manage potentially immediate threats to long-term viability (Table 5-6). Obviously, when the cause of coma, such as trauma, intracerebral hemorrhage or tumor, is known, directed therapy is begun.

Many clinicians administer *thiamine* 100 mg intramuscularly or intravenously immediately. Severe thiamine deficiency may be the result of malnourishment or dietary indiscretion as seen in chronic alcoholics. This particular vitamin deficiency can lead to a type of stupor and coma called Wernicke's encephalopathy. The process is thought to be driven by glucose administration. As most of these patients will receive intravenous fluids and glucose, thiamine should be administered early in their treatment.

After the thiamine administration, blood for laboratory tests should be drawn and the patient given 50 ml of *50% dextrose solution* (25 g). Besides oxygen, the brain uses glucose as a requisite energy substrate. Blood is drawn before glucose administration to document whether hypoglycemia was present. The CNS manifestations of hypoglycemia are myriad and may include focal findings, such as hemiplegia, on the neurologic examination.

Once adequate cerebral oxygen and glucose delivery have been attained, *seizures,* if present, must be treated. Convulsions result in massive increases in cerebral oxygen consumption and delivery. However, cerebral oxygen delivery may not be able to keep up with the need. Thus status epilepticus or even repeated grand mal seizures should be treated. Diazepam 3 to 10 mg intravenously has received widespread clinical acceptance because of its rapid onset. Alternatively, lorazepam 1 to 4 mg intravenously may be used with a maximum dose of 8 mg. Once the convulsions are under control, phenytoin 15 mg/kg should be administered. A rate of no

TABLE 5–6. Immediate Support for Coma of Unknown Origin

Thiamine 100 mg IM or IV
Draw blood; then give 50 ml 50% glucose
Treat seizures
Empiric intracranial hypertension therapy
Treat acid-base abnormalities
Normalize body temperature
Administer specific antidotes to drugs and toxins

more than 50 mg/min is recommended to prevent potentially lethal arrhythmias. If seizures recur, more diazepam is given. The doses required of diazepam and other anticonvulsives are likely to depress respiration and consciousness sufficiently to necessitate intubation and mechanical ventilation. If diazepam and phenytoin do not stop the seizures, continuous intravenous infusion of barbiturates may be necessary (see Chapter 10).

Mild *hyperventilation* to a partial carbon dioxide arterial pressure ($Paco_2$) of 30 mm Hg and administration of *mannitol* are suitable empiric treatments for the patient in whom raised intracranial pressure may be contributing to coma (see Intracranial Pressure, p. 115).

Coma may be caused wholly or partially by abnormal levels of electrolytes and other substances. Blood should be drawn and sent for determinations of sodium, glucose, calcium, phosphorus, magnesium, blood urea nitrogen, bilirubin, and arterial blood gas levels. Appropriate treatment for these and other electrolyte disorders can be found in Chapter 16.

Profound hyperthermia and hypothermia may decrease level of consciousness. The body temperature should be adjusted to between 35° and 38° C.

Various *antidotes* may be tried, such as naloxone or physostigmine, depending on evidence from the history. Specific recommendations are covered in Chapter 17.

ADVANCED MONITORING AND IMAGING

After initial cardiopulmonary and neurologic stabilization, tests may be needed as a basis for the diagnosis and to estimate the severity of disease.

Lumbar puncture is useful in the diagnosis of CNS infections that may be found in the critically ill. Besides the measurement of opening pressure, minimal cerebrospinal fluid (CSF) analysis consists of Gram stain, bacterial culture, cell count, glucose, and protein determinations. The CSF is normally sterile and should reveal no organisms on Gram stain and no growth on cell culture. Normal CSF is clear. Xanthochromia occurs when red blood cells (RBCs) have lysed in the CSF, which usually requires that the RBCs have been in the CSF for at least 4 hours. Normally CSF contains fewer than 5 white blood cells (WBCs)/cu mm, all lymphocytes. The presence of more than 1 granulocyte/cu mm should raise suspicion of bacterial infection. CSF glucose is a function of the plasma glucose level, and the CSF value is normally 65% to 80% of the serum glucose. A CSF glucose level less than 35% of the serum level suggests increased consumption induced by infection. The CSF protein concentration normally is less than 45 mg/dl. Elevated CSF protein levels may be due to infection, blood in the CSF, spinal cord block of CSF, or demyelinating disease. Normally the CSF contains no RBCs. Bloody CSF implies subarachnoid hemorrhage. However, occasionally a blood vessel is punctured during the tap and blood contaminates the CSF sample. Bloody CSF can be interpreted in a number of ways. If the amount of blood decreases from the first to the last tube collected, subarachnoid hemorrhage is unlikely. If the CSF is bloody, a cell count may determine whether an inappropriate WBC count exists. This is determined by taking the ratio of RBCs to WBCs found in the peripheral smear and comparing the ratio found in the CSF, or the clinician can empirically state that there are 700 RBCs per WBC in blood. If the CSF contains fewer than 700 RBCs per WBC, a pleocytosis exists and infection is suspected (see Chapter 12).

Skull roentgenograms are of little use in the comatose patient. Although they may reveal evidence suggesting the cause, invariably further radiographic investigation is necessary.

Cervical spine roentgenograms are necessary in the comatose patient to rule out concomitant cervical vertebral fracture. Anteroposterior and lateral films should clearly image from the foramen magnum down to the top of T1. If doubt exists, the neck should be protected by either collar or sandbags until radiographic imaging is sufficient to rule out cervical spine injury.

Computed tomography (CT) has revolutionized neuroradiology. CT scans allow the content of the calvarium to be directly visualized. Besides details of bony structure and CSF spaces, white matter can be distinguished from gray. The use of intravenous contrast medium gives highly detailed information concerning intracerebral vascular structures. Newer CT scanners allow three-dimensional reconstruction of otherwise hard-to-image locations such as the sella turcica. The main advantage of CT scans in comatose patients is the ability to diagnose a mass or masslike lesion that is amenable to surgery. Hematomas, hydrocephalus, tumors, and abscesses are examples of lesions visible on CT that may require surgical

intervention. Although certain subacute subdural hematomas and tumors appear isodense and therefore are not apparent, mass effect is usually evident because of the shift of adjoining structures. In contemporary practice it is a rare patient with decreased level of consciousness who does not receive a CT scan.

Magnetic resonance imaging (MRI) is a relatively new form of cerebral imaging that relies on the response of hydrogen atoms to a fluctuating radiofrequency signal while under the influence of a powerful magnetic field. The advantage of MRI over CT is the former's remarkable improvement in resolution of cerebral architecture. In a comparison study of patients with head injury, MRI characterized the extent of injury to a better degree than CT. However, MRI did not reveal any surgically significant lesions that had not been visualized with CT. Because of cost and time to image, MRI will probably not replace CT scanning for the evaluation of acutely comatose patients.

Cerebral angiography is performed either via direct carotid injection or by way of catheter advancement from a femoral artery. Cerebral angiography allows evaluation of the extracranial and intracranial vasculature. It is used for the precise localization of aneurysms, arteriovenous malformations, and arterial injury.

With the emergence of CT scanning and MRI, use of *cerebral radionuclide scan* with its low resolution has decreased. Its main function in critically ill patients is for confirmation of brain death.

Electrophysiologic Monitoring

The physiologic monitors of preference in critically ill patients assess function. The neurologic examination is an example; sequential neurologic examinations can assess the progress and location of neurologic disease. However, physical examination has drawbacks in the critically ill. Decreased level of consciousness reduces the patient's cooperation. As the patient sinks deeper into coma, the breadth of responses that can be elicited becomes smaller. Furthermore, pharmacologic intervention, such as muscle relaxation and sedation, may invalidate neurologic examination. Regardless, it is preferable to identify a correctable pathologic process before it results in neurologic dysfunction. Thus optimal care of critically ill patients requires CNS monitoring that is more sensitive than physical examination. This section presents two types of cerebral electrical function monitoring, electroencephalography and evoked potential testing.

Electroencephalography

Electroencephalography (EEG) is monitoring of the brain's spontaneous electrical activity recorded from the scalp. The major use for EEG in the critically ill is in patients with an altered state of consciousness. By noting the predominant frequencies as well as particular waveforms, the clinician obtains diagnostic and prognostic information. The ranges of frequency are named with Greek letters and correlate loosely with level of consciousness (Table 5-7). The presence of bilateral and symmetric alpha activity (8 to 13 Hz), which is blocked by eye opening, implies an awake adult who is at least somewhat alert. This makes the EEG a valuable tool in diagnosing psychiatric causes of coma. Alpha activity can also be seen in some patients with cerebral anoxia or brainstem infarction. The alpha pattern appears more diffuse in these patients and is not inhibited by eye opening. Controversy exists as to whether the alpha pattern in these patients is associated with a poor outcome.

As a patient becomes less awake for either physiologic or pathologic reasons, the predominant frequency slows into the theta (3 to 7 Hz) or delta (1 to 3 Hz) ranges. Metabolic encephalopathy is associated with a similar diffuse slowing of the EEG, which correlates with clinical severity. In fact, the EEG changes may precede clinical signs. Triphasic or paroxysmal waves are said to be characteristic of hepatic encephalopathy. The EEG is helpful in the diagnosis of various seizure disorders associated with a decreased level of consciousness, especially if the convulsive activity does not exhibit clinically recognizable tonic-clonic movements.

Use of EEG in the critical care setting has several drawbacks. At the paper speeds used, the amount of data generated in a short time is enormous. Continuous recording hour after hour becomes prohibitive. Furthermore, EEGs are complex, and interpretation requires significant training and experience. Hence, efforts have been made to manipulate the raw EEG into a format that not only reduces the data

TABLE 5–7. Electroencephalogram

Alpha	8-13 Hz
Theta	3-7 Hz
Delta	1-3 Hz

TABLE 5–8. Electroencephalogram Interpretation

Raw EEG
Compressed spectral array
Cerebral function monitor

generated but also is more easily interpreted (Table 5-8).

The first commercially available attempt to simplify the EEG was the Cerebral Function Monitor (CFM). This device takes the electrical signal from two parietal electrodes and, through filtering and logarithmic amplitude compression, plots a line that is a nonlinear function of both amplitude and frequency. A criticism is that it may simplify the EEG too much. On the other hand, CFM is capable of displaying transients in the EEG that may be missed by other forms of processed EEG.

One difficulty with EEG interpretation is the complexity of the EEG waveform. Interpretation may be simplified if the raw EEG is broken down into its constituent simple frequencies. Compressed spectral array (CSA) subjects a short (usually 4 to 8 seconds) epoch of EEG to fast Fourier transformation and plots power (amplitude squared) against frequency. The plot of each sequential epoch is drawn close behind the previous trace, giving a three-dimensional display (Fig. 5-4). The main advantage of this type of processed EEG is that little information is lost. However, transients may be missed and artifacts, such as movement, are included in the display.

The usefulness of processed EEG monitoring in directing clinical management of critically ill

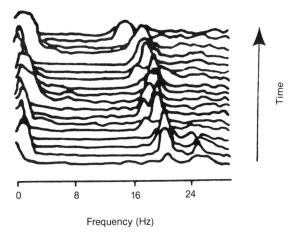

Frequency (Hz)

Figure 5–4. Example of output of compressed spectral array monitor. (From Levy WJ, Shapiro HM, Maruchak G, Meathe E: Anesthesiology 1980;53:223-236. With permission.)

patients is being evaluated. Most of the work has been performed in the operating suite where the threat to neuronal integrity is only a few hours in duration. In the ICU there are two areas in which CNS monitors would be useful. First, an early warning system could signal the occurrence of a reversible pathologic event before any clinical deterioration takes place. Second, care would be more rationally delivered if a CNS monitor could predict outcome early in the clinical course. The efficacy of continuous monitoring of processed EEG in the ICU as an early warning system has not been documented. However, a number of studies suggest the potential value of processed EEG for predicting outcome.

Evoked potentials

The EEG and its derived tests are based on the diffuse and spontaneous activity of the cerebral cortex with some influence from deeper centers (Table 5-9). Evoked potential testing is pathway specific. A particular pathway is chosen, the sensory receptor stimulated, and the response recorded in the scalp over the appropriate cortex. The amplitude of the evoked response is small compared with the background activity. Therefore evoked potential monitoring is performed by serial stimulation of a sensory receptor while the recorded response is time triggered to the stimuli. The electrical responses to many stimuli are averaged. In this fashion the part of the signal that is not time locked to the stimulus averages out and the evoked response becomes defined. An advantage of evoked potentials is the ability to accurately and quantitatively determine the functional state of a particular part of the CNS. Evoked responses are not affected as markedly as the EEG is by decreased level of consciousness or pharmacologic agents, such as sedation or general anesthesia. Thus abnormal evoked potentials imply that some process is directly affecting the sensory pathways monitored.

BRAINSTEM AUDITORY EVOKED POTENTIALS. Brainstem auditory evoked potentials (BAEPs) are elicited by presenting a series of clicks to the ears and monitoring the response at the vertex and on the earlobe of the stimulated

ear. The BAEP has five characteristic peaks (Fig. 5-5) that correlate with specific anatomic sites. Information concerning the integrity of the auditory pathway and presumably the surrounding brainstem is gleaned from the amplitude of the peaks and even more so from the latency (time) between peaks. An increasing latency between peaks I and V has been associated with a deteriorating clinical course. The part of the brainstem monitored by the BAEP appears to be hardy, and abnormalities occur only when a severe situation has developed. Thus the therapeutic and prognostic value of BAEP appears limited. Some clinicians use the BAEP to determine whether a confirmatory brain death study, such as cerebral radionuclide scanning, should be performed.

SENSORY EVOKED POTENTIALS. Sensory evoked potentials (SEPs) monitor the electrical response to stimulation of a peripheral nerve, usually the median nerve. An electrode is placed over C2 (Erb's point) to determine when the response has entered the spinal cord. Electrodes over the appropriate somatosensory cortex allow determination of the conduction time within the CNS, called the central conduction time (CCT). The CCT is prolonged by ischemia and may be of some prognostic use in comatose patients. Although SEPs are used frequently in the operating suite, their role in continuous monitoring of critically ill patients has not been defined.

VISUAL EVOKED POTENTIALS. Visual evoked potential (VEP) testing is performed in comatose patients by flashing bright stimuli through the eyelids with the use of goggles. The electrical response is monitored over the occipital cortex. Only a few studies of VEPs have

TABLE 5–9.   Evoked Responses

Brainstem auditory evoked potentials
Somatosensory evoked potentials
Visual evoked potentials
Motor evoked potentials

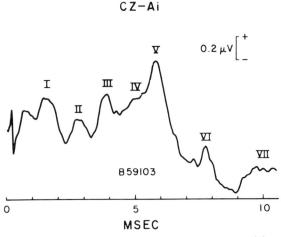

Figure 5–5. Normal brainstem auditory evoked potential tracing.

been reported in critically ill patients, and its place in critical care practice has yet to be determined.

MOTOR EVOKED POTENTIALS. The motor function of the CNS often holds more interest than the state of the sensory pathways. Thus efforts have been made to monitor motor evoked potentials. Initial techniques attempted to monitor retrograde conduction over the cortex. More recently, antegrade stimulation has been pursued by stimulation through the scalp. The motor cortex can be stimulated noninvasively. However, the use of electric stimuli to elicit a motor response is uncomfortable for awake patients. A recent technique uses magnetic fields to induce neuronal discharge in the motor cortex. With electrodes over appropriate points along the motor pathway, conduction can be measured both centrally and peripherally. The technique has been used intraoperatively.

Cerebral Blood Flow

Cerebral blood flow (CBF) is determined clinically by measuring the relative wash-in rate of some inert tracer. These techniques do not allow calculation of the total CBF. Rather, flow is expressed in terms of milliliters of blood flow per 100 g of brain tissue per minute. Under normal awake conditions CBF is about 50 ml/min/100 g brain when measured by several techniques. Simultaneous measurements of arterial and jugular venous oxygen contents allow the calculation of cerebral oxygen consumption ($CMRo_2$) by the equation

$$CMRo_2 = CBF \times (Cao_2 - Cjvo_2) \qquad (1)$$

where Cao_2 and $Cjvo_2$ represent the arterial and jugular venous oxygen contents, respectively. Under normal awake conditions, $CMRo_2$ is 3.3 ml O_2/100 g brain/min.

CBF can be measured with nitrous oxide (N_2O) or ^{133}Xe as the inert tracer. N_2O is administered via inhalation while N_2O concentrations in the arterial and jugular venous blood are monitored. This technique provides a global measurement of CBF. When ^{133}Xe is used, detectors are placed over the scalp and the rate of rise in radioactivity correlates with CBF. This technique allows regional measurements of CBF in the cortex. Because ^{133}Xe may be given intravenously or by inhalation, invasive lines are not required.

The measurement of CBF provides a direct assessment of cerebral oxygen delivery. Since CBF is normally coupled to the underlying cerebral oxygen consumption, decreases in met-

abolic activity, such as in coma, should be associated with a decrease in CBF. Thus there is no ideal CBF for a critically ill patient. The CBF should be relatively adequate for the underlying cerebral oxygen consumption.

Transcranial Doppler Monitoring

When used by a trained individual, transcranial Doppler monitoring provides information on the *velocity* of blood in the middle cerebral artery. The main application for the device has been for patients with vasospasm secondary to subarachnoid hemorrhage. As the effective vessel lumen becomes smaller, velocity increases, although flow may decrease. Clinical experience is limited.

Intracranial Pressure

Physiologic considerations support the prevention and treatment of raised intracranial pressure (ICP). Thus control of ICP is part of the management of several neurologic diseases. Intracranial hypertension (ICH) is believed detrimental because it may reduce the cerebral perfusion pressure (CPP), as expressed by the equation

$$CPP = MAP - ICP \qquad (2)$$

where MAP is the mean arterial blood pressure. Increasing ICP may lead to cerebral hypoperfusion with subsequent ischemia and edema. Edematous brain causes the ICP to rise even further, resulting in a spiraling process (Fig. 5-6). In experiments acute reductions of CPP to less than 50 mm Hg have been associated with

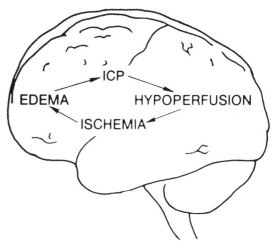

Figure 5–6. Increases in intracranial pressure may result in ischemia-induced edema, which may lead to further increases in intracranial pressure.

ischemia. The underlying cerebral disease process may distort the cerebral architecture. Elevated ICP may exacerbate these distortions and compress local blood supply and herniation. The location of the intracerebral disease may add to the morbidity of raised ICP. Because of anatomic proximity a masslike lesion in the temporal lobe, such as a tumor or hematoma, may result in brainstem compression with only a small rise in ICP. Studies in head-injured patients suggest that the ability to reduce ICP correlates with improved outcome.

Total reliance on the ICP as an indicator of brain disorder in a critically ill patient is unwise. Although an elevated ICP may contribute to coma, patients may have a low ICP and still be in coma. In essence, ICP is a mechanical measurement used for a crude estimate of the degree of brain disease. Because of compensatory mechanisms, volume may be added to the cranial vault without significantly increasing ICP. When the ICP is elevated, it indicates that a sufficient volume has been added to overwhelm these mechanisms. Furthermore, ICP measures only the state of the supratentorial compartment. Disastrous events may occur in the posterior fossa and not be reflected by the ICP measurement. ICP is but one parameter to monitor in a critically ill patient with a CNS problem and cannot replace physical evaluation.

Measurement of intracranial pressure

Indications for inserting an ICP monitor include any clinical situation in which ICP is increased and its treatment is expected to alter outcome. The use of ICP monitors is most widespread in patients with head injury. Generally an ICP monitor is placed when the GCS score is less than 8, the CT reveals a midline shift greater than 0.5 cm, or the basal cisterns are compressed. A number of ICP monitoring techniques are used (Table 5-10). As all the techniques are invasive, the risk of meningitis or ventriculitis is introduced. Numerous studies place the risk of CNS infection at about 10%. Meticulous sterile technique should be used with any ICP monitor to keep the infection rate as low as possible. After placement the monitors should be attached to a closed system that

TABLE 5–10. Intracranial Pressure Monitors

Ventriculostomy
Subarachnoid bolt
Fiberoptic catheter

includes the transducer, flush solution, manometer, and drainage bag if appropriate.

VENTRICULOSTOMY. The placement of a catheter into a frontal horn of one of the lateral ventricles is the gold standard method for ICP measurement. The technique allows reliable ICP waveform tracing and the removal of CSF for diagnostic and therapeutic purposes. The presence of massively shifted or collapsed ventricles or a coagulopathy may be a contraindication for placement of a ventriculostomy.

SUBARACHNOID BOLT. The desire to develop a simpler, less invasive device led to the development of the subarachnoid bolt. The monitor is essentially a threaded hollow bolt seated into a twist drill hole in the skull so that the bolt end is in contact with the dura. The dura and arachnoid membranes are opened below the bolt to create a continuous fluid path. Disadvantages of the subarachnoid bolt are that CSF cannot be drained significantly and that the bolt may underestimate the actual ICP at elevated levels.

FIBEROPTIC CATHETER. Transducer-tipped catheters are available for ICP monitoring. These devices contain a pressure-sensitive membrane that alters light transmission in response to changes in pressure. The fidelity of the waveforms is excellent, and satisfactory pressure measurements can be obtained within almost any intracranial compartment.

Treatment

In the normal supine patient, ICP is less than 15 mm Hg. An ICP greater than 20 mm Hg is thought to reflect a pathologic condition. The ICP is determined by the volume of the intracranial contents. If the cranium behaved as a completely closed and nondistensible container, any increase in volume would rapidly increase ICP, since fluid is noncompressible. However, in the normal brain this does not appear to be the case (Fig. 5-7). A certain amount of volume can be added slowly to the intracranial contents without much increase in ICP. As the volume increases, compensatory mechanisms prevent a rise in ICP by translocating CSF out of the foramen magnum and into the spinal canal. Furthermore, the dural venous sinuses are compressible. Once these mechanisms play out, however, small additions to intracerebral volume markedly increase ICP. Figure 5-7 displays the classic concept of a single compliance curve for the calvarium. Although this probably represents an oversimplification of the complex interaction among CSF production, intracranial

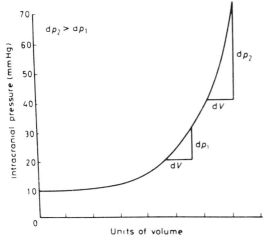

Figure 5–7. Intracranial pressure/volume curve demonstrating the difference in pressure elevations ($dp_1 < dp_2$) for the same volume change (dV) at two separate locations. (Redrawn from data presented in Figure 1 of Langfitt TW, Weinstein JD, Kassell NF: Neurology 1965;15:622-641. With permission of the publisher. From Allen SJ: In Barash PG (ed): American Society of Anesthesiologists' Refresher Courses in Anesthesiology. Philadelphia, 1987, JB Lippincott.)

TABLE 5–11. Intracranial Contents

Cerebrospinal fluid
Cerebral blood volume
Brain parenchyma

compliance, venous outflow resistance, and intradural sinus pressure, it does convey the concept of decreasing compliance as intracerebral volume increases.

The intracranial vault is made up of three compartments: CSF, cerebral blood volume, and cerebral parenchyma (Table 5-11). ICP may rise when the volume of one of these compartments increases or when a mass lesion, such as an abscess, hematoma, or tumor, increases intracranial volume. Thus intracranial hypertension (ICH) may be the result of a number of processes. Each of these processes has its own treatment. Therefore the appropriate management of ICH includes diagnosis of its cause and institution of specific therapy.

INCREASE IN CEREBRAL BLOOD VOLUME. Elevated jugular venous pressure may result in passive expansion of the cerebral vasculature, contributing to raised ICP on the steep part of the pressure/volume curve shown in Figure 5-7. Elevation of the head is a simple maneuver to enhance jugular venous outflow. Head rotation may occlude the ipsilateral internal jugular vein with a subsequent rise in venous pressure. Thus keeping the head in midposition appears to aid in ICP control. Similarly, turning the patient for routine nursing care may elevate ICP even if the head and neck are supported. In selected incidences we have found that a rotating platform turns the patient without unduly exacerbating ICH. Finally, comatose patients may exhibit

posturing behavior. This activity may elevate ICP by increasing intrathoracic pressure. The use of muscle relaxants has been shown to reduce ICP in such patients. For duration of action and economic reasons most medical centers use pancuronium or metocurine. The sympathomimetic side effects of the former drug may be undesirable in some patients.

The optimal management of blood pressure is not clear in patients with intracranial disorders. Normally, the CBF is essentially the same between mean arterial blood pressures of 50 and 150 mm Hg in previously normotensive individuals. The ability to maintain CBF relatively independent of blood pressure is called auto regulation. Intracranial disorders are associated with altered autoregulation. For example, 50% of patients with severe head injury have altered autoregulation. Thus even otherwise clinically insignificant decreases in CPP may result in CBF decreases, possibly contributing to ischemia. Conversely, increases in arterial blood pressure may be accompanied by increases in the CBV and contribute to ICH. Maintenance of blood pressure in the normal range appears the most desirable approach. Patients with long-standing hypertension exhibit an autoregulatory curve that is shifted to the right. Their range of autoregulation may be 70 to 180 mm Hg. Although they tolerate higher blood pressures, they are susceptible to cerebral ischemia if their "normal" blood pressure is not maintained.

CBF is linearly related to $Paco_2$ between 20 and 75 mm Hg. Each rise in $Paco_2$ of 1 mm Hg is associated with a 3% increase in CBF. Thus hypercarbia dramatically exacerbates ICH. Conversely, hyperventilation causes cerebral vasoconstriction and reduces ICP. In the patient with suspected or measured ICH, $Paco_2$ is typically lowered to 25 to 30 mm Hg, which results in a 30% decrease in CBF. However, the use of hypocarbia creates an anomalous situation in the care of the critically ill. Patients with suspected ICH are treated with hyperventilation, which decreases oxygen delivery to the injured organ. Although hyperventilation may improve the mechanical CNS measurement (ICP), it may also compromise metabolism.

Arterial oxygen partial pressure has little effect on CBF unless hypoxemia develops, at which point CBF rises dramatically. Thus hypoxemia is bad for two reasons. First, the injured brain is deprived of a vital nutrient. Second, the rise in CBF may result in an ICP increase. This is of particular relevance to the critically ill because patients with intracranial disorders often have impaired pulmonary gas exchange.

Hyperthermia may increase CBF sufficiently to exacerbate ICH. The patient's body core temperature should be kept below 39° C (102.2° F). Seizures cause a massive increase in $CMRo_2$ that may outstrip cerebral oxygen delivery. The potential arises for both cerebral ischemia and ICH because of the seizure-induced increase in CBF. Diagnosis of seizure activity in critically ill patients may be difficult because of the use of muscle relaxants and requires a high index of suspicion. Sudden, otherwise unexplained rises in ICP in paralyzed comatose patients may represent seizure activity. Appropriate treatment should be instituted and electrophysiologic investigation ordered.

CEREBROSPINAL FLUID.   ICH may develop or become exacerbated by increases in the CSF compartment. In a 70 kg adult, CSF is produced at a rate of 21 ml/h (about 500 ml/d) with 100 to 150 ml present at any given time in the subarachnoid space. Increase in CSF volume (hydrocephalus) is almost always due to decreased reabsorption rather than increased production. Hydrocephalus is characterized as noncommunicating hydrocephalus when a mechanical obstruction to CSF exists between the lateral and fourth ventricles. Such an obstruction is most often caused by a mass or masslike lesion compressing or distorting the aqueduct of Sylvius. Communicating hydrocephalus occurs when absorption of CSF by the pacchionian granules (subarachnoid villi) is decreased. Blood in the subarachnoid space, produced by trauma or subarachnoid hemorrhage, may slow CSF absorption sufficiently to produce hydrocephalus. CSF drainage is the immediate treatment of ICH caused by either form of hydrocephalus. Before hydrocephalus or any other surgically correctable lesion can be treated, it must be diagnosed. As with any other neurosurgical lesion, some form of imaging is necessary to make the diagnosis. CT is a reasonably reliable technique for identifying surgically correctable causes of ICH and should be performed as expeditiously as the clinical course allows.

CEREBRAL PARENCHYMA.   Increases in the volume of the cerebral parenchyma are due to edema formation. Two types of cerebral edema exist: vasogenic and cytogenic. The junctions between the cerebral capillary endothelial cells form the blood-brain barrier. Normally these junctions are very tight, and relatively little fluid can leak out of the capillaries and pass into the brain interstitium. In disease states these endothelial cell junctions may loosen, allowing more fluid out of the capillaries. This type of edema is called vasogenic. Systemic arterial hypertension may contribute to this mechanism because, once capillary permeability has increased, the higher vascular pressure may cause more fluid to leak out. Hyperosmolality may also play a role in the development of vasogenic edema. Raising the blood osmolality causes the endothelial cells to shrink away from each other. Most clinicians therefore limit the use of osmotic diuretics once the serum osmolality rises to 320 mOsm/L.

When cerebral tissue is deprived of adequate blood flow and oxygen delivery, cells become ischemic and, no longer able to maintain their internal integrity, begin to swell. This type of edema is referred to as cytogenic. Obviously, prevention is the goal for this form of ICH. Avoidance of hypotension, low cardiac output, hypoxemia, or any other factor that may adversely affect the balance of cerebral oxygen delivery to consumption requires vigilance.

STEROIDS.   Steroids have been advocated for the treatment of cerebral edema. Patients with cerebral tumors, especially of metastatic origin, often have a profound amount of peritumoral edema. The administration of high doses of steroids, such as dexamethasone, dramatically affects clinical findings in as little as 8 hours. For other types of cerebral edema the evidence is less compelling. High doses of steroids have been advocated for the treatment of cerebral edema after head injury. However, four double-blind randomized controlled studies have failed to show any beneficial effect of steroids on outcome from head injury. A recent study compared dexamethasone 100 mg/d versus no steroids. The overall amount of ICP therapy required, the peak ICP attained, and the outcome at 6 months were identical between the groups. However, if severe ICH was present, the group receiving steroids did significantly worse. Thus the evidence does not support the continued use of steroids in the treatment of head injury.

MANNITOL.   Since the turn of the century, osmotic agents have been known to decrease brain volume. Mannitol in 20% to 25% solutions has become the most commonly used osmotic diuretic in patients with ICH. The exact mechanism by which mannitol reduces ICP is not clear. Paradoxically, it seems to increase CBF as the ICP is decreasing. Unfortunately, mannitol does not decrease edema fluid. It appears to reduce brain volume by removing water from normal parts of the brain instead. The clinical use of mannitol may be associated with two problems. First, hyperosmolality may develop with aggravation of cerebral edema as mentioned previously. Second, the diuresis may result in hypovolemia. As with any critically ill patient, hypovolemia severe enough to decrease cardiac output and thus oxygen delivery should be avoided.

INITIAL MANAGEMENT OF PATIENTS WITH SUSPECTED INTRACRANIAL HYPERTENSION. The initial management of any patient with suspected raised ICP requires attention to a number of factors. Foremost is protection of cerebral oxygen delivery by correction of hypotension and hypoxemia. The patient should be mildly hyperventilated to a $Paco_2$ of 30 mm Hg. Mannitol in doses of 25 to 100 g may be administered intravenously. The neck should be stabilized until cervical injury can be ruled out. After initial stabilization the patient should undergo CT scanning and then any indicated surgical procedures. Once an ICP monitor has been placed, therapy can be titrated. Motor activity that contributes to ICH is controlled with muscle relaxants. Patients are hyperventilated to a $Paco_2$ 25 to 30 mm Hg. Mannitol is administered 12.5 g every 5 minutes until either the ICP is less than 20 mm Hg or the serum sodium level is greater than 150 mmol/L. CSF may be drained from the ventriculostomy. Seizures and hyperthermia are controlled. Lidocaine 1.5 mg/kg intravenously is effective for preventing ICP elevations associated with patient care maneuvers such as turning and suctioning. The treatment of specific diseases can be found in Section II.

SUGGESTED READING

Anziska B, Cracco RQ: Short latency somatosensory evoked potentials in brain dead patients. Arch Neurol 1980; 37:222-225

Becker DP, Miller JD, Ward JD, et al: The outcome from severe head injury with early diagnosis and intensive management. J Neurosurg 1977;47:491-502

Cooper KR, Boswell PA: Reduced functional residual capacity and abnormal oxygenation of patients with severe head injury. Chest 1983;84:29-35

Dearden NM, Gibson JS, Gibson RM, Cameron MM: Effect of high-dose dexamethasone on outcome from severe head injury. J Neurosurg 1986;64:81-88

Hecox K, Galambos R: BAEPs in human infants and adults. Arch Otolaryngol 1974;99:30-33

Hume AL, Cant BR, Shaw NA: Central somatosensory conduction time in comatose patients. Ann Neurol 1979; 5:379-384

Jennett B, Teasdale G, Galbraith S, et al: Severe head injuries in three countries. J Neurol Neurosurg Psychiatry 1977;40:291-298

Miller JD, Leech P: Effects of mannitol and steroid therapy on intracranial volume-pressure relationships in patients. J Neurosurg 1975;42:274-281

Obrist WD, Langfitt TW, Jaggi JL, et al: Cerebral blood flow and metabolism in comatose patients with acute head injury. J Neurosurg 1984;61:241-253

Plum F, Posner JB: The diagnosis of stupor and coma, ed 4. Philadelphia, 1982, FA Davis Co

Ropper AH, Kennedy SF: Neurological and neurosurgical intensive care, ed 2. Rockville, Md: Aspen Publishers. 1988

Saul TG, Ducker TB: Effect of intracranial pressure monitoring and aggressive treatment on mortality in severe head injury. J Neurosurg 1982;56:498-503

Snow RB, Zimmerman RD, Gandy SE, Deck MDF: Comparison of magnetic resonance imaging and computed tomography in the evaluation of head injury. Neurosurgery 1986;18:45-52

Sorensen K, Thomassen A, Wernberg M: Prognostic significance of alpha frequency EEG rhythm in coma after cardiac arrest. J Neurol Neurosurg Psychiatry 1978;41: 840-842

Westmoreland BF, Klass DW, Sharborough FW, et al: Alpha coma: electroencephalographic, clinical, pathologic and etiologic correlations. Arch Neurol 1975; 32:713-718

6

TECHNOLOGY OF INTENSIVE CARE UNIT MONITORS

GORDON L. GIBBY, MD

NONINVASIVE BLOOD PRESSURE MEASUREMENT

Arterial blood pressure is one of the most basic parameters measured in the ICU. Taking into account any evidence of drastic alteration in systemic vascular resistance (for example, cool, clammy extremities), clinicians generally infer the adequacy of circulation to the vital organs from the measurement of arterial blood pressure. Whenever possible, blood pressure is measured noninvasively to minimize risk of complication. Measurement devices may yield either discrete or continuous output readings; continuous measurements are preferable but cannot always be achieved. In either case the equipment interacts physically with the artery to measure the artery's internal pressure.

The simplest way of interacting with the artery is to compress it. When the constricting pressure applied to the artery exceeds the distending pressure inside it, the artery collapses and the flow is impeded. The blood pressure cuff was invented to perform this task by Riva-Rocci in 1896 and Hill and Barnard in 1897. Blood flow has been detected in many ways. The oscillometric method of observing the pulsations in the manometer caused by the inrush of blood was developed in 1890. Korotkoff in 1905 pointed out that a stethoscope could be used to hear the pulsations over a compressed artery. Simple palpation of the return of the pulse can also be used, or the return of visible pulsations may be noted on the screen of a pulse oximeter.

All these methods are based on an assumption that the constricting pressure at the artery is related to the pressure inside the cuff. Actually, a rounded "pressure front" created by the cuff extends into the encircled limb (Fig. 6–1). The depth of this pressure gradient front is related to the cuff width; a narrow cuff has a shallow pressure gradient front. If the cuff is too narrow, the pressure zone does not include the deeper artery and an artifactually high cuff pressure will be required to occlude the artery. Conversely, if the cuff is too wide, a somewhat lower pressure than ideal is measured, although the error is not as great as with an excessively narrow cuff. For the greatest accuracy the cuff

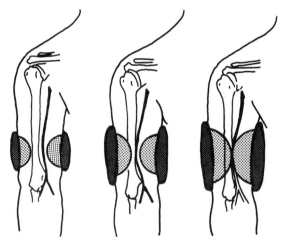

Figure 6–1. Rounded pressure fronts created by blood pressure cuffs. If the cuff is too narrow *(left)*, the full pressure front does not include the artery and the cuff must be inflated artifactually above systolic to occlude the artery. The error is less marked in the opposite direction with too large a cuff *(right)*. (From Gravenstein JS, Paulus DA: Clinical monitoring practice, ed 2. Philadelphia, 1987, JB Lippincott Co.)

should be 20% wider than the diameter of the arm; the cuff bladder must be no shorter than half the arm circumference and should be located over the artery in which the pressure is being measured.

The definitions of the Korotkoff sounds describe the succession of sounds auscultated as the cuff pressure is lowered from above systolic to below diastolic:

- Phase 1: First sound, faint, clear, and tapping
- Phase 2: Swishing sound
- Phase 3: Crisp, loud sounds
- Phase 4: Sound abruptly muffled with a soft, blowing character
- Phase 5: All sound lost

Although phase 1 is accepted as the systolic pressure, exactly which phase determines the true diastolic pressure is controversial. The muffling of the Korotkoff sounds occurs at a cuff pressure 3 to 4 mm Hg higher than invasively measured diastolic pressure, and the Korotkoff sounds disappear at 7 mm Hg lower than the invasively determined diastolic pressure. Thus some clinicians recommend that both phase 4 and phase 5 be recorded when possible; often only phase 5 (loss of sound) can be determined in the clinical situation. Some risk of misinterpreting the systolic pressure also exists. An auscultatory gap may separate phases 1 and 2 and may range up to 40 mm Hg; thus when measuring the pressure the clinician must be certain to palpate to ensure that the pulse has indeed been abolished before beginning to listen for the true phase 1.

In the common mercury manometer attached to the cuff, the pressure to be measured raises a column of mercury drawn from a reservoir. The manometer is accurate when it is operated at the angle or attitude for which it was designed, nothing obstructs the rising of the column, and the mercury content is such that with no pressure applied the device indicates zero pressure. The aneroid manometer makes use of the pressure to change the shape of a resilient piece of metal, usually the diaphragm of an enclosed volume. The movement of the diaphragm is then mechanically converted to movement of the instrument dial (Fig. 6–2). These devices should be protected from excessive shock to avoid deformation of the diaphragm. To accurately check or calibrate them, the operator should check at least two pressures in the range of interest.

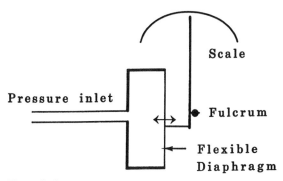

Figure 6–2. Anaeroid manometer mechanically amplifies small movements of a flexible diaphragm moved by the pressure to be measured.

Many automated noninvasive blood pressure measurement systems operate the cuff and make measurements by themselves, usually by the oscillometric method. A few examples illustrate the mechanisms used. The Ohmeda series 2100 and 2200 noninvasive blood pressure monitors (Ohmeda, Madison, Wisc.) use an eight-bit microprocessor to analyze oscillometric pressure changes in the cuff as the distending pressure is reduced in a stepwise fashion. At each step of cuff pressure the microprocessor accurately measures the cuff pressure many times per second and searches for a transient bump upward of the pressure (oscillometric pulsation). To confirm that oscillometric pulsations exist at that cuff pressure, the microprocessor requires that two similar pulsations be found. Systolic pressure is defined as the highest pressure at which such oscillometric signals are found; mean arterial pressure is the cuff pressure at which the oscillations are of greatest magnitude; and diastolic pressure is the cuff pressure at which the oscillations no longer decrease in amplitude. Quoted accuracy is the larger of ±3 mm Hg or 2% full scale.

The Sentry Model 400 automated blood pressure monitor (Automated Screen Devices, Costa Mesa, Calif.) also uses oscillometry. Mean pressure is determined from the cuff pressure giving maximum amplitude of the cuff pressure oscillations, whereas systolic and diastolic pressures are determined by an algorithm.

The Dinamap Model 1846 SX Adult/ Pediatric Vital Signs Monitor (Critikon Inc., Tampa, Fla.) also looks for two pulsations of relatively equal amplitude at each pressure step. If unable to find two pulsations within 1.6 seconds, the system lowers the cuff pressure another step. This system includes a "stat mode" in which artifact rejection is relaxed so that systolic pressure can be displayed as soon as it is determined.

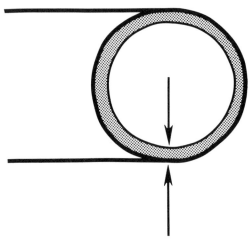

Figure 6–3. Distending pressure of artery wall. As long as pressure tending to expand artery exceeds pressures tending to collapse it, the artery remains open. At the point of "unloading," these two pressures are equal and the artery is on the verge of collapsing.

Several problems are common to all these automated systems:

- They may malfunction if a leak is present in the cuff or connections.

- They may function erratically in the presence of dysrhythmias (because they cannot find the required pulsations at the time periods expected).

- They are vulnerable to external jostling of the cuff, mistaking this for oscillometric pulsations.

- Inappropriately sized cuffs result in errors just as they do with manual measurements.

With automated devices that compress the artery, blood pressure measurements should not be repeated at close intervals (for example, every minute) for an extended time because nerve injury may result.

Penaz in 1969 presented the technique of continuously adjusting an applied cuff so that an underlying artery remains at a constant volume to allow continuous calculation of arterial blood pressure. This technique relies on the fact that the arterial diameter is a function of the distending pressure applied to the wall of the artery (Fig. 6–3). The distending pressure is equal to the internal pressure (that is, arterial blood pressure) minus the encircling pressure (from a cuff). As long as the distending pressure is positive or even zero, the artery remains patent and to a point its diameter (and hence internal volume) increases with increasing distending pressure. At zero distending pressure the artery is said to be unloaded. At some small negative pressure the artery buckles and collapses.

The commercial device (Finapres, Ohmeda) operates as follows: The system's first goal is to identify the amount of infrared light passed through the finger from a light-emitting diode (LED) at the point of unloading, just before collapse of the artery. A pneumatic bladder, controlled by a microprocessor, is placed around the proximal portion of the thumb or the middle portion of a finger. An infrared LED and photodetector are incorporated, on opposite sides of the thumb or finger, distal to the cuff. By stepwise inflation of the cuff and analysis of the resulting plethysmogram, the system can place the cuff pressure so that the artery collapses during part of the cardiac cycle. For example, the system may first raise the pressure above systolic and then decrease it, noting first the development of a short dip in transmission right at systole as the artery expands and blocks the light (Fig. 6–4). As the cuff pressure continues to decline slowly, the artery opens for longer periods surrounding the systolic peak. During diastole the artery collapses each time its internal pressure falls below that of the bladder, causing the transmitted infrared light to plateau at maximum. From these measurements the microprocessor can identify the percentage of light transmitted just as the artery is beginning to collapse. A control algorithm (proportional-integral-derivative type) then adjusts the bladder pressure moment by moment to maintain the artery just at the point of collapse. Thus the bladder pressure is continuously maintained exactly equal to the internal artery pressure.

Maintaining the precarious balance between cuff bladder pressure and internal artery pressure requires an electronic-pneumatic system with a high bandwidth (greater than 50 Hz), no overshoot, no steady state error, and little time delay (less than 10 ms).

Published testing of this device by comparisons with ipsilateral radial artery measurements has shown that when it works, it is essentially accurate within a few millimeters of mercury. The highest accuracy has been found by measuring the thumb with specially developed thumb cuffs; in this case the mean error for systolic was 4.81 mm Hg (reported value lower than correct) and for diastolic 1.49 mm Hg (reported value higher than correct). These errors may result from the tiny pressures required to maintain patency of the artery and establish forward flow. In 18% of the patients studied, however, the Finapress device was unable to find the correct pressure at some

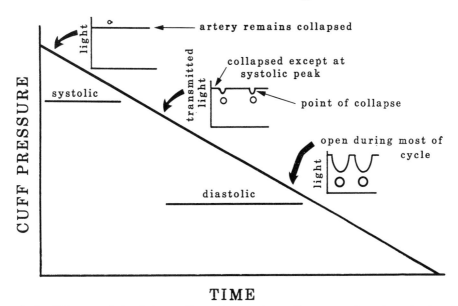

Figure 6–4. Light transmission during cardiac cycles at various cuff pressures allows determination of the exact amount of light transmitted when the artery is at the point of collapse. This measurement is needed to allow the Finapress to instantaneously control the cuff pressure to keep the artery at the same state.

point. A large number of these failures were probably secondary to the insertion of the radial arterial catheter required for the study and thus may not be real errors of the method. However, in patients receiving a vasoconstrictor drug and in 40% of patients undergoing intraoperative one-lung ventilation, the device gave wildly erroneous results. Thus the usefulness of the Finapress device may be limited in critically ill patients.

PRESSURE TRANSDUCERS AND INVASIVE MEASUREMENT OF VASCULAR PRESSURE

Invasive measurement of vascular pressures may be required in several ICU situations, especially when rapid and continuous updating of hemodynamic variables is required for moment-by-moment care of the patient. Some variables, such as central venous pressure or pulmonary artery pressure, are relatively difficult to measure noninvasively.

The first invasive measurement of arterial blood pressure was by the French physician Faivre, in the leg of an amputee. However, invasive measurement was not used clinically until 1947, after the discovery of heparin. The development of the modern catheter-over-needle intravenous access, which came much later, made easy percutaneous measurement of arterial pressures widely available.

Although fluid-filled manometer systems can measure invasive pressures, electronic transducers have allowed much greater frequency response, accuracy, and ease of use. The electronic transducer may use any of several methods to convert the pressure into an electronic signal. The pressure may deflect a mechanical spring or diaphragm (offering a dimensional movement as a function of applied pressure) to change inductance, capacitance, or resistance of a device. The resulting electrical change is then measured by its effect on an applied voltage or current.

The most common transducers in use today monitor changes in resistance. The movement of a diaphragm causes a narrow film of conducting material bonded to its surface to be stretched ("strain gauge"). This decreases the cross-sectional area of the conductor. The narrow film is connected as one of the legs of the traditional Wheatstone bridge circuit that allows electronic measurement of the pressure distending the diaphragm.

Earlier versions of these transducers were expensive (hundreds of dollars) and were thus equipped with sterile disposable protective diaphragms interposed between the actual strain gauge diaphragm and the fluid pressure to be measured. However, sterility was a continuing concern. Newer manufacturing techniques have made the price of disposable units competitive with the older devices when the costs of sterilization are considered. A bonus has been factory precalibration of the strain gauges (by such techniques as computer-controlled laser

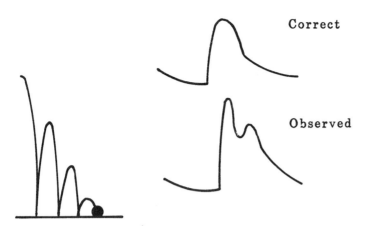

Correct

Observed

Figure 6–5. Second-order response of tennis balls and arterial line transducer systems. Just as the tennis ball bounces instead of merely falling to the floor and stopping, the arterial line measurement "bounces" when trying to follow the systolic pulse.

trimming of the film), which has made these disposable transducers far more convenient.

The most popular configurations involve voltage applied to the transducer, a fraction of which is returned for measurement to the electronic pressure module. Sensitivities have been somewhat standardized so that with appropriate cable and connector conversions, transducers from one manufacturer can be used with a wide range of monitoring equipment.

The frequency response of the transducer itself is typically better than 150 Hz, leaving the fluid connection to the patient's vasculature as the major culprit in the loss of fidelity of the pressure waveform. This mechanical system has inertia, elasticity, and resistance. The mass is that of the fluid within the tubing; the elasticity is the flexibility of the transducer diaphragm, any trapped air bubbles, and compliance in the tubing; the resistance is the friction of the fluid moving in the tubing with each new pulse.

The response of the transducer system to a systolic pulse may be compared to the bouncing of a tennis ball dropped on the floor, each bounce smaller and smaller until it reaches equilibrium (Fig. 6–5). The same sort of "ringing" can occur in the waveform of the system trying to follow a systolic pulse. Mathematically, it can be modeled as a second-order system, one with components related to the instantaneous position of a molecule in the fluid path, and to both its first (velocity) and second (acceleration) time derivatives. The magnitude of the inertia, elasticity, and resistance are reflected in the three coefficients of these three terms in the mathematical model. This type of analysis has allowed the performance of different transducer and fluid connection systems to be described in terms of a "critical frequency" (above which the response of the system takes a dramatic downward change) and a "damping coefficient" that describes whether the system overresponds or underresponds to sinusoidal pressure waves in the range of the critical frequency. Thus only two numbers must be known instead of three mechanical values. All systems of this type respond accurately to frequencies well below the critical frequency, may overshoot the correct response near the critical frequency, and respond poorly to frequencies much higher than the critical frequency (Fig. 6–6). Therefore a first rule of thumb is to purchase a system with the highest possible critical frequency.

If the critical frequency is much higher than any of the frequencies of the pressure waveform to be measured, as occurs with a Millar catheter tip transducer, the system responds accurately and the damping coefficient is unimportant.

Unfortunately, the use of tubing to allow the transducer to be mounted at a distance from the patient drastically lowers the critical frequency so that it overlaps the frequencies of the typical waveforms to be measured. A tradeoff is then required between better speed of response (resulting from a low damping coefficient, such as 0.2) and lack of overshoot (resulting from a higher damping coefficient, greater than 1.0). The optimal damping coefficient in clinical systems may be approximately 0.7. Critical frequency of a typical system declines from 33 Hz (cycles per second) with a 6-inch length of tubing to 6.45 Hz with 5 feet of tubing. Measured damping coefficients are between 0.1 and 0.3, resulting in an average systolic error of 16%.

The difficulty of the problem can vary. The frequency response required differs depending on the vascular location to be monitored. In the arterial tree, left ventricle and proximal aorta waveforms have lower frequency content and are therefore more easily accurately measured than brachial or radial arterial waveforms. In general, the farther along the arterial tree, the

Figure 6–6. The response of a second-order system changes dramatically to signals at or beyond the critical frequency. A variable frequency fluid pressure generator is connected to an arterial pressure-monitoring system, and the resulting trace is recorded while applied sinusoidal frequency is increased. With constant actual fluid amplitude, the system begins to exaggerate waveform as frequency approaches critical frequency; beyond this, the response falls off dramatically. This system is adequate for most clinical uses. (From Gravenstein JS, Paulus DA: Clinical monitoring practice, ed 2. Philadelphia, 1987, JB Lippincott Co.)

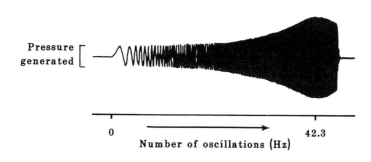

greater the frequency response of the system required for accuracy. Although not as high in frequency content as brachial or radial waveforms, the left atrium has a higher frequency content than the left ventricle and is thus more difficult to accurately measure.

Thus the typical clinical situation of radial artery pressure measured by a transducer mounted 48 inches from the artery represents the highest frequency signal monitored by a less than optimal system. Noncompliant tubing is essential, and reducing the tubing length by mounting the transducer on the patient results in greater accuracy. The clinician can objectively evaluate the performance of a system by performing the "fast flush" test advocated by Gardner: A very short flush is performed during diastole (which is quite easy with current continuous flow/press-to-flush systems) and the continuous pressure oscillation response is observed. Ideally, at the end of the flush spike the pressure quickly decays back to the arterial waveform pressure without ringing – a response seldom observed. If ringing is present, the critical frequency can be measured by inverting the period of one oscillation. Measuring the

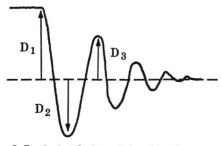

Figure 6–7. In the "flush test," the critical frequency of an arterial line transducer system can be found from the period of one oscillation, while the ratio of peak height from one oscillation to the previous (for example, D3/D2) allows calculation of the damping coefficient. (From Gravenstein JS, Paulus DA: Clinical monitoring practice, ed 2. Philadelphia, 1987, JB Lippincott Co.)

ratio of one peak to the previous peak in the opposite direction (Fig. 6–7) gives a ratio that can be converted (Fig. 6–8) into the damping coefficient. The worst response is many cycles of slow ringing. This indicates an underdamped, low-frequency response system. The clinician should then remove all air bubbles, use shorter, stiff tubing, and repeat the tests.

CARDIAC OUTPUT

The most historical method of measuring cardiac output is the Fick method, developed in 1870. The theory behind the method is simple. By conservation of mass, the rate of uptake to an area (from the outside) of any substance is equal to the outflow of the substance from the area minus its inflow to that area.

$$dV/dt = (Q_{out} \cdot C_{out}) - (Q_{in} \cdot C_{in}) \qquad (1)$$

where

dV/dt = Rate of uptake of any measurable substance
Q_{out} = Rate of blood flow out of area of interest
Q_{in} = Rate of blood flow into area of interest
C_{out} = Concentration of substance in outflow
C_{in} = Concentration of substance in inflow

Integrating over time and assuming the outflow equals the inflow (true for the heart over reasonably long periods),

$$Q = \frac{\text{Total uptake of substance}}{C_{out} - C_{in}} \qquad (2)$$

In clinical practice the substance measured may be oxygen and the area of interest is the heart plus lung. The output concentration is the arterial concentration of oxygen, and the input concentration is the mixed venous concentration; the uptake of oxygen may be measured by volume change in a supply

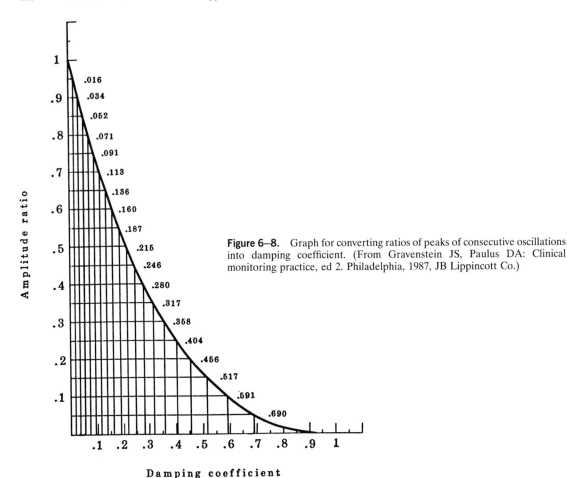

Figure 6–8. Graph for converting ratios of peaks of consecutive oscillations into damping coefficient. (From Gravenstein JS, Paulus DA: Clinical monitoring practice, ed 2. Philadelphia, 1987, JB Lippincott Co.)

container. Thus measuring arterial and mixed venous oxygenation and measuring the gaseous oxygen uptake over a time period make it possible to calculate the average cardiac output easily.

When applied with ideal conditions, measurements of cardiac output by the Fick method are within 4% of the "true value" 95% of the time. However, the following requirements must be met:

- Absolute equality between rate of oxygen uptake measured from inspired/expired (I/E) air ratio and transfer rate of oxygen transfer in pulmonary capillaries
- Arterial oxygen saturation (SaO_2) and arterial partial pressure of oxygen (PaO_2) must be constant
- No significant changes in right and left ventricle outputs
- No cardiac, pulmonary, or hepatopulmonary shunts
- Technical precision of blood and gas analysis

The obvious disadvantages of the method involve:

- The requirement for relative stability of the patient (precluding its use in rapidly changing situations)
- The complexity required to make extremely accurate volumetric measurements of the amount of oxygen taken up by the patient
- The requirement of invasive blood measurements

The indicator dilution method (Fig. 6–9) is probably the most commonly used in ICUs because of the development of the thermistor-equipped Swan-Ganz catheter. The method is simply an extension of the Fick method. A known uptake of a cold substance is determined by injection into the right atrium; the inflow of cold otherwise from the body is zero, and the outflow from the right ventricle is measured by a thermistor. All the elements of the Fick equation are then provided. The thermistor measures the time curve of the decrease in

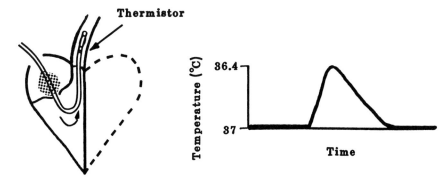

Figure 6–9. Indicator dilution method most commonly used for clinical cardiac output measurement. A bolus of cold fluid injected at "input" of the heart is sensed as a moving wave of cold by a thermistor placed distally. (From Gravenstein JS, Paulus DA: Clinical monitoring practice, ed 2. Philadelphia, 1987, JB Lippincott Co.)

downstream temperature brought about by a known injection of cool saline. With greater cardiac output the dip in temperature flows more quickly past the thermistor, and with lower cardiac output its passage is more prolonged. From these measurements,

$$\text{Cardiac output} = \frac{\text{Amount of indicator added}}{\text{Integral of concentration over time}} \quad (3)$$

The theoretical requirements for accuracy are as follows:

- Instantaneous injection
- Small volume of indicator
- Rapid and complete mixing of indicator
- No loss of indicator
- Single channel at some part of the system
- Uniformity of volume flow
- No change in volume
- Constant distribution of indicator traversal times
- Equal distribution of traversal times for indicator and blood
- Representative sample curve
- Lack of recirculation in sample curve
- Lack of concentration distortion or time smearing in measurement methods

With all these caveats the representative accuracy of the method when dye is used is thought to be less than 6% error in 95% of measurements, but when cold injectate is used, the variability may range from 1.6% to 12.3%, depending on circumstances.

Suggested causes of poor accuracy of temperature dilution measurements include poor signal/noise ratio caused by inadequately cold solution, poor mixing of the solution or changes in the blood pressure, changes in heart rate during measurement, and contact between the thermistor and the vessel wall, which prevents the thermistor from responding well to the blood temperature. This last problem has been decreased by placing the thermistor a few centimeters back from the tip of the catheter. Also, the injection must be made in less than 4 seconds. Most users average several measurements made at the same phase of respiration (usually end expiration) and may throw out earlier values before averaging.

One of the best-known noninvasive techniques for measuring cardiac output is impedance cardiography. This technique was conceived as early as 1930 but first received widespread interest in the late 1960s as a monitoring technique during the Apollo space flight. It is still not completely understood. The impedance (the generalized alternating current equivalent of direct current resistance) of the thorax, measured cephalad to caudad, depends on the conductors within the thorax. Air does not appreciably conduct, whereas the blood in the heart and great vessels does. Thus, as these volumes change during the cardiac cycle, the thoracic impedance also changes. In practice, a tiny current at a high frequency is injected by an outer pair of contacts to the neck and abdomen, and the resultant voltage drop is measured by an inner pair of electrodes. Because of this configuration and the use of high-impedance amplification, the measurement is relatively robust against changes in electrode-skin resistance. Equations have been developed to calculate the stroke volume from the resulting phasic changes in thoracic impedance that are superimposed on larger changes related to lung expansion during breathing. One example is the Nyboer equation:

$$\text{Stroke volume} = \frac{\rho \times L^2 \times \Delta Z}{Zo^2} \quad (4)$$

where

ρ = Specific resistivity of blood
L = Length in centimeters between sensing electrodes
Zo = Basal impedance measured
ΔZ = Pulsatile impedance component

Variations of this formula have included the derivative of the impedance change with respect to time. Typical correlation coefficients of 0.7 to 0.8 were found when the technique was compared with thermodilution values in a cardiac catheterization laboratory. When the NCCOM-3 commercial bioimpedance cardiac output measurement device (Bomed Medical Mfg., Irvine, Calif.) was used, a correlation coefficient of 0.65 was found in patients shortly after bypass surgery. However, tachycardia of greater than 120 beats/min is associated with a decrease in the correlation coefficient (to 0.60). These devices have a place in the noninvasive measurement of an important variable, but they have not achieved sufficient accuracy to make them first-line measurement instruments.

Ultrasound has been used in two ways to measure cardiac output noninvasively. Transesophageal echocardiography with Doppler can be used to image the mitral valve, measure its area (usually taken at maximal opening), and measure the velocity profile of blood passing through it. Integrating the flow measurements and multiplying by the area gives a measurement of cardiac output. This technique when compared with thermodilution has a correlation coefficient of 0.68, with a standard error of the estimate of 0.92 L/min. It tends to overestimate the cardiac output, perhaps because of the use of the maximal value area measurement.

A commercial device has been developed in which a Doppler probe on the tip of a probe is introduced as an orogastric tube and directed at the descending aorta by listening to the Doppler sounds. The theory is that the Doppler flow measurements in the descending aorta reflect cardiac output after the device is initially calibrated with a suprasternal probe directed at the ascending aorta. The descending aortic blood flow is a constant (k factor) of the initial stroke volume after the loss to the head and arms. Studies comparing this device with thermodilution have given correlation coefficients of 0.65 to 0.74, declining considerably with increased pulse rates.

Finally, for intubated patients, a newly developed device with a Doppler probe on the end of the endotracheal tube measures both the aortic diameter (thus possibly avoiding the significant sources of error in earlier machines) and the aortic flow in the ascending aorta. Data are not yet available on the performance of this semi-invasive device.

GASEOUS OXYGEN ANALYZERS

When patients are administered a gas mixture different from room air, the amount of oxygen in the inspired gases must be measured. At least four techniques are used clinically for this purpose, including oxygen electrodes, mass spectrometry, paramagnetic analyzers, and Raman scattering.

Polarographic analyzers, a version of oxygen electrode analyzers, may be the most common technique. A platinum cathode is separated from a silver anode in an electrolyte with a battery or other source of approximately 0.7 V connected between the two electrodes. In the presence of oxygen the following reaction proceeds:

$$O_2 + 2\ H_2O + 4\ e^- \rightarrow 4\ OH^- \qquad (5)$$

resulting in a flow of current in the circuit.

Clark's addition of a thin membrane (such as polyethylene or Teflon) separating the cathode from the oxygen to be measured caused the current to be related to the oxygen partial pressure (Po_2), separated the electrolyte from the gases, and made faster measurements possible. However, the accuracy of polarographic analyzers may be influenced by the presence of nitrous oxide or halothane, an effect the designer can minimize by carefully selecting polarization voltage and using a Teflon membrane. The response time of these devices is usually measured in tens of seconds. Batteries must be checked periodically if used, and the measurement cell must be replaced periodically.

Galvanic analyzers ("fuel cells") act as batteries, developing a voltage proportional to the oxygen tension. The accuracy of the analyzer is good, but response time is still relatively slow. These devices are not affected by nitrous oxide. Some brands give erroneous measurements in the presence of helium.

An unusual type of oxygen electrode analyzer is the solid electrolyte fuel cell, which consists of a cylinder of calcia-zirconia with porous platinum electrodes attached, maintained at 750° C. At these high temperatures the calcia-zirconia acts as an electrolytic conductor of oxygen ions. A commercial device exhibits extreme accuracy (0.01%) and extraordinary speed (90% of a step change is observed within 100 ms). The cell does not require replacement as frequently as polarographic or galvanic sensors.

Mass spectrometers are expensive ($20,000 to $100,000) pieces of equipment that accurately measure multiple gas concentrations by ionizing gas molecules in a high vacuum and then observing their endpoint in a trajectory within a magnetic field. The ratio of charge to mass determines which of several electronic collectors records a current produced by a certain gas. Typically, both helium and the propellants used in aerosolized beta-agonist inhalants for asthmatics impair the accuracy of the mass spectrometer. A specialized ion source may allow the unit to function in the presence of helium.

Paramagnetic oxygen analyzers are based on oxygen's attraction by a magnetic field. The Pauling oxygen analyzer included a glass dumbbell suspended in a magnetic field, whose position was affected by changes in Po_2. With more rugged design, the Datex PB254 anesthetic gas monitor (Datex Div., Instrumentarium OY, Helsinki, Finland) uses a small modular paramagnetic oxygen sensor that operates with a rise time measured in hundreds of milliseconds (although, because of the design of this sidestream analyzer, the analyzer lags the airway gases by several seconds).

Raman scattering has been used in research laboratories for 50 years but has become practical for clinical use only recently because of the availability of cheap laser sources and computers. An argon laser floods the gas sample with monochromatic light that interacts with the molecules of the gases present. Although the majority of the photons are transmitted or scattered, a few contribute energy to individual gas molecules with the result that a lower-energy, lower-frequency photon is scattered. Gratings and photon counters are used to achieve accurate counts of the shifted-frequency photons at each frequency that is specific for each gas in the sample. The results are reported as the partial pressure of each gas present. Commercial units are competitive in price with dedicated mass spectrometers, can calibrate from long-lasting internal argon gas sources and room air, and can identify all clinically useful gases. In addition, the commercial units perform well in the presence of helium.

TRANSCUTANEOUS OXYGEN MEASUREMENT

Transcutaneous oxygen measurement offers a noninvasive method of continuously measuring skin oxygen tension. The measurement is made by using miniaturized versions of the original Clark polarographic electrodes used for gaseous measurement of oxygen. The major differences in the construction of electrodes designed for transcutaneous use are that they are:

- Smaller
- Designed to be applied to the skin surface
- Heated to 43° to 45° C
- Equipped with a smaller reservoir for the electrolyte
- Designed to use an electrolyte base with a low vapor pressure (such as ethylene glycol) to make the electrolyte last longer

The membrane separating the electrolyte and electrodes from the skin must be permeable to oxygen. The sensor reads the tissue oxygenation at the point of application. The stratum corneum of the skin, through which the oxygen must diffuse outward to the applied sensor, is made up of keratin filaments that are in lipid and protein. Heating this material vastly improves the diffusion of oxygen; above 41° C the crystalline structure of the stratum corneum disappears, a process thought to allow oxygen to diffuse outward 100 to 1000 times faster.

Because of the different skin consistencies, the transcutaneous monitor works best in neonates, whose percutaneous measurement is ±10% of the arterial value. The ratio of percutaneous Po_2 to arterial Po_2 declines in the pediatric age group and in adults when the electrode is heated to only 42° C, and the ratio reaches an average of 34.7%. However, the trend given by the instrument can be followed for as long as 24 hours (although calibration every 8 to 12 hours is suggested). In general, the sensor functions best when used to measure Pao_2 in the very young. In the older population it has been shown to measure skin oxygen tension rather than arterial; as such it is a general indicator of peripheral perfusion and may rise and fall with the status of the critically ill patient.

In practical use, 43° C heating can be used with premature infants and the location can be changed every 2 hours. With children and adults a temperature of 44° to 44.5° C can be used for up to 8 hours, with an incidence of minor skin burns of less than 1%.

TRANSCUTANEOUS CARBON DIOXIDE MEASUREMENT

An electrode for the measurement of carbon dioxide pressure (Pco_2) was developed in 1957 by Stow. It was based on the pH electrode, which used an electrode in an acidic buffer solution separated from the test solution by a very thin glass bulb, permeable to hydrated hydrogen ions. Stow's modification was to enclose the glass bulb of the pH electrode with a rubber membrane permeable to CO_2. This measurement tool was improved by several investigators, most notably Severinghaus and Bradley. In 1973 Huch reported forming this electrode into a heated type for transcutaneous measurement of Pco_2, similar to the development of the transcutaneous Po_2 sensor. The transcutaneously measured values are always higher than those of the arterial blood. Reasons for this are that the tissue Pco_2 is usually higher than the Pco_2 of the blood perfusing it and that the heating of the tissue required increases the metabolic activity and thus the tissue Pco_2. Two formulas have been proposed to deal with the differences; in one the measured value is divided by 1.37 and then reduced by 4 mm Hg further; in the other the measured value is simply divided by 1.61. Comparison between transcutaneous Pco_2 values corrected by the second method and arterial values in adults has yielded a correlation coefficient of 0.87. Accuracy is similar to measurements of end-tidal CO_2.

MIXED VENOUS OXIMETRY

Mixed venous oxygen saturation can be measured in blood samples obtained from the pulmonary artery. It gives a crude guide to the oxygen reserve and cardiac output of the cardiovascular system. With constant arterial oxygenation and oxygen consumption, mixed venous oxygen saturation varies directly with cardiac output. An elevated mixed venous oxygen saturation may be noted in left-to-right shunt or in conditions of damaged cellular respiration, such as sepsis or cyanide poisoning (as may occur with nitroprusside administration). However, drawing multiple blood samples for measurement is time consuming and expensive and gives only discontinuous information.

Therefore a type of Swan-Ganz catheter was developed with two fiberoptic filaments running to the tip. In a commercial version (Oximetrix, Inc., Mountain View, Calif.) three different wavelengths of light from LEDs enter one filament and are carried through the catheter to illuminate the pulmonary artery blood flowing past the tip. The different light wavelengths are sequenced at 244 times per second. The reflected light is carried back to the measurement head by the second fiberoptic filament. The use of three wavelengths allows sufficient information to remove the effect of hemoglobin concentration from the measurement of oxygen concentration.

The catheter system allows continuous measurement of the mixed venous saturation in the pulmonary artery. Calibration is accomplished either in vivo by comparing separately analyzed blood samples or in vitro by inserting the tip into a sterile calibration cap with a known reflective surface.

Potential difficulties with this system include the following:

- Damage to the fiberoptics by excessive bending of the catheter, which causes low light return
- Excessive light return caused by transient positioning of the catheter tip against a vessel wall
- Obstruction of the fiberoptics by the development of small clots over the tip
- Spontaneous wedging of the catheter, which causes the system to read the saturation of pulmonary venous rather than arterial blood.

RESPIROMETERS

A wide variety of noninvasive methods are used to detect respiration. The simplest technique is to place belts around the thorax and electronically measure the stretch with respiration. A commercial example of such a monitor, the Monitron System (American Health Products, Orange, Calif.), also monitors the electrocardiogram (EKG) with pads attached to the belt and provides telemetric data and even alarms. Other devices have evaluated the respiratory changes in impedance across the chest with tiny injected currents. Thermistors have been placed in the airstream to detect the movement of air, and at least one commercially available instrument aspirates and detects carbon dioxide in the patient's facial area.

In general, airway monitoring of carbon dioxide and pulse oximetry have been used rather than these techniques, except in the home infant apnea monitor, but the recent interest in epidural narcotics may spur further developments.

SPIROMETERS

Spirometers allow measurement of the flow of gas in or out of the patient's lungs. In the most common type, spinning vanes moved by airflow are mechanically connected to a dial. The Wright spirometer has an accuracy of $\pm 5\%$ at relatively high flow rates. At low flow rates the vanes may not move because of inertia and mechanical resistance, and secretions may reduce accuracy. At high flow rates inertia may cause overreadings. The Ohmeda Model 5410 and 5420 volume monitors use a flat, thin spinning rotor (with low inertia) placed in the rotating gas flow created by curved vanes proximal and distal to the rotor. The rotation of the rotor is measured by counting the times the rotor interrupts two light beams produced by a clip-on measurement module that also heats the expendable inline rotor assembly to reduce condensation. This system has the advantages that all moving parts can be seen at all times and the rotor-stator cartridge can be easily changed if necessary. The Model 5410 volume monitor also has the ability to measure and display forced vital capacity, forced expiratory volume, and peak flow.

Alternative systems include ultrasonic detectors using a vortex, such as the Bourns LS-75 (Bear Medical Systems, Inc., Riverside, Calif.), and the simpler volume displacement systems with a bellows assembly that traps the gas to be measured.

Pneumotachometers are widely used to make flow measurements. Partial obstruction with a screen, heated mesh, fixed orifice, or Pitot tube creates a known resistance in the airway. Measurement of the pressure differential caused by flow through the tubing can be converted to an indication of the flow, although the conversion may be highly nonlinear. Integration (perhaps by a small built-in microprocessor system) yields volume measurements. Because the resistance is highly dependent on the gas characteristics, these systems are sensitive to changes in gas composition and density, as well as humidity and pressure. An error of up to 10% may occur because of the change from 21% to 100% oxygen.

TEMPERATURE MEASUREMENT

Temperature is one of the easier physiologic variables to measure. Two major temperature measurement techniques are in wide use. The first is the thermistor, a device whose resistance changes with temperature and can be indicated on a meter. Typical thermistors are made of semiconductors, substances whose electrical resistance is intermediate between that of conductors (metals) and insulators (such as glass). Metals slightly increase their resistance with an increase in temperature, but the resistance change in a semiconductor is many times that of a metal, which makes a sensitive system easier to develop. Semiconductor oxides, such as nickel oxide, manganese oxide, or cobalt oxide, are sintered into small packages, and electrical leads are attached. Combinations of thermistors and fixed resistors in series and parallel are used in older equipment to cancel out the nonlinearities in the thermal response. In newer equipment a linearizing equation may be stored in the microprocessor memory or a "look-up table" used by the microprocessor to change the measured resistance into the correct temperature. Thermistors may be made small enough to fit onto the pulmonary artery catheter; smaller thermistors can respond quickly to changes in temperature during a single cardiac cycle.

The other major temperature measurement technique is the thermocouple. The atomic difference between two metals causes development of a temperature-dependent voltage when they are twisted or connected together. Component metals are selected to maximize the potential developed, which is on the order of millivolts.

Thermistors and thermocouples can be heated by the very currents they carry, which interferes with their ability to measure. Modern designs avoid these effects by passing only small currents through the sensing device. Drift with age of the device can be a problem, but damage to the sensor wiring is more common. Both thermistors and thermocouples must be adequately insulated to protect the patient, particularly if the sensor is to be intracardiac (where 10 μA leakage current may cause ventricular fibrillation), but excessive insulation slows the response.

A recent development of microthermocouples allows accurate measurement of the temperature of any object via the characteristic infrared radiation resulting from its temperature. The infrared heats the microthermocouples aimed at the object. This technique has been used to produce a device that can measure skin or tympanic membrane temperature with excellent speed, accuracy, and resolution.

ELECTROCARDIOGRAPHY

The EKG is a signal representing the sum of countless individual action potentials in the myocardium. The individual cell maintains a resting potential of -60 to -90 mV by preserving transmembrane concentration gradients of sodium, potassium, chloride, and calcium. During an action potential, permeability to sodium and then permeability to calcium increase suddenly, generating a transmembrane change of as much as 100 mV. However, the "far field" (meaning a distance large with respect to the size of individual cells) summation of these individual changes reflects cancellation effects of potentials oriented in different directions, as well as resistive shunting and a resultant decrease in the signals. The clinically used leads are attempts at detecting specifically directed components of the EKG signal. The limb leads detect components in the coronal plane of the body at various angles. The unipolar V leads detect components directed anteriorly from the chest by placement of the "positive" lead at various points on the chest and use of a combination of the limb leads as the reference lead.

Developing a usable display of the signal requires sophisticated amplification. Even with optimal lead selection to maximize the EKG voltage available to the monitoring equipment, the voltage is on the order of 1 mV. However, standard U.S. line voltage is 120 V (AC), which is 120,000 times greater, and this voltage is often capacitively and inductively coupled through the air into the EKG electrode wiring. Thus 60-cycle interference is one of the most common problems in accurately recovering and viewing the EKG. To succeed, the EKG equipment must meet the following requirements:

- Adequate amplification ("gain") to make the millivolt signal visible on the oscilloscope or strip chart
- Faithful reproduction of the true EKG signal
- Ability to reject outside interference

The EKG amplifier is built with several characteristics to meet these requirements. It has multiple stages of amplification to multiply the signal sufficiently. Through either the effect of feedback or the use of devices with inherent input insulation (such as MOSFET transistors and, oddly enough, the older vacuum tube) it is built to have a high input impedance. That is, the 1 mV signal applied to it causes only a small current to flow into the amplifier, which is another way of saying that the amplifier does not load down the EKG signal appreciably.

The ability of the EKG amplifier circuitry to reproduce the signal faithfully is quantified in terms of the frequency and phase response of the amplifier. The frequency response refers to how the amplifier responds to sine wave signals of varying frequencies. The EKG signal itself contains frequencies from approximately 0.5 Hz to perhaps 75 Hz. To amplify such a signal properly, the EKG amplifier must have nearly identical gains ("flat response") to all frequencies from 0.5 Hz to 75 Hz. Discrepancies from the ideal are measured in decibels, a logarithmic measure of the ratio of the measured performance to the ideal performance. The American Heart Association requirements state that the gain of the amplifier must be flat to within 0.5 dB from 0.14 Hz to 50 Hz and that the response at 0.05 Hz must not be more than 3 dB down than that at 0.14 Hz.

In recent years it has become evident that in addition to amplifying all these frequencies identically, the amplifier must not delay any of them compared with the rest. This is expressed in specifications as phase linearity. A linear phase response with frequency is identical to a constant time lag for signals of all frequencies. Because different portions of the EKG signal have inherently different frequencies (the sharp QRS complex has a much higher frequency than the long ST segment), it is important that all frequencies have the same total time delay through the entire amplifier of the EKG machine, or odd smearing and changes may result. Typical filters used in EKG machines to restrict the lower frequency response, in an attempt to reduce respiratory or electrocautery interference, may introduce phase nonlinearities and severely change the time delays applied to some frequencies. This results in artifactually abnormal ST segments, typically misinterpreted as ischemic changes. Therefore a primary requirement before use of any EKG machine to analyze a patient's ST segments is to verify that the frequency response of the system meets the American Heart Association requirements given previously and that the system has (perhaps within 6% of ideal) a linear phase response between 0.5 and 50 Hz.

To reject the inductively coupled 60-cycle signals that are one of the largest interference signals, the EKG equipment takes advantage of the fact that the interference is likely to add a nearly identical interference voltage to each wire attached to the patient (at least as long as the wires are reasonably close to one another). Amplifiers that respond far more to differences in the voltages of the different wires than to the (common) interference signal present on all the wires are used. These amplifiers are said to have a high common mode rejection ratio.

Finally, to protect the patient, the amplifier must not inject any appreciable electrical current into the patient. This requirement is often met by isolating the first stage of the amplifier from the remainder by optical or transformer coupling.

A typical commercially available EKG instrument is the Datascope 2000A (Datascope Corp., Paramus, N.J.). Its frequency response is measured from the lower and higher frequencies where the amplification falls to 0.707 of the optimum, or midfrequency amplification; these are known as 3 db bandwidth measurements. Although the frequency response of the EKG amplifiers to the rear panel diagnostic output jack is 0.05 to 150 Hz, the frequency response of the signal displayed on the cathode ray tube is only 0.5 to 40 Hz; with an electrocautery filter installed, the frequency response is 0.5 to 25 Hz. The relatively high lower frequency cutoffs improve the rejection of respiratory and other low-frequency artifacts but raise concern over the phase linearity that is not specified.

EKG equipment is typically equipped with an audible signal to indicate each QRS complex. If so, the equipment must be equipped with an algorithm (as in the Datascope 2000A) to avoid erroneously detecting both QRS and T waves. In addition, some provision must be made to avoid counting the typical sharp, fast pacer spike as a QRS complex.

Automated measurement of ST segment changes is a valuable asset in detecting ischemia. It is now available as an algorithm on commercial EKG machines. In one system, the Marquette Series 7000 Monitor (Marquette Electronics Inc., Milwaukee, Wis.), the reference point is set 40 ms before the QRS onset and the ST segment's voltage is measured 80 ms after the QRS.

ECHOCARDIOGRAPHY

Ultrasound echocardiography offers the ability to visualize, in real time and without any risk from radiation, the beating heart with sufficient clarity to make diagnoses previously possible only in a catheterization laboratory. Furthermore, all of this can be done at the bedside. Despite the high cost of this monitor (currently $100,000 to $200,000), its advantages indicate that it will become increasingly important in the care of ICU patients.

Ultrasound is a sound wave (that is, a vibrational wave requiring a medium) as distinct from an electromagnetic wave (which propagates even in a vacuum). The waves used in diagnostic medicine have frequencies in the megahertz range. Higher frequencies (with smaller wavelengths on the order of fractions of a millimeter) offer greater resolution, whereas lower frequencies have lower attenuation and thus better penetration into body structures. Ultrasound waves are generated by electronic oscillators similar to radio transmitters but are connected to piezoelectric transducers instead of antennae. The piezoelectric transducers convert the electronic oscillations into sound vibrations. The transmission of sound waves through the body is affected by attenuation, scattering, and reflection, which occur at interfaces between structures of differing acoustic impedance. It requires some adjustment at first to realize the returning echoes are generated by *interfaces* between areas of different acoustic impedance, unlike x-ray images, which show *volumes* of different density. At some interfaces (such as tissue to air) the reflection is almost total and thus structures beyond air interfaces cannot be visualized. To avoid this problem, the interface between the transducer and the patient is a jelly that allows good passage of the sound waves and easy movement of the transducer over the skin surface.

Whereas earlier devices allowed only an "ice pick" view of the varying acoustical impedances encountered by the sonarlike repetitive ultrasound pulses, newer systems present two-dimensional views that are far more understandable. By use of either mechanical rotation or electrical phased arrays of many transducers, the ultrasound beam is repetitively steered in a quadrant, and the resulting image is displayed on a screen, appearing similar to a slice from a CT scanner. Orienting the transducer in different directions allows the slice to show any desired region. By keeping in mind that the echoes viewed are caused by reflections, the viewer recognizes that the left ventricle appears as circular echoes from the endocardial wall and epicardial wall, and a variably dense region representing the wall itself. The papillary muscles in the left ventricle in the short axis view help orient the viewer. The motion of the ventricle is obvious on the two-dimensional monitor. Signals from the transesophageal probes may be even clearer than signals from a precordial probe.

The resolution of the two-dimensional image is on the order of 1 to 2 mm. Because ultrasound, like laser light, is coherent (all waves are in exact step), it suffers from a speckle quality on the image, similar to that seen with laser beams. Other limitations to image resolution are transducer reverberation artifacts, acoustic shadowing (behind ribs), and sidelobes of the transducer beam (which has some sensitivity at angles other than the desired one). The thickness of the slice visualized may be on the order of several millimeters.

Echocardiography detects ischemia by regional changes in contraction of the ventricular wall during systole. It is considered the most sensitive indicator of ischemia. It may also find use in evaluating the care of patients after myocardial infarction. Treatment plans eventually may be based on end-diastolic ventricular volume, evaluated by echo rather than by the more indirect measurement of pressure.

A major advance would be the development of automated systems to evaluate the size and regional contractility of the ventricle continuously from echo images. Several groups have developed "edge detection" algorithms that can electronically determine the position of the ventricular wall, making electronic comparisons across time possible. However, these systems have been far too slow for clinical use and require sensitive adjustment. Further developments are needed in this area.

SUGGESTED READINGS

Invasive and Noninvasive Blood Pressure Measurement

Blitt CD: Monitoring in anesthesia and critical care medicine. New York, 1985, Churchill Livingstone

Boehmer RD: Continuous, real-time, noninvasive monitor of blood pressure: Penaz methodology applied to the finger. J Clin Monit 1987;3:272-287

Gardner RM: Direct blood pressure measurement—dynamic response requirements. Anesthesiology 1981; 54:227-236

Geddes LA: The direct and indirect measurement of blood pressure. Chicago, 1970, Year Book Medical Publishers

Cardiac Output Measurements

Gravenstein JS, Paulus DA: Clinical monitoring practice, ed 2. Philadelphia, 1987, JB Lippincott Co.

Taylor SH, Solke B: Is the measurement of cardiac output useful in clinical practice? Br J Anaesth 1988;60:90S-98S

Gas Mixture and Transcutaneous Gas Tension Measurements

Sergejev IP: Monitoring of respiratory function during anesthesia. Int Anesthesiol Clin 1981;19:31-59

Westenskow DR, Coleman DL: Can the Raman scattering analyzer compete with mass spectrometers: an affirmative reply. J Clin Monit 1989;5:34-36

Tremper KK: Transcutaneous Po_2 measurement. Can Anesth Soc J 1984;31(6):664-677

Electrocardiography

Lambert CR, Imperi GA, Pepine CJ. Low-frequency requirement for recording ischemic ST-segment abnormalities in coronary artery disease. Am J Cardiol 1986;58:225-229

Taylor DI, Vincent R: Artefactual ST segment abnormalities due to electrocardiograph design. Br Heart J 1985;54:121-128

Echocardiography

De Bruijn NP, Clements FM: Transesophageal echocardiography. Norwell, MA, 1987, Martinus Nijhoff Publishing

7

CLINICAL AND TECHNICAL ISSUES IN PULSE OXIMETRY AND CAPNOMETRY

DAVID B. SWEDLOW, MD, AND SHARON M. IRVING

SAFETY MONITORING IN CRITICAL CARE

Many critical care practitioners believe that no serious safety problem exists in critical care. If a previously healthy patient experiences an accident during anesthesia, there is a cry of outrage. In the critical care unit, however, the patient is already critically ill and assumed to be at great risk; an injury or death is thought to be attributable primarily to the patient's illness, rather than to a preventable accident.

In fact, the practice of critical care is fairly safe. However, mishaps do occur, sometimes with devastating results. An early quantitative study by Osborn of critical care risk explored factors leading to sudden unexplained arrhythmia in postthoracotomy patients. Over a 16-month period, adequate records were obtained for 150 patients, representing 320 patient days. Sixteen potentially serious respiratory abnormalities were discovered, 11 of which were associated with life-threatening arrhythmias. In each case the house officer or nurse gave a similar story: "The patient was doing well and it just happened all of a sudden without warning." These data suggest that about 10% of the patients in a critical care unit may have some form of respiratory accident, and more than two thirds of these accidents may result in serious cardiac arrhythmias. Significantly, in all patients in this study the relationship between the cardiac arrhythmia and the preceding respiratory difficulty was not recognized by the health care professionals on the scene.

Two recent advances in safety-monitoring technology address preventable causes of patient injury in the critical care unit: pulse oximetry, which measures patient oxygenation, and capnography, which assesses ventilation. The clinical utility of oximetry and capnography are reviewed elsewhere.

Safety monitoring using pulse oximetry and capnography is now a published standard of care. Professional societies concerned with the quality of medical care and patient safety have embraced these safety monitors in routine care. In October 1986 the American Society of Anesthesiologists promulgated monitoring standards that call for continual monitoring of patient oxygenation and ventilation and in 1989 mandated the use of pulse oximetry and capnometry for all patients. The Society of Critical Care Medicine published monitoring guidelines for critical care units in 1988. These guidelines call for pulse oximetry or transcutaneous monitoring of the partial pressure of oxygen ($Ptco_2$) for all patients receiving supplemental oxygen, and they call for all units to provide capnography. Several states mandate the use of pulse oximetry and capnography during anesthesia. In 1988 the Joint Commission on Accreditation of Hospitals issued guidelines requiring that the same monitoring standards be used in the operating room and whenever patients receive sedation or analgesia capable of interfering with airway-protective reflexes.

Choosing a Safety Monitor

Accidental hypoxia is a major accompaniment of preventable disaster in critical care. Hypoxia often results from the failure to provide adequate ventilation. To minimize preventable injury, which physiologic variable should be monitored—oxygenation via pulse oximetry or ventilation via capnography?

TABLE 7–1. Critical Events Initially Detectable by Pulse Oximetry, Capnography, or Both

CONDITION	OXIMETRY	CAPNOGRAPHY
Hypoxic gas mixture	Yes	No
Severe atelectasis	Yes	No
Inadequate positive end-expiratory pressure therapy in adult respiratory distress syndrome	Yes	No
Bronchial intubation	Yes	Maybe
Bronchospasm	Yes	Yes
Cardiac arrest	Yes	Yes
Large pulmonary embolus	Yes	Yes
Malignant hyperthermia	Maybe	Yes
Laryngospasm	Maybe	Yes
Partial airway obstruction	Maybe	Yes
Esophageal intubation	Delayed	Yes
Complete airway disconnection	Delayed	Yes
Accidental extubation	Delayed	Yes
Breathing circuit leaks	Delayed	Yes
Partial rebreathing	No	Yes
Moderate hypoventilation	No	Yes

On the surface, oxygen saturation seems an ideal safety-related variable to monitor, since virtually all patients experience hypoxemia before irreversible injury, regardless of the cause of the injury. However, monitoring alveolar ventilation and carbon dioxide excretion via capnography provides early warning of some clinical situations that may ultimately lead to hypoxia and injury. Capnography is unique in its ability to monitor the integrity of the patient's cardiopulmonary system, airway function, and the function of life support equipment used to ventilate the patient.

Table 7–1 summarizes critical events that initially may be detected by pulse oximetry, capnography, or both techniques. Because the clinician never knows in advance what critical event may occur in a specific patient, it seems prudent to take the "belt and suspenders" approach, using pulse oximetry to monitor oxygenation and capnography to monitor ventilation.

PULSE OXIMETRY

Pulse oximetry provides a definitive warning of hypoxemia in patients with compromised cardiopulmonary status, as well as those at risk for impaired ventilation. The pulse oximeter noninvasively and continually monitors the oxygen saturation of arterial hemoglobin, facilitating detection of hypoxemia before clinical signs are apparent and enabling prompt correc-

tion. The abbreviation SaO_2 designates oxygen saturation of arterial hemoglobin. When SaO_2 is measured by pulse oximetry, it is often identified as SpO_2.

In many clinical settings pulse oximetry offers significant advantages over the other commonly available means of assessing blood oxygenation: invasive blood gas measurements and $PtcO_2$ monitoring. Pulse oximeters provide continual data, respond rapidly, are portable and easy to use, and require no calibration. They require no warmup or equilibration time, which is particularly important during emergencies or short procedures. Because pulse oximetry is noninvasive, its measurements are more likely to reflect the patient's true level of oxygenation. In contrast, the arterial sampling required for in vitro blood gas measurements often produces significant physiologic disturbances, particularly in infants and small children. In addition, the pulse oximeter's sensor, unlike the $PtcO_2$ monitor's electrode, is easily applied, does not generate significant heat, and can remain in place for a long time.

Operating Principles

Pulse oximetry is based on the differential absorption of red and infrared light by the two dominant forms of hemoglobin, oxyhemoglobin and reduced hemoglobin (Fig. 7–1). If red light (660 nm) is shone through reduced hemoglobin, most of the light is absorbed; when the same light is shone through oxyhemoglobin, less is absorbed. The opposite is true with an infrared light source (approximately 900 to 1000 nm): oxyhemoglobin absorbs more infrared light than

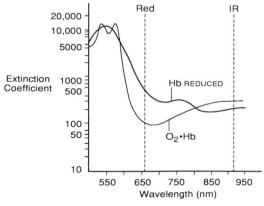

Figure 7–1. The absorption spectra of oxyhemoglobin and reduced hemoglobin. Note the differential absorption of red and infrared light by the two forms of hemoglobin. These differences in absorption are used by the pulse oximeter to determine the relative amount of each form of hemoglobin. The result is expressed as oxygen saturation.

reduced hemoglobin. The optical term that describes this tendency for blood to absorb light is the extinction coefficient (ϵ). Blood with a higher extinction coefficient at a particular wavelength of light (that is, color) absorbs more light of that wavelength than blood with a lower extinction coefficient. A pulse oximeter uses this differential absorption to determine the ratio of the two types of hemoglobin in blood.

A pulse oximeter has two light-emitting diodes (LEDs) that serve as light sources (one red and one infrared) and a photodiode as a photodetector. The LEDs are placed on one side of a pulsing arterial bed, with the photodetector opposing them across the tissue. The red and infrared light that shines through the tissue passes through constant, nonpulsatile tissue components and pulsatile arterial blood. The nonpulsatile tissue components normally include venous and capillary blood, tissue, bone, skin, hair, and other elements such as dirt and nail polish. The pulsatile tissue component is assumed to consist solely of arterial and arteriolar blood — a key assumption in pulse oximetry. The photodetector measures the amount of red and infrared light transmitted through the tissue.

Assuming that the only pulsatile light-absorbing substance is the arterial and arteriolar blood, the difference between the minimum light transmittance (which occurs at maximum blood volume, or systole) and the maximum light transmittance (which occurs at minimum blood volume, or diastole) is the light absorbed by the pulsatile component. Figure 7–2 is a schematic representation of the transmittance of light through tissue components, yielding the maximum and minimum light transmittance measurements that form the basis of Sp_{O_2} determinations.

Absorption results in two plethysmograms, one generated by the red light and one by the infrared. The amplitude of the waveforms, or the changes in light transmittance at each wavelength, results from the blood volume changes during the arterial pulse and the concentrations of oxyhemoglobin and reduced hemoglobin. Oxyhemoglobin absorbs less red and more infrared light than reduced hemoglobin. Consequently, if a patient's hemoglobin is 100% saturated, the inflowing pulsatile blood absorbs relatively little red light and more infrared. The pulsatile portion of the raw signal is compared with the light intensity at minimum transmission to account for light absorption by the constant, nonpulsatile layer. As shown in Figure 7–3, at 100% saturation this red waveform is relatively small because little change occurs in red absorption, while the comparable infrared waveform is large because of the large change in infrared absorption. If most of the hemoglobin is reduced, the inflowing pulsatile blood absorbs a larger amount of red light and less infrared. The resulting red waveform is fairly large and the infrared is small. When the saturation percentage is in the low 80s, the relative amplitudes of the red and infrared waveforms are equal.

Red and infrared absorption is measured many times each second. In some pulse oximeters, each optical pulse signal is analyzed to determine whether it has the specific characteristics of an arterial pulse waveform. The maximum and minimum pulse interval, the amplitude and variability of the signal, and other signal characteristics are analyzed. If the signal fulfills these requirements, it is accepted as a true pulse waveform and used in saturation measurement. If signal anomalies are present (for example, excessively high or low signal

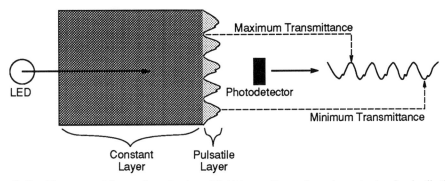

Figure 7–2. Measurement, by a pulse oximeter, of light transmittance through constant and pulsatile tissue components. During an arterial pulse the maximum amount of light is transmitted through the tissue at diastole and the minimum amount is transmitted at systole. The changes in light transmittance during the pulse result in the optical plethysmogram.

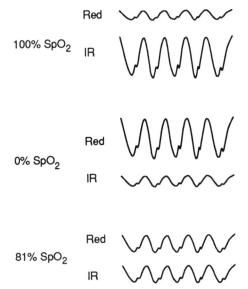

Figure 7—3. The red and infrared plethysmograms are used by a pulse oximeter to measure oxygen saturation.

amplitude, excessively narrow or wide pulse interval, or wildly erratic peak and trough values), the signal is rejected as a probable artifact and is not used to measure saturation. In other devices saturation is calculated from every sampled point in the signal, regardless of whether artifact is present. These oximeters depend on averaging of the sampled points to smooth the values and compensate for artifact.

Once a signal has been accepted as an arterial pulse, saturation for that pulse is measured: the pulse oximeter computes the logarithm of the ratio of the maximum to the minimum red signal amplitude, yielding value A; it next computes the logarithm of the ratio of the maximum to the minimum infrared signal amplitude, yielding value B; and it then determines the ratio of value A to value B. The oximeter then applies this ratio to a calibration curve that relates A/B to saturation (Fig. 7–4). This calibration curve was developed through empiric calibration studies of normal volunteers and was validated in clinical trials involving patients in a variety of clinical settings.

When the amplitude of the pulsatile signal is adequate to allow reliable detection by pulse oximetry, the instrument generally is accurate over the commonly encountered saturation range of 50% to 100%. The clinician should realize that pulse oximeters are designed to reliably detect hypoxemia, not to serve as precision measuring devices at some arbitrary saturation value. From the perspective of patient safety, the important issue is that the pulse oximeter reliably detect dangerous decreases in oxygen saturation. At very low saturations the clinician's attention should be directed toward correcting the hypoxemia, not worrying about the instrument's accuracy and precision.

Clinical and Technical Issues

Although pulse oximetry is reliable, clinical and technical factors affect its application.

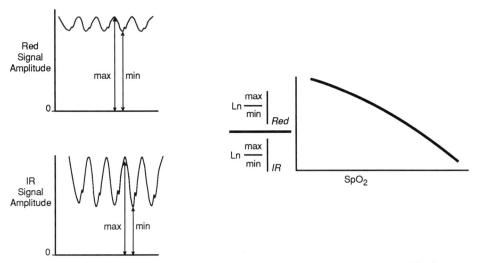

Figure 7—4. The computations used by a pulse oximeter to determine oxygen saturation. The instrument determines the ratio of the natural logarithms of the maximum and minimum red and infrared signal amplitudes. It then uses this ratio to determine oxygen saturation, based on empiric calibration studies.

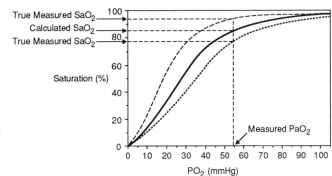

Figure 7–5. Errors in calculated oxygen saturation values that are attributable to shifts in the oxyhemoglobin dissociation curve.

Differences Between Measured and Calculated Saturation

Saturation may be measured by a pulse oximeter or a laboratory CO-oximeter, or it may be estimated by calculation from blood gas data. Although significant differences can be seen when measured saturation is compared with calculated saturation, they are not properly attributable to measurement errors by the oximeter. Discrepancies most commonly arise because the calculated saturation has not been appropriately corrected for factors that shift the oxyhemoglobin dissociation curve. This curve relates the partial pressure of oxygen (Po_2) in blood to the saturation of that blood, and its position is a complex function of such variables as acid-base balance, temperature, partial pressure of carbon dioxide in the blood (Pco_2), and concentration of 2,3-diphosphoglycerate (2,3-DPG). Blood gas machines calculate an approximate saturation level based on measured Po_2, using a normal adult curve corrected for measured pH and Pco_2 at a fixed temperature.

In the presence of abnormal hemoglobins such as fetal hemoglobin, or in situations in which blood levels of 2,3-DPG are decreased, the curve is shifted to the left. Deficiencies of 2,3-DPG are common in clinical practice. Transfusion of banked blood (which often contains little or no 2,3-DPG) and phosphate depletion caused by malnutrition decrease the 2,3-DPG concentration. Almost by definition, any patient who has been in an ICU for more than 3 days is malnourished.

The effect of a left-shifted curve can be seen from the example of a patient who has a left-shifted curve because of low 2,3-DPG and has a partial pressure of oxygen in arterial blood

(Pao_2) of approximately 55 mm Hg (7.3 kPa). When this patient's saturation is calculated from a blood gas measurement, the laboratory uses the normal curve that is built into the blood gas machine. That curve, which assumes a normal concentration of 2,3-DPG, may yield a calculated saturation percentage in the mid-80s. In contrast, because this is a left-shifted curve, the measured saturation is in the mid-90s. In this situation the measured saturation, whether it is from a laboratory CO-oximeter or a pulse oximeter, is the true saturation. The calculated blood gas saturation is in error because it is based on a normal curve whereas this patient has a left-shifted curve (Fig. 7–5).

The oxyhemoglobin dissociation curve can also be shifted to the right. This occurs when patients have an increased 2,3-DPG concentration. Sickle cell hemoglobin and chronic hypoxia caused by chronic obstructive pulmonary disease, cyanotic heart disease, severe chronic asthma, or high-altitude living result in a right-shifted curve. The right shift leads to the opposite discrepancy between the calculated and the measured saturation. From the normal curve a Pao_2 of about 55 mm Hg generates a calculated saturation percentage in the 80s. But the true measured saturation percentage is in the high 70s. In this situation the measured saturation is once again correct and the calculated saturation is in error (Fig. 7–5).

Carboxyhemoglobin

Carboxyhemoglobin (CoHb), an abnormal hemoglobin that results when carbon monoxide binds to hemoglobin, is commonly present in the blood in low concentrations (less than

10%). Carboxyhemoglobin has two significant effects in pulse oximetry: it results in a discrepancy between functional and fractional saturation measurements, and it produces a measurement artifact because of its spectral absorption characteristics.

EFFECT ON FUNCTIONAL AND FRACTIONAL SATURATION

An understanding of carboxyhemoglobin's effects on saturation requires an understanding of the difference between functional and fractional saturation. Functional, or physiologic, saturation is the ratio of oxyhemoglobin (O_2Hb) to the sum of oxyhemoglobin and reduced hemoglobin (Hb reduced):

$$\text{Saturation (functional)} = \frac{O_2Hb}{O_2Hb + Hb_{reduced}}$$

Functional saturation is measured by two-wavelength pulse oximeters. These instruments assume that only two types of molecules are present — oxyhemoglobin and reduced hemoglobin — and they operate at wavelengths that optimally distinguish those forms of hemoglobin.

Fractional, or chemical, saturation is the ratio of oxyhemoglobin to the sum of the four molecules that are measured by a four-wavelength CO-oximeter — oxyhemoglobin, reduced hemoglobin, carboxyhemoglobin, and methemoglobin (MetHb):

$$\text{Saturation (fractional)} = \frac{O_2Hb}{O_2Hb + Hb_{reduced} + COHb + MetHb}$$

Functional and fractional saturation measurements are often but not always equal. If 60 oxygen molecules are mixed with 15 hemoglobin molecules, the result is 15 oxyhemoglobin molecules, with each hemoglobin molecule binding four oxygen molecules. In this situation the functional oxygen saturation is 100% (15 oxyhemoglobin divided by the sum of 15 oxyhemoglobin plus zero reduced hemoglobin). The fractional saturation is also 100% (15 oxyhemoglobin divided by the sum of 15 oxyhemoglobin plus zero reduced plus zero carboxyhemoglobin plus zero methemoglobin). Consequently, in this situation, functional and fractional saturations are equivalent.

Adding four carbon monoxide molecules to the preceding mixture changes the outcome. Hemoglobin has 200 to 250 times greater affinity for carbon monoxide than it does for oxygen, and consequently most hemoglobin that is exposed to carbon monoxide binds to it, forming carboxyhemoglobin. Therefore, when 60 oxygen molecules, four carbon monoxide molecules, and 15 hemoglobin molecules are mixed, the four carbon monoxide molecules bind to one hemoglobin molecule. Four oxygen molecules remain unbound, existing as dissolved oxygen. When this happens, functional and fractional saturations are no longer equal. Functional saturation is 100% (14 oxyhemoglobin divided by the sum of 14 oxyhemoglobin plus zero reduced). However, fractional saturation is 93% (14 oxyhemoglobin divided by the sum of 14 oxyhemoglobin plus zero reduced plus one carboxyhemoglobin plus zero methemoglobin).

Both the functional and the fractional saturations are correct because they measure different attributes of blood. And both may be clinically valuable, as demonstrated in the following example. Fire rescue personnel give oxygen by mask to an 18-year-old man found unconscious in a burning house. On arrival in the emergency room his PaO_2 is high, his $PaCO_2$ is somewhat low, and his hemoglobin concentration is reasonable. If the major concern is his cardiopulmonary function, functional saturation, measured by pulse oximetry, is the best variable to monitor. It reveals, on a moment-to-moment basis, how much of the available hemoglobin is occupied by oxygen. On the other hand, if the major concern is whether the patient suffered significant carbon monoxide exposure, pulse oximetry is not sufficient. Measuring fractional saturation using a laboratory CO-oximeter is important because it estimates what fraction of his total hemoglobin is occupied by carbon monoxide. With this patient a pulse oximeter may yield a functional saturation of 98% to 100%. That means that the lungs and the heart are working well, there is no major intrapulmonary shunt, and pulmonary edema has not yet occurred. A laboratory CO-oximeter may yield a fractional saturation of only 68%, indicating a major carbon monoxide exposure.

Fractional saturation from a laboratory CO-oximeter may be converted to functional saturation for comparison with data from a pulse oximeter by means of the following formula:

$$\text{Saturation (functional)} = \frac{O_2Hb_{(fractional)}}{1 - (COHb + MetHb)}$$

SPECTRAL EFFECT

In the presence of a significant level of carboxyhemoglobin, a spectral error is introduced into the measurements obtained by a pulse oximeter. This spectral error occurs because the attenuation of infrared light by carboxyhemoglobin is only approximately one-tenth that of normal hemoglobin. This causes an artifactually low saturation measurement, reducing saturation by approximately 1% for every 10% carboxyhemoglobin. In most clinical situations, in which the carboxyhemoglobin concentration is less than 10%, this error in saturation is not clinically meaningful and may be safely ignored. In heavy smokers carboxyhemoglobin levels do not commonly exceed 10%.

In a study that provided empiric evidence of this spectral error, investigators exposed animals to increasing carbon monoxide levels. As a result, the blood concentration of carboxyhemoglobin rose. The composition of the breathing mixture ensured that hemoglobin not bound to carbon monoxide would be fully saturated. Saturation was measured by pulse oximetry, and concurrent samples were obtained for laboratory measurement of carboxyhemoglobin. Because the gas mixture ensured that the reduced hemoglobin level would not increase, functional saturation should have remained 100% if pulse oximetry were insensitive to carboxyhemoglobin. In fact, the study demonstrated an error in the pulse oximeter's saturation measurement of approximately 1% for every 10% carboxyhemoglobin (Fig. 7–6).

Ambient Light Interference

Because pulse oximetry relies on the absorption of red and infrared light, interference from ambient light must be controlled. Steady and variable light sources present different challenges to a pulse oximeter, and their effects are expressed differently.

STEADY AMBIENT LIGHT

When steady sunlight or room light reaches the pulse oximeter's photodetector, this ambient light combines with the pulsatile light signal from the tissue. The combined signal does not accurately reflect tissue absorption; it is offset by a baseline shift that is attributable to the steady ambient light. Depending on the wavelengths of the ambient light, the level of the red signal, the infrared signal, or both may be affected. Saturation is determined from the ratio of the natural logarithm of the maximum and minimum red light intensity to the natural logarithm of the maximum and minimum infrared light intensity. If one of the waveforms is offset by ambient light, a different maximum

and minimum result. If the pulse oximeter could not suppress the effect of this ambient light, the saturation measurements would be incorrect.

Pulse oximeters use "synchronous demodulation" of the signal to eliminate the effect of steady ambient light. The oximeter coordinates its absorption measurements with the activity of the LEDs, sampling once when each LED is on and once when it is off. The LED-off sample measures ambient light. The pulse oximeter subtracts this LED-off signal from the LED-on signal, eliminating the contribution of ambient light. This sampling typically occurs approximately 3000 times each second. Figure 7–7 schematically illustrates the effect of ambient light interference and the elimination of its effect by synchronous demodulation.

Two limits on the ability of synchronous demodulation to correct ambient light interference must be kept in mind. First, when the ambient light is extremely bright, it saturates the oximeter's photodetector, preventing detection of the pulsatile signal. Second, when the ambient light is rapidly changing, it can interfere with the oximeter's pulse detection algorithms, described in more detail in the next section. In both of these instances interference may be controlled by shielding the oximeter's sensor with opaque material.

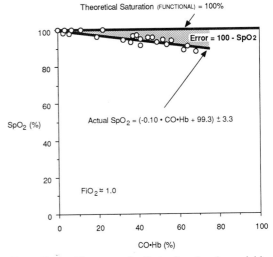

Figure 7–6. The spectral effect of carboxyhemoglobin introduces an error into oxygen saturation measurements obtained by pulse oximetry. Ideally, as the carboxyhemoglobin level increases during breathing of carbon monoxide, functional saturation should remain 100%. Note the progressively increasing error in the measured saturation level as the carboxyhemoglobin concentration increases. This error, a decrease in saturation of approximately 1% for each 10% increase in carboxyhemoglobin , is due to the spectral properties of carboxyhemoglobin. (Modified from Barker SJ, Tremper KK: Anesthesiology 1987;66(5):677-679, with permission.)

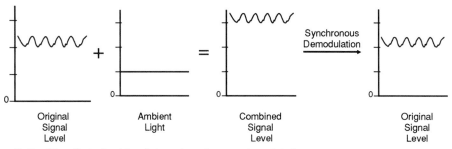

Figure 7–7. The effect of ambient light and synchronous demodulation on oxygen saturation measurements by pulse oximetry. Steady or slowly changing ambient light displaces the signal by some amount. Synchronous demodulation subtracts the ambient light signal from the combined signal and restores the original signal level.

RAPIDLY CHANGING LIGHT

Rapidly changing external light sources, such as the light from a surgical xenon arc lamp, a fluorescent light, or the LEDs in the sensor of another pulse oximeter, produce a type of optical interference that is more complex than that produced by steady light sources. The patient's true pulsatile signal is superimposed on the rapidly changing external light.

Many apparently pure alternating light sources have a great deal of high-frequency noise, which is composed of harmonics and other high-frequency components. This noise often reaches 10,000 to 20,000 cycles per second, whereas a pulse oximeter's synchronous demodulation sampling rate does not normally exceed 3000 samples per second. When the pulse oximeter samples at a rate slower than the frequency of the noise, information is missed in the sampling. Figure 7–8 illustrates the result. The pulse oximeter may connect individual samples to produce a "waveform," the frequency of which may approximate a normal heart rate. When this happens, the pulse oximeter may interpret this artifactual waveform as a real pulse, an error known as aliasing. Aliasing causes actual errors in the pulse oximeter's measurements. This type of ambient light interference is eliminated by covering the sensor with an opaque barrier to shield it from excess light and by applying the sensor snugly.

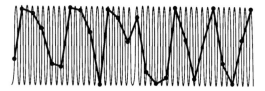

Figure 7–8. Aliasing occurs in the presence of very high frequency noise when samples are connected to form an artifactual waveform that is confused with an acceptable pulse signal.

Optical Shunting

Another common light-related problem is optical shunting, in which light from the LEDs reaches the photodetector without traveling through the pulsing tissue bed. Light may travel around the surface of the sensor site or pass through edematous tissue. Optical shunting is usually caused by loosely or incorrectly applied sensors, exhausted sensor adhesive, or sensors that are too big or too small for the patient. During optical shunting the true pulsatile signal is combined with the light signal that reaches the photodetector after passing through air or edema fluid.

The absorption spectrum of air is flat at the wavelengths used by a pulse oximeter. Consequently, when light from the pulse oximeter's LEDs passes through air, the resulting red and infrared signals have approximately equal amplitudes. When their amplitudes are equal, the measured saturation percentage is in the low 80s, as shown in Figure 7–3. When this shunt signal is added to the real pulsatile signal, a low saturation artifactually rises toward the low 80s and a high saturation artifactually falls toward the low 80s.

Because optical shunts occur at the sensor site, sensor design and application are crucial in preventing optical shunting. The sensor must be appropriately sized for the patient and the application site. The ideal sensor is one that closely adheres to the skin. This eliminates air gaps that provide alternate pathways for light, and it helps ensure correct alignment of the LEDs and photodetector.

Motion Artifact and Low Perfusion

Patient movement and low perfusion present similar challenges to a pulse oximeter. In both situations the instrument may have difficulty differentiating the pulsatile signal from background noise and, as a result, may be unable to track the patient's pulse. With patient motion the nonpulsatile layer is moving and even may be effectively pulsing (for example, when the patient is shivering). Consequently, although the amplitude of the pulse signal may be normal, superimposed motion artifacts may obscure the true signal. With low perfusion the volume changes of pulsatile blood in the periphery may be so small that the pulse is obscured by background noise of equal or larger amplitude, and the oximeter cannot identify the real pulse. Performance in the presence of movement or low perfusion can be a significant limitation of conventional pulse oximetry.

Several approaches have been developed to address the challenge of low perfusion. Oximeters should have a pulse strength indicator that reflects the amplitude of the pulsatile signal at the sensor site. If the pulse is too weak for reliable detection, the sensor may be moved to a site where the pulse is stronger. Also, sensors have been designed for application to sites at which blood flow is preserved during low peripheral perfusion. For example, a nasal sensor, which is applied across the nasal septal anterior ethmoid artery supplied by the internal carotid artery, may allow the oximeter to detect "central" pulses even when peripheral perfusion is relatively poor.

In addition, advanced signal processing algorithms may be incorporated to enhance performance during patient movement or low perfusion. In one type of signal processing the oximeter is provided with an independent timing signal that is related to the pulse. This timing signal defines a window of time within which the pulsatile signal is analyzed, enhancing the oximeter's ability to differentiate the true pulse from noise.

C-LOCK electrocardiographic (EKG) synchronization (Nellcor, Inc., Hayward, Calif.) is one such signal-processing method, using the EKG QRS complex as a timing signal. Figure 7–9 provides a conceptual overview of EKG synchronized signal processing. Figure 7–9, *A,* is the unprocessed optical pulse signal from a poorly perfused patient. In Figure 7–9, *B,* the position of each QRS complex is identified on that optical signal. Figure 7–9, *C,* is a schematic representation of EKG synchronization. The oximeter positions each segment of the optical pulse signal so that each QRS complex aligns. Then, for each point of the segment, the oximeter computes a normalized and weighted sum. This sum is computed by "exponential smoothing": the amplitude of the most recently acquired raw pulse signal segment is reduced by a fraction (less than 1), and that fractional signal segment is then added to the product of 1 minus that fraction times the value of the old composite pulse signal segment. This yields the new composite pulse signal, represented in Figure 7–9, *D.* The new composite signal is the weighted average of the components of the optical pulse signal that are synchronous with the EKG, and it is the clean signal from which

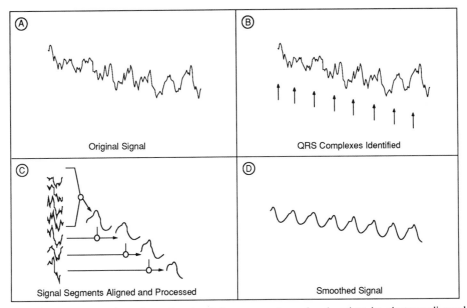

Figure 7–9. The processing of a pulse signal from a poorly perfused patient by electrocardiographic synchronization. Using the QRS complex as a timing signal enables the oximeter to greatly improve the quality of the pulse signal. This cleaner signal is then used to compute saturation.

saturation is measured. With this type of signal processing, events that are synchronous with the QRS complex are passed through relatively unaltered, while those that are not synchronous with the EKG are attenuated. Therefore the optical pulse signal, which is the result of cardiac activity, is passed unchanged, while noise, which is random with respect to the EKG, is attenuated.

The effectiveness of EKG synchronized signal processing in the presence of motion artifact is demonstrated in Figure 7–10. During a desaturation study in a normal volunteer, the subject moved one hand and kept the other stationary. Two pulse oximeters, one of which used EKG synchronized signal processing while the other used conventional pulse oximetry, were attached to the moving hand. Two conventional oximeters were attached to the stationary hand. If motion artifact did not affect the measurements, data from all four oximeters should have been equivalent. EKG synchronized processing enabled the oximeter to track the pulse accurately despite movement, producing saturation measurements that were comparable to those obtained from the nonmoving hand. In contrast, the oximeter that did not use EKG synchronized technology yielded erratic saturation measurements during movement because of the effect of motion artifact.

Summary

Effective use of pulse oximetry requires an understanding of key issues that affect the application of the technology and the interpretation of saturation measurements. Relevant physiologic parameters, such as factors that shift the oxyhemoglobin dissociation curve or the

presence of dysfunctional hemoglobins, must be considered. To control optical factors that can interfere with oximetry measurements, appropriate sensor design and application, as well as shielding the sensor from bright external light, are important. Finally, in situations that challenge signal detection, such as the presence of motion or low perfusion, it is important to use mechanisms that enhance the oximeter's ability to identify and track the pulse.

CAPNOMETRY AND CAPNOGRAPHY

The measurement of carbon dioxide (CO_2) is a second significant safety monitoring technology available to the critical care practitioner. *Capnometry* is the measurement of the partial pressure (or concentration) of CO_2 in the patient's airway during the entire ventilatory cycle. A capnometer provides a numerical measurement of inspired and end-tidal CO_2. *Capnography* is the graphic display of the partial pressure or concentration of CO_2 as a waveform, usually plotted as CO_2 versus time. When the waveform display is calibrated, capnography includes capnometry. Capnography provides the means to assess alveolar ventilation, the integrity of the airway, the functioning of the breathing circuit, ventilator function, patient cardiopulmonary function, and the subtleties of rebreathing. Thus it provides an early warning system for problems that could lead to disaster if left uncorrected.

The term "capnometry" is used throughout the following discussion, except when the discussion refers to capabilities available only through capnography.

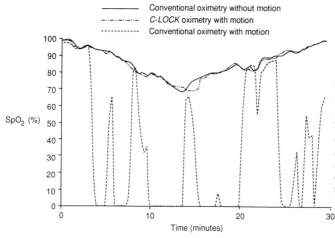

Figure 7–10. Electrocardiographic (EKG) synchronized signal processing enables a pulse oximeter to obtain accurate oxygen saturation measurements despite motion artifact. Ideally, during this motion study all four oximeters should have produced equivalent data. However, the conventional oximeter without EKG synchronization was unable to follow the pulsatile signal and consequently was unable to measure saturation accurately, while the oximeter using EKG synchronized processing tracked the pulse and measured the true saturation.

Operating Principles

The partial pressure of CO_2 (Pco_2) in the airway is measured by respiratory gas sampling. In the most common sampling method, gas is diverted from the airway and aspirated through a tube to the CO_2 monitor. Diverting capnometers allow true zero-CO_2 reference measurements, which tend to produce dependable, drift-free performance and thus accurate CO_2 measurements. An alternative to the diverting instrument is the nondiverting, or mainstream, capnometer in which a special flow-through adapter and CO_2 monitor are placed on the patient's airway.

In the majority of stand-alone capnometers, CO_2 concentration is measured by infrared spectroscopy. These measurements are obtained in the "optical bench" of the CO_2 monitor, in which a beam of infrared light is passed through the sample gas and light absorption by that gas is measured. Ideally, infrared light is also passed through gas in a reference chamber and absorption by that gas is measured. By comparing absorption by the sample gas with that by the reference gas, the capnometer determines the amount of CO_2 in the sample gas, and it then displays the CO_2 concentration. Raman scattering and mass spectrometry are alternative methods of CO_2 measurement.

Normal Respiratory Gas Exchange
Normal Capnogram

CO_2 rapidly moves across the endothelial membrane from the capillary to the alveolus. By the time blood leaves the alveolar lung unit, the Pco_2 in the end-capillary blood and the alveolus are equal, as shown in Figure 7–11. The end-capillary blood ultimately becomes arterial blood after mixing with blood from other perfused lung units. In general, the alveolar Pco_2 ($Paco_2$) and the arterial Pco_2 ($Paco_2$) are equal.

The capnogram displays the CO_2 concentration at the patient's airway over time. During the early phase of exhalation, CO_2-free gas from the tracheal dead space is exhaled. This corresponds to segment *A-B* of the capnogram illustrated in Figure 7–11. As exhalation continues, CO_2-rich alveolar gas begins to percolate out of the patient's airway, displacing the CO_2-free dead space gas. In the capnogram this is reflected in a CO_2 level that rises with a sharp upstroke (segment *B-C*). If all ventilated lung units emptied simultaneously with equal time constants, segment *B-C* would be vertical. To the extent that the emptying is uneven, the upstroke becomes less vertical and more slurred. Eventually alveolar gas dominates the exhaled gas and the rate of change in the CO_2 level dramatically decreases. Because little additional gas is exhaled during this latter part of the breath, the CO_2 concentration remains fairly constant. This is the alveolar plateau, the relatively horizontal segment of the capnogram at the end of exhalation (segment *C-D*). The maximum level of exhaled CO_2 usually occurs at the end of the tidal breath, at point *D*. This maximum is thus called end-tidal CO_2. In most conditions, end-tidal CO_2 is a good approximation of the $Paco_2$, which under ideal conditions closely approximates the $Paco_2$ (represented by the dotted line in Fig. 7–11). Finally, as the patient again inhales CO_2-free fresh gas, the CO_2 concentration at the airway drops abruptly. Normally, in the absence of rebreathing, no measurable CO_2 is present in the inspired gas,

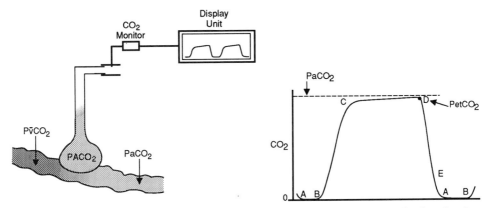

Figure 7–11. The components of the normal capnogram reflect changes in the CO_2 level at the airway throughout the ventilatory cycle. The dotted line represents $Paco_2$. Under ideal conditions $Petco_2$ closely approximates $Paco_2$.

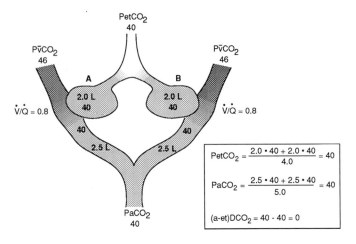

$$PetCO_2 = \frac{2.0 \cdot 40 + 2.0 \cdot 40}{4.0} = 40$$

$$PaCO_2 = \frac{2.5 \cdot 40 + 2.5 \cdot 40}{5.0} = 40$$

$$(a\text{-}et)DCO_2 = 40 - 40 = 0$$

Figure 7–12. Ideal matching of ventilation and perfusion results in an $(a\text{-}et)DCO_2$ value of zero.

and thus the capnogram abruptly falls to zero (segment *D-E*). The cycle then repeats itself with the next exhalation.

Therefore the essentials of a normal capnogram are a zero baseline during early exhalation, a sharp upstroke during midexhalation, a relatively horizontal alveolar plateau during late exhalation, and a sharp downstroke and return to a zero baseline during inspiration. A capnogram that does not have these normal attributes suggests an anomaly in the patient's cardiopulmonary system, a malfunction in the airway, or a malfunction in the gas delivery system.

Ideal Ventilation-Perfusion Matching

When ventilation and perfusion are well matched throughout the lung, $PaCO_2$ and the partial pressure of end-tidal CO_2 ($PetCO_2$) are equal. In the hypothetical two–lung unit model shown in Figure 7–12, both lung *A* and lung *B* have a normal ventilation/perfusion ratio ($\dot{V}/\dot{Q}$) of 0.8 (2.0 L/min of ventilation and 2.5 L/min of perfusion delivered to each lung unit). In this model the PCO_2 in the mixed venous blood ($P\bar{v}CO_2$) that returns to each lung unit is 46 mm Hg. As the blood traverses the lung unit, CO_2 diffuses through the capillary-alveolar membrane and enters the alveolus. When the blood has finished traversing the lung unit, the PCO_2 of the alveolus and of the end-capillary blood is the same, 40 mm Hg. The blood leaving the lung units ultimately becomes arterial blood after mixing in the left atrium and left ventricle. The resulting mixed $PaCO_2$ is 40 mm Hg. The gas leaving the alveoli also mixes, and the resulting mixed $PetCO_2$ is 40 mm Hg. Thus, when ventilation and perfusion are ideally matched, the difference between

the $PaCO_2$ and $PetCO_2$, also known as the $(a\text{-}et)DCO_2$, is zero.

In most patients ventilation and perfusion are reasonably well matched and end-tidal and arterial CO_2 are remarkably close together. The data in Figure 7–13 are from a clinical study of 39 children, aged 3 months to 17 years, whose $PetCO_2$ measurements were compared with simultaneously measured $PaCO_2$ values after correction of the $PaCO_2$ measurements for actual body temperature. The solid line is the line of identity, on which all data should lie if $PetCO_2$ and $PaCO_2$ are identical. Note the close agreement between the two measurements, with $PetCO_2$ typically a few millimeters of mercury lower than the simultaneously measured $PaCO_2$. This finding—that end-tidal values closely approximate arterial values, with $PetCO_2$ slightly underestimating $PaCO_2$—is typical of capnometric studies in patients with normal matching of ventilation and perfusion.

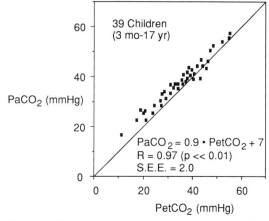

Figure 7–13. In patients with normal ventilation-perfusion matching, $PetCO_2$ closely approximates $PaCO_2$

Clinical and Technical Issues

When a capnometer is used in clinical practice, the complaint is often heard that *"the monitor is not working!"* Of course, in some cases the instrument truly is not working; perhaps it is miscalibrated or dirt, water, or mucus is interfering with the reference measurement in the optical bench. But typically this complaint actually means that $Petco_2$ and $Paco_2$ are not equal.

Both physiologic anomalies and technical factors can result in $Petco_2$ values that do not approximate $Paco_2$. For $Petco_2$ to closely approximate $Paco_2$, two physiologic assumptions must be met: the lung units must empty fully with approximately equal time constants (resulting in $Petco_2$ measurements that closely approximate $Paco_2$), and ventilation and perfusion must be well matched in the lung units (resulting in $Paco_2$ measurements that closely approximate $Paco_2$). When these assumptions are not valid because the patient's physiology is not normal, $Petco_2$ may differ significantly from $Paco_2$. In addition, technical variables can produce $Petco_2$ values that do not closely approximate $Paco_2$. These include the design of the gas sampling system, the distance the gas must be transported, and the instrument's calibration methods. Proper interpretation of the readings from a capnometer requires an understanding of these physiologic and technical issues.

Ventilation-Perfusion Maldistributions
DEAD SPACE VENTILATION

Wasted ventilation, or the ventilation of dead space, is a clinical problem that produces differences between end-tidal and arterial CO_2 levels. Dead space is gas volume in the respiratory tract and lung that participates in tidal breathing but not in gas exchange. Obvious examples are the volume of the endotracheal tube (apparatus dead space) and the volume of the tracheal lumen and large bronchi that do not have lung acini (anatomic dead space). Less obvious, but especially important in critically ill patients, is alveolar dead space, which is attributable to lung units that receive ventilation that greatly exceeds perfusion. Since perfusion to these lung units is inadequate, gas exchange in these overventilated, underperfused lung units is less efficient than normal. This high ventilation/perfusion ratio increases the $(a\text{-}et)Dco_2$.

An example of dead space ventilation can be seen in the two-lung unit model in Figure 7–14. Lungs *A* and *B* each receive half of the normal alveolar ventilation, 2 L/min. However, because of a massive pulmonary embolus, lung *A* receives no perfusion. Therefore the ventilation to lung *A* is wasted, or dead space ventilation. In this model the alveolar and end-pulmonary capillary Pco_2 in lung *A* is 8 mm Hg. (The nonzero alveolar Pco_2 in lung *A* is attributable to rebreathing into lung *A* of some of the gas previously exhaled from lung *B*.) The $Petco_2$ is 26 mm Hg and the $Paco_2$ is 43 mm Hg, with a resulting $(a\text{-}et)Dco_2$ of 17 mm Hg. In this case the capnometer indicates a $Petco_2$ of 26 mm Hg, while a simultaneous arterial blood gas yields a $Paco_2$ of 43 mm Hg. Both are correct—the large $(a\text{-}et)Dco_2$ is not an indication of instrument malfunction, but rather of *patient malfunction*. The $(a\text{-}et)Dco_2$ reflects dead space ventilation, and the size of the difference provides valuable information about the amount of wasted ventilation.

Dead space ventilation is an appreciable fraction of tidal breathing in many common clinical situations, including severe respiratory failure, pulmonary hypoperfusion, pulmonary thromboembolism, lateral decubitus position, systemic hypoperfusion, air embolism, and cardiac

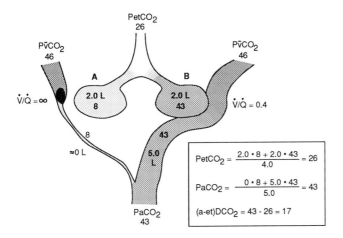

Figure 7–14. Dead space ventilation typically results in a large $(a\text{-}et)Dco_2$ value.

$$PetCO_2 = \frac{2.0 \cdot 8 + 2.0 \cdot 43}{4.0} = 26$$

$$PaCO_2 = \frac{0 \cdot 8 + 5.0 \cdot 43}{5.0} = 43$$

$$(a\text{-}et)DCO_2 = 43 - 26 = 17$$

arrest. In these conditions the clinician using a capnometer may see a large $(a-et)Dco_2$ (typically greater than 10 mm Hg).

Figure 7–15, *A*, is redrawn from a study that compared $Paco_2$ and $Petco_2$ measurements in 17 adults with severe acute respiratory distress syndrome. The solid line is the line of identity; if there were perfect agreement between $Petco_2$ and $Paco_2$, all data pairs would lie on this line. The $Petco_2$ measurements underestimated $Paco_2$, with $(a-et)Dco_2$ values ranging from zero to 38 mm Hg. This does not indicate that the capnometer was malfunctioning, but rather that the patient's physiology was malfunctioning.

The size of the $(a-et)Dco_2$ has considerable clinical significance, as demonstrated when the data from the preceding study are replotted as $(a-et)Dco_2$ versus an independent measure of lung function, the ratio of dead space ventilation

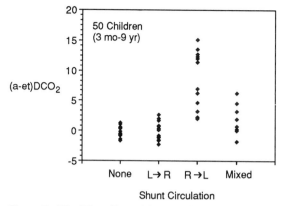

Figure 7–16. The effect of intracardiac shunts on the $(a-et)Dco_2$ value. $Petco_2$ was a good estimator of $Paco_2$ in all patients *except* those with right-to-left shunts. (Modified from Fletcher R: Anesth Analg 1988;67[5]:442-447, with permission.)

to tidal volume (VD/VT) (Fig. 7–15, *B*). The patient who had an $(a-et)Dco_2$ of zero had a normal VD/VT (less than 0.3). As VD/VT increased in progressively sicker patients, the $(a-et)Dco_2$ also increased. Thus the $(a-et)Dco_2$ was a good estimator of VD/VT. Since VD/VT values greater than 0.5 are generally considered diagnostic of severe respiratory failure, the clinician may wish to use the more easily measured $(a-et)Dco_2$, rather than the more difficult dead space measurement, as an indicator of the severity of respiratory failure. In any case the $(a-et)Dco_2$ measurement yields valuable information about respiratory physiology. Generally, as the patient's pulmonary function improves, the $(a-et)Dco_2$ decreases.

In most cases the $(a-et)Dco_2$ is relatively small, usually less than 5 to 7 mm Hg, even when significant cardiopulmonary dysfunction is present. However, in some patients the $(a-et)Dco_2$ may increase dramatically because of dead space ventilation. In patients with right-to-left intracardiac shunts, such as tetralogy of Fallot or pulmonary atresia, the blood entering the right side of the heart tends to traverse the ventricular or atrial septum and cross directly to the left side without first entering the pulmonary circulation. Such right-to-left shunts effectively result in dead space ventilation because pulmonary perfusion is reduced. A study of the $(a-et)Dco_2$ measurements in 50 children with congenital heart disease confirmed that patients with right-to-left shunting defects had the largest $(a-et)Dco_2$ measurements (Fig. 7–16). A more typical $(a-et)Dco_2$ of approximately 5 mm Hg did not rule out significant right-to-left shunting.

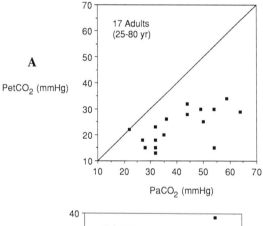

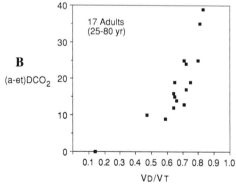

Figure 7–15. **A,** In patients with severe respiratory failure, large $(a-et)Dco_2$ values were commonly seen. **B,** A widened $(a-et)Dco_2$ was seen in respiratory failure. When the data from **A** were replotted against VD/VT, a close relationship emerged between wasted ventilation and the $(a-et)Dco_2$ measurement. (Modified from Yamanaka MK, Sue DY: Chest 1987; 92[5]:832-835, with permission.)

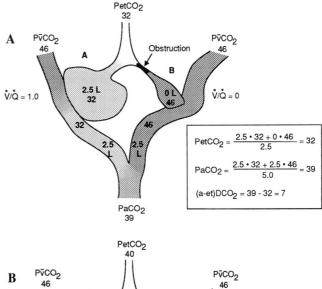

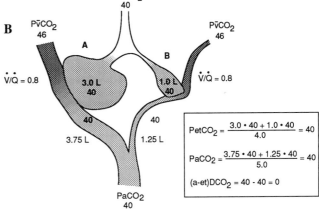

Figure 7–17. **A,** The effect of shunt perfusion on the (a-et)Dco_2 value. Shunt perfusion increases the (a-et)Dco_2, but to a much smaller extent than dead space ventilation. **B,** Full compensation via hypoxic pulmonary vasoconstriction returns the (a-et)Dco_2 to a value near zero.

SHUNT PERFUSION

Shunt perfusion is at the opposite end of the ventilation/perfusion spectrum from dead space ventilation. Unlike dead space ventilation, however, in shunt perfusion the (a-et)Dco_2 is usually small and $Petco_2$ fairly accurately reflects $Paco_2$. Shunt perfusion occurs whenever lung units receive excessively high perfusion relative to the amount of ventilation they receive. In the two–lung unit model in Figure 7–17, *A*, the airway in lung *B* is obstructed and the ventilation to lung *A* is increased in an attempt to compensate. Both lungs continue to receive the same perfusion, 2.5 L/min. The $\dot{V}/\dot{Q}$ ratio for lung *A* is elevated slightly, but not enough to cause significant problems, while the $\dot{V}/\dot{Q}$ ratio for lung *B* is reduced to zero, since there is no ventilation and normal perfusion. In this model the $Petco_2$ is 32 mm Hg and the $Paco_2$ is 39 mm Hg. The resulting (a-et)Dco_2 is 7 mm Hg.

Shunt perfusion is the dominant respiratory abnormality in many clinical conditions, in-

cluding atelectasis and pneumonia. Although such conditions may produce profound hypoxia, the elevation in the (a-et)Dco_2 is usually small and the end-tidal value can often be used to estimate the arterial CO_2 value. An explanation for this may be found in the lung's ability to adjust perfusion to match ventilation via a reflex called hypoxic pulmonary vasoconstriction. When a lung unit becomes hypoxic, as occurs when its ventilation is greatly diminished, this reflex constricts the pulmonary arterial vessels supplying that lung unit. This ameliorates the effect of shunt perfusion, moving oxygenation back toward normal. A second effect of hypoxic pulmonary vasoconstriction is that blood flow is shunted from hypoxic lung units to ones that are well ventilated, bringing the elevated $\dot{V}/\dot{Q}$ toward a more normal value. As a result, the $Petco_2$ values come closer to the $Paco_2$ measurements, allowing convenient estimation of $Paco_2$ from $Petco_2$, even in patients with significant cardiopulmonary disease (Fig. 7–17, *B*).

Gas Sampling

The gas sampling method used by a capnometer affects the accuracy of the capnogram and $Petco_2$ measurements. Relevant factors include the portion of the ventilatory circuit from which the gas is sampled, the distance over which the gas is transported before analysis, and the sample flow rate of the instrument. Figure 7–18 diagrams the three major capnometric gas sampling configurations.

With a nondiverting, or mainstream, device, the CO_2 monitor is placed on the airway so there is no need to divert gas from the airway. This sampling configuration is typically available only in infrared capnometers, because only infrared CO_2 monitors are small enough to fit on the airway.

A second, newer sampling configuration is seen in the proximal-diverting device. A lightweight, low-profile airway adapter is placed on the patient's airway, and gas is sampled from the airway and transported to the optical bench, which is placed near the patient but not on the airway itself. This proximal optical bench is the actual CO_2 monitor; the sample pump and the data processing and display electronics are housed in the larger display unit that is located distal to the patient, near the operator.

A third sampling configuration is found in the distal-diverting device, the classic "sidestream" capnometer. In a distal-diverting system, gas is sampled from the airway and transported to the CO_2 monitor, which is located distal to the patient, in the display unit.

SAMPLING LOCATION

In some breathing circuits, especially those with a constant flow bypassing the patient, the accuracy of the $Petco_2$ measurements may be affected by the location of the sampling site in the breathing circuit.

In the breathing circuit shown in Figure 7–19, constant flow is provided to the patient, with forced positive-pressure ventilation by intermittent occlusion of the expiratory valve. In this type of circuit the accuracy of the capnogram, the $Petco_2$ measurements, and hence the displayed values depends on the sampling site. Sampling near the endotracheal tube results in the most accurate values because there is little contamination with fresh gas from the breathing circuit (point *A*). The **Y** connector of the breathing circuit is the next best sampling site (point *B*). However, if the fresh gas flow is large compared with the expiratory flow rate of the

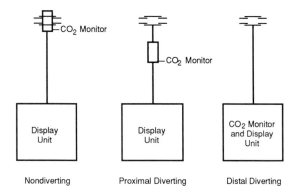

Nondiverting   Proximal Diverting   Distal Diverting

Figure 7–18. Nondiverting, proximal-diverting, and distal-diverting capnographic gas sampling configurations.

patient (as may be the case in neonates and small children), the capnogram and the $Petco_2$ values may be distorted because of dilution with the fresh gas flowing through the **Y** connector. If gas is sampled "downstream" from the patient, the waveform and $Petco_2$ are increasingly diluted by fresh gas from the circuit (points *C* and *D*). If gas is sampled "upstream" from the patient in the fresh gas supply, none of the exhaled CO_2 is detected and the measured $Petco_2$ is zero (point *E*).

The best sampling site is within the patient's endotracheal tube or at the airway, as far as possible from the **Y** connector of the breathing circuit. When such a sampling location is used, significant dilution is seen only in children and in adults in whom bypass circuits with a high fresh gas flow are used.

The location from which the sample is obtained is especially important when Mapleson D or Bain circuits are used, whether in the operating room during anesthesia, in the ICU, or during transport. The CO_2 concentration in a

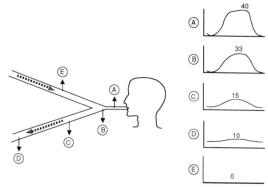

Figure 7–19. The effect of sampling location on the accuracy of the capnogram and $Petco_2$ measurements during continuous-flow positive-pressure ventilation. The best sampling location is one that is closest to the endotracheal tube.

Figure 7–20. The effect of sampling location on the accuracy of the capnogram and $Petco_2$ measurements in a Mapleson D or Bain circuit. The best sampling site is one that is close to the endotracheal tube and far from the fresh gas input.

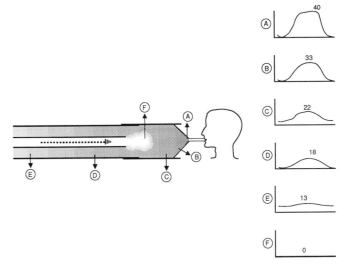

Mapleson D circuit depends highly on the location from which the sample is obtained, the fresh gas flow rate, the patient's exhaled tidal volume, and the expiratory flow rate.

Figure 7–20 shows typical capnograms and $Petco_2$ values that result when gas is sampled at various locations in a Mapleson D circuit. The most reliable sampling point is as close to the endotracheal tube as possible. Immediately adjacent to the endotracheal tube, the capnogram and $Petco_2$ values generally are free from the influence of fresh gas from the circuit (point A). As the sample site moves away from the endotracheal tube, dilution by CO_2-free fresh gas becomes greater (points B and C). As the sample site is farther from the patient and closer to the exhalation valve of the breathing circuit, the waveform assumes a steady-state value that reflects a mixture of expired gas from the patient and fresh gas from the circuit (points D and E). At a sample site immediately adjacent to the fresh gas inflow, the sampled gas is dominated by CO_2-free fresh gas and the capnogram and $Petco_2$ values are greatly distorted (point F).

In breathing circuits with intermittent flow (demand valve ventilators) and in adults with large exhaled tidal volumes, the capnogram and $Petco_2$ values usually are unaffected by the subtleties of sampling location.

SAMPLE FLOW RATE

If the tidal volume is small, as in infants and children, and the sample flow rate is large (greater than 150 ml/min), the capnogram and $Petco_2$ measurements may be significantly diluted by the entrainment of fresh system gas (Fig. 7–21). Using a system designed for a low sample flow rate, typically less than 75 ml/min, usually restores the waveform and $Petco_2$ readings to more accurate values. Consequently, choosing a capnometer designed for a low sample flow rate is especially important when monitoring neonates or small children.

SAMPLE TRANSPORT

Even if errors caused by sampling site and sample flow rate are minimized, sample transport can introduce errors in the measurement of CO_2. Three gas sampling configurations are currently available: the nondiverting system, with the CO_2 monitor mounted on the airway; the proximal-diverting system, with the CO_2

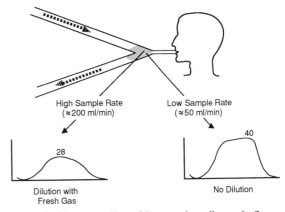

Figure 7–21. The effect of large and small sample flow rates on the capnogram and $Petco_2$ measurements from a patient with a small tidal volume. Small sample flow rates (typically less than 75 ml/min) provide better waveforms and more accurate measurements than do large sample flow rates.

monitor mounted proximal to the patient, separate from the display unit; and the distal-diverting system, with the CO_2 monitor incorporated in the display unit.

A key advantage of a nondiverting instrument is that sample transport is not an issue. Because the CO_2 monitor is mounted on the airway, the system has no sample tube that can become plugged, cause waveform distortion, or induce delay. A CO_2 monitor mounted on the airway also has disadvantages: it is bulky and heavy; because its size must be minimized, the additional optics required to measure nitrous oxide (N_2O) or anesthetic agent are usually not incorporated; and if its optical windows become contaminated with material from the airway, reference measurements and therefore CO_2 measurements become unreliable.

With a proximal-diverting instrument the CO_2 monitor is removed from the airway. This eliminates the size restriction imposed on an airway-mounted CO_2 monitor, allowing incorporation of the optics required for measuring N_2O and correcting the CO_2 measurements for the effects of N_2O. However, this system design results in sample transport issues: it requires a sample tube that introduces a delay time and can clog or cause waveform distortion. However, an incorporated filtering system and filter-purging mechanism minimize clogging problems and protect the optical windows of the CO_2 monitor from contamination. Also, because the CO_2 monitor is adjacent to the patient rather than in the display unit, the length of the sample tube and the resulting waveform distortion and delay time are minimized.

Like the proximal-diverting instrument, a distal-diverting capnometer eliminates the size restriction imposed on an airway-mounted monitor by placing the CO_2 monitor in the display unit. This allows incorporation of N_2O-measuring optics and helps protect the optical windows of the CO_2 monitor from contamination. However, sample transport is a greater challenge in this system than in the proximal-diverting system. Because the CO_2 monitor is distal to the patient, the sample tube generally must be longer than in a proximal-diverting system. Consequently, delay time and waveform distortion may be more significant with the distal-diverting capnometer.

Summary

To use capnometry effectively, the clinician must understand a range of issues that affect its application and the interpretation of CO_2 mea-

surements. Ventilation-perfusion maldistributions such as dead space ventilation, intracardiac shunts, and shunt perfusion may affect the accuracy with which $Petco_2$ measurements reflect $Paco_2$ levels. A number of technical factors relating to system design and application are important in ensuring that the capnogram accurately reflects changes in CO_2 levels. These include the design of the gas sampling system, the point in the breathing circuit from which the gas is sampled, the sample flow rate, the sample transport system, and the calibration methods incorporated into the instrument.

CONCLUSION

Because of the increasing use of pulse oximetry and capnometry in critical care, it is important to understand key clinical and technical issues that determine the most effective use of these instruments. Both technologies provide early warning of potentially catastrophic events and thus permit early intervention. Therefore they are rapidly becoming part of standard-of-care monitoring for critically ill patients.

SUGGESTED READINGS

American Society of Anesthesiologists: Standards for basic intra-operative monitoring. ASA Newsletter 1986;50(12)

Barker SJ, Tremper KK: The effect of carbon monoxide inhalation on pulse oximetry and transcutaneous Po_2. Anesthesiology 1987;66(5):677-679

Comroe JH: Matching of gas and blood. In Physiology of Respiration. Chicago, 1974, Year Book Medical Publishers

Fisher DM, Swedlow DB: Estimating $Paco_2$ by end-tidal gas sampling in children. Crit Care Med 1981;9(3):287

Fletcher R: Invasive and noninvasive measurement of the respiratory deadspace in anesthetized children with cardiac disease. Anesth Analg 1988;67(5):442-447

Gandhi SK, Munshi CA, Kampine JP: Early warning sign of an accidental endobronchial intubation: a sudden drop or sudden rise in $Paco_2$? Anesthesiology 1986; 65(1):114-115

Gravenstein N, Lampotang S, Beneken JEW: Factors influencing capnography in the Bain circuit. J Clin Monit 1985;1(1):6-10

Harris AP, Sendak MJ, Donham RT: Changes in arterial oxygen saturation immediately after birth in the human neonate. J Pediatr 1986;109(1):117-119

Joint Commission on Accreditation of Hospitals: Accreditation manual for hospitals. 1988;287-289

Keenan RL, Boyan CP: Cardiac arrest due to anesthesia. JAMA 1985;26;253(16):2373-2377

Linko K, Paloheimo M, Tammisto T: Capnography for detection of accidental oesophageal intubation. Acta Anaesthesiol Scand 1983;27(3):199-202

Murray IP, Modell JH: Early detection of endotracheal tube accidents by monitoring carbon dioxide concentration in respiratory gas. Anesthesiology 1983;59(4):344-346

Nellcor: C-LOCK; ECG synchronization principles of operation. Pulse Oximetry Note Number 6, 1988

Nellcor: Measurement of functional and fractional oxygen saturation. Pulse Oximetry Note Number 2, 1987

Osborn JJ, Raison JCA, Beaumont JO, et al: Respiratory causes of "sudden unexplained arrhythmia" in postthoracotomy patients. Surgery 1971;69(1):24-28

Ozanne GM, Young WG, Mazzei WJ, Severinghaus JW: Multipatient anesthetic mass spectrometry: rapid analysis of data stored in long catheters. Anesthesiology 1981;55:62-70

Sendak MJ, Harris AP, Donham RT: Accuracy of pulse oximetry during arterial oxyhemoglobin desaturation in dogs. Anesthesiology 1988;68(1):111-114

Severinghaus JW, Naifeh KH: Accuracy of response of six pulse oximeters to profound hypoxia. Anesthesiology 1987;67(4):551-558

Smalhout B, Kalenda Z: An atlas of capnography, vol I. The Netherlands, 1983, Kerckebosch-Zeist

Swedlow DB: Capnometry and capnography: the anesthesia disaster warning system. Semin Anesth 1986;5(3):194-205

Task Force on Guidelines: Recommendations for critical care unit design. Crit Care Med 1988;16(8):796-806

Task Force on Guidelines: Recommendations for services and personnel for delivery of care in a critical care setting. Crit Care Med 1988;16(8):809-811

Westenskow DR, Smith KW, Coleman DL, et al: Clinical evaluation of a raman scattering multiple gas analyzer for the operating room. Anesthesiology 1989;70(2):350-355

Yamanaka MK, Sue DY: Comparison of arterial-end-tidal PCO_2 difference and dead space/tidal volume ratio in respiratory failure. Chest 1987;92(5):832-835

Yelderman M, New W: Evaluation of pulse oximetry. Anesthesiology 1983;59(4):349-352

SECTION II

ORGAN SYSTEM FAILURE

8

RESPIRATORY FAILURE

STEVEN J. ALLEN, MD

ATELECTASIS

Perioperative Atelectasis

Although not necessarily a life-threatening problem by itself, atelectasis enhances the development of detrimental conditions, including pneumonia and hypoxemia. Atelectasis is a common finding in postoperative patients. The collapse appears to occur in the dependent lung regions during general anesthesia and is proportional to the decrease in functional residual capacity (FRC). This type of atelectasis is most commonly not lobar and resolves spontaneously within hours after the anesthetic is terminated.

Elderly patients present additional problems in the perioperative period. Not only do they have a lower preoperative pulmonary artery partial pressure of oxygen (Pao$_2$) when breathing room air than younger patients, they also suffer a greater fall in their postoperative Pao$_2$. Again, the decrease in Pao$_2$ correlates with the decrease in FRC in these older patients.

Postoperative atelectasis and hypoxemia may also develop in patients with decreased pulmonary compliance. Typical operating room ventilators are generally unable to deliver an adequate tidal volume if the inflation pressures needed are in excess of 40 cm H$_2$O. Thus a patient with poor pulmonary compliance may develop diffuse atelectasis and hypoxemia, both of which resolve when the patient receives ventilation with a standard ICU mechanical ventilator.

Prophylaxis is as important as treatment in postoperative atelectasis. Secretion clearance and lung expansion maneuvers as described in Chapter 3 are the mainstays of management. Besides suctioning, chest physiotherapy, cough-ing, and deep breathing exercises, control of pain that may limit cooperation should be addressed.

Lobar Atelectasis

The mechanism of lobar atelectasis involves obstruction of a bronchus with distal absorption atelectasis. ICU patients are generally nursed in the supine and head up position, and thus the atelectasis tends to occur in the posterior and inferior segments. Right upper lobe atelectasis occurs when the endotracheal tube is advanced sufficiently to obstruct the right upper lobe bronchus. Diagnosis of lobar atelectasis generally requires a chest roentgenogram. Commonly, a critically ill patient has a number of densities on chest roentgenogram, the causes of which may be varied. Radiographic diagnosis of atelectasis includes evidence of consolidation and volume loss. Although solitary lobar collapse has a variable effect on Pao$_2$, these areas do form an excellent site for pneumonias. Once they are recognized, efforts should be made to reexpand the segment. Appropriate maneuvers, discussed in Chapter 3, include suctioning and positioning the patient so that the atelectatic segment is nondependent. If pain impairs the patient's ability to inspire deeply, one of the several available analgesic techniques (parenteral narcotics, intercostal blocks, pleural catheter or epidural infusion of narcotic or local anesthetic agents) should be considered. Chest physiotherapy is as effective as fiberoptic bronchoscopy in the resolution of atelectasis. However, fiberoptic bronchoscopy is occasionally helpful in the reexpansion of atelectasis in immobile patients with impaired cough ability, such as chemically paralyzed, head-injured, and quadriplegic patients. Atelectasis may also be due to causes that may not respond to the preceding maneuvers. For example, a patient with an elevated diaphragm caused by massive ascites may demonstrate compressive atelectasis. These patients may have no trouble with secretions, but the pressure on the diaphragm may interfere with maintenance of a normal FRC. The presence of a large pleural effusion, pneumothorax, or other intrathoracic mass may also create compressive atelectasis. Chest physiotherapy would not be expected to have beneficial effects for these conditions.

PULMONARY EDEMA

Pulmonary edema is defined as an abnormal amount of fluid in the pulmonary extravascular compartment. It occurs when fluid enters the pulmonary interstitium faster than it is removed. A number of disease processes, many of which are covered in this chapter, may result in the formation of pulmonary edema. All disorders that produce pulmonary edema do so in a fashion that may be described by equations concerning fluid movement. Understanding how pulmonary edema might arise requires some knowledge of the Starling equation (Eq. 1).

$$J_v = K_f[(P_c - P_t) - \sigma(\pi_c - \pi_t)] \qquad (1)$$

where

J_v = Rate of fluid flux
K_f = Filtration coefficient
P_c = Capillary hydrostatic pressure (not the pulmonary capillary wedge pressure)
P_t = Tissue hydrostatic pressure
σ = Reflection coefficient
π_c = Plasma osmotic pressure due to proteins
π_t = Tissue osmotic pressure due to proteins

Despite its apparent complexity, the equation essentially says that the amount of fluid that enters the interstitium is determined by the hydrostatic gradient ($P_c - P_t$), tending to push fluid out of the capillary, and the colloid osmotic gradient ($\pi_c - \pi_t$), acting to hold fluid inside the capillary. Anything that changes one of these factors with respect to the others changes the amount of fluid that leaves the capillary. A reduction in π_c, which occurs frequently in response to disease, or an increase in P_c as a result of fluid infusion, causes J_v to rise. The fraction of the protein molecules that are reflected by the capillary membrane is represented by σ. A value of 1 means that the membrane is impermeable, and zero indicates completely permeable. The normal σ for albu-

TABLE 8–1. Antiedema Safety Factors

Increased tissue hydrostatic pressure
Decreased tissue colloid osmotic pressure
Increased lymph flow rate

min in the lungs is 0.7. If a disease process decreases σ, the osmotic gradient has less effect retarding the egress of fluid out of the capillary and edema occurs with lower P_c elevations.

Although no edema is present under normal conditions, there is a net positive amount of fluid leaving the capillary. In fact, J_v can rise a certain amount before edema starts to occur. The reason is that antiedema safety factors (Table 8–1) oppose the formation of edema. P_c can be raised to levels that overwhelm the antiedema safety factors and result in pulmonary edema. This occurs when the rate at which fluid enters the interstitium is greater than the lymph flow rate removing it.

The risk to the patient with pulmonary edema is ventilatory failure. Fluid in the interstitium appears to cause reflex tachypnea. Once lung weight has increased 40%, alveolar flooding occurs, resulting in ventilation/perfusion mismatching and decreased FRC. Pulmonary compliance may decrease, increasing the patient's work of breathing. As pulmonary edema increases, ventilatory compromise worsens, resulting in cyanosis and respiratory acidosis.

Tests that are helpful in the diagnosis of pulmonary edema are largely limited to the physical examination, chest roentgenogram, and arterial blood gases. No laboratory test can detect the presence of small amounts of pulmonary edema. The first sign may be tachypnea, which may induce hypertension, peripheral vasoconstriction, diaphoresis, and restlessness. Generally the patient is more comfortable in a sitting position, which shifts the edema fluid to the lung bases. At this stage, end-inspiratory rales may be present. In some patients expiratory wheezes (cardiac asthma) may be the predominant auscultatory finding. PaO_2 may be normal initially, but $PaCO_2$ may be low, reflecting the edema-induced tachypnea. On a portable chest roentgenogram, edema is evidenced by vascular congestion, blurred vessel edges, peribronchial cuffs, which represent fluid around the bronchi, and fluffy consolidation. If the patient has been lying on one side, the edema may appear to be unilateral.

As the amount of edema increases, work of breathing increases because of increased airway resistance and decreased lung compliance.

TABLE 8–2. Pulmonary Edema Reduction

Decrease tissue hydrostatic pressure
  Reduce fluid administration rate
  Reduce intravascular volume with diuretics
  Vasodilators
Increase tissue colloid osmotic pressure with
  colloid solutions
Facilitate lymph flow

Increased airway resistance is caused by mucosal edema, which narrows the caliber of the airways, and decreased lung compliance is caused by vascular engorgement and edema. When alveolar flooding develops, pink frothy sputum may be produced and gas exchange worsens. Pao_2 is low unless treated with an increased fraction of inspired oxygen (Fio_2). $Paco_2$ may be elevated, reflecting the patient's inability to maintain adequate alveolar ventilation. Patients should be treated with mechanical ventilation when acidosis develops.

Treatment consists of supportive steps to treat the ventilatory failure (described in Chapter 3), as well as maneuvers to reduce the amount of pulmonary edema. Management of associated respiratory failure may include positive airway pressure, oxygen, intubation, and mechanical ventilation. The application of positive end-expiratory pressure (PEEP) improves oxygenation by increasing the FRC and correcting ventilation/perfusion mismatches. At one time PEEP was incorrectly thought to "push" pulmonary edema fluid out of the lungs.

Approaches to reducing the amount of pulmonary edema are based on the Starling equation. Pulmonary edema occurs because fluid enters the interstitium faster than it can be removed. Thus, J_v needs to be decreased (Table 8–2). In the most straightforward cases, such as congestive heart failure or fluid overload, pulmonary edema exists because P_c is greatly elevated. Thus P_c should be lowered, so fluid enters the interstitium more slowly than the lymph flow rate removing it. P_c in this situation is most easily lowered by giving a diuretic such as furosemide. Diuretics reduce pulmonary edema by decreasing the intravascular volume sufficiently to reduce capillary pressures. Furosemide also is beneficial in pulmonary edema because it acts as a venodilator, further lowering P_c. Diuresis should be performed carefully in a brittle patient to prevent a sudden decrease in left ventricular filling pressure and subsequent fall in cardiac output. Treatment of other causes of pulmonary edema is covered with their specific causes in this chapter.

ADULT RESPIRATORY DISTRESS SYNDROME

Originally described by Petty in 1967, adult respiratory distress syndrome (ARDS) has become a major challenge to intensivists. ARDS is a diffuse process that includes pulmonary edema on chest roentgenogram, decreased pulmonary compliance (stiff lungs), refractory hypoxemia, and in late stages pulmonary hypertension. ARDS represents a stereotypic response to a wide variety of insults, both direct and indirect. Thus ARDS appears to be the result of some inherent process that does not depend on a specific disease. Table 8–3 lists many of the conditions that have been associated with ARDS. Conditions in which ARDS is most likely to develop include sepsis, aspiration, pulmonary contusion, toxic substance inhalation, long bone fractures, and near drowning.

The pathophysiology of ARDS has yet to be elucidated. Proposed mediators have included activated complement, proteases, arachidonic acid, free radicals, platelet-activating factor, and other, less well-defined compounds. The neutrophil has been indicted because it contains many of these mediators. However, neutropenic patients have been reported to have the syndrome. Investigators have suggested that other cellular elements, such as macrophages, may be the source of the responsible mediators.

Interstitial pulmonary edema is the earliest pathologic finding in ARDS. This is followed by the movement of inflammatory cells into the interstitium, as well as the development of proteinaceous alveolar fluid. Type I alveolar

TABLE 8–3. Conditions Associated with Adult Respiratory Distress Syndrome

Direct Injury

Pulmonary contusion
Aspiration
Pneumonia
Air embolism
Fat embolism
Oxygen toxicity
Toxic inhalation
Smoke inhalation
Cardiopulmonary bypass
Near drowning
Amniotic fluid embolism

Indirect Injury

Sepsis
Multiple transfusions
Pancreatitis
Head injury

epithelial cells, which make surfactant, are replaced by type II cells. Hyaline membranes may then form on the alveolar surfaces as the inflammatory process continues. Eventually fibrosis develops with obliteration of alveoli. Capillary thrombosis becomes more apparent and may be the reason for the pulmonary hypertension common in late ARDS. In survivors, remodeling and reduction of the fibrosis occur with time.

Clinical Course.   Tachypnea is the first clinically apparent sign of ARDS. Tachypnea is caused by the increased work of breathing, which initially results from a decrease in FRC as well as the disease process itself, and by respiratory stimulation from hypoxia. As the lungs become stiffer, respiratory distress is evident. Generally, sputum production is slight and auscultation of the chest reveals little. Arterial hypoxemia may develop anytime during the course of the disease. Chest roentgenograms reveal a nonspecific pulmonary edema pattern without evidence of fluid overload. As the disease progresses, pulmonary hypertension may develop. Because of the stiffness of the lungs and the high inflation pressures needed to ventilate these patients, catastrophic pneumothorax is a potential problem. If the course of the disease cannot be altered, the patient has progressive difficulty in maintaining adequate oxygenation. However, it is the rare patient who dies of hypoxemia. Most commonly patients die of concomitant multiple system organ failure. Although right ventricular dysfunction is at least in part due to pulmonary hypertension, the role of overt right ventricular failure in the death of these patients is not known.

Diagnosis.   The severity of pulmonary dysfunction in affected patients varies widely; only the most severe cases are classified as ARDS. The currently accepted criteria for ARDS include (1) refractory hypoxemia, (2) pulmonary infiltrates on chest roentgenogram, (3) decreased pulmonary compliance, and (4) no cardiac failure (pulmonary capillary wedge pressure less than 18 mm Hg) or other basis for the observed pulmonary findings. Unfortunately, ARDS has no specific marker and diagnosis must be based on clinical criteria.

Recognition of the patient at risk for ARDS is as important as diagnosing the disease once it has started. Patients at risk should have their respiratory rate and arterial oxygen saturation (Sao_2) monitored. Tachypnea and hypoxemia may respond to mask CPAP. However, many patients with ARDS will require intubation and mechanical ventilation. Most important, the cause should be ascertained and treated directly.

Treatment

Positive End-Expiratory Pressure. PEEP is a mainstay in the management of severe ARDS. PEEP does not reduce pulmonary edema or force alveolar fluid back into the interstitium, although it may cause a redistribution of fluid within the alveoli. Prophylactic PEEP does not prevent or ameliorate ARDS, nor does it alter the natural history of ARDS. PEEP is instituted to maintain acceptable Sao_2 while preventing toxic concentrations of inspired oxygen. The oxygenation defect in ARDS is thought to be due to a significantly increased number of perfused lung units that are collapsed and not ventilated. PEEP improves oxygenation in ARDS by reexpanding these collapsed alveoli.

The application of PEEP is associated with a number of adverse effects, some of which may be life threatening. The main concerns of PEEP are those associated with any form of positive-pressure ventilation: barotrauma and cardiovascular depression. The mechanisms involved with the development of these problems are discussed in the section on complications of mechanical ventilation in Chapter 3. Cardiovascular depression is monitored by observation of trends in hemodynamic parameters, such as blood pressure, heart rate, central venous pressure, cardiac output, pulmonary capillary wedge pressure, and pulmonary artery pressure. The risk of barotrauma is reduced by monitoring of static compliance. Compliance should increase or remain unchanged as FRC is inflated with PEEP. However, if the lung becomes overinflated, the flat part of the lung pressure/volume curve is reached and compliance decreases with further increases in PEEP, increasing the risk of barotrauma. Other adverse effects of PEEP are due to increased central venous pressure and include increased intracranial pressure, hepatic congestion, and renal dysfunction.

PEEP therapy should be considered when a patient requires potentially toxic concentrations of oxygen to maintain acceptable arterial saturation. This may be expressed by a Pao_2/Fio_2 ratio (P/F ratio) less than 150 or, if a pulmonary artery catheter is present, the shunt fraction ($\dot{Q}s/\dot{Q}t$) is greater than 20%.

The only absolute contraindication to the application of PEEP is the presence of an undrained pneumothorax. Relative contraindications include risk or presence of increased intracranial pressure, hypovolemia, marginal cardiovascular function, emphysema, cavitary pneumonias, and unilateral lung disease. PEEP may be applied to selected patients with these conditions if they are carefully monitored (physician at the bedside) so PEEP can be immediately decreased if adverse effects arise. In patients with unilateral lung disease or even heterogeneous involvement, PEEP causes areas of compliant lung to expand more than stiff lung. Thus, as PEEP is increased, compliant lung overdistends and begins to compress diseased lung, exacerbating the poor ventilation to these lung units. In this situation the application of PEEP results in worsening blood gas concentrations. Selective bronchial intubation with a double-lumen tube and differential application of PEEP may be effective in this situation (see "Independent Lung Ventilation," Chapter 3).

Because of the complexity of PEEP application and monitoring of adverse effects, a standardized approach is favored. An advantage of such a technique is that the nurse, respiratory technician, and physician become familiar with what should be done next. Furthermore, a standardized approach reduces errors in clinical management. If the patient's condition requires the application of PEEP higher than 10 cm H_2O, placement of a pulmonary artery catheter should be considered.

The application of PEEP should always be considered a trial. Some patients who seem to be excellent candidates may exhibit unexpected hemodynamic deterioration. Assessment should follow every increment in PEEP to titrate therapy optimally. PEEP should be titrated over a short time to minimize the exposure to high concentrations of inspired oxygen and prevent further collapse of alveoli. The PEEP trial is continued until either a desirable physiologic endpoint is attained or an unacceptable condition occurs. Whenever a PEEP trial is instituted, a physician should be in attendance to evaluate the patient's response. The following method incorporates the monitoring of oxygen delivery and lung mechanics necessary for optimal care:

1. Establish baseline status by documenting data.
   a. Pulmonary data
      (1) FIO_2
      (2) PEEP level
      (3) Peak inspiratory pressure
      (4) Inspiratory plateau pressure
      (5) Tidal volume (Compliance = Tidal volume/(Inspiratory plateau − PEEP)
      (6) Respiratory rate
      (7) Arterial blood gases and CO-oximetry
      (8) Mixed venous blood gases and CO-oximetry*
   b. Cardiovascular data
      (1) Heart rate
      (2) Mean arterial blood pressure
      (3) Central venous pressure
      (4) Pulmonary artery pressure*
      (5) Pulmonary capillary wedge pressure*
      (6) Cardiac output*

2. Increase PEEP by a 2.5 to 5 cm H_2O increment without altering any other ventilator setting. Observe the patient for immediate adverse effects such as hypotension or increased intracranial pressure.

3. Allow approximately 15 minutes for stabilization to the new PEEP, and repeat measurements.

4. Analyze the response to PEEP to determine the next step.
   a. If PaO_2 has improved, the FIO_2 is lowered. The goal is to have acceptable oxygenation on FIO_2 less than 0.5. Generally, acceptable oxygenation is defined as an SaO_2 greater than 88%. However, some proponents believe that PEEP should be increased until the $\dot{Q}s/\dot{Q}t$ is less than 20%. Once the goal of acceptable oxygenation has been achieved, the PEEP trial is stopped.
   b. If the PaO_2 has decreased, it may be due to either overdistention of lung or decreased cardiac output. PEEP should be decreased to its previous level and the problem corrected, if possible.
   c. Regardless of the PaO_2, if the cardiac output decreases by more than 20% or the venous oxygen saturation (SvO_2) decreases by 10% or more in actual saturation, the PEEP should be reduced to the previous level. Hemodynamic support with either fluids or inotropic agents, as appropriate, should be instituted and the PEEP trial reattempted.
   d. If the pulmonary compliance decreases, overdistention is likely to be present. The improvement of oxygenation may not justify the risk of barotrauma at this level of PEEP.
   e. PEEP is increased in 2.5 to 5 cm H_2O steps until one of the preceding situations occurs. There is no maximum level of PEEP, but the incidence of complications rises as PEEP reaches 25 cm H_2O.

---

* Requires pulmonary artery catheter.

Once an optimal level of PEEP has been determined, close monitoring should continue because progress of the underlying disease may require adjustments. The patient should be weaned from PEEP only when the need for the PEEP has resolved. Premature reduction in PEEP is defined as an unacceptable decrease in Pao_2. In one study 42% of patients required an increase in PEEP above the level of the preweaning PEEP to achieve adequate oxygenation. Thus guidelines for PEEP reduction are helpful to prevent losing ground. First, the patient should no longer have sepsis and should demonstrate a stable clinical course for at least 12 hours with a Pao_2 of 80 mm Hg or more on an Fio_2 of 0.4 or less. When weaning starts from the higher levels of PEEP (greater than 12 cm H_2O), the oxygenation response to a very short trial of decreased PEEP should be considered. The PEEP is decreased for 3 minutes, at the end of which an arterial sample is sent for analysis and the PEEP is immediately returned to its previous level while results are awaited. Investigators have demonstrated that if the Pao_2 decreases less than 20% with the 3-minute trial, a more prolonged interval should be tolerated. This technique has the advantage of not leaving the patient at a potentially inadequate level of PEEP until the blood gas values are received. Oxygenation is monitored for several hours, and if the patient is stable, another PEEP weaning trial is instituted. Obviously this protocol is directed at the sickest ARDS patients. Patients with more transient forms of acute lung injury may be weaned over a shorter time.

FLUID THERAPY.   Fluid therapy in ARDS is controversial. Starling equation (Eq. 1) considerations dictate that to minimize pulmonary edema, P_c is kept low and π_c is maintained. Crystalloid solutions decrease π_c, filter more quickly into the interstitium, and because of the relatively greater volume needed, increase P_c and result in more pulmonary edema than colloid solutions. Proponents of crystalloid solutions in ARDS believe that the colloid molecules become lodged in the interstitium and exacerbate edema formation. No studies have conclusively associated one type of solution with a better outcome than another. Regardless, even in a situation of increased permeability, maintaining P_c as low as is hemodynamically possible minimizes pulmonary edema fluid.

Outcome.   In the patients with ARDS who die, cause of death is frequently sepsis and multiple system organ failure, not ventilatory failure. This may explain why, despite the interest and investigation over the past 20 years, out-

come from ARDS is little improved. Patients who survive ARDS commonly have residual pulmonary disease, including dyspnea at rest or on exertion, restrictive or obstructive defect on pulmonary function studies, increased diffusion capacity, persistent abnormalities on chest roentgenogram, and airway hyperreactivity.

ASPIRATION

Pulmonary aspiration of gastric contents occurs in a wide variety of clinical settings. Certain factors increase the risk of aspiration (Table 8–4). The severity of the resultant pneumonitis depends on the pH, volume, and particulate nature of the aspirated material. It is commonly accepted but has never been proven that aspirates with a pH less than 2.5 and a volume greater than 25 ml are more likely to produce severe aspiration pneumonitis. Acidic fluid causes necrosis of the bronchial epithelial cells, atelectasis, edema, and hemorrhage.

Clinical presentation is variable and often characterized by nonspecific findings. The clinical picture also depends on the severity of the pneumonitis. Patients may have only wheezing or a full-blown syndrome consisting of cyanosis, tachypnea, and hypotension. Usually tachypnea occurs first.

Since the clinical findings are often nonspecific in aspiration, a high index of suspicion is required to make the diagnosis. Identification of gastric material in the lower airways by observation or suctioning makes the diagnosis easy. The diagnosis should be entertained when unexpected wheezing or acute respiratory failure develops in a patient with risk factors, especially when the level of consciousness is depressed. Arterial hypoxemia occurs early, and arterial blood gases should be drawn for analysis. Chest roentgenography may be misleading early in the course of the disease. The chest roentgenogram may be normal initially and lag behind the clinical picture by 12 hours. Alter-

TABLE 8–4.   Aspiration Risk Factors

Decreased level of consciousness
Inadequate cough
Regurgitation
Artificial airway
Increased perioperative risk
Increased gastric contents
    Pregnancy
    Upper gastrointestinal hemorrhage
    Ileus
Nasogastric tube

natively, it may reveal what appears to be severe consolidation (atelectasis), which clears after a few hours of positive-pressure ventilation. In an erect patient the right lower lobe is more likely to be involved. However, many hospitalized patients are in other positions when they aspirate and the distribution may be diffuse. Gastric or pharyngeal pH testing is of little value because the results do not assist in diagnosis. Fluid aspirated from the trachea can be tested for glucose with a dipstick to confirm the occurrence of aspiration because glucose is not present in pulmonary secretions.

Treatment of aspiration pneumonitis is similar to management of other forms of acute respiratory failure. The initial maneuver in a witnessed aspiration is to suction the trachea. Following removal of possible offending material, oxygen should be administered and the airway protected. Airway protection is important both to provide positive-pressure ventilation and to prevent further aspiration. Lavage of the bronchial tree is not indicated. Aspirated acid causes damage immediately on contact with the respiratory system. Furthermore, the buffering capacity of the bronchial epithelial cells neutralizes the acid within seconds.

Some investigators believe that positive-pressure ventilation shortens the course of aspiration pneumonitis. Whether to intubate the patient and begin positive-pressure ventilation is determined by the severity of the gas exchange abnormality. A patient who is awake, not hypoxic when breathing room air, and not likely to continue to aspirate is a candidate for careful observation. However, because deterioration can occur rapidly, many patients with aspiration should be managed with mechanical ventilation. The principles of respiratory support are outlined in Chapter 3.

Corticosteroids have not been shown to improve the outcome from aspiration. Unless the aspirate is grossly infected, prophylactic antibiotics should not be used. If bacterial pneumonia develops after the aspiration episode, cultures should be used to guide antibiotic therapy.

Because of the potentially catastrophic nature of aspiration, prevention offers the best outcome. Thus a cuffed endotracheal or tracheostomy tube should be placed if the patient's level of consciousness is depressed (Glasgow Coma Scale score less than 10) or airway reflexes are obtunded. The clinician can rarely be sure that a critically ill patient has an empty stomach. Therefore the airway should be protected as described in earlier chapters if intubation is required.

Aspiration is always a risk, even when appropriate precautions are taken. A number of prophylactic drugs have been suggested for reducing the severity of the potential aspiration. Reducing the acidity of gastric contents has been approached from several angles. Traditionally, particulate antacids, such as Maalox, Mylanta, and Amphojel, have been administered every 1 to 4 hours to maintain gastric pH above 4.5. However, experimental work has revealed that aspiration of these particulate antacids causes a pneumonitis indistinguishable from acid aspiration. This finding has generated interest in a nonparticulate antacid, 0.3 M sodium citrate (Bicitra). Another approach has involved blocking the H_2 receptors that stimulate the gastric parietal cells to secrete acid. Cimetidine, raniditine, and famotidine are the common H_2 blockers in current practice. Because of the number of significant interactions with other drugs, cimetidine has dropped in popularity in recent years. Increasing gastric pH may create other problems. Alkalinizing gastric contents results in bacterial overgrowth, which may increase the incidence of nosocomial pneumonias.

Metoclopromide is used to enhance gastric emptying by decreasing pyloric sphincter tone. Its antiaspiration efficacy has not been proved.

Particulate aspiration presents specific problems. The clinical impact is determined by the size, composition, and location. Large foreign bodies that obstruct the trachea may produce asphyxia, cyanosis, and death. More commonly, aspirated particles are smaller and become lodged in either of the main bronchi. If the foreign body completely obstructs an airway, distal atelectasis may develop. Such atelectasis usually results in pneumonia. Foreign bodies lodged in the bronchial tree tend to form granulomas and should therefore be removed by bronchoscopy as soon as the patient's condition allows.

Hydrocarbon aspiration can be depressingly difficult to manage. It is associated with a profound pneumonitis that may progress to sterile abscesses, ARDS, bronchopleural fistulas, and other problems. Hydrocarbon aspiration usually occurs secondary to accidental or suicidal ingestion. Immediate protection of the airway is crucial.

ASTHMA

The American Thoracic Society defines asthma as "a syndrome characterized by increased responsiveness of the tracheobronchial tree to a variety of stimuli." Bronchospasm produces increased work of breathing, air trapping, and gas exchange impairment. Its diagnosis and treatment are important components of optimal critical care practice. Asthma may occur in a variety of situations in critically ill patients. In a patient with a progressive history of wheezing, asthma may embarrass ventilatory function sufficiently to require admission to an ICU. Conversely, in a critically ill patient bronchospasm may develop as a response to the presence of an endotracheal tube, pneumonia, or inhalation of toxic fumes.

Recent work has greatly expanded understanding of the pathophysiology of asthma. Triggers of asthma include antigens (extrinsic asthma) and nonspecific agents (intrinsic asthma) that do not act through immunologic mechanisms. The nonspecific triggers include a wide variety of unrelated substances, such as aerosols of distilled or hypertonic water, sulfur dioxide, ammonia, aspirin and other nonsteroidal antiinflammatory agents, sulfites, beta blockers, exercise, and emotional disturbance. The extent to which any trigger can induce asthma depends largely on the intensity of airway reactiveness. Airway reactiveness may vary in an asthmatic patient depending on concurrent problems, and therapy adequate on one day may be insufficient on another.

The mast cell appears to be involved with allergic triggers of asthma. Mast cells may also be stimulated by nonallergic triggers such as hypoxia, opiates, neuropeptides, and changes in local osmolarity. Degranulation of mast cells increases vascular permeability, smooth muscle contraction, mucus secretion, and leukocyte chemoattraction. Late changes include mucosal edema, cellular infiltration, and desquamation of epithelial cells.

Airway narrowing produces most of the clinically significant effects of asthma. Recent evidence suggests that the airway narrowing involves the entire bronchial tree. Early in the attack, airway narrowing is due primarily to bronchial smooth muscle contraction, which is relatively easy to reverse with beta agonists. However, airway narrowing is probably exacerbated by mucus and mucosal edema in the late phases and is more resistant to pharmacologic intervention.

Clinical Presentation. Patients with asthma have a prolonged expiratory phase and may or may not have audible wheezes. Pulmonary function testing reveals an obstructive pattern. Air trapping, increased residual volume, and increased functional residual capacity may de-

velop from the airway obstruction. Distribution of ventilation tends to be uneven, reducing the efficiency of breathing. Hypoxic pulmonary vasoconstriction (HPV) reduces blood flow to poorly ventilated lung units. If enough lung units are poorly ventilated, HPV may induce pulmonary hypertension. Mild hypoxemia and hypocapnia are common findings in asthmatic attacks. As the patient becomes fatigued, normocapnia replaces hypocapnia and is thus an ominous sign of impending ventilatory failure. Cardiovascular effects of a severe asthma attack are due to the more negative pleural pressure, HPV, hyperinflation of the lung, and acidosis. The most serious cardiovascular problem is pulmonary hypertension, which may result in right ventricular overload as evidenced by a decrease in cardiac output. Pulsus paradoxus occurs with severe asthma, although its exact mechanism is not clear.

Diagnosis. Asthma is an unusual disease in contemporary critical care practice because the diagnosis can be based only on history and physical examination. No laboratory or radiologic test diagnoses wheezing; it must be heard. However, not all wheezing is due to asthma. Wheezing may be also associated with endobronchial intubation, aspiration of gastric contents, kinked endotracheal tube, extrinsic airway compression, pulmonary edema, and pneumothorax. Bronchospasm results in end-expiratory musical rales. Inspiratory rales alone suggest pulmonary edema as a cause.

Treatment. Management of asthma has evolved over the past few years away from methylxanthine derivatives (theophyllines) and toward selective beta$_2$-adrenergic agonists and earlier use of steroids. Bronchial smooth muscle exhibits beta$_2$ receptors that, when stimulated, cause relaxation. Older beta agonists, such as isoetharine and isoproterenol, have undesirable side effects, particularly cardiac arrhythmias, which result from concomitant beta$_1$ receptor activity. Newer agents are more selective for beta$_2$ receptors (less cardiac stimulation) and have a longer duration. The available agents may be given by inhalation, intravenously, subcutaneously, or orally. The inhalation method offers several advantages for delivery of drug in the critically ill. Delivery to the site of action is immediate, and side effects are minimized. Inhalation may be accomplished with a metered dose inhaler or by nebulization either with a mask or in line with a mechanical ventilator. However, patients may exhibit airflow restriction of such magnitude that effective delivery of the drug is impossible. These patients require

TABLE 8–5.   Beta Agonists

DRUG	BETA$_2$ SELECTIVE	ROUTE
Epinephrine	No	Inhalation, subcutaneous
Isoetharine (Bronkosol)	No	Inhalation
Isoproterenol (Isuprel)	No	Inhalation (intravenous for children)
Metapro-terenol (Alupent)	No	Inhalation
Albuterol (Proventil, Ventolin)	Yes	Inhalation
Terbutaline (Brethine)	Yes	Inhalation, subcu-taneous, oral
Bitolterol (Tornalate)	Yes	Inhalation

parenteral administration of bronchodilator. Table 8–5 displays the beta agonists, their route of administration, and their beta$_2$ selectivity.

Corticosteroids are now administered as soon as an inadequate response to beta-adrenergic drugs has been demonstrated. These drugs are given in high doses but for less than 2 weeks to prevent complications. Corticosteroid administration has been assisted by the availability of metered dose inhalers of beclomethasone (Vanceril), flunisolide (Aerobid), and triamcinolone (Azmacort).

Bronchoconstriction may also be mediated by cholinergic receptors. Nebulized atropine and ipratropium (Atrovent) often improve bronchospasm when combined with beta-adrenergic drugs, especially in patients with chronic obstructive pulmonary disease. Ipratropium has been shown to be as effective as beta-adrenergic agonists in bronchospasm associated with COPD. Ipratropium does not cause demonstrable change in mucus viscosity and is not associated with tachycardia.

Sodium cromolyn (Intal) is a mast cell stabilizer. Although it is an excellent prophylactic drug in compliant patients, it has no role in the treatment of an acute asthmatic attack.

Theophylline has become less popular in recent years because of its inherent narrow therapeutic index and the effectiveness of the newer beta-adrenergic agents. Studies have failed to find any benefit of administering theophylline to patients already receiving beta-adrenergic therapy. Furthermore, theophylline enhanced cardiac toxicity. The loading dose of theophylline is 5 to 6 mg/kg given over 20 to 30 minutes followed by an infusion of 0.5 to 5

mg/kg/h depending on whether the patient is a rapid or slow acetylator. Blood levels should be monitored. At concentrations less than 10 μg/ml, toxic side effects are unusual but so is bronchodilation. Therapeutic levels, believed to be 10 to 20 μg/ml, are often associated with jitteriness. Levels above 20 μg/ml may result in severe and life-threatening complications, including diarrhea, tachyarrhythmias, seizures, and death.

Status Asthmaticus

Status asthmaticus is defined as life-threatening bronchospasm that is unresolved with routine therapy. Patients with this condition should be observed in an ICU. Generally the patient continues to wheeze despite beta-adrenergic agents and theophylline. Attempts are made to identify and treat the precipitating event, such as bacterial infection, exposure to irritant or antigenic substances, and emotional stress. ICU management includes humidified oxygen administration for the associated hypoxemia. The patient should be monitored with a pulse oximeter and frequent arterial blood gas tests.

Rehydration is thought to assist with mobilization of secretions. Patients frequently decrease their fluid intake with onset of acute dyspnea.

Diagnostic studies, such as peak expiratory flow to monitor effect of therapy, arterial blood gases, hematocrit, hemoglobin, electrolytes, chest roentgenography, sputum Gram stain and culture, and electrocardiography, are performed.

Intubation is performed, and mechanical ventilation is instituted as soon as the patient shows evidence of fatigue or gas exchange deterioration. Mechanical ventilation may be difficult because of the need for extremely high inflation pressures to get the tidal volume in and prolonged expiratory times to allow the tidal volume to come back out. Clinicians must watch for air trapping and auto-PEEP because they would further compromise the patient.

Administration of corticosteroids, such as hydrocortisone 1 g intravenously with 4 mg/kg every 4 hours, is begun. Atropine or ipratropium may be tried. Antibiotics are administered for documented infection.

As a last resort, general anesthesia may be instituted. All of the volatile anesthetic agents are potent bronchodilators. However, halothane may interact with beta$_2$ agonists and theophylline to produce adverse cardiac effects.

Thus enflurane and isoflurane are better choices. Ketamine has also been used successfully to treat refractory asthma. However, simultaneous administration of theophylline may result in life-threatening cardiac arrhythmias.

Bronchial lavage is a controversial technique for the treatment of status asthmaticus. Segmental bronchi are lavaged with a bronchoscope to remove inspissated material while the rest of the lung maintains gas exchange.

Extracorporeal removal of carbon dioxide has been reported in the management of hypercarbia in a patient with status asthmaticus.

ACUTE RESPIRATORY FAILURE RELATED TO CHRONIC OBSTRUCTIVE PULMONARY DISEASE

Chronic obstructive pulmonary disease (COPD) is a term that covers a variety of disease processes, such as chronic bronchitis, emphysema, cystic fibrosis, and asthma, although common usage generally excludes the latter two. The accepted definition of chronic bronchitis is based on clinical presentation. The patient must have a chronic productive cough for at least 3 months in at least 2 consecutive years. Excessive production of mucus and mucus gland hypertrophy occur, although the physiologic significance of these findings is unknown. Emphysema is an anatomic definition for disruption of alveolar septa. The major effect of emphysema is destruction of the structural support of the lung with a decrease in elastic recoil. This change increases pulmonary compliance.

COPD can alter the lung's mechanical characteristics in a variety of ways. Characteristic changes in the lung's architecture result in two processes, abnormally high FRC and intrinsic PEEP, which contribute to increased work of breathing in patients with COPD. The decrease in elastic recoil of the pulmonary parenchyma results in an increased FRC. Increased end-expiratory lung volumes push the diaphragm down, flattening the muscle. This decreases the efficiency of the diaphragm by two mechanisms. First, because the diaphragm is shortened, it is at a less efficient point on the length-contractility curve. Second, the amount of force generated is directly related to the degree of curvature, which is less when the diaphragm is flattened. Because of the abnormal lung architecture, gas flow during expiration is impeded. In a tachypneic patient, expiration may not be long enough to allow the alveolar pressure to reach zero. The resulting alveolar pressure is called intrinsic PEEP. Intrinsic PEEP increases work of breathing because the patient must generate a pleural pressure sufficiently negative to overcome the alveolar positive pressure before inspiratory flow occurs. This amount of work is in addition to the elastic and resistive elements of work of breathing discussed at the end of Chapter 3.

Increases in work of breathing increase oxygen consumption and carbon dioxide production. If patients cannot expend the necessary energy, alveolar hypoventilation may develop with hypercarbia and hypoxemia, which lead to decreases in oxygen delivery to the respiratory muscles. Thus a vicious cycle begins. On the other hand, if the patient does increase ventilatory work, the increased carbon dioxide production may offset the increased minute ventilation with the result that the $Paco_2$ does not decrease or even rises.

COPD is also associated with increased venous admixture, which may result in hypoxemia. Areas of affected lung may exhibit HPV in response to the hypoxia. The effect of this reflex is to reduce blood flow to poorly ventilated lung units and decrease the venous admixture. If enough lung units are involved, however, vasoconstriction results in pulmonary hypertension and may progress to cor pulmonale, which consists of right ventricular failure, jugular venous distention, and peripheral edema (see below). Improvement of the hypoxemia with either increased alveolar ventilation or small increases in Fio_2 may reduce the HPV sufficiently to improve right ventricular function.

The key point to understand about COPD is that these patients have diminished pulmonary reserve under normal conditions. Therefore any insult that places demands on their ventilatory function may result in abrupt respiratory failure. Common insults that increase oxygen demand beyond ventilatory capacity are listed in Table 8–6.

Clinical Presentation. A history usually reveals a long exposure to tobacco, dyspnea on mild exertion, and perhaps productive cough. Some patients also have a history of wheezing. Physical examination may reveal the barrel chest appearance of emphysema, prolonged expiratory phase with or without expiratory wheezing, cyanosis, basilar rales, or coarse rhonchi. Laboratory findings may include polycythemia and hypoxemia, hypercarbia, and a compensatory metabolic alkalosis. Typical arterial blood gas findings are a pH of 7.35, a Pco_2 of 55 mm Hg, and a Po_2 of 50 mm Hg. Chest roentgenograms in a critically ill patient with a

TABLE 8–6. Common Precipitants of Acute Respiratory Failure in Chronic Obstructive Pulmonary Disease

CONDITION	TREATMENT
Hypoxia	Administer oxygen
Bronchospasm	Administer beta agonists, ipratropium, aminophylline, steroids; pulmonary toilet
Cardiac disturbance	Administer antiarrhythmics, inotropes, calcium entry blockers, diuretics; correct metabolic derangements
Infection	Administer antibiotics empirically while awaiting culture results
Pulmonary embolism	Diagnose; consider heparin, inferior caval interruption, thrombolytics
Anatomic precipitant	Treat pneumothorax, pleural effusion, rib fractures, upper airway obstruction
Metabolic derangements	Correct hypophosphatemia, hypocalcemia, hypomagnesemia, hypokalemia

Modified from Schmidt GA, JB Hall: Acute on chronic respiratory failure. JAMA 1989; 261:3444-3453. Copyright 1989, American Medical Association.

history of COPD are almost always difficult to interpret. COPD is associated with evidence of hyperlucency and flattened diaphragm (from hyperinflation), or increased densities probably secondary to fibrotic changes in the parenchyma. Films taken when the patient was reasonable healthy may help. However, in these patients life-threatening deterioration of pulmonary function can develop with surprisingly little radiographic change. Pulmonary function tests generally reveal an obstructive pattern. Testing before and after the administration of bronchodilators, if feasible, should be performed even in the absence of audible wheezing. Results of pulmonary function and arterial blood gas studies obtained during a "normal" or baseline period are useful to determine the level to which the patient can be expected to improve.

Diagnosis.   Most clinicians agree that a Pa_{O_2} of 55 mm Hg or less or Pa_{CO_2} of 50 mm Hg or more represents respiratory failure. However, whether these values necessitate admission to a critical care unit depends on several factors, including whether the values actually represent baseline condition, the severity of the underlying pulmonary disease, and patient's prognosis. The pH may be helpful in determining whether hypercarbia is chronic. The pH decreases by 0.05 to 0.08 unit for an acute increase in Pa_{CO_2} of 10 mm Hg, but only 0.03 unit for a chronic increase in Pa_{CO_2} of the same magnitude.

Acute hypercarbia is associated with evidence of sympathetic stimulation, such as diaphoresis, tachycardia, occasionally hypertension, and dyspnea. However, the immediate physiologic threat of increased Pa_{CO_2} may be appreciated by reviewing the alveolar air equation (Eq. 7 in Chapter 3). Increases in Pa_{CO_2} must eventually result in decreases in Pa_{O_2}. For example, assuming a respiratory quotient of 0.8, for each increase in Pa_{CO_2}, the Pa_{O_2} decreases by 1.25 mm Hg. Thus, to achieve a Pa_{O_2} of only 40 mm Hg, Pa_{CO_2} must remain below 90 mm Hg while the patient is breathing room air.

Treatment.   Correction of the exacerbating condition offers the best chance of returning the patient to baseline status. Drainage of a pneumothorax, antibiotic treatment of pneumonia or bronchitis, aggressive application of lung-clearing techniques in the presence of copious secretions, analgesics for rib fractures, correction of congestive heart failure, and adequate nutrition may aid in management. Because the benefit of bronchodilators may not be detected by standard pulmonary function tests, these patients should receive a course of therapy and be subjectively judged for effect.

Acute respiratory failure in patients with COPD may result in hypoxemia. Although hypoxemia poses unacceptable risks, clinicians have been reluctant to administer oxygen to these patients for fear of inducing respiratory depression. Some patients with COPD have had hypercarbia for a sufficient time that their ventilatory drive is not influenced by further increases in Pa_{CO_2}. Hypoxemia in these patients appears to be the major influence on ventilation, and relief of hypoxemia by supplemental oxygen has been thought to cause a decrease in minute ventilation and a significant increase in Pa_{CO_2}. However, studies have demonstrated that most of these patients are able to maintain minute ventilation when administered oxygen. Although Pa_{CO_2} increases, the slight decrease in minute ventilation is insufficient to explain the observed rise in Pa_{CO_2}. Regardless, the level of supplemental oxygen must be carefully titrated to increase Pa_{O_2} to at least 60 mm Hg (90% arterial saturation) to prevent further physiologic embarrassment.

These patients have an increased work of breathing even at their best. When attempting to wean them from mechanical ventilation after an acute exacerbation, the clinician should make every effort not to increase the work of breathing by the ventilation technique. As airway resistance is increased with smaller airway diameter, the largest endotracheal tube that can be safely placed should be used. Bronchospasm should be minimized without inducing toxicity. Precise management of nutrition may make an otherwise unweanable patient with COPD weanable. A normal postprandial respiratory quotient (RQ) is 0.8, meaning that the amount of carbon dioxide produced is 80% of the amount of oxygen consumed. However, if glucose is used as the sole source of nonnitrogen calories, the RQ increases to 1.0 and more carbon dioxide is produced for the same amount of oxygen consumption. Furthermore, if glucose is administered in excess of caloric needs, it is converted to triglyceride and stored as fat. The RQ associated with lipogenesis is 8.0. The RQ of overfed patients may rise to 1.2, representing a 50% increase in carbon dioxide production. Thus excessive glucose administration should be avoided. This may be most easily achieved by delivering up to 50% of the nonnitrogen calories as fat. A more detailed discussion of the management of the difficult-to-wean patient appears in Chapter 3.

COR PULMONALE

Cor pulmonale is right ventricular failure induced by pulmonary hypertension. Pulmonary hypertension arises in a number of lung disorders, including COPD. Its major circulatory effect is the impedance to right ventricular ejection. The thin-walled right ventricle is poorly constructed to generate high systolic pressures. Thus pulmonary hypertension can cause right ventricle hypertrophy or dilatation and eventually failure.

Early in the disease, right ventricular hypertrophy may develop with the maintenance of a normal cardiac output and a normal cardiovascular response to exercise. However, as the disease progresses, exercise intolerance evolves in association with markedly elevated right ventricular end-diastolic pressure. Decreased cardiac output causes salt and water retention, which exacerbates the venous and pulmonary hypertension.

Clinical Presentation. Physical examination may reveal evidence of the underlying lung

disorder. As pulmonary hypertension progresses, the right ventricle becomes hypertrophic and dilated. The second heart sound may be enhanced by pulmonary hypertension and may even be palpable. As the right ventricle dilates, pulmonary valve insufficiency develops. The onset of central venous hypertension heralds tricuspid insufficiency.

Diagnosis. Cor pulmonale is underdiagnosed in critically ill patients. Low cardiac output is generally attributed to dysfunction of the left side of the heart. However, the left ventricle depends on the right ventricle for adequate filling. A number of signs suggest cor pulmonale, including electrocardiographic evidence of right ventricular hypertrophy, increased central venous pressure, increased right ventricular end-diastolic pressure, and right ventricular dilatation detectable by echocardiography or chest roentgenography.

Treatment. By definition, pulmonary hypertension is the culprit in cor pulmonale. Thus management is directed at decreasing the pulmonary artery pressure. One potentially reversible component is hypoxic pulmonary vasoconstriction, which is corrected by oxygen administration. Acute infection should be aggressively treated with appropriate antibiotics and chest physiotherapy as indicated. Acidosis worsens pulmonary hypertension and should be corrected. Diuretics such as furosemide are administered to correct the salt and water retention. However, hypovolemia should be avoided because it has a deleterious effect on right ventricular function. Controversy surrounds the use of cardiac glycosides in these patients. In the ICU patient, other inotropes, such as dobutamine, can be used more effectively in the acute situation with less risk of toxicity. Although a direct pulmonary vasodilator is the specific agent needed in the care of these patients, no drug of this category has yet shown efficacy.

PULMONARY THROMBOEMBOLISM

Clinically important thromboemboli usually arise from large veins of the lower extremity or pelvis. Thromboembolism is a common complication in hospitalized patients but is often difficult to diagnose. Ten percent of patients with the disease die too quickly for diagnosis and treatment. Thus prevention in high-risk groups is important.

Several risk factors for pulmonary thromboembolism have been identified and are

TABLE 8–7. Predisposing Factors for Pulmonary Thromboembolism

Immobility (paralysis)
Advanced age
Major surgery (orthopedic)
Trauma
Oral contraceptives
Malignancy
Obesity
Congestive heart failure
Myocardial infarction
Shock
Hypercoagulable states

presented in Table 8–7. The most important of these is immobility.

The pathophysiology of pulmonary thromboembolism is not clearly understood. An embolus large enough to obstruct the pulmonary artery (saddle embolus) can produce acute pulmonary hypertension, right ventricular failure, and sudden death. In milder forms of the disease, the degree of pulmonary hypertension is inappropriately high for the amount of pulmonary circulation that has been occluded. As yet unknown neurohumoral mediators have been implicated in the purported pulmonary vasoconstriction to explain the pulmonary hypertension. The mechanism for observed gas exchange abnormalities is also unknown. Mechanical obstruction of segmental pulmonary blood flow should result only in increased dead space. This might lead to an increased $PaCO_2$ if tachypnea and increased minute ventilation did not invariably develop. However, hypoxemia (low $\dot{V}/\dot{Q}$ units and shunt) is common in severe cases, possibly because of recruitment of arteriovenous shunts, atelectasis, and edema often seen in pathologic specimens. The cause of the atelectasis and edema is not clear.

Clinical presentation is variable and nonspecific. An unknown number of pulmonary thromboembolisms are clinically inapparent. Sudden onset of dyspnea may be the only finding. At the other end of the spectrum, the patient may have right ventricular failure and shock with cyanosis and systemic hypotension. Patients with pulmonary infarction are more likely to have the classic triad of dyspnea, pleurisy, and hemoptysis along with fever, tachycardia, and pleural friction rub. Because of the presence of a second arterial circulation (bronchial), pulmonary thromboembolism does not generally cause infarction unless there is underlying lung disease.

Recognizing even minor pulmonary thromboembolism is important to prevent a subsequent and potentially fatal episode. Because the disease often is evidenced by nonspecific and seemingly minor signs and symptoms, a high index of suspicion must be maintained when tachypnea develops in high-risk patients. The most common clinical situation is peripheral pulmonary embolism without infarction. Besides tachypnea and tachycardia, few abnormalities may be found on physical examination. The patient may complain of pleuritic chest pain, or migratory expiratory wheezes may be found in some instances of multiple emboli. The electrocardiogram may show evidence of right ventricular strain, such as right axis deviation and incomplete right bundle branch block. Massive embolism can produce the classic Q wave in lead I and inverted T wave in lead III. Chest roentgenographic abnormalities are subtle and are often noticed only in retrospect. Segmental decrease in vessel markings (Westermark's sign) may be seen. However, the electrocardiogram and chest roentgenogram in many instances are normal, and more specific diagnostic tests should be performed. Arrhythmias, especially supraventricular, are common.

Arterial blood gas analysis may document an unexpected decrease in PaO_2, which, although nonspecific for embolism, may raise suspicion further. Hypocapnia is an expected finding in spontaneously breathing patients, but hypercapnia may occur in patients with fixed minute ventilation.

Radionuclide lung perfusion scans have achieved remarkable popularity, largely because of their simple, quick, and safe nature. In normal lungs a negative scan rules out emboli and a positive is diagnostic. In patients with underlying pulmonary or cardiac disease, interpretation of the scan may be difficult. A good-quality chest roentgenogram is necessary to interpret the perfusion scan, and a ventilation scan may be performed to clarify which parts of the lung are ventilated but not perfused. COPD, pneumonia, and left ventricular failure are some of the conditions that may make accurate interpretation of the perfusion scan difficult if not impossible. Ventilation scans improve the specificity of the scanning technique. If both ventilation and perfusion are diminished in the same lung segment, embolism is unlikely. Pulmonary angiography is the test of choice if the perfusion scan is questionable, underlying pulmonary disease precludes interpretation of the perfusion scan, or surgery for pulmonary embolism is required. Angiographic findings diagnostic of embolism are pulmonary vessel filling defects and cutoffs. However, small emboli may completely occlude small pulmonary artery branches, which may not be appreciated on angiography. When pulmonary embolism is suspected but not identified by lung studies, the leg veins should be studied for presence of thrombus. Impedance plethysmography is a noninvasive test that estimates blood volume changes in the calf by measurement of electrical resistance while a thigh cuff is inflated and deflated. The presence of venous thrombus reduces the magnitude of blood volume changes. If the impedance plethysmogram shows abnormalities, radioisotope or contrast venography should be performed.

The first line of treatment of pulmonary thromboembolism is anticoagulation with continuous intravenous heparin. Patients are loaded with 5000 to 10,000 units followed by 500 to 2000 units/h continuous infusion. Conventionally, the heparin infusion is titrated to keep the activated partial thromboplastin time (aPTT) 1½ to 2 times the preheparin value. The incidence of major bleeding with this technique is 1%, which appears to be less than with intermittent heparin anticoagulation. Thrombocytopenia often develops because of the heparin infusion, which may have to be discontinued. Heparin-induced thrombocytopenia may occur by either of two mechanisms. In 10% to 15% of patients a mild decrease in the platelet count occurs, which resolves despite continuation of heparin. This nonidiosyncratic thrombocytopenia is of little clinical significance. Idiosyncratic thrombocytopenia occurs in less than 5% of patients receiving heparin. The mechanism appears to be aggregation of platelets in the microcirculation mediated by immunoglobulin G antibodies. The risk of this process is arterial thrombosis. The diagnosis is confirmed by demonstrating heparin-dependent platelet serotonin release. Warfarin is used for the long-term prophylaxis of pulmonary thromboembolism and should be started soon after heparin institution. Recommendations are to prolong the prothrombin time to 1¼ times the control value.

Thrombolytic agents such as streptokinase and urokinase have undergone numerous trials. However, their use has been associated with many problems, the most significant of which is major bleeding. They may find their greatest benefit in nonoperative treatment of massive pulmonary embolism associated with hemodynamic instability.

Pulmonary thromboembolectomy has been performed less frequently as medical management has improved. Because the operative mortality rate is high, surgery is reserved for severely affected patients who are not likely to survive with medical management alone.

Migration of clots from the pelvis and legs may be retarded by two types of surgical procedure: those in which an obstruction, such as a filter, is placed within the cava, and those in which the diameter of the inferior vena cava is reduced. These techniques are generally used in patients with angiographically proven pulmonary embolism and in whom anticoagulation is contraindicated.

Prophylaxis with subcutaneous heparin 5000 units twice a day has been effective in several population groups at risk. However, the occasional episode of major bleeding is probably the major impediment to wide-scale acceptance of this practice.

PNEUMONIA

The management of pneumonia is discussed in Chapter 12.

BRONCHOPLEURAL FISTULA

Bronchopleural fistula (BPF) is defined as a communication between the tracheobronchial tree and the pleural space. Thus the presence of an air leak in a chest tube is a BPF by definition. However, the term is generally reserved for air leaks that result in loss of a significant portion of each tidal volume. BPF may result from penetrating or blunt trauma to the tracheobronchial tree, leakage from a bronchial stump following lobectomy or pneumonectomy, the presence of high airway pressures, or necrotizing processes, such as abscess, acid aspiration, or pneumonia. BPF arises in ARDS because of the combination of high airway pressures and derangement of the pulmonary architecture.

Pathophysiology. BPF represents a low-resistance pathway for gas flow. Thus part of the tidal volume is diverted out the BPF rather than into alveoli. Although carbon dioxide is present in the gas that exits the BPF, its concentration is low. BPF represents an increase in dead space ventilation. Unless minute ventilation is increased, hypercarbia develops.

Clinical Presentation. BPF should be suspected when tension pneumothorax develops quickly or when a large or continuous air leak is present through a tube thoracostomy. If the BPF is not drained, the immediate risk is lethal tension pneumothorax. Once it is drained,

TABLE 8–8. Proposed Techniques for Bronchopleural Fistula Management

Removal of mechanical ventilation and positive end-expiratory pressure
Intermittent occlusion of chest tubes
Selective positioning of endobronchial plug
Increasing negative pressure in pleural space
Application of positive pressure to pleural space
Extracorporeal membrane oxygenation
Differential ventilation through double-lumen tube

hypercarbia may become a significant management problem.

Treatment. The management of BPF is determined by the size of the leak and the degree to which gas exchange is impaired. In a trauma patient with massive BPF on admission, bronchoscopy is indicated to locate the air leak. Clinically significant BPF resulting from bronchial or tracheal disruption by blunt trauma is generally proximal to the fifth bronchial division (90% within 2 cm of the carina) and should be visible with a bronchoscope. Once the airway disruption is identified, surgical treatment by primary repair or lung resection is considered.

Management of milder forms of BPF consists of tube thoracostomy with suction. However, progressive hypercarbia occasionally develops despite optimal conventional ventilation. A number of techniques are used for management of BPF, since none is routinely effective. These are listed in Table 8–8. High-frequency jet ventilation (HFJV) is effective in decreasing $Paco_2$ only in the occasional patient with BPF. Paradoxically, gas flow through the fistula is increased when HFJV is instituted. A recent technique that shows promise for treating BPF is the administration of fibrin glue to seal the air leak. This has been used successfully in BPF involving third and fourth division bronchi.

INHALATION INJURY

The management of inhalation injury is discussed in Chapter 19.

FAT EMBOLISM

Fat embolism is defined as the clinical syndrome of recent long bone fractures, decreased level of consciousness, thrombocytopenia, and ARDS. The pathophysiology is thought to involve the release of fat from the marrow of fractured bones. The fat embolizes into the pulmonary circulation and creates a mechanical obstruction. Lipases digest the embolus, releasing reactive fatty acids that stimulate an intense inflammatory reaction and may produce profound hypoxemia. Some of the fat does not lodge in the lungs but rather passes through to embolize to other organs, producing the classic petechiae in various cutaneous areas, mucous membranes, and the retina. Although embolization of the brain has been proposed as the mechanism for the mental status changes, focal neurologic deficit is rare.

The clinical progression of fat embolism is thought to occur over the 72 hours after the fracture. However, patients may exhibit a decreased Pao_2 while breathing room air on admission. The severity of the syndrome may vary from only the presence of petechiae to a catastrophic situation that includes coma, cardiovascular instability, severe ARDS, and coagulopathy.

Diagnosis. No test specifically diagnoses fat embolism. The presence of fat in the blood, sputum, or urine is nonspecific. Generally the diagnosis is made after other possible causes have been excluded.

Treatment. Fat embolism has no specific treatment. Efforts should be made to stabilize fractures to prevent recurrent embolization. Therapies that have been proposed and discarded because of lack of demonstrated benefit include steroids, alcohol infusion, heparin, and dextran. Evidence suggests that steroids given prophylactically may reduce the incidence of the development of the syndrome. Thus fat embolism is treated by supporting the particular organs that are failing.

NEAR DROWNING

The variety of pathologic processes that may develop in a victim of near drowning has been appreciated only recently. Salinity of the water in which near drowning occurs can greatly influence electrolyte and intravascular volume status at the time of hospital admission. Salt water aspiration results in osmotic flooding of the pulmonary interstitium and hypovolemia. Fresh water immersion is associated with hypervolemia, transient hyponatremia, hemolysis, and pulmonary edema. The volume of fluid that leaks into the lung may be sufficient to cause eventual hypovolemia. However, some patients aspirate little water because of laryngospasm or breath holding. The major pathophysiologic problem of these patients is cardiac and cerebral hypoxia. Near drowning in cold water can prolong the time before permanent neurologic damage occurs. However, the clinician is then faced with the medical complications of hypothermia (see Chapter 20). Patients may suffer near drowning because of an unrelated medical problem such as acute alcohol intoxication, myocardial infarction, or epilepsy.

Any patient who has lost consciousness while swimming, is found lying near water after trauma, or appears to have aspirated a significant amount of water should be observed for near-drowning sequelae. Immediate therapy includes cardiopulmonary resuscitation if the patient is pulseless and apneic. Even if spontaneous ventilation appears adequate, oxygen should be administered until arterial saturation can be assessed. As soon as feasible, chest roentgenography and serum electrolyte and arterial blood gas measurements should be performed.

Treatment. Management of the near-drowning victim in the hospital is guided mainly by the patient's level of consciousness and the severity of gas exchange impairment. In patients who do not regain consciousness quickly, severe cerebral hypoxia should be suspected. Some clinicians have advocated aggressive cerebral resuscitation of these patients, including intracranial pressure monitoring, hypothermia, and barbiturate-induced coma. Little data exist to suggest that such therapy improves outcome. Regardless, the presence of coma requires certain interventions, such as control of the airway, assurance of adequate ventilation and nutrition, physical therapy to prevent contractures, and frequent position changes to prevent decubitus ulcers.

Severity of respiratory failure depends on the amount and nature of the aspirate. Sequential physical examinations, chest roentgenograms, and arterial blood gas studies should be monitored to assess the course of the pulmonary insult. Continuous positive airway pressure with or without mechanical ventilation has been reported effective in restoring the PaO_2 to acceptable levels while administering nontoxic concentrations of inspired oxygen. However, most patients with hypoxemia require mechanical ventilation and PEEP. The guidelines for PEEP application in the ARDS section of this chapter are appropriate in this situation as well. As with aspiration pneumonia, prophylactic antibiotics and corticosteroid administration are not recommended.

VENTILATORY PUMP FAILURE

A number of conditions spare the lungs but impair the bellows apparatus sufficiently to cause alveolar hypoventilation or impair pulmonary toilet. These conditions may be divided into four categories (Table 8–9).

Depressed respiratory drive is most commonly due to narcotic drugs administered orally, parenterally, or intrathecally. This condition responds to intravenous naloxone, which should be administered to any patient with respiratory acidosis in which narcotic overdose is suspected. In patients with depressed respiratory drive caused by disease of the brainstem ventilation centers, a number of stimulants, such as aminophylline, amphetamines, and acetazolamide, have been attempted with little success.

Flail chest is the most common acute chest wall deformity in critically ill patients. Although it is the underlying pulmonary contusion that accounts for the observed hypoxemia, the presence of a flail segment probably worsens the patient's ventilatory performance. Current therapy includes adequate analgesia to prevent splinting in response to pain.

The pulmonary management of patients with progressive muscle and neurologic diseases is directed at maintaining pulmonary toilet to

TABLE 8–9. Categories of Inadequate Ventilatory Bellows Activity

Depressed Respiratory Drive

Narcotic or sedative overdose
Hypothyroidism
Starvation
Brainstem injury

Chest Wall Compromise

Rib fractures/flail segment
Kyphoscoliosis
Increased abdominal pressure (ascites, bowel distention)

Impairment of Neuromuscular Transmission

Muscle relaxants, aminoglycosides, botulinum toxin
Myasthenia gravis
Guillain-Barré syndrome
Amyotrophic lateral sclerosis
Spinal cord injury

Muscle Weakness

Myopathies, inherited and acquired
Hypocalcemia, hypophosphatemia, hypomagnesemia, hypokalemia
Starvation
Shock (cardiogenic, hypovolemic, septic, and hypoxemic)

prevent or delay the development of atelectasis and pneumonia with attendant risk of intubation and mechanical ventilation. In some of these diseases the patient does not improve, and long-term ventilatory support must be planned. However, in some diseases, such as myasthenia gravis and Guillain-Barré syndrome, the respiratory muscle weakness may be transient.

Pulmonary management of Guillain-Barré syndrome. Patients with Guillain-Barré syndrome should be brought to an ICU whenever the disease threatens to result in alveolar hypoventilation. In patients destined to have respiratory failure, respiratory function declines slowly and then decreases abruptly. Thus the goal of ventilatory monitoring is to identify patients in whom respiratory failure will develop and institute mechanical ventilation before a crisis situation develops. One suggested method is to measure vital capacity and negative inspiratory force (NIF) every 8 to 12 hours or more frequently. Vital capacity of 15 ml/kg or less and NIF greater than -25 cm H_2O are evidence of such marginal ventilatory function that intubation and mechanical ventilation should be considered. Some clinicians recommend intervention when a rapid downward trend is present even if pulmonary mechanisms appear adequate. If required, mechanical ventilation should be adjusted to prevent patient fatigue until muscle strength has increased sufficiently to allow weaning and extubation. Tracheostomy is not necessary in many patients with Guillain-Barré syndrome, since the need for mechanical ventilation is often less than 2 weeks. Regardless of the need for intubation, these patients have impaired cough because of weak expiratory muscles. Retained secretions should be prevented by appropriate application of pulmonary toilet techniques as discussed in Chapter 3.

SUGGESTED READINGS

Atelectasis

Mackenzie CF: Chest physiotherapy in the intensive care unit, ed 2. Baltimore, 1989, Williams & Wilkins, Chapters 1 and 7

Pulmonary Edema

Allen SJ, Drake RE, Williams JP, et al: Recent advances in pulmonary edema. Crit Care Med 1987;15:963-970
Staub NC: Pathophysiology of pulmonary edema. In: Staub NC, Taylor AE (eds): Edema. New York, 1984, Raven Press, pp 719-746

Adult Respiratory Distress Syndrome

Petty TL: Adult respiratory distress syndrome: definition and historical perspective. Clin Chest Med 1982;3:3-7
Luterman A, Horovitz JH, Carrico CJ, et al: Withdrawal from positive end-expiratory pressure. Surgery 1978; 83:328-332

Aspiration

Wynne JW: Aspiration pneumonitis: correlation of experimental models with clinical disease. Clin Chest Med 1982;3:25-34

Asthma

FitzGerald JM, Hargreave FE: The assessment and management of acute life-threatening asthma. Chest 1989;95:888-894
MacFadden ER: Therapy of acute asthma. J Allergy Clin Immunol 1989;84:151-158

Acute Respiratory Failure Related to Chronic Obstructive Pulmonary Disease

American Thoracic Society: Standards for the diagnosis and care of patients with chronic obstructive pulmonary disease (COPD) and asthma. Am Rev Respir Dis 1962; 136:225-244
Schmidt GA, Hall JB: Acute on chronic respiratory failure. JAMA 1989;261:3444-3453

Pulmonary Thromboembolism

Collins R, Scrimgeour A, Yusuf S, et al: Reduction in fatal pulmonary embolism and venous thrombosis by perioperative administration of subcutaneous heparin: overview of results of randomized trials in general, orthopedic, and urologic surgery. N Engl J Med 1988;318:1162-1173

Bronchopleural Fistula

Powner DJ: Pulmonary barotrauma in the intensive care unit. J Intensive Care Med 1988;3:224-232
Regel G, Sturm JA, Neumann C, et al: Occlusion of bronchopleural fistula after lung injury. J Trauma 1989; 29:223-226

Fat Embolism

Chan KM, Tham KT, Chnow YN, et al: Posttraumatic fat embolism: clinical and subclinical presentations. J Trauma 1984;24:45-49
Eddy AC, Rice CL, Carrico CJ: Fat embolism syndrome: monitoring and management. J Crit Illness 1987; 2:24-37

Near Drowning

Modell JH: Near drowning and pulmonary aspiration. ASA Refresher Course No. 156. ASA Refresher Course Lectures, 1989

Ventilatory Pump Failure

Tobin MJ: Respiratory muscles in disease. Clin Chest Med 1988;9:263-286.

9

CARDIOVASCULAR DISORDERS

JOHN W. HOYT, MD, RAM E. RAJAGOPALAN, MB, BS, AND JOSEPH A. WAPENSKI, MD

The initial and secondary evaluation and stabilization of critically ill patients with cardiovascular disease are covered in Chapters 2 and 4. This chapter deals with specific cardiac problems encountered in the critical care environment, be it a medical, surgical, coronary, or postanesthesia recovery critical care unit. Cardiac problems, particularly those relating to coronary artery disease, affect many aspects of health care delivery and all ICUs. This chapter looks at electrophysiologic, muscular, valvular, and vascular disorders as they pertain to the care of critically ill patients with cardiac disease.

ELECTROPHYSIOLOGIC DISORDERS

Arrhythmia recognition and management is an important part of ICU care. Intensivists often have the disadvantage of not possessing all the tools required to make an accurate diagnosis of the nature of the arrhythmia, especially in the face of time constraints. Although electrophysiologic testing may help identify an abnormal rhythm with greater accuracy, an intensivist armed with a single-channel electrocardiographic (EKG) monitor, a 12-lead surface EKG, a clinical history, and simple diagnostic maneuvers can make an excellent appraisal of the nature of the arrhythmia.

"Knee-jerk" therapy for arrhythmias in the ICU is potentially dangerous. Except in life-threatening situations characterized by severe hemodynamic compromise, time must be taken for accurate identification of the pathologic rhythm. Failure to do so may result in inappropriate therapy and significant morbidity.

Differentiating broadly between tachyarrhythmias and bradyarrhythmias and further subdividing the tachyarrhythmias into narrow and broad complex types may be useful. This allows an algorithmic approach to identifying most of the common arrhythmias and the formulation of a therapeutic approach that avoids inappropriate remedies.

Tachyarrhythmias

Errors in the diagnosis and treatment of tachyarrhythmias are common. For example, the erroneous identification of ventricular tachycardia as a supraventricular rhythm with aberrant conduction could lead to inappropriate therapy with verapamil. The resulting vasodilatation in the presence of a persistent arrhythmia could have disastrous consequences.

Narrow complex tachyarrhythmias

Diagnosis. Tachycardia with a narrow complex (less than 120 ms duration) is always supraventricular in origin. Although abnormal automaticity may be the cause, reentrant mechanisms are more likely (Figs. 9–1 and 9–2). The diagnostic value of the readily available single-channel strip recording can be augmented by a 12-lead surface EKG. Since identification of P waves is essential, modified EKG leads that magnify P wave amplitude may be advantageous. Toward this end, noninvasive examination of the precordium with Lewis leads (a lead I signal recorded with the left arm electrode in V_1 position and right arm electrode in the first right intercostal space) is an attractive alternative to the use of esophageal leads. If P waves are difficult to identify, vagal maneuvers may be useful in unmasking atrial activity. The Valsalva maneuver, although highly effective, is difficult to perform in many ICU patients. Carotid sinus massage may be a valuable alternative. All other

174

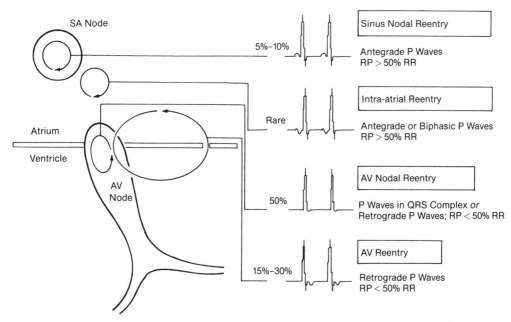

Figure 9–1. Reentrant supraventricular tachycardia. The arrhythmia may originate at sites ranging from the sinus node to the atrioventricular junction and use accessory pathways. The classic electrocardiographic pattern and frequency of each arrhythmia are indicated.

techniques may either be inconvenient to perform (for example, the diving reflex) or unpleasant to the patient (as with ocular pressure) and should be avoided. Pharmacologic interventions may be useful in diagnosis. Although verapamil and short-acting beta blockers can be used, the very short half-life and atrial, sinoatrial, and atrioventricular (AV) node selectivity of adenosine make it ideal for this purpose. Adenosine is a purine nucleoside that slows AV nodal

conduction and dilates peripheral and coronary vessels. The drug has a half-life in seconds and is indicated in paroxysmal supraventricular tachycardia. It is given as a rapid intravenous bolus in doses of 6 to 12 mg.

The EKG rhythm strip may provide valuable clues if examined systematically. Once an adequate lead has been selected, the rate, regularity, P wave to QRS association, and PR and RP intervals must be carefully assessed. If the initial

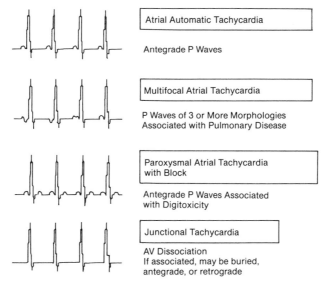

Figure 9–2. Automatic supraventricular tachycardia with classic electrocardiographic patterns depending on the site of origin of the automatic focus. Realization of the importance of digitalis toxicity as a cause will modify the therapeutic approach to these arrhythmias.

ART=85/43(56)

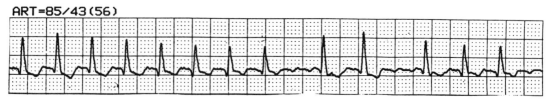

Figure 9–3. Atrial flutter. This regular supraventricular tachycardia is a consequence of a 2:1 atrioventricular (AV) conduction of atrial flutter. Flutter waves cannot be identified until a vagal maneuver unmasks it by further blocking AV conduction.

and terminal portions of a run of arrhythmia are available, they must be examined in detail.

Identification of P waves allows analysis of the activation sequence. Upright P waves in leads II, III, and aVF indicate a normal or high atrial focus of origin. Negative P waves in these leads demonstrate low atrial or junctional foci. In atrial flutter the typical pattern is a saw-toothed rhythm occurring at 250 to 350 beats/min (Fig. 9–3). Atrial activity in atrial fibrillation is difficult to identify. Its existence is suspected with an irregularly irregular ventricular rhythm in the absence of identifiable atrial activity. Occasionally, irregular, low-amplitude fibrillatory waves are noted on a surface EKG (Fig. 9–4).

An irregular RR interval suggests atrial fibrillation or the presence of a supraventricular tachycardia with a variable AV block. Tachycardias associated with abnormal automaticity have periods of acceleration (warm-up) and deceleration (cool-down) that may be mistaken for irregularity.

Although an atrial pace of 250 to 300 beats/min is characteristic of atrial flutter, the rate by itself seldom provides clues to the arrhythmia's origin. However, in the presence of atrial fibrillation, a short RR interval with a rate of more than 280 beats/min strongly suggests antegrade conduction over an accessory pathway because the AV node cannot conduct impulses at this rapid rate. The rhythm is usually of the wide complex type, but varying degrees of fusion due to simultaneous conduction across AV nodal and accessory pathways may confuse identification (Fig. 9–5). This is extremely useful in making a decision about the treatment of atrial fibrillation.

Initiation or termination of an arrhythmia by an atrial or ventricular premature beat is highly suggestive of a reentrant mechanism (Fig. 9–6). In reentrant tachycardias the initiating P wave is likely to be morphologically distinct from that seen during the arrhythmia, since it originates at a site not associated with the reentrant circuit.

Besides helping to unmask atrial activity, vagal stimulation can be used to differentiate between automatic and reentrant mechanisms. Abrupt termination suggests reentry. Automatic foci, on the other hand, slow down with stimulation and accelerate after the cessation of the stimulus. Sensitivity to such stimuli also indicates the involvement of myocardial conducting tissue that is under autonomic influence such as the sinus and AV nodes. Vagal stimulation maneuvers are more likely to be successful when applied soon after the onset of the dysrhythmia, before the onset of the adrenergic response to the tachycardia, which is likely to make it refractory to such manipulation.

0 LEAD V1 HR =73 A=0 RESP=87   ART=165/51(85)

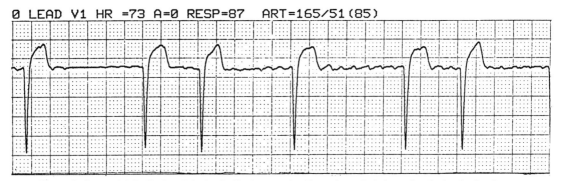

Figure 9–4. Atrial fibrillation. It is classically characterized by an irregularly irregular rhythm in the absence of P waves. In this example coarse atrial fibrillatory waves of varying morphology, amplitude, and frequency are seen.

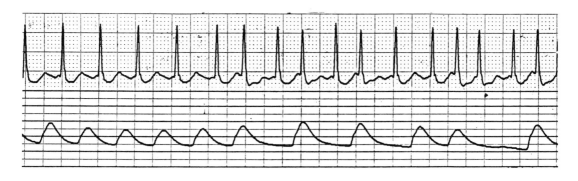

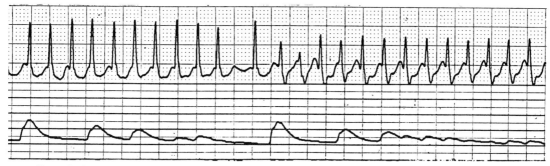

Figure 9–5. In this case atrial fibrillation with stable hemodynamics abruptly deteriorates into atrial flutter *(lower panel)* with 1:1 conduction at a rate of 270 beats/min. Because hemodynamic compromise exists, the patient was treated with cardioversion. If the patient had been stable, the rapid rate should have provided a clue to the existence of a fast accessory pathway and would have contraindicated the use of digitalis and verapamil.

If AV dissociation is naturally observed or can be induced without affecting the persistence of the arrhythmia, a reentrant mechanism involving the AV node can be excluded.

In about 60% of AV nodal reentrant tachycardia, P waves are not visible because they are buried in the QRS complex. Retrograde P waves with an RP interval less than 50% of the RR interval typify AV reciprocating tachycardias and 30% of AV nodal reentrant tachycardia. Long RP (more than 50% of RR) intervals are seen in the rare "atypical" AV nodal reentrant tachycardias. Long RP intervals are also seen in atrial tachycardias (sinus node reentry, intraatrial reentry, and atrial automatic tachycardias), but they can be differentiated by the presence of antegrade P waves.

Based on the preceding principles, algorithms have been developed for the noninvasive identification of narrow complex tachycardias. A modification of one scheme developed by Bar is provided in Figure 9–7.

Management. Regardless of the cause of the arrhythmia, management of narrow complex tachyarrhythmias begins with the recognition that either reentrant or automatic mechanisms are responsible. Treatment attempts to

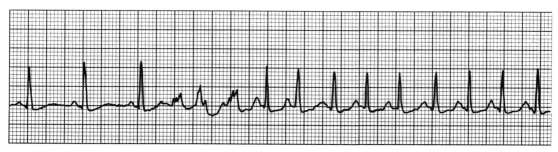

Figure 9–6. A relatively abrupt transition of sinus rhythm to a regular supraventricular tachycardia is preceded by three wide complex ectopic beats. A reentrant mechanism is likely.

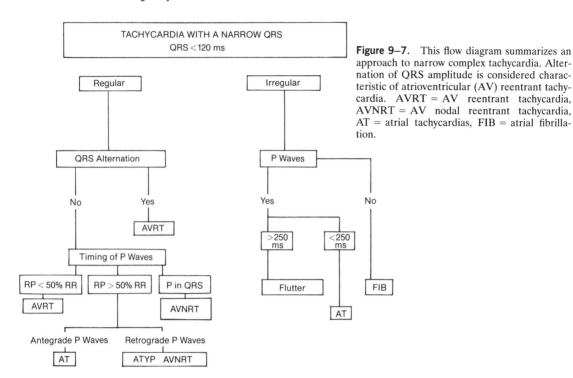

Figure 9–7. This flow diagram summarizes an approach to narrow complex tachycardia. Alternation of QRS amplitude is considered characteristic of atrioventricular (AV) reentrant tachycardia. AVRT = AV reentrant tachycardia, AVNRT = AV nodal reentrant tachycardia, AT = atrial tachycardias, FIB = atrial fibrillation.

terminate the arrhythmia, or if this cannot be achieved, to control the heart rate (Table 9–1).

All life-threatening arrhythmias should be treated by emergency cardioversion while an attempt is made to identify the origin of the rest.

Vagal maneuvers sometimes terminate reentrant tachycardias. Recalcitrant rhythms respond to intravenous verapamil or short-acting beta blockers, such as esmolol, or to a repetition of vagal maneuvers after treatment with these drugs. The recent availability of adenosine has proved a major boon. Although it has deleterious side effects, they are brief and the drug is equal in efficacy to verapamil, making it a useful addition to the armamentarium for the diagnosis and treatment of supraventricular tachycardia (Fig. 9–8).

At this point, if the arrhythmia has not been terminated, a careful attempt at identification of the rhythm may be needed. The impact of drug-induced or vagally mediated AV block on the arrhythmia and on the atrial rhythm is particularly relevant. With the exclusion of atrial flutter and fibrillation, a significant fraction of the unresponsive tachycardias are likely to be automatic. Therapy with type Ia antiarrhythmics, such as procainamide,

TABLE 9–1.   Summary of Drugs Used in Treatment of Supraventricular Tachycardias

DRUG	CLASS	DOSE	MECHANISM	SIDE EFFECTS
Verapamil	Calcium channel blocker	5-10 mg IV	AV nodal block	Hypotension; bradycardia
Adenosine	Nucleoside	6-12 mg IV	SA/AV node block; decreased atrial automaticity	Facial flushing; chest pain, dyspnea
Esmolol	Beta-adrenergic blocker	500 µg/kg load + 50 µg/kg/min/ drip	AV nodal block	Hypotension; bradycardia
Procainamide	Type Ia antiarrhythmic	10-20 mg/kg at 100 mg over 1-3 min	Accessory pathway block; decreased automaticity	Hypotension; proarrhythmia
Digitalis	Glycoside	0.5 mg then 0.25 mg q2-4 h to 1.25 mg total	AV nodal block	Arrhythmias; GI symptoms

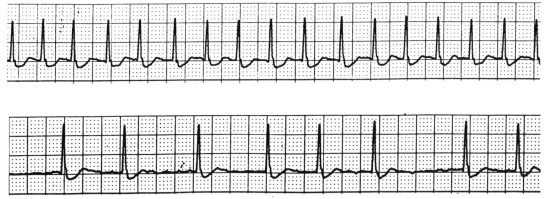

Figure 9–8. The seemingly regular tachycardia seen in the upper panel responded to 6 mg of adenosine by demonstrating the existence of atrial fibrillation. Although adenosine is not used therapeutically for atrial fibrillation, this example demonstrates its value in diagnosis.

may be the best option at this juncture. These drugs not only suppress the automatic activity but also delay the impulse conduction along the accessory AV pathways, effectively terminating refractory reentrant dysrhythmias. Type IA agents are never the first-line agents for supraventricular tachycardia and should be used only when AV node–slowing drugs have been ineffective.

Since digitalis toxicity is an important contributor to automatic rhythms, arrhythmias characteristic of this condition should be identified. Paroxysmal atrial tachycardia with AV block and junctional ectopic tachycardia are two rhythms that should be recognized. A normalization of the irregularity of atrial fibrillation should raise suspicion of the latter rhythm. Treatment with digoxin withdrawal, potassium to correct hypokalemia, dilantin, lidocaine, and antidigoxin fab antibodies must be considered.

Multifocal atrial tachycardia (Fig. 9–9), another automatic rhythm seen in the ICU, is usually associated with significant pulmonary disease. This arrhythmia, which is characterized by the presence of at least three distinct atrial foci, is treated with verapamil or beta blockers. Digitalis may be ineffective. If the above-mentioned arrhythmias are excluded, digitalis may be used for control of ventricular rates when other maneuvers have failed.

Digitalis is also the treatment of choice in the control of the ventricular response in atrial flutter and fibrillation when the clinical evidence of antegrade conduction along an accessory AV pathway (Wolff-Parkinson-White syndrome) is considered unlikely. Digitalis therapy does not result in cardioversion, which may be achieved with type Ia agents and DC cardioversion. Overdrive pacing at 10% to 15% above the intrinsic rate may terminate atrial flutter.

Wide complex tachyarrhythmia

A wide complex beat (QRS greater than 120 ms) occurs when the normal conduction of a ventricular impulse down the bundle of His into the bundle branches is precluded. Consequently the impulse may originate above the bundle of His (atrial or junctional) and be blocked at a refractory bundle branch or bypass it, or it may

SAO2=98 NIBP=08:33   90/ 55(61)

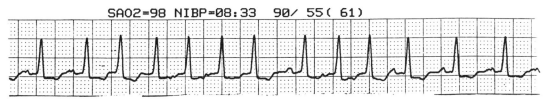

Figure 9–9. This irregular tachycardia may be mistaken for atrial fibrillation on a casual examination of the strip. The presence of P waves of three different morphologies preceding QRS complexes leads to the real diagnosis of multifocal atrial tachycardia. This rhythm responds poorly to digitalization.

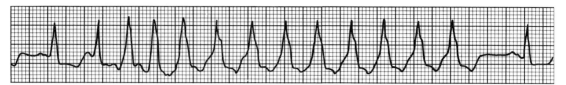

Figure 9–10. A single-channel recording provides few clues to the origin of this wide complex tachycardia rhythm. Although atrioventricular dissociation may clinch the diagnosis of ventricular tachycardia, its absence, as in this example, is of no value diagnostically. A 12-lead electrocardiogram would be useful.

originate distal to the bifurcation of the bundle branches.

Incorrect diagnosis and treatment of wide complex tachycardia is of greater significance than a similar mishandling of a narrow complex rhythm. This is because treating a potentially lethal arrhythmia of ventricular origin as a supraventricular tachycardia results in disastrous hemodynamic decompensation.

Diagnosis. Noninvasive differentiation between ventricular and supraventricular foci (Figs. 9–10 and 9–11) poses a challenge that has been extensively studied. It may occur when supraventricular tachycardia is associated with a preexisting bundle branch block, a functional aberrancy (Ashman phenomenon), or antegrade conduction over an accessory pathway and ventricular tachycardia.

Although three of the preceding mechanisms are easily comprehended, the principles involved in functional aberrant ventricular conduction may need elaboration. The refractory period of the conducting tissue of the bundle branch depends on the heart rate and the cycle length of the immediately preceding complex. The refractory period therefore shortens with fast heart rates and increases with slowing of the rate. Consequently the refractory period is lengthened by a long cycle beat (longer RR interval, slower rate) so that a subsequent premature beat is faced with a blocked bundle branch and is conducted aberrantly (Fig. 9–12).

Because recognition of the pattern of bundle branch block plays an important part in the differential diagnosis of wide complex tachycardias, characteristics of these configurations are described in the following paragraphs.

Under normal conditions the septum is activated from left to right, a fact that remains unchanged in right bundle branch block. With left bundle branch block, however, the direction of septal activation is reversed. This is followed by a normal activation of the ventricle associated with the unblocked bundle branch, while depolarization of the opposite ventricle proceeds along contiguous myocardium. Because the conduction is slow along nonspecialized myocardium, the QRS is significantly prolonged. By convention, the block is termed complete when the QRS duration is greater than 120 ms and incomplete when it is less than 120 ms.

In right bundle branch block, characteristic findings are seen in right-sided leads such as V_1. The initial normal septal activation results in a small R wave followed by a deep S wave, indicating left ventricular depolarization. Subsequent right ventricular activation results in an R´ wave.

Left bundle branch block is characterized by slurring of the R wave in leads I and V_6, indicating the right-to-left myocardial activation sequence (Fig. 9-13). Reversed septal activation is reflected by a small R wave in the inferior aVF lead. With the altered direction of septal activation, Q waves fail to register, making the clinician "electrocardiographically blind" to acute myocardial infarction.

In view of the complexity of the situation and the importance of accurate diagnosis, several criteria for distinguishing between ventricular and supraventricular beats have been established (Fig. 9–14).

In one subpopulation of patients with wide complex tachycardia referred for electrophysiologic evaluation, the presence of structural

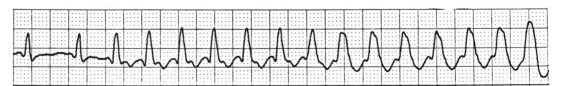

Figure 9-11. A QRS duration of greater than 0.16 second is a sensitive indicator of ventricular tachycardia. This patient required cardioversion because of hemodynamic deterioration.

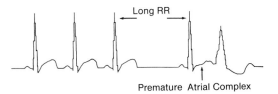

Figure 9–12. The long cycle preceding the premature beat sets up the conditions required for blockade of a bundle branch, resulting in the aberrant pattern of ventricular conduction. This classic pattern is useful in differentiating it from a ventricular complex and is known as the Ashman phenomenon.

heart disease or a clinical history of myocardial infarction strongly suggested ventricular tachycardia, with greater than 95% positive predictive value. However, even in the absence of such history, about one third of the patients had a ventricular focus.

Hemodynamic stability is commonly but incorrectly thought to suggest a supraventricular origin of the wide complex rhythm. In a recent analysis of hemodynamically stable patients with wide complex tachyarrhythmias, about 80% of patients referred for electrophysiologic

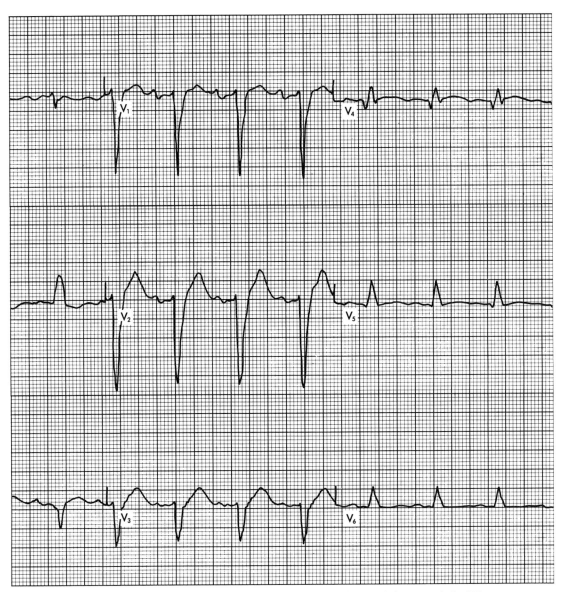

Figure 9–13. The widened QRS complex of 0.12 second and the characteristic pattern in lead V_6 suggests a complete left bundle branch block. The ST/T demonstrates an axis opposite to that of the QRS. This patient also demonstrates a first-degree atrioventricular block.

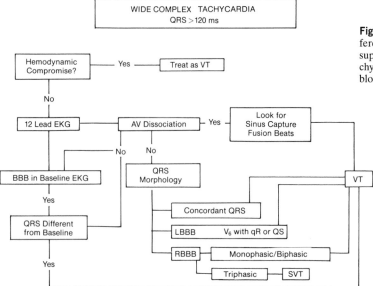

Figure 9–14. An algorithm for the differentiation between ventricular (VT) and supraventricular (SVT) wide complex tachycardias. RBBB = right bundle branch block, LBBB = left bundle branch block.

evaluation of this condition had ventricular tachycardia. Thus such patients must be evaluated more carefully, preferably by a 12-lead EKG during the tachyarrhythmia. This should be analyzed using the following rules, proposed initially by Wellens and associates and modified by other investigators.

Wellens suggested that rates above 170 beats/min with a right bundle branch block pattern indicated aberrant conduction of a supraventricular rhythm. However, more recent studies do not substantiate this claim. Because of the large overlap of rates, this criterion cannot be used reliably.

Although AV dissociation is a reliable indicator of ventricular tachycardia, it is detected by surface EKG in only about 25% of such cases. If present, it establishes the diagnosis of ventricular tachycardia. The existence of sinus capture and fusion beats corroborates this conclusion, although their absence has no diagnostic significance.

Wellens' original study suggested that a QRS width greater than 140 ms indicated ventricular tachycardia. This must be viewed in light of the nature of the bundle branch block pattern. A QRS greater than 160 ms with a left bundle branch block or greater than 140 ms with a right bundle branch block is a more accurate criterion for the identification of ventricular tachycardia.

The distribution of normal, left, and right axes is too similar in patients with ventricular or supraventricular tachycardias to have diagnostic value. However, extreme axis deviation (− 90 to

± 180 degrees) aids the diagnosis of ventricular tachycardia.

A number of features have been analyzed to enhance noninvasive differentiation between ventricular and supraventricular wide complex rhythms. A concordant pattern in the precordial leads with positive QRS complexes suggests ventricular tachycardia. In the presence of a right bundle branch block, monophasic or biphasic QRS complexes in V_1 are characteristic of ventricular tachycardia while a triphasic pattern is seen in supraventricular tachycardia with aberrancy. With a left bundle branch block a qR or QS pattern in V_6 is seen only in ventricular tachycardia.

If the baseline EKG demonstrates a preexisting bundle branch block and it remains unchanged during the tachycardia, a supraventricular focus of origin is likely to exist. Patients with ventricular tachycardia, on the other hand, have a QRS morphology distinctly different from that seen at baseline.

Collectively the preceding features have reasonable diagnostic value, but individually they lack sensitivity, specificity, or both (Table 9–2). The value of these tests must be assessed prospectively in a primary care population rather than in highly selective referral groups. Unfortunately, the relative proportions of ventricular and supraventricular tachycardias among patients with wide complex rhythms in a primary care situation (emergency room or ICU) is unknown. Based on current evidence in referral populations, arguments can be made that ventricular tachycardia is the most

TABLE 9–2. Features Useful for Differential Diagnosis of Wide-Complex Tachycardia

EKG CRITERION	VENTRICULAR	SUPRAVENTRICULAR	COMMENTS
Atrioventricular dissociation	Yes	No	Very specific for VT
QRS duration	>160 ms with LBBB > 140 ms with RBBB	< 140 ms	Low specificity for VT
QRS axis	Varies, but -90 to ± 180 is diagnostic	Variable	Low sensitivity and specificity
QRS morphology: V lead concordance	Positive concordance	–	
QRS morphology: V_1 with RBBB	Monophasic or biphasic	Triphasic	Low specificity for VT
QRS morphology: V_6 with LBBB	QR or QS	–	

VT = ventricular tachycardia, RBBB = right bundle branch block, LBBB = left bundle branch block.

common cause of wide complex tachycardia. The use of a highly sensitive diagnostic criterion (QRS greater than 140 ms or QRS morphology) and consequent overdiagnosis of ventricular tachycardia may lead to safer therapeutic decisions.

Management. All unrecognizable patterns should be treated as ventricular tachycardia. Administration of verapamil to a patient with undiagnosed broad complex tachycardia is a common error that can be disastrous. A recent study evaluated the value of adenosine in differentiating between ventricular and supraventricular foci. The drug was successful in terminating most supraventricular broad complex tachycardias and did not result in unfavorable hemodynamic outcome in patients with ventricular tachycardia. If this lack of adverse effects can be confirmed on a large scale, an adenosine trial may be a valuable addition to the diagnostic algorithm for broad complex tachycardias.

Hemodynamic stability is the major factor that determines the mode of therapy for ventricular tachycardia. All unstable or unconscious patients are treated with immediate cardioversion. Patients demonstrating no compromise may respond to pharmacologic therapy. Once the diagnostic protocol identifies the rhythm as ventricular tachycardia, lidocaine (a type Ib antiarrhythmic) is the treatment of choice. Negative inotropy is the major adverse effect of this agent in the acute treatment of ventricular tachycardia. Procainamide (type Ia) is occasionally effective when lidocaine is not. This drug may be ideal in a situation of diagnostic uncertainty because it can terminate both ventricular tachycardia and reentrant supraventricular rhythms with aberrant conduction. However, the loading dose must be administered over 30 to 45 minutes to avoid causing serious hypotension, and the patient's stability during this period is crucial. Bretylium tosylate (type III antiarrhythmic) is effective in ventricular tachycardia, especially with acute myocardial infarction. Alternative drugs such as beta blockers or phenytoin may be tried if these agents are not successful (Table 9–3).

IRREGULAR BROAD COMPLEX RHYTHMS

Irregular broad complex rhythms are most likely to be atrial fibrillation with a bundle branch block or accessory pathway conduction. The clinical importance of atrial fibrillation and flutter in the presence of a preexcitation syndrome, such as Wolff-Parkinson-White syndrome, must be recognized. The wide complexes seen are a result of antegrade conduction over the accessory pathway, accounting for maximum preexcitation of the ventricles. This arrhythmia has a tendency for triggering hemodynamic collapse and ventricular fibrillation. Cardioversion is the only form of therapy that should be used in hemodynamically compromised patients. In a stabler patient, verapamil and digitalis, which block the AV node without affecting the accessory pathway, may accelerate the tachycardia and therefore should not be used. Procainamide is the treatment of choice under these circumstances. Irregularity of rhythm is extremely unusual in ventricular tachycardia. This could occur in polymorphic ventricular tachycardia but is infrequent and unsustained.

ACCELERATED IDIOVENTRICULAR RHYTHM

A regular broad complex rhythm that causes much concern to the novice in the ICU is accelerated idioventricular rhythm or slow

TABLE 9–3. Pharmacotherapy of Ventricular Tachycardias

DRUG	CLASS	DOSE	COMMENTS
Lidocaine	Type Ib antiarrhythmic	1 mg/kg loading dose; 1-4 mg/min drip	Serum level <5 μg/ml; negative inotrope
Procainamide	Type Ia antiarrhythmic	10-20 mg/kg at 50 mg/min; then 1-5 mg/min drip	Serum Procan + NAPA <20 μg/ml; hypotension; proarrhythmia
Bretylium Tosylate	Type III antiarrhythmic	5-10 mg/kg loading dose; then 1-2 mg/min drip	Effective in myocardial infarction; hypotension
Propranolol	Beta blocker (type II)	1 mg over 1 min IV observing response and blood pressure	Hypotension; bradycardia; bronchospasm
Quinidine	Type Ia	10 mg/kg loading at a rate of 0.5 mg/kg/min	Hypotension; atrioventricular block
Phenytoin	Type Ib antiarrhythmic	250 mg over 10 min; repeat until effective to a total of 15 mg/kg	Hypotension; ideal for digitalis toxicity and torsades de pointes

ventricular tachycardia (Fig. 9–15). This is an escape rhythm originating distal to the bundle of His. Although the usual rate of this escape focus is less than 40 beats/min, it may exceed this physiologic rate and override the slower sinus pacemaker. This rhythm, which has a rate of 60 to 100 beats/min, appears ominous because of its broad complex nature. It is usually benign and need not be treated unless the patient's hemodynamic status deteriorates. In such a case, conventional type Ib antiarrhythmics would be inappropriate. Acceleration of the patient's sinus rate by 0.5 mg of atropine may be all that is required. It is common in patients with acute myocardial infarction and is claimed to be an indicator of successful thrombolysis.

POLYMORPHIC VENTRICULAR TACHYCARDIA

A special situation that needs to be identified in the ICU is the polymorphic ventricular tachycardia associated with prominent late diastolic U waves and bradycardic pauses. This entity, commonly called torsades de pointes, may be difficult to manage and consequently must be distinguished from other forms of ventricular tachycardia. The ventricular tachycardia demonstrates a progressive change in QRS amplitude, making the tracing appear to twist around the isoelectric line. Its association with prominent U waves and prolonged QT intervals has led to the hypothesis that the U waves may represent late repolarization of areas of the myocardium. This results in spatial and temporal heterogeneity of myocardial repolarization, which sets up an excellent milieu for reentry. This tachycardia has a wide range of causes, including the use of types Ia and Ic antiarrhythmic agents, hypokalemia, hypomagnesemia, bradyarrhythmias, and congenital prolonged QT syndromes. When torsades de pointes is recognized, the best response is obtained by treatment with 1 to 2 g of intravenous magnesium sulfate or acceleration of the underlying bradycardia by pacing or pharmacologic means. The U wave becomes less prominent under these circumstances. Correction of

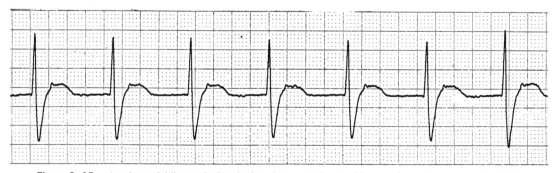

Figure 9–15. Accelerated idioventricular rhythm demonstrating a wide complex pattern at a rate of 70 beats/min. Retrograde P waves can be identified on each T wave. No treatment is required in a hemodynamically stable patient.

provocative factors such as hypokalemia is essential. Phenytoin and other type Ib antiarrhythmics may be useful in the acute and long-term management of this condition.

ISOLATED PREMATURE VENTRICULAR COMPLEXES

Although isolated premature ventricular complexes do not carry the prognostic significance of the arrhythmias discussed previously, they are commonly encountered in the ICU. Recognition is aided by the presence of bizarre wide complexes, no preceding P wave, and a classic compensatory pause. When these complexes alternate with normal sinus beats, it is termed bigeminy. A sequential pair is called a couplet, and a run of three or more ventricular beats is ventricular tachycardia. A ventricular ectopic beat can be distinguished from an aberrant premature atrial contraction using the criteria developed for the differential diagnosis of ventricular tachycardia. A compensatory pause may not be seen after a premature atrial contraction. Therapy is not required for premature ventricular contractions in patients without organic heart disease or in the absence of short runs or frequent multiform beats. For the premature complexes that do require therapy, management may begin with correction of hypoxia or hypokalemia that may predispose the patient to this problem. If the arrhythmia persists, treatment with lidocaine or other antiarrhythmics may be warranted in the acute situation.

Bradyarrhythmias

Pacemaker activity can originate in any portion of the cardiac conduction system from the sinus node to the bundle of His. However, since the rate of the sinus pacemaker exceeds that of the distal conduction system, it determines the basal heart rate. Any pathologic process that slows the sinus pacemaker or blocks impulse conduction to the ventricle may result in an "escape" of distal pacemaker activity and a junctional or idioventricular rhythm with an intrinsically slow rate.

Diagnosis. Bradycardia therefore may result from slowing of intrinsic pacemaker activity or from conduction blocks. In either case the clinician should follow an algorithmic approach to identify the mechanisms of bradycardia, looking for atrial activity on the surface EKG or with intraatrial and esophageal electrodes (Fig. 9–16).

If P waves are not identifiable, two possible rhythms should be considered. Atrial fibrillation with an AV block is likely, especially if an irregular ventricular response is noted. A regular rhythm with unidentifiable P waves may indicate a junctional rhythm. A complete sinoatrial block also does not demonstrate P waves.

When atrial activity is detected and demonstrates a slow response, a sinus node dysfunction or sinoatrial block should be suspected. Sinus bradycardia demonstrates a slow regular atrial rate with normal P wave morphology. It may be a physiologic rhythm in athletes. This rhythm may also be seen in patients receiving beta blockers or with hypothyroidism or acute myocardial infarction. Sinoatrial blocks may be first, second, or third degree (Fig. 9–17). First-degree blocks are not identifiable with a surface EKG. Second-degree blocks may simulate the Wenckebach AV block. This is identified by a progressive narrowing of the PP interval until a complete block results in a pause. A type II second-degree block may be difficult to identify

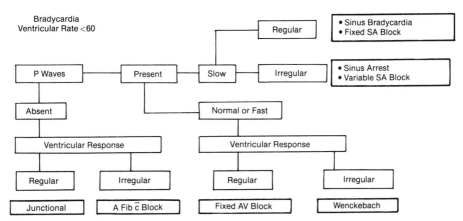

Figure 9–16. This algorithm for the differential diagnosis of bradyarrhythmias stresses the importance of identification of P waves and its relationship to the QRS.

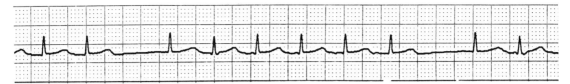

Figure 9–17. Although P waves are difficult to identify in this strip, this patient demonstrates a pattern characterized by an abrupt doubling of the RR interval, suggesting sinoatrial block. This differentiates sinoatrial block from a sinus arrest, which does not demonstrate a variation of RR intervals, which is a multiple of the basal rate.

if it has a 2:1 pattern. In such a situation it cannot be differentiated from a sinus bradycardia. A third-degree sinoatrial block causes a complete absence of normal P waves. Sinus arrest is a failure of sinus node depolarization (Fig. 9–18). It may be difficult to differentiate from sinoatrial block, but a pause that is not a multiple of the PP interval would help make the diagnosis. Sinoatrial block is most commonly associated with digitalis excess, but quinidine, acute myocardial infarction, myocarditis, and hyperkalemia may also be etiologic factors.

A slow ventricular rate in the presence of a normal or even accelerated sinus rate suggests AV block, which may be classified as first, second, or third degree.

First-degree AV block is characterized by a prolongation of the PR interval beyond the physiologic range of 0.2 second. The usual site of the block is above the bundle of His. Etiologic factors are the same as for sinoatrial blocks.

In second-degree AV block, conduction of atrial impulses to the ventricle fails intermittently (Fig. 9–19). In a Mobitz type I second-degree block a progressively increasing conduction delay ends in a completely blocked impulse. On a surface EKG this is characterized by progressive increase of PR intervals until a dropped ventricular beat occurs. As the PR interval increases, the RR interval appears to shorten and the PP interval remains fixed. The block is usually at the level of the AV node (supra-Hisian). However, if associated with a

bundle branch block or symptoms, a less benign infra-Hisian process may exist. In a Mobitz type II second-degree block, no variation occurs and a fixed proportion of atrial impulses are conducted to the ventricle. This type of block is usually infra-Hisian.

With third-degree AV block no atrial impulses are conducted to the ventricle (Fig. 9–20). An escape rhythm may originate in the AV junction or ventricle. Although this type of block is usually infra-Hisian, when it occurs in association with an inferior myocardial infarction, the block may be higher and spontaneous resolution is common.

Management. The presence of symptoms is an indication for therapeutic intervention in bradycardia. Syncope, hemodynamic compromise, or anginal symptoms associated with bradycardia warrant acceleration of the heart rate. Atropine is the treatment of choice in an acute situation. An intravenous dose of 0.5 to 1 mg usually accelerates the heart rate and improves AV conduction. Although isoproterenol (1 to 4 μg/min) may be administered to patients with blocks refractory to atropine, temporary transvenous pacing is probably a better alternative (Table 9–4).

The decision to provide a temporary transvenous pacer for treatment of AV block depends on the suspected level of the block. Supra-Hisian blocks, at the level of the AV node, are usually well tolerated because the escape rhythm arises in the high AV junction and is faster (40 to 60 beats/min) and stabler

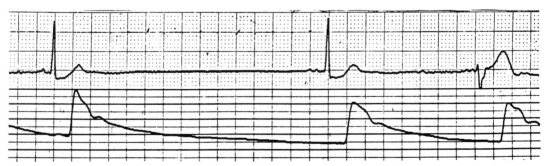

Figure 9–18. The long pauses without any atrial activity and the absence of any relationship to the basal heart rate suggest sinus arrest. A ventricular escape beat is observed during one of the pauses.

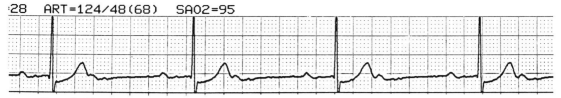

:28   ART=124/48(68)   SAO2=95

Figure 9–19. In second-degree atrioventricular (AV) block every other P wave is conducted to the ventricle with a fixed PR interval. This pattern with a 2:1 conduction does not allow the differentiation between Mobitz type I and type II AV block.

than a ventricular escape pattern. Since the AV node and inferior wall are supplied by the right coronary artery, a third-degree block associated with an inferior wall myocardial infarction is most likely to be supra-Hisian. Besides, complete recovery of the node is the rule, and an asymptomatic patient may not need even temporary pacing.

In contrast, an infra-Hisian block is poorly tolerated because of the slowness and unreliability of ventricular escape rhythms. This type of block is typically a third-degree block with an anterior wall myocardial infarction. Because the slow rate is likely to be associated with hemodynamic instability, a pacemaker is required.

Subtle clues pointing to the site of the block may be encountered. A wide QRS complex suggests an infra-Hisian block. Changes in the PR interval, on the other hand, point to a supra-Hisian block.

Once a decision to provide pacer support has been made, the mode used depends on the clinical situation. The urgency of an asystolic or bradycardic arrest prompts initial stabilization with a transcutaneous pacer. Transvenous pacers may be placed in less urgent circumstances. If the patient has undergone cardiac surgery, epicardial pacer leads may be available. Transesophageal and transthoracic approaches are less popular.

Transcutaneous pacing is achieved by passing a current between two large chest pads placed over the precordium and posterior chest wall. A long pulse duration of the electrical stimulus ensures preferential activation of cardiac over skeletal muscle. Successful pacing can be achieved in more than 40% of patients without fear of inducing ventricular tachycardia or fibrillation. Obesity, poor electrode contact, and large pleural and pericardial effusions promote pacing failure. Although transcutaneous pacing has been used long term, a more reliable pacing alternative should be sought soon after stabilization of the patient. Significant pain from muscle activation and skin abrasions is reported in conscious patients, and sedation must be considered.

Transvenous pacing of right atrial or ventricular endocardium is the most dependable emergency technique available. Central venous access is needed; any contraindication to cannulation of a central vein, such as the presence of coagulopathy, must be evaluated. Pacing is traditionally performed by bipolar ventricular catheters, which may be balloon tipped to facilitate "blind" placement. AV sequential and atrial pacing may also be possible, and single-pass catheters are being developed for the former mode.

In most emergency situations, asynchronous (VOO) or demand (VVI) pacing of the ventricles is used. In the VOO mode the pacer fires at a fixed rate without sensing the heart's electrical activity. The QRS complex is sensed

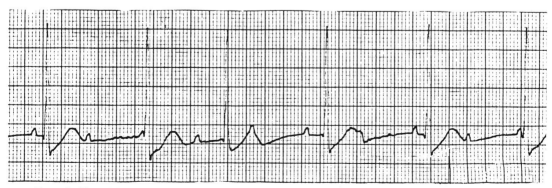

Figure 9–20. Third-degree atrioventricular block is characterized by the lack of any relationship between the atrial and ventricular complexes. The atrium has a rate of about 100 beats/min, while the unrelated ventricle depolarizes at a frequency of fewer than 60 beats/min.

TABLE 9–4. Indications for Emergency Pacemaker Placement in ICUs

CLINICAL STATUS	INDICATION	COMMENT
Acute myocardial infarct	Third-degree AV block with anterior wall MI	Infra-Hisian site
	Mobitz II AV block	
	Mobitz I, wide QRS, anterior MI	
	New RBBB plus left hemiblock	High risk for high-grade block
	Alternating BBB	
	New first-degree plus LBBB	
	Sinus node dysfunction	Symptoms
No myocardial infarct	Symptomatic first-, second-, or third-degree AV block	Symptoms
	Third-degree block with wide QRS and <50 beats/min ventricular rate	Infra-Hisian block
	Mobitz II with wide QRS	Infra-Hisian block
	Symptomatic sinus node dysfunction	Symptoms
Prophylaxis	Right heart catheter with LBBB	Prevention of complete heart block
	Suppression of bradycardia-related arrhythmia; torsades	Prevention of lethal arrhythmia
	Cardioversion; pharmacologic treatment of sick sinus syndrome	Bradycardia may be exacerbated

Any bradycardic patient who remains symptomatic or unstable on pharmacologic therapy requires a pacemaker.

in the demand mode, and a pacemaker potential is suppressed when such activity is detected. This allows the pacemaker to function only when the heart fails to produce an impulse.

Pacing catheter placement may be blind but can be confirmed by observing surface EKG evidence of capture, when the pacer is advanced after being set in the asynchronous mode. Otherwise, a precordial EKG lead may be connected to the electrode and advanced until evidence of an injury (ST elevation) is observed.

In asystolic patients the pacemaker is set in an asynchronous mode, and pacing is initiated at the maximum output. This is gradually reduced to establish a threshold at which consistent pacing occurs. The output is then set at three times this threshold to allow for an increase in threshold that is to be anticipated with continued pacing and shifts of catheter position. If the patient has an underlying rhythm, synchronization is needed and the sensitivity of the sensing electrode is adjusted to establish adequate pacing.

The occasional patient who relies significantly on atrial contribution for cardiac output may need atrial pacing, if reliable AV conduction is present, or AV sequential pacing to improve hemodynamic parameters.

Complications include venous thrombosis, catheter infection, arrhythmias, and myocardial perforation. Septal perforation, as indicated by a paced complex with right bundle branch block and cardiac tamponade, is relatively rare. Poor lead contact, lead displacement, myocardial fibrosis, and metabolic problems (hyperkalemia, acidosis) may account for poor sensing and pacing.

MUSCLE DISORDERS

Cardiac muscle particularly depends on the delivery of oxygenated blood for the maintenance of function. Under baseline conditions, blood flow to cardiac muscle is 60 to 90 ml/min/100 g of heart tissue via the right and left coronary arteries. If a person has a normal hemoglobin level of 15 g/dl, a hemoglobin oxygen saturation of 95% to 98%, and a hemoglobin oxygen carrying capacity of 1.34 ml oxygen per gram of hemoglobin, cardiac muscle requires oxygenation of 10 to 20 ml/min/100 g of tissue.

The right coronary artery supplies the right ventricle and the apex of the heart. The left coronary artery supplies the septum and the left ventricular wall. This vessel divides into two large and dominant vessels, the left anterior descending and the left circumflex arteries. These vessels run in the epicardial fat and send penetrating branches through the muscle to the endocardium to deliver oxygenated blood to the muscular and conduction areas of the heart. An occlusion of the right coronary artery commonly leads to an inferior wall infarction, significant problems with bradycardia, and types of second-degree heart block because of loss of blood flow to conduction areas of the heart. An occlusion of the left coronary artery leads to an anteroseptal myocardial infarction. Conduction problems in the left coronary artery are usually bundle branch blocks or complete heart block because of blood supply problems to the septum and the His-Purkinje system.

Myocardial Oxygen Consumption

When myocardial oxygen consumption ($M\dot{V}O_2$) needs are not met by the delivery of oxygenated blood through the coronary arteries, ischemia occurs. Ischemia is nothing more than the oxygen deprivation of heart muscle, but it has many causes, most of which are seen in a critical care unit at one time or another.

Four determinants of $M\dot{V}O_2$ are commonly manipulated to restore balance to cardiac oxygen supply and demand. They are heart rate, systolic blood pressure, contractility, and myocardial wall tension (Table 9–5).

Heart Rate

Heart rate is of particular importance because it affects both the demand side and the supply side of the oxygen equation. Slow heart rates of 60 to 70 beats/min provide significantly more time for diastole than systole. Since coronary blood flow occurs largely during diastole, low heart rates tend to preserve diastolic time and coronary blood flow. When the heart rate reaches 90 beats/min, systole and diastole are approximately equal in duration. At heart rates above 90 beats/min, and particularly above 100 beats/min, which meets the definition of tachycardia, diastolic time is compromised and coronary flow is reduced. Increasing the number of contractions per minute increases oxygen consumption and lowers availability of coronary flow. For the critically ill patient, heart rates between 60 and 90 beats/min seem to strike the best balance between myocardial oxygen consumption and delivery. This physiologic fact is the basis for the important role of beta blockers in critical care of ischemic patients.

Systolic Blood Pressure

Systolic blood pressure is the second determinant of $M\dot{V}O_2$. For some time anesthesiologists were interested in the rate × pressure product (heart rate × systolic blood pressure) as an indicator of cardiac oxygen demands. Other investigators noted that the area under the arterial systolic pressure curve, called the time tension index (TTI), correlated with $M\dot{V}O_2$ and that the area under the arterial diastolic pressure curve, called the diastolic pressure time index (DPTI), correlated with cardiac oxygen supply. The TTI and DPTI can be used to calculate the endocardial viability ratio (EVR) as an index of supply and demand abnormalities. Excesses of systolic pressure and heart rate could be shown to create subendocardial myocardial infarctions at certain EVR measurements because of oxygen delivery problems. Whether one is a proponent of rate × pressure product or EVR, a number of models show that systolic pressure is important to $M\dot{V}O_2$.

Wall Tension

Wall tension is a third and commonly manipulated determinant of $M\dot{V}O_2$. An enlarged, dilated, tense ventricle, as might be seen in congestive heart failure, has elevated oxygen demands. Manipulation of preload and afterload to reduce ventricular size reduces cardiac demands for oxygen. This is always a balance in critical care. Increasing the left ventricular end-diastolic volume (LVEDV) stretches the cardiac muscle and improves contractility via the Starling mechanism. On the other hand, this can tip a heart with borderline oxygenation into ischemia. The heart is an aerobic organ that is intolerant of ischemia.

Contractility

Contractility is the final determinant of $M\dot{V}O_2$. Depending on the state of catecholamine stimulation, calcium level, preload, and use of cardiac glycosides, contractility of cardiac muscle in an ICU can vary tremendously. In the past, clinicians hesitated to use catecholamine therapy in acute myocardial infarction for fear of extending the infarct by increasing $M\dot{V}O_2$. That concern remains but clearly applies much more to the use of epinephrine or norepinephrine. It applies somewhat to the use of dopamine depending on the dose. Newer agents for the manipulation of contractility, such as dobutamine or amrinone, have little effect on $M\dot{V}O_2$. The reason for that lies in the balance between oxygen supply and demand. Both agents increase $M\dot{V}O_2$ because of their impact on contractility. Both agents also decrease $M\dot{V}O_2$

TABLE 9–5. Determinants of Myocardial Oxygen Consumption

OXYGEN DEMAND	OXYGEN SUPPLY
Heart rate	Diastolic time
Systolic blood pressure	Driving pressure
Contractility	Hemoglobin
Wall tension	Oxygen saturation

because of their effect on preload and afterload. The result is the safe use of both agents in the management of low cardiac output syndromes without excessive concerns about augmented $M\dot{V}o_2$.

Myocardial Oxygen Delivery

On the other side of the equation are an equal number of determinants of myocardial oxygen delivery. They include diastolic time, diastolic pressure, hemoglobin concentration, and oxygen saturation of hemoglobin. The importance of diastolic time in permitting coronary blood flow has already been discussed. Diastolic pressure and coronary driving pressure are also critical. At a coronary driving pressure of 40 mm Hg or less, coronary flow ceases. Depending on the degree of coronary vascular disease, this driving pressure becomes more significant. Ischemia may occur with minimal hypotension if flow is significantly obstructed. Coronary arteries attempt to vasodilate to permit a matching of oxygen supply and demand, but in the presence of an obstructing atheromatous plaque this autoregulation may be insignificant to improving flow.

Other determinants of oxygen supply are hemoglobin levels and oxygen saturation of hemoglobin. In the operating room and critical care unit anesthesiologists commonly maintain a hemoglobin level of 9 to 10 g/dl and 90% oxygen saturation for optimal oxygen delivery. The individual validity of this rule varies tremendously and depends on all the other factors already discussed that regulate the balance of cardiac oxygen supply and demand. In some situations with normal blood pressure and heart rate and minimal coronary obstruction, hemoglobin levels of 6 to 7 g/dl are more than adequate. In other clinical situations, such as aortic stenosis with a fixed cardiac output, 9 g/dl may be inadequate and lead to ischemia.

Ischemia

Ischemia damages the heart. Both chronic ischemia and acute ischemic episodes cause significant systolic and diastolic abnormalities. In the acute situation ischemia leads to wall motion abnormalities. Two-dimensional echocardiography can demonstrate poorly contracting cardiac muscle or hypokinesis in the presence of ischemia. An 80% reduction in blood flow causes akinesis or an absence of contraction, and a 95% reduction of flow causes dyskinesis or a bulging of the ischemic area

during contraction. Ischemia also affects diastolic function, leading to a noncompliant ventricle. During episodes of ischemia, left ventricular end-diastolic pressure (LVEDP) may rise sharply with no change in LVEDV.

Diastolic function is commonly altered during ischemic episodes in critically ill patients with pulmonary artery catheters. When ischemia begins, pulmonary artery systolic and diastolic pressure and pulmonary capillary wedge pressure (PCWP) increase rapidly. V-shaped waves may appear suddenly on the wedge tracing, signaling the onset of functional mitral insufficiency.

The EKG is the most common ICU monitor of ischemia. Changes in the precordial or limb leads may show ST depression early in the course of ischemia. Many ICU EKG signals are inadequate for the early detection of ischemia. Chest pain may or may not be present. Many diabetic patients with significant ischemia have little or no chest pain during significant ischemia. One other monitor of ischemia, the fiberoptic pulmonary artery catheter, may be useful in predicting altered cardiac function. With this catheter the continuous trend of mixed venous oxygen saturation ($S\bar{v}o_2$) from the pulmonary artery can be monitored. As ischemia occurs, wall motion changes lead to a decline in cardiac output. In compensation, extraction of oxygen from hemoglobin increases throughout the body to meet metabolic needs. $S\bar{v}o_2$ declines with increased extraction, indicating a fall in cardiac output.

Congestive Heart Failure and Pulmonary Edema

Sudden unexpected episodes of congestive heart failure and pulmonary edema are common in patients with ischemic cardiac problems, as may be seen with atherosclerotic cardiovascular disease. When this occurs in the ICU or recovery room, fluid overload is commonly thought to be present. In fact, most episodes of cardiac pulmonary edema in hospitalized patients are probably due to alterations in diastolic function caused by ischemia. The clinical preoccupation with fluid overload leads to the aggressive diuresis of patients with a normal intravascular volume. Resultant hypovolemia can precipitate hypotension, worsening the balance of cardiac oxygen supply and demand. The role of ischemia should be considered in the clinical management of acute pulmonary edema. Such interventions as controlling blood pressure and heart rate, reducing preload and afterload with nitrates or calcium channel blockers, such as nifedipine, or dilating coronary arteries with agents to reduce coronary vascular resistance may be a wiser approach to managing acute congestive heart failure.

Hibernating Myocardium

Chronic ischemia is now known to cause a chronic malfunctioning heart known as hibernating myocardium. Chronic ischemia causes low cardiac output and high risk for infarction. This malfunctioning cardiac state is reversible with revascularization by angioplasty or after coronary artery bypass graft. The diagnosis of hibernating myocardium is difficult and involves assessing wall motion abnormalities and potential improvement with nitrates. A patient admitted for abdominal aortic aneurysm repair with a hibernating myocardium caused by chronic ischemia might be considered for a coronary artery bypass graft to improve cardiac function before the aortic operation.

Stunned Myocardium

Short but frequent episodes of ischemia do not damage the cellular structure of cardiac muscle but rather impair myocardial function. Longer episodes of ischemia can cause cardiac muscle cell damage without leading to necrosis. This process, called stunning, is associated with subcellular electron micrograph abnormalities that are reversible within 7 to 10 days of the ischemic episode if the imbalance of myocardial oxygen supply and demand is corrected. During the stunned state, myocardial function is decreased, commonly with reduced cardiac output and poor peripheral perfusion. A common clinical example is an intraoperative ischemic episode associated with anesthesia induction, hypertension, and tachycardia. If ischemia persists long enough, cells are in an injured but reversible state. Postoperatively this patient may require a week of hemodynamic support to guarantee adequate organ perfusion.

The stunning process seems related to abnormalities of cardiac intracellular calcium. Ischemia depletes intracellular adenosine triphosphate (ATP) stores. This interferes with transsarcolemma $Na^+ - K^+$ exchange. Intracellular Na^+ increases, leading to elevated $Na^+ - Ca^{++}$ exchange. With decreased ATP stores, Ca^{++} removal from the cell is diminished. These various processes lead to high intracellular calcium concentrations in the cardiac cell and mitochondrial calcium overload. Calcium overload further depresses ATP production, leading to stunned cardiac cells that function poorly from a systolic and diastolic standpoint. With restoration of myocardial oxygen supply and demand balance, necrosis is avoided and eventually the cell returns to its previous level of function. Calcium channel blockers and beta blockers, both of which affect movement of calcium into the cell, are thought to reduce the calcium overload on the cardiac cell during ischemia. Some investigations have shown significant protection from ischemia by agents such as nifedipine during ischemic episodes.

When dealing with reduced myocardial function after a stunning episode, the clinician must pay close attention to myocardial oxygen supply and demand. The stunned cardiac cells maintain responsiveness to beta-adrenergic stimulation, but improper treatment can increase $M\dot{V}o_2$ and cause recurrent ischemia. The patient with a stunned myocardium is best managed with control of heart rate, blood pressure, and preload to minimize oxygen consumption. Contractility can be improved with dobutamine or amrinone to provide optimal organ perfusion if other determinants of oxygen consumption and delivery are in balance. Such agents as epinephrine and high-dose dopamine (greater than 10 µg/kg/min), which increase heart rate, blood pressure, and PCWP, are contraindicated.

Unstable Angina

Persistent and unrelieved ischemia in most patients leads to the clinical syndrome of unstable angina. This is associated with EKG changes of ST depression, marked agitation, catecholamine release, and poor cardiac output. This life-threatening situation must be halted to prevent cardiac muscle necrosis. Over the past 10 to 15 years, trauma critical care centers have become aware of the clinical significance of the "golden hour," the time from injury to resuscitation and restoration of adequate peripheral perfusion. In the case of an ischemic patient with cardiac disease there is also a "golden hour" or "critical interval" for the correction of myocardial oxygen supply and demand balance.

Management

The basis of ischemia correction includes nitrates, such as topical nitrates or intravenous nitroglycerin (Table 9–6). Nitrates cause vascular smooth muscle relaxation. This leads to arterial vasodilatation resulting in afterload

TABLE 9–6. Therapy for the Ischemic Myocardium

Nitroglycerin
Calcium channel blocker
Beta blocker
Improved oxygenation
Red blood cell transfusion
Cardiac output support
Blood pressure support
Intraaortic balloon

reduction and venous dilatation resulting in preload reduction. These effects reduce myocardial oxygen consumption. In addition, coronary artery vasodilatation increases cardiac oxygen delivery. Calcium channel blockers have a similar preload, afterload, and coronary artery effect. Nifedipine, which can be administered orally to the critically ill patient by emptying a 10 mg capsule into the mouth, acts quickly in ischemia and is the drug of choice. Diltiazem can be given orally but is not a liquid in a capsule, so the time to effect is increased. Verapamil can be given intravenously but usually is used for arrhythmia management. It has potent negative inotropic effects and has not achieved popularity as ischemia therapy in critical care.

Beta blockers should also be considered for ischemia therapy, particularly if the patient has a heart rate of 90 beats/min or above. Intravenous propranolol in 0.5 mg doses has been used commonly in anesthesia for control of heart rate. It is a nonselective beta blocker with rapid onset when given intravenously and a 4- to 6-hour half-life. Intravenous propranolol has been largely replaced by intravenous metoprolol for use in cardiac disease, since metoprolol is a cardioselective beta blocker with onset of action and half-life similar to those of propranolol. Intravenous doses of 1 to 5 mg are commonly used in acute myocardial infarction.

In an ischemic patient when left ventricular failure is a concern, esmolol may be a better choice. Esmolol is an ultrashort-acting cardioselective beta blocker that must be given intravenously. It has a 7- to 9-minute half-life with a rapid onset of action. This agent must be given by continuous intravenous infusion for the control of tachycardia associated with ischemia because of its short half-life. Doses of 100 to 200 μg/kg/min are generally effective in restoring heart rate to a more normal level. If the patient shows any worsening of congestive failure or hypotension, the agent can be stopped and is essentially cleared from the bloodstream in 30 minutes.

Oxygen saturation of hemoglobin, hemoglobin concentration, and adequate diastolic pressure are all considerations for the patient with unstable angina. If chest pain or signs of ischemia are not corrected within 30 to 60 minutes of institution of the preceding recommendations, the patient should be considered for the urgent insertion of an intraaortic counterpulsation balloon (IACB). In the past the IACB was limited to assisting patients who could not be separated from cardiopulmonary bypass. This indication was expanded to cardiogenic shock and to patients with left main artery disease who were candidates for cardiac catheterization and coronary artery surgery. Now the indications for the use of IACB are expanding to unstable angina and stunned myocardium, in which IACB reduces afterload to restore myocardial oxygen supply and demand balance. Many patients have an almost magical relief of chest pain with the insertion of the IACB, largely because of the prominent afterload reduction. The sudden deflation of a 30 ml balloon in the thoracic aorta during systole markedly assists with ejection of stroke volume and relieves ischemia.

Myocardial Infarction

Ischemia that progresses beyond angina, stunning, and reversible injury causes myocardial muscle necrosis that is commonly known as infarction. In the last 30 years medical understanding of myocardial infarction has greatly increased. In the late 1960s and early 1970s coronary thrombosis was emphasized as the cause of infarction and it was common to administer anticoagulants to all patients with a new myocardial infarction. In the late 1970s and early 1980s the emphasis shifted from thrombosis to vascular disease. In the last 5 years these philosophies have merged, and infarction is now considered to be related to both thrombosis and vascular obstruction from atheromatous disease.

Pathophysiology. This new pathophysiology of myocardial infarction allows for thrombotic and nonthrombotic causes. Nonthrombotic causes are discussed previously in the chapter because they are caused by imbalances in myocardial oxygen supply and demand. In these situations episodes of hypertension, tachycardia, and ventricular dilatation increase myocardial oxygen consumption above the ability of the coronary arteries to deliver oxygenated blood. If this persists, infarction occurs. Because of the anatomy of the coronary arteries in their path from the epicardial area to the subendocardial area, subendocardial infarction is common with excessive myocardial oxygen consumption. Patchy nontransmural areas of muscle necrosis, unrelated to thrombosis, are also possible. Many postoperative myocardial infarctions that occur within 72 hours of surgery are related to postoperative pain, hypertension, tachycardia, and persistent ischemia that becomes infarction (Table 9–7).

Diagnosis. The diagnosis of infarction is based on the EKG and cardiac enzyme concentrations, as well as physical signs and symptoms. From an EKG standpoint myocardial infarctions are sometimes classified as Q wave, referring to transmural necrosis usually of thrombotic origin, and non–Q wave, referring to a nontransmural necrosis of nonthrombotic or only partially thrombotic origin. With a Q wave infarction the EKG traditionally progresses from early ST depression with T wave inversion to ST elevation to loss of R wave and new Q wave. In the case of a non–Q wave infarction the EKG diagnosis is much more difficult and may be limited to signs of ischemia, ST depression, and an elevation of cardiac enzyme concentrations. Many postoperative infarctions are in that category.

Cardiac enzymes are significant indicators and discriminators of infarction when the EKG is questionable. The first enzyme to become elevated in infarction is creatine kinase (CK) which exceeds normal limits within 4 to 8 hours after necrosis of myocardial cells begins. A reliable relationship exists between the amount of CK rise and the size of the infarction. CK levels peak in 24 hours after infarction and then decline to normal within 3 to 4 days after infarction. The three types of CK enzyme are CK-MM, largely from skeletal muscle, CK-BB from the brain and kidney, and CK-MB from the heart. Therefore, in addition to monitoring total CK rise, the physician must monitor total CK-MB rise and percentage of CK as CK-MB to confirm the presence of myocardial necrosis.

A second cardiac enzyme, lactate dehydrogenase (LDH), can be helpful in diagnosing myocardial infarction, particularly if blood samples are drawn late after suspected infarction or

TABLE 9–7. Non Q Wave Myocardial Infarction Management

Nitroglycerin
Calcium channel blockers
Arrhythmia control
Cardiac oxygen supply/demand

if significant skeletal muscle damage from surgery has produced a markedly elevated total CK level. Of the five LDH isoenzymes, LDH1 is of cardiac origin. The ratio between LDH1 and LDH2 is helpful in differentiating the cause of an increased total LDH. A ratio exceeding 1, is a helpful diagnostic criterion for myocardial infarction. LDH rises more slowly than CK, starting at 24 to 48 hours after infarction. It reaches a peak in 3 to 6 days and then slowly declines to normal.

The predominant cause of myocardial infarction is not imbalances of myocardial oxygen supply and demand because of excesses of heart rate and blood pressure. In the last 5 to 10 years thrombosis of an epicardial vessel, usually proximal, in a left anterior descending or circumflex artery has become accepted as the cause of transmural Q wave myocardial infarction.

The epicardial thrombosis is thought to be related to the rupture of an atheromatous plaque. As coronary vascular disease progresses, narrowing often occurs in a proximal epicardial vessel where plaque formation is excessive. If this plaque ruptures, the site of endothelial damage is flooded with fat and interstitial fluid. This activates the coagulation chain, leading to the formation of fibrin from fibrinogen. The fibrin network accumulates platelets and red blood cells, leading to a total occlusion of the vessel. Many times a vasospastic response takes place in the area of the thrombosis, worsening ischemia and necrosis in adjacent areas of myocardium. The clot can propagate in the vessel and enlarge, involving more branches of the primary vessel.

With the onset of thrombosis, ischemia occurs quickly, ST depression takes place and is soon replaced by ST elevation on the EKG, and most patients have the onset of chest pain. This pain or angina differs among patients. It can be burning or pressurelike and commonly radiates to the left arm and into the neck or jaw. Within 6 to 8 hours of the onset of thrombosis, necrosis of involved cardiac muscle is complete and irreversible. If left untreated, this condition evolves to a completed Q wave myocardial infarction.

Management. The use of thrombolytic agents has largely changed the preceding scenario and promotes reperfusion of the myocardium (Table 9–8). Agents such as tissue plasminogen activator (tPA) convert inactive plasminogen to active plasmin. The attachment of plasmin to fibrin breaks down the fibrin structure of the clot, leading to a dissolution of the clot and formation of fibrin degradation products. If tPA is given within 6 hours of the

TABLE 9–8. Thrombolysis

Indications
Less than 6 hours chest pain
New electrocardiographic (EKG) ST elevation

Contraindications
Recent surgery
Bleeding
Age greater than 75 years
Stroke
Cardiopulmonary resuscitation

Reperfusion Evidence
Relief of pain
Arrhythmias
Normal ST segement on EKG

onset of chest pain, approximately 70% to 80% of vessels are reopened and cardiac muscle is reperfused. Other thrombolytic agents, such as streptokinase and anistreplase, are now available.

The longest and largest clinical experience is with streptokinase, which was first given by the intracoronary route. Comparisons of streptokinase and tPA show similar long-term mortality statistics and similar left ventricular function data, suggesting that the less expensive drug streptokinase may be as good as the newer and much more expensive tPA. A closer analysis of that information shows that intravenous tPA causes a higher percentage of coronary artery reperfusion than does streptokinase. Some of these vessels reocclude if heparin is not started concomitantly with the tPA. Heparin appears to keep the extra vessels opened by tPA patent. Whether that will result in a lower mortality rate or better ventricular function in some patients is unclear.

Only preliminary information is available on anistreplase, which is almost as expensive as tPA. Its major advantage is that it can be given as a bolus without a continuous infusion. The usual dosage of tPA is a 10 mg bolus, 50 mg infused over the first hour, and 20 mg infused over each of the next 2 hours for a total dose of 100 mg. Some interest has been expressed in front loading this dose more than is already recommended, but little information justifies that change.

Indications for thrombolysis include chest pain of less than 6 hours' duration and new ST elevation on EKG. A thrombolytic agent should be started immediately after a diagnosis has been made to minimize the "critical interval" of oxygen-deprived myocardial muscle. Reperfusion can be diagnosed if the patient has relief of chest pain, reperfusion arrhythmias, which are usually ventricular in nature, return of the elevated ST segment to an isoelectric position, and a rapid rise in serum CK enzyme level caused by a washout of enzymes during the reperfusion process. If reperfusion occurs, the patient may well have 7 to 10 days of ventricular dysfunction from the stunning process of temporary occlusion.

Urgent cardiac catheterization is unnecessary in this patient population if the vessel opens and stays open. This procedure can be done electively. There is also no need to perform balloon angioplasty of the partially occluded atheromatous vessel that initiated the clotting process. Emergency angioplasty actually seems to increase deaths among patients with acute myocardial infarction who respond to thrombolysis.

Contraindications to thrombolysis include recent surgery, recent bleeding, such as gastrointestinal or intracerebral, and old age, particularly when associated with an inferior wall infarction. Patients older than 75 years with an inferior wall infarction seem less likely to benefit and at much greater risk for spontaneous hemorrhage from thrombolysis. Relative contraindications might include cardiac arrest with chest compression or previous instrumentation with bleeding such as attempted insertion of a pulmonary artery catheter with puncture of the carotid artery.

If a patient fails to respond to intravenous thrombolysis or the vessel occludes again after reperfusion, cardiac catheterization is indicated. Instrumentation of the vessel may restore flow. In such a situation angioplasty may save a vessel and permit reperfusion. If this fails and the infarction process is in an early stage, emergency coronary artery bypass grafting may be attempted to restore blood flow to cardiac muscle.

The use of thrombolysis has revolutionized the practice of cardiology and the critical care of patients with cardiac disease. As mentioned previously, speed and expertise have suddenly become as relevant to cardiology as they are to trauma management. Cardiac catheterization laboratories must be open 24 hours a day with technicians on call. Emergency medicine departments must act quickly and be prepared to begin thrombolysis within minutes of the diagnosis of new myocardial infarction. Air medical evacuation systems, started largely to speed trauma patients to trauma centers, are now swamped with cardiac patients being urgently transported to cardiac centers to stop the ischemia and necrosis of myocardial muscle. Community rescue squads must be vigilant for signs of myocardial infarction. Some rescue squads are attempting to use thrombolytic agents in prehospital care to speed up the thrombolytic process. Portable facsimile machines allow physicians in the emergency department to diagnose ST elevation so that paramedics in the field can administer a thrombolytic agent as the patient is transported to the hospital.

Heparin plays an important role in the management of patients with unstable angina and those given thrombolysis. In unstable angina, heparin should be initiated on admission to the ICU with a 5000 unit bolus and 1000 units/h, with adjustment of the hourly dose to keep the partial thromboplastin time at 2 to 2½ times normal. This reduces the subsequent incidence of infarction. Heparin should also be started during the administration of the thrombolytic tPA. Full heparinization, as used in unstable angina, helps to keep vessels open and prevent reocclusion by further thrombosis. This is particularly true with tPA; early use of heparin seems to preserve tPA's advantage over streptokinase by maintaining the patency of the additional 10% of vessels tPA reperfuses.

Human denial of disease being what it is, many patients still arrive in emergency rooms 12 to 24 hours after the onset of chest pain with a completed Q wave myocardial infarction. The management of these patients continues to be based on the physiologic principles already elaborated in this chapter (Table 9–9). Arrhythmias must be controlled with lidocaine, heart rate must be controlled with beta blockers, and extension of the infarct should be prevented with such agents as nitrates. Beta blockers are critically important to patients with completed Q wave infarcts. Numerous studies have clearly shown a reduced long-term mortality rate if beta blockers are started early and continued after discharge from the hospital. The usual agent in the critical care setting is metoprolol in 5 mg intravenous doses followed with oral doses when possible. Esmolol is equally good in this setting, but much less prospective work

TABLE 9–9. Q Wave Myocardial Infarction Therapy

Beta blockers
Nitroglycerin
Arrhythmia control
Hemodynamic monitoring
Inotropic therapy
Afterload reduction
Increase left ventricular end-diastolic volume
Intraaortic balloon

is available to demonstrate the value of this agent.

If the patient with a completed Q wave infarct does poorly and congestive heart failure, pulmonary edema, and reduced peripheral perfusion develop, invasive hemodynamic monitoring is required to ensure adequate cardiac function. A fiberoptic pulmonary artery catheter is particularly helpful, since a declining $S\bar{v}O_2$ indicates inadequate oxygen transport, a key issue in myocardial infarction. The presence of PCWP greater than 18 mm Hg and cardiac index less than 2.2 L/min/m^2 is associated with a significant mortality rate. Critical care physicians have the task of diagnosing this situation early and initiating corrective action to lower filling pressures and increase cardiac output.

As previously described, nitrates, the beta-agonist drug dobutamine, and the phosphodiesterase inhibitor amrinone are appropriate therapies to restore peripheral perfusion in cardiogenic shock. Both dobutamine and amrinone can be titrated to 20 µg/kg/min and often behave synergistically when used in combination. As a synthetic catecholamine, dobutamine has a rapid onset of action and a short half-life. It has a minimal effect on heart rate, blood pressure, and $M\dot{V}O_2$. The best monitors of patient response are $S\bar{v}O_2$ and intermittent thermal dilution measurements of cardiac output. Amrinone is not a catecholamine and has a 4- to 6-hour half-life. Like all longer-acting drugs, it requires an initial bolus to establish a blood level. A starting bolus of 0.75 to 1 mg/kg followed by a continuous infusion of 5 µg/kg/min normally causes a significant improvement in cardiac output. With both drugs preload, as monitored by PCWP, and afterload, as monitored by systemic vascular resistance index, decrease and cardiac output increases, restoring the delivery of oxygenated blood to the periphery.

Of the two drugs, amrinone is a much greater arterial vasodilator. For that reason it should not be given to hypovolemic patients. When amrinone is used, many patients with cardiac disease require some fluid resuscitation, even if they started with a PCWP greater than 18 mm Hg, because of this vasodilatation.

Calcium channel blockers, despite their beneficial effects on ischemia, coronary vasculature, preload, and afterload, are contraindicated in patients with ventricular decompensation. The marked negative inotropic effect worsened cardiac function in a large multiinstitutional study and led to higher mortality rates.

Use of beta blockers in cardiogenic shock is controversial. They clearly reduce mortality rates in patients with completed Q wave infarction, even with mild congestive heart failure. Their value to control heart rate in cardiogenic shock is unclear. Their ability in lowering heart rate to decrease $M\dot{V}o_2$ and prolong diastolic time seems attractive, but the negative inotropic response may offset these gains.

In summary, the pharmacologic pillars of therapy for cardiogenic shock include nitrates, dobutamine, and amrinone. Preload should be maintained at a PCWP of 15 to 18 mm Hg to take advantage of the Starling effect. This should restore the cardiac index to greater than 2.5 L/min/m^2, $S\bar{v}o_2$ to 65% or greater, and urine output to 0.5 to 1 ml/kg/h. If this does not occur, if poor perfusion and poor cardiac function persist, or if evidence of reversible ischemia continues, the IACB should be attempted. Initial hemodynamic monitoring and pharmacologic stabilization should be accomplished within 2 hours of the diagnosis of cardiogenic shock. If this therapy fails, there is no need for delay in starting counterpulsation. This aggressive approach to cardiogenic shock has lowered the mortality rate from between 80% and 90% in the early 1970s to between 30% and 40% in the current critical care era. Again we emphasize the need for speed and expertise to minimize the "critical interval" and its impact on the ischemic myocardium and ischemic peripheral organs.

In today's sophisticated era of critical care, physicians can often restore peripheral perfusion in cardiogenic shock with mechanical and pharmacologic support and then be unable to wean the patient from the drugs and equipment used in the ICU. In this situation the clinician must consider the desires of the patient and the family, the probability of survival and return to function, and alternative support techniques. In elderly patients with multiple chronic diseases, such as diabetes, peripheral vascular disease, and renal failure, withdrawal of life support is the only alternative. This can be done with the agreement of the patient or the patient's surrogate. In younger patients with single organ failure, artificial heart devices can serve as a bridge to cardiac transplantation, which is now a successful alternative.

Early Detection and Correction of Cardiac Disease

One of the great tasks of caring for patients with cardiac disease is the early detection and correction of problems before they progress to myocardial infarction and cardiogenic shock.

That is particularly true in the surgical ICU and in the perioperative management of patients with coronary artery disease. Myocardial infarction has a significant postoperative complication and mortality rate, which should be prevented by better preoperative preparation whenever possible.

Techniques of imaging the heart can assist with preoperative preparation by finding myocardial areas that are ischemic at rest or during exercise. Preoperative correction of this ischemia by medication, angioplasty, or coronary artery bypass graft can significantly improve the surgical ICU course of patients undergoing elective noncardiac surgery. In patients with myocardial infarction, reducing ischemia during anesthesia induction and performing surgery early in the course of the infarction reduce postoperative complications.

The use of ultrasound to image the myocardium is discussed previously in this chapter. The equipment is portable and can be used easily in the ICU to obtain some sense of wall motion abnormalities and other intracardiac problems, such as papillary muscle rupture with mitral insufficiency or ventricular septal defect associated with myocardial infarction.

Nuclear medicine employs isotopes for visualizing the heart and evaluating physiologic parameters of cardiac function. Most hospitals can provide several types of cardiac radionuclide study, including perfusion studies, radionuclide ventriculogram studies, and infarct avid studies.

Perfusion scans of the myocardium are the most widely employed radionuclide studies of the heart. These studies are usually obtained with thallium-201 chloride. Thallium is a cation whose behavior is similar to that of potassium. A patient who has been fasting for at least several hours exercises on a treadmill, usually according to a predefined study protocol. At the time of the treadmill exercise test an EKG is obtained. At 1 to 2 minutes before termination of exercise, the patient is injected intravenously with 2 to 4 mCi of thallium-201 chloride. Within the next several minutes the patient is transported to a gamma camera for immediate poststress imaging of the heart. Repeat images are obtained 4 hours later for comparison.

The thallium is distributed throughout the myocardium according to blood flow. Its deposition within the myocardium is proportional to blood flow over a wide range of flow rates. Images may be obtained either as planar views or in a tomographic format as single-photon emission computed tomography (SPECT) (Fig. 9–21).

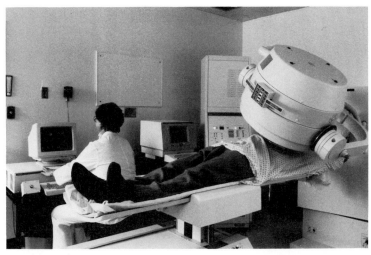

Figure 9–21. A typical single-headed rotating camera, with a technician sitting at the computer console and a patient lying on the imaging table. This device can be used for making either planar images or single-photon emission computed tomography (SPECT) images of the heart.

The planar images are usually acquired at 10-minute intervals in anterior, left anterior oblique (LAO), and steep LAO or left lateral projections (Fig. 9–22). Total imaging time is approximately 30 minutes. By comparing the distribution of activity in the immediate poststress phase with the redistribution phase 4 hours later, the physician can ascertain whether the isotope was distributed normally or some areas were deficient in distribution of isotope (Figs. 9–23 and 9–24). If a defect noted on the immediate poststress view demonstrates redistribution of the isotope on the 4-hour delayed image, that is, a normal delayed image, the tissue is considered to be ischemic and the ischemia was produced by exercise (Figs. 9–25 and 9–26). If a persistent area of decreased isotope is seen on poststress and delayed images, the area is considered to be infarcted.

At 4 hours approximately 50% of the thallium has washed out of normal myocardium, giving less isotope to image than immediately after stress. Images can be normalized so that the intensity of poststress and redistribution images is comparable. If an area of decreased perfusion is present immediately after stress, an ischemic area may actually accumulate activity from the blood pool in the intervening 4 hours, indicating reestablishment of blood flow to an area of jeopardized or ischemic myocardium. An infarcted area does not accumulate activity, since nonviable cells do not actively take up potassium or its analogs, such as thallium.

SPECT employs the same format as perfusion scanning in that a patient exercises on a treadmill according to a predetermined proto-

col. The patient usually receives 3 to 4 mCi of thallium-201 chloride intravenously 1 to 2 minutes before the termination of exercise. Tomographic images are obtained immediately after stress and again at 4 hours. In this instance the images are obtained in multiple projections. The projections range from 32 separate projections from a right anterior oblique (RAO) position to a left posterior oblique (LPO) position, covering 180 degrees, to usually 64 separate projections obtained in a complete circle around the patient's body. The time for imaging each of these projections ranges from 30 to 50 seconds. Total imaging time is therefore 20 minutes or more. Ideally imaging would be completed within 20 minutes, since redistribution of thallium may occur after that time. The images can be reconstructed by a back projection technique similar to that used in other tomographic imaging, such as computed tomography. Cross-sectional images of the heart can then be generated, which allows sections of myocardium to be examined in greater detail than is generally available with planar imaging.

Interpretation of SPECT images again matches the homogeneity of isotope distribution throughout the myocardium on the immediate poststress image with the redistribution image. If distribution is homogeneous on both sets of images, the scan is interpreted as normal. If isotope is deficient in a section of the myocardium in the immediate poststress phase, comparison with the redistribution images is necessary. Redistribution images demonstrate either uptake of isotope in an ischemic region or persistent lack of isotope in an infarcted region.

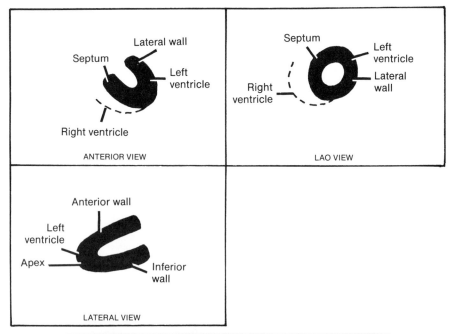

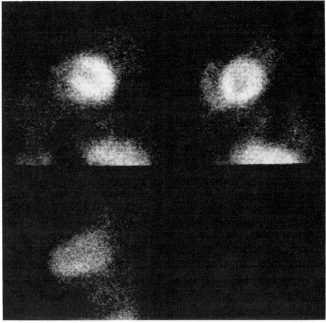

Figure 9–22. A normal planar thallium scan of the heart. The image in the upper left-hand corner is an anterior view. The image in the right upper corner is a left anterior oblique (LAO) view, and the image in the lower left-hand corner is a left lateral view or steep LAO view. The normal distribution of activity throughout the heart can be noted on this study. The redistribution study obtained 4 hours later (not shown) was virtually identical and is consistent with a normal thallium scan of the heart.

Recent attention has been given to reinjection techniques. After the 4-hour period of waiting for redistribution, the patient may receive a second injection of 1 mCi of thallium-201 chloride. The reinjection provides superior counting statistics in evaluating areas of severely ischemic myocardium that would otherwise be interpreted as infarcted. Newer perfusion agents that employ technetium-99m-labeled compounds are also undergoing rapid development. Such compounds are likely to improve resolution and evaluation of the myocardium, since technetium-99m has better imaging characteristics than thallium-201 chloride.

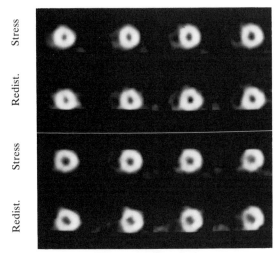

Stress

Redist.

Stress

Redist.

Figure 9–23. A series of tomographic images through the heart. This is along the short axis, which would cut the left ventricle in cross-sectional views, so that it would resemble a doughnut. The top row is immediately after stress and starts from the apex on the left and moves toward the base on the right. The second row is matched redistribution images that were obtained 4 hours later. The third row is continuation of the stress images extending farther up to the base of the heart, and the fourth row represents matched redistribution images.

Radionuclide ventriculograms are another method of evaluating cardiac function. A carrier such as the patient's red blood cells or human serum albumin is labeled with technetium-99m pertechnetate. This allows visualization of the blood pool within the heart. Images can be obtained for specific segments of the cardiac cycle ranging from diastole to systole. The RR interval, as on the EKG, can be broken into 20 to 24 equal time segments. These segments have images of the heart in various phases of contraction and relaxation. The effect is to collect a series of images with the heart in various stages of beating. This gating of the RR interval for collection of multiple images results in a film of the heart beating, an image reminiscent of a ventriculogram obtained during cardiac catheterization. Ejection fraction, chamber volumes, rate of relaxation, and rate of contraction can be calculated, the distribution of contraction over a segment of the myocardium can be observed, and wall motion can be evaluated for areas of akinesis or dyskinesis.

Infarct avid imaging techniques have been available for about 20 years. Technetium-99m pyrophosphate binds to infarcted myocardial cells. In the 24 to 72 hours after infarction, calcification in infarcted tissue (on a microscopic level) is responsible for binding technetium-99m pyrophosphate. This allows confirmation and localization of a myocardial

infarction. This test is less reliable than other methods of evaluating myocardial infarction and thus is relatively unused. A method still in early development uses monoclonal antibodies labeled with iodine radioisotopes to image infarcts.

A future consideration for cardiac evaluation is positron emission tomography (PET). This tomographic technique is used for imaging various organs, such as the heart. PET takes advantage of a different form of radioactive decay. When technetium-99m decays, it emits a single photon that is used for imaging, hence the name single-photon emission computed tomography. PET employs isotopes that emit positrons. Positrons subsequently decay into two photons that are emitted in opposite directions. By employing a ring of detectors around the body, one can locate the line of emission of these photon pairs. This ring of detectors can be arranged in a pattern similar in appearance to the CT scanner. PET scanning has better imaging characteristics than SPECT imaging and permits quantitation.

Many of the isotopes used in PET, such as carbon-11, nitrogen-13, oxygen-15, and fluorine-18, may be incorporated into analogs of molecules that take part in normal human biochemistry. For example, carbon may be incorporated into glucose, amino acids, or fatty acids, such as palmitate or acetate. Fluorine-18 may be incorporated into fluorine-18-2-fluoro-deoxyglucose (FDG) for monitoring glucose metabolism. These isotopes require the presence of a cyclotron and a radiochemistry laboratory. They have short half-lives ranging from seconds to several hours. Other isotopes, such as rubidium-82 (a potassium analog), which may be used for perfusion, also have short half-lives but can be obtained from a generator that can be shipped to the hospital from a production facility elsewhere.

PET scanning is the basis for the myocardial viability test. This test identifies myocardial segments that demonstrate hypoperfusion but viable nonfunctional tissue. If a perfusion defect is demonstrated, a compound such as FDG is administered to the patient. If the FDG is taken up by the apparently underperfused or nonperfused myocardial segment, those cells are judged to be alive. The myocardial segment that shows decreased perfusion but the persistence of basic glucose metabolism may be judged as infarcted on the basis of other tests such as an EKG or echocardiogram. The segment may be hypokinetic or dyskinetic. Such segments have been shown to recover function when

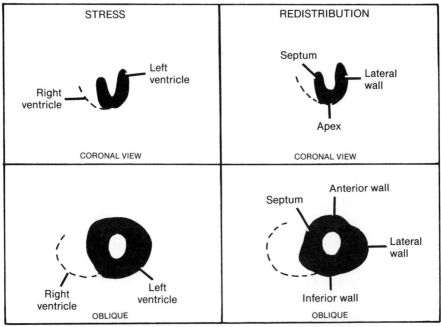

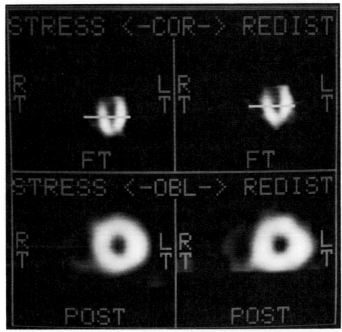

Figure 9–24. A comparison of stress and redistribution images along the short axis. Stress images are on the left, and redistribution images are on the right. A coronal (horizontal) slice through the heart is used as a reference to show the level of the heart that is displayed on the short axis or oblique images as noted in Figure 9–22. This is a normal study.

revascularized. Chronically akinetic depressed segments showing this type of recovery are referred to as hibernating myocardium because this myocardium is still viable and capable of functioning if perfusion is restored. The availability of this technology is restricted, however, because of its complexity.

Other Cardiac Abnormalities

A variety of cardiac abnormalities other than acute coronary artery disease can cause marginal or inadequate delivery of oxygenated blood to the peripheral tissues. These include chronic congestive heart failure, myocarditis, myocardial contusion as occurs in trauma,

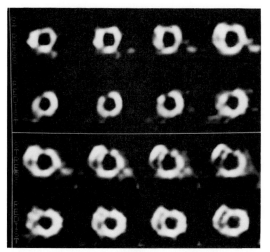

Figure 9–25. A montage of stress and redistribution images similar to those in Figure 9–23. This is an abnormal study that demonstrates irregular uptake of activity throughout the heart on both stress and redistribution images. An area of decreased perfusion in the midseptum can be seen in the third row of images, which are stress images. The redistribution images that match the stress images are in the fourth row, immediately below. Redistribution is occurring in the midseptum, which is indicative of exercise-induced ischemia. The right ventricle is hypertrophied and appears prominent in this patient, who has a history of left ventricular failure. Other abnormalities are also present.

pericardial tamponade, cardiomyopathy, and various forms of valvular disease.

Chronic Congestive Heart Failure

Chronic congestive heart failure is commonly caused by chronic coronary artery disease. Many patients survive a first myocardial infarction and have a progression of coronary artery disease. Subsequent infarctions encroach on viable contracting myocardium and reduce cardiac reserve.

The best measures of cardiac function in patients with chronic congestive heart failure is ejection fraction, usually measured by a radioactive isotope technique. Normal hearts eject 60% to 70% of the blood in the ventricle at the end of diastole. As cardiac muscle is lost because of chronic coronary artery disease, this number approaches 30%, which is associated with exercise limitation and admissions to the ICU because of episodes of congestive heart failure. Preoperative patients with an ejection fraction less than 30% are likely to have a difficult postoperative course if they have lengthy surgery with significant fluid shifts. Repeated admissions to the ICU for episodes of congestive heart failure and pulmonary edema are associated with a poor prognosis and low 1-year survival.

Historically outpatient management has been based on the use of cardiac glycosides, such as digoxin, and diuretics, such as furosemide. Many clinicians attempt to use the same management during episodes of postoperative or in-hospital congestive failure.

The hemodynamics of chronic congestive heart failure is difficult to interpret without the use of a pulmonary artery catheter. Hemodynamic monitoring should be instituted if the patient does not respond in the first few hours to standard pulmonary edema therapy (oxygen, furosemide, morphine, and nitrates) (Table 9–10). Many patients in chronic congestive heart failure have an elevated wedge pressure but are normovolemic or hypovolemic. Patients with a low ejection fraction have a poor tolerance of afterload, and small amounts of vasoconstriction without evidence of hypertension can lead to pulmonary edema.

Correction of congestive heart failure after initiation of hemodynamic monitoring is based on inotropic support and afterload reduction with an agent such as dobutamine. The patient can then be transferred to orally administered afterload reducers such as captopril or hydralazine. The converting enzyme inhibitor enalaprilat can be given intravenously in doses of 0.625 to 2.5 mg every 6 to 8 hours to replace beta-agonist drugs. The combined use of converting enzyme inhibitors or hydralazine with digoxin and diuretics has replaced previous therapy for chronic congestive heart failure and improved survival. The role of digoxin in this entity is unclear. It has been used in the past and seems to help with systolic function but is probably of little use in diastolic dysfunction.

Myocarditis

A variety of infectious and noninfectious agents can lead to myocarditis or inflammation of cardiac muscle. Symptoms of myocarditis are fatigue, dyspnea, palpitations, and sometimes chest pain or discomfort. Inflammation of the heart causes cardiac dilatation and congestive heart failure with poor peripheral perfusion.

TABLE 9–10. Congestive Heart Failure Therapy

Oxygen
Diuretic
Morphine
Nitroglycerin
Ace inhibitor
Hydralazine
Digoxin

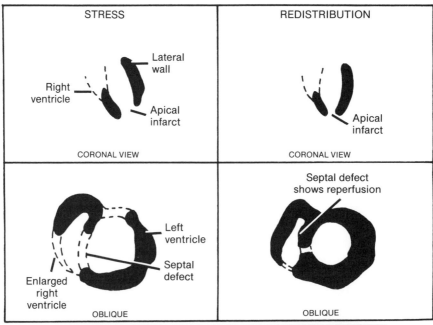

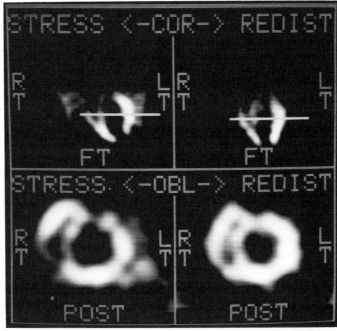

Figure 9–26. Magnification of the abnormal study demonstrated in Figure 9–25. In this case the immediate poststress image appears in the lower left-hand view. The midseptum has decreased isotope in comparison with the rest of the left ventricle. The right ventricle is also abnormally prominent on this image, which indicates right ventricular hypertrophy. A cross-sectional reference can be made with respect to the coronal image through the heart, which is immediately above the short axis images. Redistribution images demonstrate significant redistribution, indicating that the patient has exercise-induced ischemia involving the septum. The coronal images show a fixed defect at the apex, consistent with an area of infarction.

Physical findings include heart murmur, friction rub, gallop, faint heart sounds, and distended neck veins. Many patients have an exceedingly low ejection fraction when first examined. Hemodynamic studies show a persistent tachycardia.

Myocarditis can be caused by bacteria, viruses, rickettsiae, fungi, and parasites. In the

United States the most likely cause is a virus. In the past, myocarditis was associated with diphtheria, tuberculosis, and typhoid.

Hemodynamic management of patients with myocarditis, as in the case of chronic congestive heart failure from coronary artery disease and multiple infarctions, is based on afterload reduction. No oral inotropic agents to augment contractility can be used by outpatients. Use of intermittent infusions or home infusions of dobutamine or amrinone to help such patients has attracted interest but is not standard therapy with known long-term benefits.

Cardiac Contusion

Chest trauma can lead to low cardiac output from cardiac contusion and pericardial tamponade. Cardiac contusion behaves similarly to myocardial infarction from coronary artery disease. The diagnosis can be confirmed by elevation of the cardiac enzymes CK-MB and LDH1. The magnitude of the contusion can be evaluated by the cardiac imaging techniques discussed previously. Hypokinesis is commonly found but may be reversible as the patient recovers from the trauma. If the patient has low cardiac output, pharmacologic afterload reduction with converting enzyme inhibitors or hydralazine or mechanical afterload reduction with an IACB may be helpful. Inotropic therapy with dobutamine or amrinone may be needed to sustain cardiac output.

As in all the previous discussions of cardiac function, blood pressure should not be the target for correcting cardiac function in myocardial contusion. Blood pressure is a function of systemic vascular resistance and cardiac output. In heart failure caused by cardiac contusion or other cardiac problems, blood pressure may be normal even though cardiac output is very low and systemic vascular resistance is very high. Hemodynamic monitoring is needed to titrate cardiac output to an acceptable level while afterload is reduced and inotropic support is provided. Agents with alpha activity, such as dopamine and epinephrine, may put significant stress on the contused myocardium.

Cardiac Tamponade

Cardiac tamponade can be associated with trauma and hemopericardium or with other medical entities, such as myocardial infarction, myocarditis, and renal failure. The accumulation of fluid in the pericardium puts pressure on the heart and reduces filling. This creates hypotension and poor cardiac output. Depending on the cause, the therapy should be fluid resuscitation and drainage of the pericardial fluid.

Patients with pericardial fluid need an elevated venous pressure to force blood into the heart. As a result, fluid resuscitation is first-line management. If trauma is associated with the tamponade, an immediate pericardial tap may be needed to correct problems with cardiac output. This can be done by a subxiphoid approach with a spinal needle. The removal of as little as 100 ml of fluid can significantly improve cardiac function.

Cardiomyopathy

Cardiomyopathy refers to noninflammatory disease of the myocardium, which can be divided into dilated, hypertrophic, and infiltrative categories. These two entities are not related but are sometimes mentioned together as cardiac diseases that impede performance.

DILATED CARDIOMYOPATHY

The term "dilated cardiomyopathy" refers to a pathologic entity that causes enlargement of both ventricular chambers. This dilatation can be caused by chronic coronary artery disease with repeated small infarcts, producing progressive muscle loss, chamber dilatation, and systolic dysfunction. Likewise, chronic alcoholism can be toxic to the myocardium, leading to a dilated cardiomyopathy. Often this diagnosis is not obvious, so the clinical problem is labeled idiopathic dilated cardiomyopathy. Many toxins can cause a slow and progressive deterioration of cardiac function that falls into the category of dilated cardiomyopathy, but the etiologic diagnosis may not be readily apparent even at autopsy.

HYPERTROPHIC CARDIOMYOPATHY

Hypertrophic cardiomyopathy is an increase in muscle mass with small ventricular cavities. This was known as idiopathic hypertrophic subaortic stenosis (IHSS) until it was found that not all patients with this entity had obstruction. Whereas systolic dysfunction characterizes dilated cardiomyopathy, diastolic dysfunction characterizes hypertrophic cardiomyopathy. The huge muscle mass of the heart is stiff and fills poorly, leading to elevated chamber pressures and pulmonary capillary pressure. These patients are short of breath because of chronically elevated wedge pressure. The cause of hypertrophic cardiomyopathy appears to be genetic with variable penetrance. Medical management is different from that of dilated cardiomyopathy. Here the problem is excessive contracting muscle mass, and agents with negative inotropic effects such as beta blockers and calcium channel blockers work best. Surgical procedures attempt to open the blood outflow tract obstructed by muscle mass.

INFILTRATIVE CARDIOMYOPATHY

Infiltrative cardiomyopathy is the third category. Amyloid is a frequent example. These patients have both conduction and muscle problems.

VALVULAR DISORDERS

This chapter has dealt so far with inadequacies of perfusion created by electrophysiologic and muscular problems. Of equal importance are perfusion inadequacies created by valvular problems. The heart is an electrically active muscular organ that is responsible for circulating oxygenated blood to meet the metabolic needs of all body tissues including itself. To accomplish that task it creates pulsatile flow by intermittently filling and emptying as electrophysiologic stimuli cause the cardiac muscle mass to contract and shorten. The cardiac chambers continually fill and empty to propel a stroke volume of 30 to 80 ml of blood into the vasculature. Valves are present to maintain forward flow within this pulsatile system. When these valves are damaged, forward flow is compromised and peripheral perfusion is reduced.

Two valves commonly affected by disease are the mitral and aortic, the inlet and outlet valves for the left ventricle. Damage to these valves leads to clinically significant disturbances of perfusion. The inlet and outlet valves of the right ventricle, the tricuspid and the pulmonary, are certainly important clinically but cause problems less frequently in the critical care environment.

Mitral Valve

The mitral valve is between the left atrium and the left ventricle and is composed of four components: mitral annulus, mitral leaflets, chordae tendineae, and papillary muscles. As with most valves in a fluid system, two types of problems can occur, obstruction to flow and valvular incompetence.

Mitral Stenosis

The clinical example of valvular obstruction is mitral stenosis usually caused by rheumatic fever. In the stenosis process the valve components fuse so that the valve moves poorly and obstructs flow and ventricular filling. This causes blood to back up into the left atrium and reduces left ventricular volume. The greatest clinical impact is on the pulmonary system, with elevated pulmonary artery pressures and PCWP. Lung water increases and lung compliance decreases. Forced vital capacity is reduced, and dyspnea, orthopnea, and ultimately pulmonary edema occur.

Progressive enlargement of the left atrium leads to abnormal electrical activity with the occurrence of atrial fibrillation. The loss of active atrial emptying in the face of atrial fibrillation creates further difficulties moving blood across the stenotic mitral valve, with as much as a 20% decrease in cardiac output. In addition, atrial fibrillation leads to coagulation in the left atrium with mural thrombi and systemic embolization of clot. Patients with mitral stenosis and atrial fibrillation are generally given anticoagulants to prevent this complication.

The mitral valve area is 4 to 6 cm^2 and represents no obstruction to flow. With progressive mitral stenosis the valve size decreases, and at 2 cm^2 a significant gradient in pressure from left atrium to left ventricle is required to permit forward flow. Further decrease in valve size leads to the requirement for higher pressure gradients between the left atrium and the left ventricle and greater backup of blood into the lungs.

Management. Mitral stenosis is difficult to manage in the critical care environment. Control of heart rate with atrial fibrillation is essential to guarantee adequate cardiac output. The use of cardiac glycosides, such as digoxin, is required to maintain a ventricular response rate of 100 beats/min or below. This improves ventricular filling and cardiac output. It is doubtful that the inotropic effect of digoxin is helpful in this setting. Patients with mitral stenosis are likely to have fluid retention, right ventricular failure, and peripheral pulmonary edema. Diuretics are helpful in managing fluid status. Other therapies normally directed at improving cardiac output are of little benefit. Ultimately surgical correction of mitral stenosis is the solution to improving forward flow.

Mitral Regurgitation

Mitral regurgitation is a more common clinical entity in critical care. This condition has both anatomic and functional causes. As mentioned earlier in this chapter, functional mitral regurgitation is seen commonly in patients with cardiac disease when there is cardiac dilatation. During hemodynamic monitoring with a pulmonary artery catheter, bedside nurses commonly report inability to wedge the balloon-tipped catheter. Investigation by the ICU physician shows that the catheter actually wedges, but on inflation large V waves represent functional mitral regurgitation and come and go with the occurrence of left ventricular failure.

The four causes of mitral regurgitation relate to the four parts of the mitral valve. Regurgitation can be caused by damage to the mitral valve leaflets, usually from rheumatic fever. Regurgitation can also be caused by problems with the mitral valve annulus. The annulus can expand and contract with the size of the ventricle. An episode of acute ventricular dilatation associated with an ischemic episode causes the annulus to expand and permits regurgitation — a functional form of mitral regurgitation. Calcification of the annulus from hypertension, diabetes, aortic stenosis, Marfan's syndrome, or Hurler's syndrome can also cause mitral regurgitation. In addition there is idiopathic calcification of the mitral annulus. Damage to the chordae tendineae, as from trauma, infective endocarditis, or rheumatic fever, can cause mitral regurgitation.

One of the more common causes of acute mitral regurgitation in the critical care setting is damage to the papillary muscle. Since blood flow to the myocardium goes from epicardium to endocardium, the papillary muscle is supplied by an end vessel in the coronary circulation. Papillary muscle ischemia leads to malfunction of the muscle and mitral regurgitation. Most likely the V waves seen intermittently on PCWP tracing during ischemic events are a combination of papillary muscle dysfunction from ischemia and ventricular dilatation with enlargement of the mitral annulus. If ischemia persists, infarction and necrosis of the papillary muscle can occur, leading to rupture of the muscle with a free-floating chorda tendinea and wide-open mitral regurgitation.

Papillary muscle rupture is not a rare cause of acute pulmonary edema, and the patient who has pulmonary edema when first examined requires emergency life support. These patients usually need intubation and ventilation to guarantee adequate oxygenation. In addition, they need cardiac support with pharmacologic or mechanical afterload reduction to promote the forward flow of blood until the damaged valve can be corrected surgically.

Mitral regurgitation results in emptying of the left ventricle into the left atrium. This decreases the stroke volume delivered to the aorta and reduces peripheral perfusion. The heart compensates with further emptying of the ventricle. As previously noted, a normal ejection fraction is 60% to 70% of LVEDV. With mitral regurgitation this can be increased to compensate for blood loss into the left atrium. This compensation works well for the slow progressive forms of mitral regurgitation that may be associated with calcification of the mitral annulus. It works less well for acute causes of mitral regurgitation, such as papillary muscle rupture. In these cases emergency surgical correction is needed after stabilization and life support.

Aortic Valve

The second important cardiac valve in critical care is the aortic valve, which is composed of three cusps and lies between the left ventricle and the aorta. It serves as an outlet valve to prevent regurgitant flow back into the heart during diastole. As with the mitral valve, some clinical entities cause obstruction and incompetence of the aortic valve.

Aortic Stenosis

Aortic stenosis may be congenital or acquired. Unicuspid and bicuspid valves can be present at birth and lead to significant aortic obstruction. The usual causes of acquired aortic stenosis are valve damage from rheumatic fever and degenerative calcification of the valve associated with aging. Some forms of atherosclerosis involve the aortic valve, leading to stenosis and obstruction.

The physiologic response to aortic stenosis is a progressive increase in left ventricular muscle mass. A decrease in the valve size from stenosis creates a pressure gradient from the left ventricular chamber to the aorta during systole. When the valve size has decreased to 0.75 cm^2 or less, a pressure gradient of 50 mm Hg or greater is commonly present, and the patient has a critical obstruction.

To compensate for the progressive obstruction and pressure gradient, the muscle mass of the left ventricle increases. The ventricular chamber size may decrease, and the ventricle wall tends to be stiff and difficult to fill during diastole. The heart depends greatly on a sinus rhythm and atrial contraction to fill the ventricle and ensure an adequate LVEDV.

In patients with aortic stenosis, cardiac output is commonly normal at rest but increases poorly with stress because of the obstruction to flow. Digoxin does little to improve strength of contraction. Diuretics, particularly potent ones, such as furosemide, that influence the loop of Henle, can be dangerous. Potent diuretics are likely to decrease intravascular volume and reduce LVEDV. Cardiac output in patients with aortic stenosis depends on ventricular filling. Agents with a negative inotropic effect such as beta blockers or calcium channel blockers may also impair cardiac performance.

Aortic stenosis is evidenced as angina and syncope. The angina is frequently caused, not by coronary artery disease, but by an imbalance in myocardial oxygen consumption and delivery as discussed previously. The large muscle mass of the patient with aortic stenosis has a high oxygen consumption. During forceful contraction of the ventricle the coronary arteries are compressed, leading to restricted coronary flow and a myocardial oxygen deficit. This deficit causes angina. Patients' complaints of syncope are usually based on postural effects and the inability to increase cardiac output in response to position changes.

Management. Careful hemodynamic monitoring and assessment of oxygen transport are essential to the ICU management of patients with aortic stenosis. It is important to maintain a generous intravascular volume, a state of adequate contractility avoiding agents that have a negative inotropic effect, and a sinus rhythm with a heart rate of 60 to 100 beats/min to permit adequate diastolic time for coronary blood flow. Hemoglobin level is particularly important to patients with aortic stenosis because they cannot increase cardiac output to compensate for changes in oxygen consumption. A hemoglobin level of at least 10 g/dl is essential, but monitoring $S\bar{v}O_2$ best indicates the adequacy of oxygen transport. A low $S\bar{v}O_2$ is likely to indicate increased oxygen extraction because of inadequate cardiac output or hemoglobin level.

Aortic Regurgitation

The aortic valve can also demonstrate regurgitation and create quite a different clinical picture from aortic stenosis. Rheumatic fever, infective endocarditis, and trauma with damage to the valve and ascending aorta can cause insufficiency or regurgitation of the aortic valve. Some diseases affecting the ascending aorta, such as syphilis, ankylosing spondylitis, Marfan's syndrome, and Ehlers-Danlos syndrome, can destroy the vessel and damage the aortic valve, leading to regurgitation.

As in aortic stenosis, regurgitation increases left ventricular muscle mass. This mass surrounds a markedly enlarged left ventricular chamber. Cardiac output or volume of blood ejected by the left ventricle may be four or five times normal to produce a forward flow of 5 L of oxygenated blood. Eventually the ventricle fails from excessive effort, and dyspnea, orthopnea, and significant problems with exertion occur.

Management. Several physiologic points are important in managing critically ill patients with aortic regurgitation. Forward flow is important and can be augmented by afterload reduction. Agents causing peripheral vasodilatation, such as hydralazine and nitroprusside, are likely to improve peripheral perfusion. Maintaining an adequate intravascular volume is essential. Drugs with a significant negative inotropic effect usually impair some of the natural compensations the heart has developed for the regurgitant valve.

• • •

Patients with valvular disease present special situations to the critical care practitioner. Their problems can be most difficult to manage in the perioperative period. As in the case of coronary artery disease, the patient with aortic or mitral valve disease should be considered for elective repair of the heart before other types of elective surgery. A clear understanding of the physiologic differences between stenosis and regurgitation is needed to make good patient care decisions in the critical care setting.

VASCULAR DISORDERS

When many clinicians think and write about the cardiovascular system, they focus on the heart, minimizing the role of the vasculature as if it were a mere conduit for the delivery of blood to the peripheral tissues. The last 15 years of hemodynamic monitoring in critical care has clearly demonstrated that the peripheral vasculature and its degree of muscular tone or vasoconstriction have tremendous impact on tissue perfusion. Some degree of vasoconstriction is required to create a driving pressure for the movement of blood. Particularly when a person is in the upright position, vasoconstriction creates the intravascular pressure needed to ensure blood flow to the brain.

Cardiogenic and Hypovolemic Shock

The importance of vasoconstriction or systemic vascular resistance is well demonstrated in various shock states. In both hypovolemic and cardiogenic shock, blood delivery to the various organs is reduced. In hypovolemic shock this is caused by a depleted intravascular volume and a small LVEDV. In cardiogenic shock it is caused by a reduced cardiac output from a malfunctioning heart pump. In both situations the body reacts to maintain blood pressure by vasoconstriction. To preserve blood flow to the heart and brain, a marked reduction of blood flow occurs to other organs, such as skeletal muscle, kidneys, and liver. In the case of hypovolemic shock this vasoconstriction is appropriate for best use of a reduced intravascular volume until other corrective measures occur. In cardiogenic shock, however, vasoconstriction is largely defeating and further worsens the function of a damaged heart. Reversal of this vasoconstriction or afterload reduction actually improves peripheral perfusion.

Septic and Anaphylactic Shock

Vasodilatation is a vascular abnormality that by itself creates shock. The sudden wide-open vasodilatation or loss of afterload associated with septic shock or anaphylactic shock demonstrates the importance of vasoconstriction. In this situation the down-regulation of the alpha receptor in the arterioles promotes vasodilatation. The cause of down-regulation is unclear but has been thought to be endotoxin. However, since vasodilatation is seen in gram-negative, gram-positive, and fungal bloodstream infections, endotoxin may not be the only cause of vasodilatation. Other circulating products, such as interleukin lymphokines, may be responsible for this hypotensive reaction to sepsis.

Management. The management of both septic and anaphylactic shock involves the restoration of peripheral vascular resistance by the use of alpha-agonist agents, such as norepinephrine, phenylephrine, or high-dose dopamine (greater than 10 μg/kg/min). When the cause of sepsis has been corrected by drainage of pus and use of antibiotics, the alpha receptor begins to work appropriately and vasoconstricting agents can be discontinued. When vasoconstrictors are used to treat septic shock, hemodynamic monitoring is necessary. Fluid resuscitation is the first line of therapy in septic shock. If this fails to restore a mean blood pressure of 60 to 70 mm Hg, alpha-agonist drugs should be used. These agents should be titrated to restore resistance to normal, being careful to preserve cardiac output. Excessive use of vasoconstrictors damages the kidneys and greatly reduces blood flow to other vital organs. Monitoring of $S\bar{v}o_2$ can help ensure adequate cardiac output. In sepsis with a high cardiac output, $S\bar{v}o_2$ is normally greater than 70%. As alpha-agonist drugs are used, $S\bar{v}o_2$ should be maintained at 70% or more to ensure proper delivery of oxygenated blood to the tissues. Low-dose dopamine (less than 3 μg/kg/min) can be used with norepinephrine and phenylephrine to blunt the effect of alpha stimulation on the kidney. Dopamine in low doses increases blood flow to the kidney via the dopaminergic receptor in the renal vasculature.

A cardiac muscle defect in septic shock reduces the ejection fraction and increases LVEDV. This depressed contractility does not prevent extremes of cardiac performance, with thermal dilution cardiac output measurements of 10 to 16 L/min in septic shock. The role of beta-agonist drugs, such as dobutamine, is unclear in sepsis when cardiac output is high and contractility is reduced. The most important issue is restoration of perfusion pressure with alpha-agonist drugs and fluid resuscitation. If cardiac output declines or $S\bar{v}o_2$ is less than 70% with acceptable hemoglobin levels, beta-agonist drugs may be indicated. Some evidence in the management of septic shock indicates that maintaining supranormal oxygen delivery may reduce morbidity and mortality.

Aneurysms

Vascular diseases that cause deterioration of the vessel wall are encountered in critical care. The most common of these is atherosclerosis, which affects both the abdominal and the thoracic aorta. Progressive atherosclerosis of the aorta weakens the wall and leads to aneurysm formation. Of aortic aneurysms, 75% occur in the abdomen and 25% in the chest.

Abdominal Aortic Aneurysms

Aneurysms of the abdominal aorta are usually below the renal arteries and above the bifurcation of the aorta into the iliac arteries. The width of the abdominal aorta is 1.5 to 2 cm. An aneurysm of the abdominal aorta of 4 cm or greater is considered clinically significant. Aneurysms of 6 cm or greater are generally operated on to reduce the risk of sudden death from rupture. Generally the larger the aneurysm, the greater the risk of rupture. Some surgeons believe that smaller aneurysms, in the range of 4 cm, should also be considered for surgery.

Aneurysms of the abdominal aorta rupture into two parts of the body. About 80% rupture in the retroperitoneal area, which can tamponade the initial bleeding. These patients have pain and a hematoma in the flank and groin. About 20% of aneurysms rupture into the peritoneum, filling the abdomen with blood and leading to cardiovascular collapse. This is a life-threatening surgical emergency and must be corrected immediately.

The diagnosis of vascular aneurysm is based on the results of echocardiography, angiography, computed tomography, or magnetic resonance imaging. In an elective situation any of these techniques is appropriate. In an emergency situation echocardiography or abdominal computed tomography is usually fast and expedites the diagnosis before surgery. In peritoneal rupture of the aneurysm, the diagnosis is based on clinical examination and requires no other test for verification, since the patient is usually in shock.

Most patients spend several days in the ICU after elective repair of an abdominal aneurysm. This procedure is associated with a 5% to 10% mortality rate, higher than elective coronary artery bypass graft surgery, because of postoperative complications. Most patients undergoing elective repair of an abdominal aortic aneurysm have systemic atherosclerosis with involvement of the coronary arteries. Perioperative myocardial infarction is one of the most common postoperative complications from repair of an abdominal aortic aneurysm. In some medical centers an extensive preoperative workup is done to look for cardiac ischemia. Radionuclide imaging of the heart can detect areas of ischemia; their presence suggests that repair of the coronary arteries should precede abdominal surgery.

Renal failure is another significant postoperative complication. Problems with intraoperative fluid management and hypotension can precipitate postoperative renal failure. Hemodynamic monitoring, aggressive fluid management, and the intraoperative use of diuretics to improve renal blood flow and urine output have reduced the incidence of perioperative renal failure. Postoperative patients in the ICU need continued volume resuscitation to ensure good renal perfusion.

Thoracic Aortic Aneurysms

Aortic aneurysms in the chest usually occur in the aortic arch or descending aorta. The pathologic features are the same as for the abdominal aorta, but the risk of rupture is less. Aneurysms in the chest may produce unexpected symptoms resulting from compression of another organ. For example, patients with thoracic aneurysms may have respiratory complaints because of compression of the trachea. Other patients may have dysphagia because of compression of the esophagus.

Aneurysms larger than 7 cm are generally resected, depending on the patient's age and concomitant illnesses. These patients require a thoracotomy and several postoperative days in the ICU. Resection of an aneurysm of the ascending aorta or aortic arch requires cardiopulmonary bypass. Resection of an aneurysm of the descending aorta can be performed with a bypass shunt. These patients have postoperative respiratory problems and are at risk of cardiac ischemia, but the risk of renal failure is less than with abdominal aneurysms.

Thoracic Aortic Dissection

Dissection is a more common disease of the thoracic aorta. An intimal tear allows a column of blood to enter the aortic wall, destroying the media and stripping the intima from the adventitia. This life-threatening emergency occurs commonly in the critical care setting. Patients have pain that is severe from onset and does not usually intensify, unlike the pain of myocardial infarction. The pain is in the chest, front or back between the shoulder blades, and is commonly described as ripping or tearing. On admission to the emergency room these patients frequently appear vasoconstricted and mottled, have hypertension and tachycardia, and are agitated and uncomfortable.

Physical examination usually reveals some defect from occlusion of a vessel. The dissection process may cause the intima to fold over and occlude a carotid artery, producing neurologic symptoms suggestive of a stroke. Pulses may be missing in the extremities, or there may be evidence of a coronary artery occlusion, suggesting thrombosis of a cardiac vessel. The dissection process causes myocardial infarction by disruption of a coronary vessel. Aortic dissection can also cause aortic insufficiency from disruption of the aortic valve.

The two basic types of dissection are those of the ascending aorta and the descending aorta. Dissections of the ascending aorta can be limited to the ascending aorta or can extend into the arch and descending aorta. Aortic dissections are caused by degeneration of the aortic media, commonly known as cystic medial necrosis. This can be associated with a medical syndrome, such as Marfan's syndrome, or occur spontaneously for unknown reasons.

Diagnosis is based on history and physical examination with confirmation by echocardiography, computed tomography, or angiography.

Management. The ICU plays a key role in the management of aortic dissection. Unlike patients with ruptured abdominal aortic aneurysm, which is a surgical emergency, those with thoracic aortic dissection should be medically stabilized before surgery. Blood pressure control is essential and should begin immediately to prevent further dissection. Nitroprusside has been commonly used to reduce blood pressure. In addition, the strength of contraction during systole should be blunted with a beta blocker, such as intravenous propranolol, to limit the risk of extended dissection.

Recently labetalol has been used in aortic dissection because of its alpha- and beta-blocking properties. Given intravenously in boluses of 5 to 20 mg, this agent controls both systolic blood pressure and contractility. After a satisfactory blood pressure has been achieved with intravenous boluses, a continuous infusion of 0.5 to 1 mg/kg/h should be considered to maintain blood pressure reduction and limit dissection.

After stabilization, surgery can be performed on the same day or during the next several days depending on the extent of the dissection. A dissection of the ascending aorta is repaired by dividing the aorta at the site of the intimal tear and reinforcing the wall and primarily closing the vessel. Usually a vascular graft is not needed. A dissection of the descending aorta is repaired with a vascular tube graft. Cardiopulmonary bypass is generally needed for surgical repair of aortic dissections.

Postoperative care may be complicated and prolonged. Hypertension may persist, requiring ongoing control of blood pressure. Vascular disease can cause complications involving the heart, kidney, and brain.

SUMMARY

This chapter looks at the physiologic role of the cardiovascular system and the various diseases that can affect that physiology. The chapter emphasizes ICU management and provides practical guidance for the clinical care of patients with cardiovascular disease. As noted at the beginning, cardiovascular problems permeate critical care, crossing all specialty boundaries and involving different types of ICUs. Any critical care physician, whether from a background of anesthesia, surgery, internal medicine, or pediatrics, must be able to recognize and manage physiologic derangements of the cardiovascular system.

SUGGESTED READINGS

Akhtar M, et al: Wide QRS complex tachycardia, reappraisal of a common clinical problem. Ann Intern Med 1988;109:905-912

Antman EM, Stone PH, Muller JE, et al: Calcium channel blocking agents in the treatment of cardiovascular disorders. I. Basic and clinical electrophysiologic effects. Ann Intern Med 1980;93:875-904

Anulty JH, Rahimtoola SH, Murphy E, et al: Natural history of "high risk" bundle branch block. N Engl J Med 1982;307:137-143

Artucio H, DiGenio A, Pereyra M: Left ventricular function during sepsis. Crit Care Med 1989;17:323-327

Baim DS: Effect of phosphodiesterase inhibition on myocardial oxygen consumption and coronary blood flow. Am J Cardiol 1989;63:23A-26A

Bar FW, Brugada P, Dassen WRM, Wellens HJJ: Differential diagnosis of tachycardia with narrow QRS complex (shorter than 0.12 second). Am J Cardiol 1984;54:555

Beer N, Gallegos I, Cohen A, et al: Efficacy of sublingual nifedipine in the acute treatment of systemic hypertension. Chest 1981;79:571-574

Bolli R, Jeroudi MO, Patel BS, et al: Marked reduction of free radical generation and contractile dysfunction by antioxidant therapy begun at the time of reperfusion. Circ Res 1989;65:607-622

Borner N, Erbel R, Braun B, et al: Diagnosis of aortic dissection by transesophageal echocardiography. Am J Cardiol 1984;54:1157-1158

Boucher CA, Breweter DC, Darling RC, et al: Determination of cardiac risk by dipyridamole-thallium imaging before peripheral vascular surgery. N Engl J Med 1985; 312:389-394

Braunwald E: Effects of digitalis on the normal and the failing heart. J Am Coll Cardiol 1985;5:51A-59A

Braunwald E: Heart disease. Philadelphia, 1988, WB Saunders Co

Cebul RD, Whisnant JP: Carotid endarterectomy. Ann Intern Med 1989;111:660-670

Cheng DC, Chung F, Burns RJ: Postoperative myocardial infarction documented by technetium pyrophosphate scan using single photon emission computed tomography: significance of intraoperative myocardial ischemia and hemodynamic control. Anesthesiology 1989; 17:818-826

Chernow B, Roth BL: Pharmacologic manipulation of the peripheral vasculature in shock: clinical and experimental approaches. Circ Shock 1986;18:141-155

Cohen MV: Free radicals in ischemic and reperfusion myocardial injury: is this the time for clinical trials? Ann Intern Med 1989;111:918-931

Collen D: Coronary thrombolysis: streptokinase or recombinant tissue-type plasminogen activator? Ann Intern Med 1990;112:529-538

Coller BS: Platelets and thrombolytic therapy. N Engl J Med 1990;322:33-42

Colucci WS, Denniss AR, Leatherman GF: Intracoronary infusion of dobutamine to patients with and without severe congestive heart failure. J Clin Invest 1988;81:1103-1110

Coppola JT, Shaoulian EM, Rentrop P: Therapeutic options in acute myocardial infarction. Chest 1989;95:1309-1315

Cunnion RF, Parrillo JE: Myocardial dysfunction in sepsis. Chest 1989;95:941-945

DeBusk RF: Specialized testing after recent acute myocardial infarction. Ann Intern Med 1989;110:470-481

Dilsizian V, Rocco T, Freedman N, et al: Enhanced detection of ischemic but viable myocardium by the reinjection of thallium after stress-redistribution imaging. N Engl J Med 1990;323:141-146

Eagle KA, Coley CM, Newell JB: Combining clinical and thallium data optimizes preoperative assessment of cardiac risk before major vascular surgery. Ann Intern Med 1989;110:859-866

Edwards FH, Bellamy RF, Burge JR, et al: True emergency coronary artery bypass surgery. Ann Thorac Surg 1990;49:603-611

Erbel R, Pop T, Diefenbach C, et al: Long-term results of thrombolytic therapy with and without percutaneous transluminal coronary angioplasty. J Am Coll Cardiol 1989;14:276-285

Fowler MB, Alerman EL, Oesterle SN, et al: Dobutamine and dopamine after cardiac surgery: greater augmentation of myocardial blood flow with dobutamine. Circulation 1984;70:I103-I111

Freeman MR, Williams AE, Chisholm RJ, et al: Intracoronary thrombus and complex morphology in unstable angina. Circulation 1989;80:17-23

Frye RL, Gibbons RJ, Schaff HV, et al: Treatment of coronary artery disease. J Am Coll Cardiol 1989;13:957-968

GISSI-2: A factorial randomised trial of alteplase versus streptokinase and heparin versus no heparin among 12490 patients with acute myocardial infarction. Lancet 1990;336:65-71

Goldhaber SZ: Tissue plasminogen activator in cardiopulmonary disease. Chest 1989;95:243-244

Gottliev SS, Kukin ML, Yushak M, et al: Adverse hemodynamic and clinical effects of encainide in severe chronic heart failure. Ann Intern Med 1989;110:505-509

Grines CL, DeMaria AN: Optimal utilization of thrombolytic therapy for acute myocardial infarction: concepts and controversies. J Am Coll Cardiol 1990;16:223-231

Guyton RA, Arcidi JM, Langford DA, et al: Emergency coronary bypass of cardiogenic shock. Circulation 1987;76:V22-27

Hands ME, Rutherford JD, Muller JE, et al: The in-hospital development of cardiogenic shock after myocardial infarction: incidence, predictors of occurrence, outcome and prognostic factors. J Am Coll Cardiol 1989;14:40-46

Hennekens CH, Buring JE, Sandercock P, et al: Aspirin and other antiplatelet agents in the secondary and primary prevention of cardiovascular disease. Circulation 1989;80:749-756

Henning RJ, Grenvik A: Critical care cardiology. New York, 1989, Churchill Livingstone

Hindman MC, Wagner GS, JaRo M, et al: The clinical significance of bundle branch block complicating acute myocardial infarction. Circulation 1978;58:689-699

Hurst JW, et al: The heart. New York, 1978, McGraw-Hill Book Co

Jugdutt BI, Warnic JW: Intravenous nitroglycerin therapy to limit myocardial infarct size, expansion, and complications. Circulation 1988;78:906-919

Kase CS, O'Neal AM, Fisher M, et al: Intracranial hemorrhage after use of tissue plasminogen activator for coronary thrombolysis. Ann Intern Med 1990;112:17-21

Kastor JA: Multifocal atrial tachycardia. N Engl J Med 1990;322:1713-1717

Katz AM: Cardiomyopathy of overload: a major determinant of prognosis in congestive heart failure. N Engl J Med 1990;322:100-110

Koch-Weser J: Drug therapy (bretylium). N Engl J Med 1979;300:473-477

Lam JYT, Chesebro JH, Fuster V: Platelets, vasoconstriction, and nitroglycerin during arterial wall injury. Circulation 1988;78:712-716

Lee L, Bates ER, Pitt B, et al: Percutaneous transluminal coronary angioplasty improves survival in acute myocardial infarction complicated by cardiogenic shock. Circulation 1988;78:1345-1351

Lee TH, Weisber MC, Brand DA, et al: Candidates for thrombolysis among emergency room patients with acute chest pain. Ann Intern Med 1989;110:957-962

Levine JH, Michael JR, Guarnieri T: Treatment of multifocal atrial tachycardia with verapamil. N Engl J Med 1985;312:21-25

Levine SR, Crowley TJ, Hai HA: Hypomagnesemia and ventricular tachycardia. Chest 1982;81:244-247

Lytle BW, Mahfood SS, Cosgrove DM, et al: Replacement of the ascending aorta: early and late results. J Thorac Cardiovasc Surg 1990;99:651-658

Makela VHM, Kapur PA: New drugs for the treatment of heart failure: amrinone and milrinone. Semin Anesth 1988;2:92-99

Manolis AS, Estes NAM: Supraventricular tachycardia, mechanisms and therapy. Arch Intern Med 1987;147:1706-1716

McKenna TM, Martin FM, Chernow B, et al: Vascular endothelium contributes to decreased aortic contractility in experimental sepsis. Circ Shock 1986;19:267-273

McMillan M, Chernow B, Roth BL: Hepatic alpha$_1$-adrenergic receptor alteration in a rat model of chronic sepsis. Circ Shock 1986;19:185-193

Moncada R, Churchill R, Reynes C, et al: Diagnosis of dissecting aortic aneurysm by computed tomography. Lancet, January 31, 1981;238-241

Moncada S, Palmer RMJ, Higgs EA: The discovery of nitric oxide as the endogenous nitrovasodilator. Hypertension 1988;12:365-372

Moothart RW, Spangler RD, Blount SG: Echocardiography in aortic root dissection and dilatation. Am J Cardiol 1975;36:11-16

Moss AJ, Benhorin J: Prognosis and management after a first myocardial infarction. N Engl J Med 1990;322:743-753

Multicenter Diltiazem Postinfarction Trial Research Group: The effect of diltiazem on mortality and reinfarction after myocardial infarction. N Engl J Med 1988;319:385-392

Nasraway SA, Rachow EC, Astiz ME, et al: Inotropic response to digoxin and dopamine in patients with severe sepsis, cardiac failure, and systemic hypoperfusion. Chest 1989;95:612-615

Neuhaus KL, Feuerer W, Jeep-Tebbe S, et al: Improved thrombolysis with a modified dose regimen of recombinant tissue-type plasminogen activator. J Am Coll Cardiol 1989;15:1566-1569

Nevitt MP, Ballard DJ, Hallett JW: Prognosis of abdominal aortic aneurysms: a population based study. N Engl J Med 1989;321:1009-1014

Olsen KH, Kluger J, Fieldman A: Combination high dose amrinone and dopamine in the management of moribund cardiogenic shock after open heart surgery. Chest 1988; 94:503-506

Palmer RF, Lasseter KC: Sodium nitroprusside. N Engl J Med 1975;292:294-297

Parisi AF, Khuri S, Deupree RH, et al: Medical compared with surgical management of unstable angina. Circulation 1989;80:1176-1189

Parker RB, McCollam PL: Adenosine in the episodic treatment of paroxysmal supraventricular tachycardia. Clin Pharmacol 1990;9:261-271

Podrid PJ: Antiarrhythmic drug therapy: benefits and hazards (parts I and II). Chest 1985;88:452-460, 618-624

Popma JJ, Dehmer GJ: Care of the patient after coronary angioplasty. Ann Intern Med 1989;110:547-559

Przyklenk K, Kloner RA: "Reperfusion injury" by oxygen-derived free radicals? Circ Res 1989;64:86-96

Raby KE, Goldman L, Creager MA, et al: Correlation between preoperative ischemia and major cardiac events after peripheral vascular surgery. N Engl J Med 1989; 321:1296-1300

Rackow EC, Packman MI, Weil MH: Hemodynamic effects of digoxin during acute cardiac failure: a comparison in patients with and without acute myocardial infarction. Crit Care Med 1987;15:1001-1005

Rahimtoola SH: Perspective on valvular heart disease: an update. J Am Coll Cardiol 1989;14:1-23

Rahimtoola SH: The hibernating myocardium. Am Heart J 1989;117:211-221

Rahimtoola SH: The pharmacologic treatment of chronic congestive heart failure. Circulation 1989;80:693-699

Reilly JM, Cunnion RE, Burch-Whitman C, et al: A circulating myocardial depressant substance is associated with cardiac dysfunction and peripheral hypoperfusion (lactic acidemia) in patients with septic shock. Chest 1989;95:1072-1080

Reves JG, Croughwell ND, Hawkins E, et al: Esmolol for treatment of intraoperative tachycardia and/or hypertension in patients having cardiac operations. J Thorac Cardiovasc Surg 1990;100:221-227

Rinkenberger R: Cardiac rhythm in the critical care setting: treatment. In Dantzker DR (ed): Treatment in cardio-pulmonary critical care. New York, 1986, Grune & Stratton

Sane DC, Califf RM, Topol EJ, et al: Bleeding during thrombolytic therapy for acute myocardial infarction: mechanisms and management. Ann Intern Med 1989; 111:1010-1022

Schlatmann TJM, Becker AE: Pathogenesis of dissecting aneurysm of aorta. Am J Cardiol 1977;39:21-26

Schreuder WO, Schneider AJ, Groeneveld ABJ, et al: Effect of dopamine vs norepinephrine on hemodynamics in septic shock. Chest 1989;95:1282-1288

Shub C: Heart failure and abnormal ventricular function. Chest 1989;96:906-914

Smalling RW, Schumacher R, Morris D, et al: Improved infarct-related arterial patency after high dose, weight-adjusted, rapid infusion of tissue-type plasminogen activator in myocardial infarction: results of a multicenter randomized trial of two dosage regimens. J Am Coll Cardiol 1990;15:915-921

Spirito P, Chiarella F, Carratino L, et al: Clinical course and prognosis of hypertrophic cardiomyopathy in an outpatient population. N Engl J Med 1989;320:749-755

Suffredini AF, Fromm RE, Parker MM, et al: The cardiovascular response of normal humans to the administration of endotoxin. N Engl J Med 1989;321: 280-287

Sundram P, Reddy HK, McElroy PA, et al: Myocardial energetics and efficiency in patients with idiopathic cardiomyopathy: response to dobutamine and amrinone. Am Heart J 1990;119:891-898

Sung RJ, Elser B, McAllister RG, et al: Intravenous verapamil for termination of re-entrant supraventricular tachycardias. Ann Intern Med 1980;93:682-689

Topol EJ: Coronary angioplasty for acute myocardial infarction. Ann Intern Med 1988;109:970-980

Topol EJ, George BS, Kereiakes DJ, et al: A randomized controlled trial of intravenous tissue plasminogen activator and early intravenous heparin in acute myocardial infarction. Circulation 1989;79:281-286

Turner DA, Tracy J, Haines SJ: Risk of late stroke and survival following carotid endarterectomy procedures for symptomatic patients. J Neurosurg 1990;73:193-200

Van der Wall EE, Cats VM, Blokland AK, et al: The effects of diltiazem on cardiac function in silent ischemia after myocardial infarction. Am Heart J 1989;118: 655-660

VanLente F, Martin A, Ratliff NB, et al: The predictive value of serum enzymes for perioperative myocardial infarction after cardiac operations. J Thorac Cardiovasc Surg 1989;98:704-710

Vincent JL, Reuse C, Kahn RJ: Administration of dopexamine, a new adrenergic agent, in cardiorespiratory failure. Chest 1989;96:1233-1236

Waxman HL, Myerburg RJ, Appel R, et al: Verapamil for control of ventricular rate in paroxysmal supraventricular tachycardia and atrial fibrillation or flutter. Ann Intern Med 1981;94:1-6

Wellens HJJ et al: The value of the electrocardiogram in the differential diagnosis of tachycardia with a widened QRS complex. Am J Med 1978;64:27-33

White HD, Rivers JT, Maslowski AH, et al: Effect of intravenous streptokinase as compared with that of tissue plasminogen activator on left ventricular function after first myocardial infarction. N Engl J Med 1989;320: 817-821

Wolfe CL: Cardiac imaging. Cardiol Clin 1989;7:3

CRITICAL NEUROLOGIC AND PSYCHIATRIC ILLNESS

DONALD S. PROUGH, MD, AND ANTHONY R. RIELA, MD

As a specialty, critical care has historically emphasized the management of acute respiratory and cardiac dysfunction more than acute neurologic disease. Nevertheless, many patients are admitted to ICUs with, or subsequently develop, acute neurologic complications of diverse cause. Of these, a substantial proportion, such as those associated with stroke, subarachnoid hemorrhage, and the post–cardiac arrest syndrome, results from impaired cerebral perfusion. However, infection, neoplastic disease, trauma, and neurodegenerative disease also cause acute nervous system injury and result in death and long-term disability.

Until recently, little specific therapy was available for most acute neurologic diseases. However, the last several years have brought rapid advances in understanding of the pathophysiology of neurologic disease, in the ability to monitor the central nervous system, and in the range of therapeutic approaches that are available or under development. Recent clinical experience demonstrates that the outcome from several highly lethal or disabling conditions may be improved by the application of sound principles of neurologic and neurosurgical intensive care.

This chapter outlines the management of several common neurologic diseases and injuries that may result in admission to an ICU. For each condition a management strategy is suggested that is based on current practice; in addition, promising therapeutic research is noted.

CEREBROVASCULAR CRISES

The most commonly encountered cerebrovascular crises in critical care are ischemic stroke, subarachnoid hemorrhage, and intracranial hemorrhage. Although all three are associated with substantial morbidity and mortality, the prognoses of acute stroke and subarachnoid hemorrhage have improved and may progress further as recently developed treatment strategies are more widely applied.

Stroke

Pathophysiology. Stroke develops as a consequence of inadequate delivery of oxygen to a focal area of brain. Ischemia may be produced not only by decreases in cerebral O_2 delivery (CDo_2; the product of cerebral blood flow [CBF] and arterial O_2 content [Cao_2]) but also by increases in the cerebral metabolic rate for O_2 ($CMRo_2$). Normal values for cerebral oxygenation variables are displayed in Table 10–1. The normal brain receives approximately 15%

TABLE 10–1. Normal Cerebral Oxygenation Variables

CBF	50 ml $\cdot$ 100 g^{-1} $\cdot$ min^{-1}
Cao$_2$	20 ml $\cdot$ 100 ml^{-1}
CDo$_2$	10 ml $\cdot$ 100 g^{-1} $\cdot$ min^{-1}
Cjvo$_2$	13 ml $\cdot$ 100 ml^{-1}
C(a-jv)o$_2$	7.0 ml $\cdot$ 100 ml^{-1}
Sjvo$_2$	65%
Pjvo$_2$	35 mm Hg
CMRo$_2$	3.5 ml $\cdot$ 100 g^{-1} $\cdot$ min^{-1}

Relationships Among Cerebral Circulatory Variables

$$CDo_2 = CBF \times Cao_2$$
$$CMRo_2 = CBF \times C(a\text{-}jv)o_2$$
$$CPP = MAP - ICP$$

CBF = cerebral blood flow, Cao$_2$ = arterial oxygen (O_2) content, CDo$_2$ = cerebral O_2 delivery, Cjvo$_2$ = jugular bulb O_2 content, C(a-jv)o$_2$ = cerebral arteriovenous O_2 content difference, Sjvo$_2$ = jugular bulb hemoglobin saturation, Pjvo$_2$ = jugular bulb O_2 tension, CMRo$_2$ = cerebral metabolic rate for O_2, CPP = cerebral perfusion pressure, ICP = intracranial pressure, MAP = mean arterial pressure.

TABLE 10–2. Cerebral Blood Flow Thresholds

VALUE	NORMAL THRESHOLD
Normal resting flow	$50 \ ml \cdot 100 \ g^{-1} \cdot min^{-1}$
EEG slowing	$24 \ ml \cdot 100 \ g^{-1} \cdot min^{-1}$
Evoked response failure	$15\text{-}20 \ ml \cdot 100 \ g^{-1} \cdot min^{-1}$
Ca^{++} entry	$< 10 \ ml \cdot 100 \ g^{-1} \cdot min^{-1}$
Cell death	$< 10 \ ml \cdot 100 \ g^{-1} \cdot min^{-1}$

of cardiac output and requires 20% of total body O_2 consumption. O_2 extraction is high; consequently, jugular venous O_2 saturation ($Sjvo_2$) and tension ($Pjvo_2$) are lower than systemic mixed venous O_2 saturation ($S\bar{v}o_2$) and tension ($P\bar{v}o_2$). Defective uptake or utilization of O_2, as occurs in cyanide poisoning, may also produce cerebral ischemia.

The brain is uniquely susceptible to O_2 deprivation for several reasons. Preservation of neurologic function requires energy expenditure that exceeds the maximal energy produced by anaerobic metabolism. In addition, there are no cerebral O_2 stores and few if any unperfused "reserve" cerebral capillaries. Therefore ischemia quickly depletes phosphocreatine and adenosine triphosphate (ATP), increases anaerobic metabolism of glucose (thereby increasing lactate production), rapidly reduces intracellular pH, and disrupts ionic gradients. A greater CBF is necessary to maintain electrical function than to preserve cell viability (Table 10–2). Ischemia is more likely to occur in certain areas of brain, including the arterial boundary zones between major arterial branches, the cerebellum, the basal ganglia, and parts of the hippocampus.

Cerebral ischemia initiates a cascade of metabolic consequences that potentiate further destruction of brain tissue. Particularly important biochemical changes in ischemia include increases in intracellular calcium (Ca^{++}), release of thromboxane A_2, generation of free O_2 radicals, production of excitatory amino acids, and accumulation of lactic acid. Ischemic cells do not maintain the normal gradient between intracellular and extracellular cations, resulting in cytotoxic edema and translocation of Ca^{++}. The Ca^{++} concentration, normally far higher extracellularly than in the cytoplasm, rapidly increases in the cytoplasm. Ca^{++} both directly constricts the cerebral vasculature and facilitates the production of thromboxane A_2, a potent cerebral vasoconstrictor. Ca^{++} overload also stimulates proteolysis and loss of enzymatic function, which destroys cell membranes, resulting in receptor dysfunction and the failure of

intracellular transport mechanisms. Free O_2 radicals, produced as a consequence of the metabolism of free fatty acids and nucleotides, initiate lipoperoxidation, which can irreversibly damage cell membranes. Excitatory amino acids, such as glutamate, may cause further ischemic injury by stimulating cellular metabolism at a time when substrate is insufficient to meet demands. Anaerobic metabolism of glucose during ischemia produces intracellular lactic acidosis, which may perpetuate neural cell injury.

Diagnosis. The diagnosis of stroke, as with many neurologic diseases, became more precise after the introduction of computed tomographic (CT) scanning in the early 1970s. In the initial evaluation of a suspected stroke, CT scanning excludes other treatable causes of acute focal deficits, such as intracranial hemorrhage. Classically, the low-density area of tissue corresponding to a stroke is not apparent on a CT scan for several days after the event, whereas intracranial hemorrhage is visible immediately. Magnetic resonance imaging, although more expensive, is more sensitive than CT scanning in detecting early ischemic damage.

Treatment. Historically, clinicians have managed ischemic stroke with general supportive measures. These include bed rest, O_2 administration, avoidance of blood pressure extremes, and airway support and mechanical ventilation as needed. Cerebral edema after stroke, occasionally severe enough to cause herniation, has conventionally been managed with mannitol and, occasionally, intubation and hyperventilation. Unfortunately, cerebral infarction sufficiently extensive to produce intracranial hypertension is rarely associated with good functional outcome.

The most common explanations for a nonaggressive approach to stroke management are pessimism regarding the potential for improving outcome and the limited tolerance of elderly, often frail patients for invasive, aggressive treatment. Because of the rapidity with which brain tissue is irreversibly injured by lack of O_2, most focal ischemic damage is likely to have occurred before admission. However, even after a substantial interval of focal ischemia, potentially salvageable brain tissue may remain in an ischemic penumbra (Fig. 10–1), an area adjacent to devitalized tissue in which flow has been reduced to a level that produces ischemic dysfunction without producing cell death. In the penumbral area, measures designed to increase CBF or to decrease $CMRo_2$ might preserve viable tissue and improve outcome.

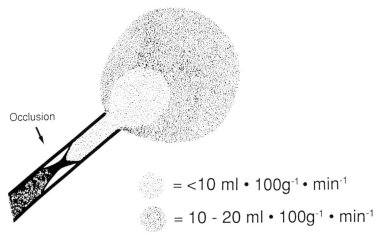

Occlusion

$= <10$ ml $\cdot$ 100g^{-1} $\cdot$ min^{-1}

$= 10 - 20$ ml $\cdot$ 100g^{-1} $\cdot$ min^{-1}

Figure 10–1.   Diagram of ischemic penumbra. In the area of brain tissue distal to an obstructing vascular legion, cerebral ischemia may be irreversible *(lightly stippled area)* or potentially reversible *(medium stippling area)*. One critical determinant of the recoverability of brain tissue is the absolute level of perfusion. Tissue receiving less than 10 ml $\cdot$ 100 g^{-1} $\cdot$ min^{-1} quickly becomes infarcted. However, in tissue with flow insufficient to support function but greater than 10 ml $\cdot$ 100 g^{-1} $\cdot$ min^{-1} (ischemic penumbra), restoration of flow may permit tissue survival.

Although conventional supportive care is still the mainstay of treatment, recent pharmacologic advances may alter management. Promising approaches to therapy include hypervolemic hemodilution, Ca^{++} entry blockers, pentoxifylline, and thrombolysis.

In animal experiments, hypervolemic hemodilution augments CBF distal to middle cerebral artery occlusion, but the clinical effects of hemodilution are less well defined. In patients with acute stroke, isovolemic hemodilution also increases CBF and improves electroencephalographic (EEG) activity; however, multicenter clinical trials of hemodilution after stroke have produced conflicting results. The Scandinavian Stroke Study Group failed to demonstrate any significant short- or long-term therapeutic benefit. In contrast, the Hemodilution in Stroke Study Group showed a possible benefit if hemodilution with pentastarch was initiated within 12 hours of stroke onset, if the hematocrit value declined at least 15%, and if cardiac output increased at least 10%. Because of the frequency with which cardiovascular disease accompanies cerebrovascular disease in this predominantly elderly population, care must be taken to prevent congestive heart failure as blood volume is expanded. Hypervolemic hemodilution also could aggravate cerebral edema and intracranial hypertension.

Ca^{++} entry blockers improve CBF and protect focally ischemic brain distal to occlusions. Nimodipine, a Ca^{++} entry blocker that preferentially dilates the cerebral vasculature, improves both CBF and intracellular pH in animals. Nimodipine also reportedly improves clinical outcome after stroke, although additional studies are necessary. However, in patients with large hemispheric infarctions, the potential value of nimodipine must be weighed against the increases in intracranial pressure (ICP) that accompany cerebral vasodilatation.

Pentoxifylline, a methylxanthine that reduces blood viscosity and improves distal circulatory flow in lower extremity claudication, increases CBF in low-flow areas in patients with chronic cerebrovascular disease. It produces clinical improvement if administered during the first few days following acute stroke but does not improve long-term outcome. Because the side effects of pentoxifylline are minimal, it may become a useful adjunct to other modalities in acute stroke.

Thrombolysis also reduces the extent of brain infarction, as has been well demonstrated in myocardial infarction. However, clinical trials have proceeded cautiously because of the obvious risks of intracranial bleeding and of distal embolization of clot fragments.

Hemodilution, Ca^{++} entry blockers, and pentoxifylline appear to have different mechanisms of action. Consequently, the maximal improvement in neurologic outcome may ultimately be achieved with a combination of agents, each of which limits injury in a specific way. Other agents, such as antagonists of the excitotoxins glutamate and aspartate, may also prove efficacious.

Subarachnoid Hemorrhage

Ten percent of all strokes, approximately 28,000 per year, result from subarachnoid hemorrhage (SAH), usually arising from a ruptured intracranial aneurysm. At least half of those patients die or are disabled as a consequence of the hemorrhage or its sequelae. The two most feared complications are rebleeding, occurring in about 7% of patients, and symptomatic vasospasm, complicating the course of 15% to 20% of patients.

Pathophysiology. Most SAH occurs when saccular aneurysms at the base of the brain rupture into the basal cisterns. The risk of rupture of asymptomatic aneurysms is a function of size. Aneurysms greater than 1 cm in diameter rupture at a rate of 1% to 2% per year. Those less than 7 mm in diameter rarely rupture. Arteriovenous malformations also rupture, producing many of the features of aneurysmal bleeding.

SAH causes neurologic symptoms in several ways. First, the acute hemorrhage may produce a transient rise in ICP to the level of mean arterial pressure. The ensuing immediate loss of consciousness persists for hours or days. Second, neurologic function may deteriorate because of acute communicating hydrocephalus, a complication of intraventricular bleeding. Third, after an interval of several days, cerebral vasospasm may produce cerebral ischemia. In some cases vasospasm may be sufficiently severe to precipitate ischemic brain infarction and intracranial hypertension. To assist in management and the recognition of complications, hospitals customarily assign patients a clinical grade on admission. The Hunt-Hess classification recognizes five grades (Table 10–3).

Cerebral vasospasm has received considerable attention because it is a delayed complication that presumably could be prevented or reversed if effective therapy were identified.

TABLE 10–3. Hunt-Hess Grading System for Subarachnoid Hemorrhage

GRADE	CLINICAL CHARACTERISTICS
1	Asymptomatic, or minimal headache and mild nuchal rigidity
2	More severe headache, nuchal rigidity, neurologic deficits limited to cranial nerve palsies
3	Drowsiness, confusion, or mild focal deficit
4	Stupor, hemiparesis, possible early decerebration
5	Deep coma, decerebrate rigidity, moribund

Although symptoms of cerebral ischemia occur in only 15% to 20% of patients, angiographic evidence of vasospasm develops in 50% to 70%. Effective therapy could lower the unacceptable morbidity and mortality of patients hospitalized with SAH. The cause of vasospasm is unclear, but it appears to require the presence of blood in the basal cisterns. The proposed mechanisms include active contraction of cerebral arteries, failure of vasorelaxation, proliferation of the arterial medial layer, luminal obstruction, and arterial inflammation. Putative mediators of spasm include Ca^{++}, O_2 free radicals, and thromboxane A_2.

Diagnosis. Diagnosis requires a high index of suspicion, particularly in the assessment of sudden, severe headache, with or without transient loss of consciousness. The CT scan establishes the diagnosis of SAH in 75% of cases by demonstrating the presence of blood in the subarachnoid space. If the CT scan fails to establish the diagnosis, lumbar puncture may reveal erythrocytes in the cerebrospinal fluid. Angiography is used to establish the diagnosis in questionable cases and to provide necessary information for planning surgical therapy. Other helpful tests include electrocardiography to seek the ST and T wave changes that commonly accompany SAH and serum electrolyte measurement to detect hyponatremia secondary to the syndrome of inappropriate antidiuretic hormone secretion (SIADH) or the cerebral salt-wasting syndrome.

Treatment. The treatment of SAH includes general supportive care, surgical obliteration of the aneurysm, and medical management of vasospasm. General supportive care includes bed rest, stool softeners, sedatives and analgesics as necessary (avoiding aspirin), and control of blood pressure. The arterial hypertension that commonly accompanies SAH must be cautiously treated. Untreated hypertension may increase the risk of rebleeding; excessive reduction of blood pressure may precipitate ischemic sequelae. Hypertension accompanied by stupor may also be a diagnostic clue to increased ICP. When stupor indicates the presence of communicating hydrocephalus, cerebroventricular drainage is used to control ICP.

A variety of pharmacologic agents have been employed, including glucocorticoids and antifibrinolytics. Glucocorticoids provide little specific benefit, but they seem to improve cerebral edema after SAH and to reduce headache severity. Antifibrinolytics such as epsilon-aminocaproic acid decrease the rate of lysis of

TABLE 10–4. Mathematical Principles Involved in Manipulation of Cerebral Blood Flow

Hagen-Poiseuille Equation

$$Q = \frac{\pi \cdot r^4 (P_2 - P_1)}{8L \cdot viscosity} \qquad \text{(Eq. 1)}$$

where

Q = Flow (CBF in this case)
r = Radius of the vessel
$P_2 - P_1$ = Pressure drop along the vessel
L = Vessel length

FACTOR	TYPICAL INTERVENTIONS
r	Ca^{++} entry blocker (nimodipine, nicardipine)
$P_2 - P_1$	Hypertension
	Hypervolemic hemodilution
Viscosity	Hemodilution

the clot surrounding the aneurysm, thereby reducing the risk of rebleeding. However, antifibrinolytics also increase the incidence of delayed ischemic complications.

Perhaps the most controversial topic of the last decade regarding therapy for SAH has been the timing of surgical intervention. Conventionally, surgery has been delayed 7 to 10 days until the risk of postoperative vasospasm begins to decline. However, the delay in surgical obliteration increases the risk of rebleeding in the interval between diagnosis and definitive treatment. Recently several groups have shown that early surgical intervention is associated with mortality and morbidity comparable to that of delayed surgery, particularly if combined with antivasospasm treatment such as hypervolemic hemodilution or Ca^{++} entry blockers.

Antivasospastic treatment has progressed substantially during the past few years. Both pharmacologic treatment and hypervolemic hemodilution are widely applied to prevent or treat the ischemic sequelae of SAH. The rationale for treatment of vasospasm can be inferred from the Hagen-Poiseuille equation. According to the equation, CBF can be increased only by increasing vessel caliber, increasing the pressure gradient along the vessel, or reducing blood viscosity (Table 10–4).

Hypervolemic hemodilution improves neurologic status in patients who have vasospasm while awaiting operation and in those in whom symptomatic vasospasm develops after surgical obliteration of an aneurysm. The principal limitation of volume expansion as treatment for vasospasm is that the accompanying increase

in blood pressure promotes rebleeding. However, after successful clipping of an aneurysm, assuming that no other aneurysms are present, hypervolemic hemodilution can be combined with induced hypertension to maximize two factors that determine CBF. Those who advocate early surgical intervention emphasize the greater safety of rheologic and blood pressure manipulation after aneurysm obliteration.

Although several pharmacologic treatments for experimental vasospasm have been investigated during the past decade, Ca^{++} entry blockers appear most likely to alter clinical outcome. An extensive multicenter study has demonstrated a prophylactic effect of nimodipine on the development of vasospasm in patients entering the hospital with acute subarachnoid hemorrhage but with minimal neurologic deficits. The combination of early surgical intervention with nimodipine prophylaxis appears to produce favorable results. Nimodipine also improves established vasospasm. Nicardipine, another Ca^{++} entry blocker, reduces vasospasm in a dose-dependent fashion. Because the Ca^{++} entry blocking drugs that antagonize vasospasm also tend to reduce blood pressure and to increase ICP, attention must be paid to the maintenance of cerebral perfusion pressure.

Primary Intracerebral Hemorrhage

Nearly 60,000 patients per year suffer nontraumatic intracranial hemorrhage unrelated to intracranial aneurysms. The mortality rate exceeds 50% in patients who become comatose. Usually related to chronic systemic hypertension, primary intracranial hemorrhage most commonly occurs in penetrating vessels in the basal ganglia, subcortical white matter, thalamus, cerebellum, and pons.

Diagnosis. Usually, primary brain hemorrhage is abrupt in onset and progresses rapidly. Although the clinical picture may suggest the cause of neurologic deterioration, CT scanning provides the definitive diagnosis.

Treatment. The treatment of primary brain hemorrhage is intubation if coma is profound, seizure prophylaxis with phenytoin, ICP reduction (if necessary) with mannitol, and control of blood pressure. Endotracheal intubation should be performed with care to prevent reflex hypertension. Systolic blood pressure should be reduced to less than 160 mm Hg, ideally by using beta-blocking drugs that reduce the impact of arterial pulsations on the

TABLE 10–5.   Mortality Rates in Traumatic and Nontraumatic Coma

CATEGORY	MORTALITY RATE (%)	↓ NEUROLOGIC FUNCTION (%)	REFERENCE
All Coma			
Coma ≥ 48 h	>77	–	Teres (1982)
Coma + shock	>95	–	"
Nontraumatic			
Coma ≥24 h	65	90	Levy (1981)
SAH, other CVA	74	95	"
Hypoxic	58	90	"
Hepatic	49	73	"
End-stage hepatic disease and acute respiratory failure	100	–	Matuschak (1985)
Postcardiopulmonary Resuscitation			
All patients	–	90	Levy (1985)
Coma and barbiturate medication	77	82	BRCT I (1986)
Traumatic			
GCS on admission: 3	83	–	Klauber (1981)
6-7	24	–	"
GCS 3 + acute subdural	74	92	Genarelli (1982)
Clinical Prognostic Indicators			
Post-CPR: no pupillary reflex	–	100	Levy (1985)
Post-CPR: posturing, ↓ motor, no spontaneous eye movement, 24 h after CPR	–	99	

SAH = subarachnoid hemorrhage, CVA = cerebrovascular accident, ARDS = adult respiratory distress syndrome, CPR = cardiopulmonary resuscitation, GCS = Glasgow Coma Scale.
References: BRCT I: N Engl J Med 1986;314:397-403. Gennarelli TA: J Neurosurg 1982;56:26-32. Klauber et al: Neurosurgery 1981;9: 236-241. Levy DE et al: Ann Intern Med 1981;94:293-301. Levy DE et al: JAMA 1985;253:1420-1426. Matuschak et al.: Am Rev Respir Dis 1985;131:A135. Teres D et al: Crit Care Med 1982; 10:86-95.

damaged arterial wall. Labetalol, a combination alpha and beta blocker, is particularly useful. The pure vasodilators nitroglycerin and nitroprusside may increase ICP. Glucocorticoids are of no benefit.

ICP pressure monitoring and control of intracranial hypertension may be useful if an altered sensorium is present at initial examination or develops later. The indications for surgical evacuation of intracranial hematomas vary with the lesion's location and size. Cerebellar hematomas exceeding 2 cm in diameter and large lobar hematomas frequently require emergency evacuation to prevent brainstem compression or herniation. Surgical evacuation of hemorrhages from the brainstem, thalamus, and putamen remains controversial.

ENCEPHALOPATHY AND COMA

Encephalopathy and coma commonly occur in critically ill patients. The prognosis of patients with traumatic or nontraumatic coma depends on the depth and cause of coma and the quality of intensive care (Table 10–5).

Hypoxic and Ischemic Encephalopathy

After the global cerebral ischemic insult associated with cardiac arrest, many patients recover adequate cardiovascular, pulmonary, and renal function but are left with profound neurologic deficits. Less than 10% of patients who have suffered out-of-hospital cardiac arrest return to their previous level of activity. Of patients who undergo cardiopulmonary resuscitation in the hospital, only 10% are alive 1 year later.

Pathophysiology. Global cerebral ischemia or hypoxia precipitates the biochemical sequences previously described. However, after adequate cerebral oxygenation is restored, neurologic injury appears to progress. Improvement in the dismal outcome of patients who have survived initial resuscitation requires a better understanding of the time course and mechanisms of what has been termed reperfusion injury. The theory underlying neurologic reperfusion injury is that ischemic injury is not

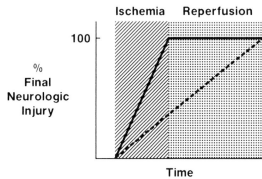

— No reperfusion injury
--- Reperfusion injury

Figure 10–2. Diagram of the concept of reperfusion injury. In brain tissue subjected to ischemia followed by reperfusion, the magnitude of final neurologic injury could be fixed at the time perfusion is restored *(solid line)* or could continue after restoration of perfusion *(dotted line)*. If neurologic injury progresses after restoration of perfusion, appropriate pharmacologic or physiologic interventions might reduce the ultimate extent of injury. (Reprinted with permission from the International Anesthesia Research Society from "Nimodipine and the 'no reflow phenomenon'—experimental triumph, clinical failure?" by Prough DS, Furberg CD: Anesth Analg 1989;68:431-435.)

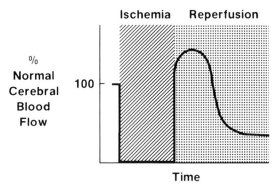

Figure 10–3. Diagram of the "no-reflow" phenomenon. After an episode of complete or nearly complete ischemia, reperfusion of brain tissue is typically associated with a transient increase in cerebral blood flow, after which cerebral blood flow falls to a fraction of baseline values. This "no-reflow phenomenon" or postischemic hypoperfusion may be responsible, in part, for progression of neurologic deficits after ischemia. (Reprinted with permission from the International Anesthesia Research Society from "Nimodipine and the 'no reflow phenomenon'—experimental triumph, clinical failure?" by Prough DS, Furberg CD: Anesth Analg 1989;68:431-435.)

complete when perfusion is restored but progresses in the subsequent minutes to hours (Fig. 10–2). The concept is therapeutically optimistic because it suggests that prompt therapy after arrest may limit or reverse the ultimate extent of neurologic disability. One of the first mechanisms proposed to explain reperfusion injury was postischemic hypoperfusion (PIH), or the "no-reflow phenomenon" (Fig. 10–3). Initially shown in animals, PIH has subsequently been demonstrated in humans. The intense, vasodilator-resistant cerebral vasoconstriction may reduce CBF to a greater extent than $CMRo_2$, perpetuating ischemic damage.

The factors contributing to PIH and to the other features of reperfusion injury include the toxic effects of increased intracellular ionized Ca^{++}, the generation of O_2 free radicals, the production of the cerebral vasoconstrictor thromboxane A_2, and the development of intracellular acidosis. However, many of the numerous biochemical reactions influenced by ischemia are thought to mediate ischemic injury or postischemic reperfusion injury. Each potential mechanism, and the therapeutic agents dependent on the validity of that mechanism, must be painstakingly evaluated. The purported mediator must be capable of generating a potentially harmful physiologic response, must be generated pathophysiologically in sufficient concentrations at the site of the response, and,

when pharmacologically antagonized, must attenuate injury.

Diagnosis. The diagnosis of hypoxic or anoxic encephalopathy is usually apparent from the clinical situation. If the cause of cardiorespiratory decompensation is uncertain, CT scanning may exclude primary central nervous system causes such as intracranial hemorrhage or trauma. The prognosis of patients with postresuscitation coma can be estimated based on serial neurologic examinations.

Treatment. The most important aspect of care of the patient with hypoxic or anoxic encephalopathy is support of the cardiac and pulmonary systems. Specific neurologic resuscitative therapy remains an elusive goal. Strategies for reducing neurologic injury are outlined in Table 10–6. Of the various interventions that have been applied in animal models, nimodipine and free radical scavengers, especially the 21-aminosteroids, offer the greatest promise. However, in a prelimi-

TABLE 10–6. Strategies for Reducing Neurologic Injury Following Cardiac Arrest

STRATEGY	EXAMPLES
Increase CBF	Ca^{++} entry blockers, free radical scavengers
Decrease $CMRo_2$	Barbiturates
Decrease cytotoxicity	Free radical scavengers, Ca^{++} entry blockers, excitotoxin antagonists

nary clinical study, nimodipine accelerated awakening after cardiac arrest but did not significantly improve neurologic outcome. Barbiturates, long a controversial form of therapy after global cerebral ischemia, also failed to improve clinical outcome in an extensive clinical trial.

In all likelihood, effective postresuscitation therapy will not be based on a single agent, but rather will consist of a combination of agents that improve microcirculatory flow, control or reduce $CMRo_2$, and block cytotoxicity.

Hypertensive Encephalopathy

Hypertensive encephalopathy is a neurologic emergency characterized by severe blood pressure elevation, headache, altered mental status, visual disturbances, and occasionally convulsions. The incidence of hypertensive emergencies (defined as a blood pressure of 200/120 mm Hg or higher in association with threatened organ system injury) has declined as medical control of chronic hypertension has improved. In addition, newer antihypertensive drugs have made acute hypertension easier to manage. Clonidine, nifedipine, labetalol, and captopril reduce blood pressure rapidly in nearly all cases.

Pathophysiology. Chronic hypertension gradually increases the upper limit of cerebral perfusion pressure autoregulation. However, when blood pressure abruptly rises much higher than the patient's accustomed levels, breakthrough of autoregulation occurs, accompanied by marked increases in CBF and, in severe cases, arteriolar necrotic changes, thrombosis of arterioles and capillaries, microinfarctions, and petechial hemorrhages. Although ICP may be elevated, cerebral edema is usually absent.

Diagnosis. The most critical aspect of the differential diagnosis of hypertensive encephalopathy is the exclusion of other causes of neurologic symptoms and hypertension. These include cerebral infarction, intracerebral hemorrhage, meningitis, intracranial tumor, and uremic encephalopathy. After emergency initiation of antihypertensive treatment, CT scanning should be performed to exclude primary intracranial disease or injury.

Treatment. Although oral drug therapy reduces blood pressure in the majority of patients, hypertensive emergencies usually require intravenous therapy. Among nonparenteral drugs commonly used in less urgent situations, nifedipine 10 mg sublingually and clonidine 0.1 to 0.2 mg orally reduce blood pressure within minutes to hours. Intravenous treatment options were limited until several years ago. Diazoxide, administered as a single 300 mg bolus, produced an unacceptable incidence of hypotension. However, smaller (50 to 150 mg) increments reduce blood pressure with little risk of excessive hypotension. Diazoxide is relatively contraindicated in patients with coronary artery disease. Sodium nitroprusside reduces blood pressure in virtually all patients, but the potential for sudden hypotension, especially in hypovolemic patients, mandates continuous blood pressure monitoring. Nitroglycerin reduces blood pressure less consistently than nitroprusside. Both nitroprusside and nitroglycerin increase ICP. Hydralazine, if given in small incremental doses of 5 to 10 mg intravenously, reduces blood pressure and increases ICP. Currently its primary indication is for the management of pregnancy-induced hypertensive emergencies. Labetalol is an alternative choice for emergency control of blood pressure. Administered in small doses, starting with 2.5 to 5 mg and progressing upward rapidly until the desired effect is achieved, labetalol controls most hypertension. Labetalol is relatively contraindicated in patients who have severely reduced left ventricular function and should be used with caution in patients with obstructive airway disease.

Reye's Syndrome

Now rare, Reye's syndrome is a puzzling metabolic encephalopathy that once affected as many as three to six children per 100,000 under the age of 17. Although the cause of Reye's syndrome has never been conclusively established, it appears to represent an interaction between acute viral illness and salicylates. A marked decline in the use of salicylates as antipyretics in childhood illnesses has been temporally associated with a dramatic reduction in the incidence of the disease.

Pathophysiology. The most lethal aspect of Reye's syndrome is intracranial hypertension. However, complete recovery is likely if ICP can be adequately controlled during the acute illness.

Treatment. In severe cases, control of ICP with intubation, neuromuscular blockade, sedation, mechanical hyperventilation, euvolemic dehydration, and osmotic diuresis are associated with a high probability of good outcome. In cases refractory to these measures, high-dose

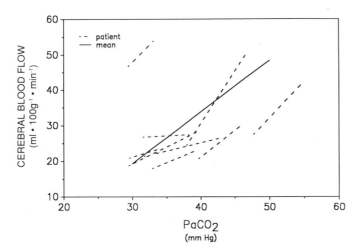

Figure 10–4. Response of cerebral blood flow to changes in arterial carbon dioxide partial pressure ($PaCO_2$) in patients with systemic sepsis. In such patients cerebral blood flow is usually less than the normal value of 50 ml · 100 g^{-1} · min^{-1} at a $PaCO_2$ of 40 mm Hg. Although this cerebral hypoperfusion could explain some of the mental status changes in patients with sepsis, the preservation of cerebrovascular reactivity to changes in $PaCO_2$ is not consistent with a primary vascular source of septic encephalopathy. (From Bowton DL, Bertels NH, Prough DS, et al: Cerebral blood flow is reduced in patients with sepsis syndrome. Crit Care Med 1989;17:399-403. © by Williams & Wilkins 1989.)

barbiturate coma may permit survival with limited neurologic sequelae. Less commonly, hypothermia and decompressive craniectomy are employed to reduce uncontrollable ICP.

Encephalopathy Associated with Renal Failure

Uremic encephalopathy complicates the course of acute and chronic renal failure. Although the most common biochemical marker of uremic encephalopathy is an elevated blood urea nitrogen (BUN) level, the mechanism of central nervous system depression probably involves other poorly defined metabolites. In general, BUN levels exceeding 100 mg/dl, especially if associated with a rapid rise, are necessary for the diagnosis. The treatment is dialysis.

Dialysis itself is associated with an encephalopathic syndrome called the disequilibrium syndrome. Usually accompanying sudden drops from high levels of BUN (greater than 150 mg/dl) and serum sodium, dialysis disequilibrium can be prevented by less rapid reduction of azotemia and serum sodium concentration.

Sepsis

Sepsis and septic shock are associated with a high incidence of encephalopathy. Encephalopathy portends a greater likelihood of death, even if the severity of other organ system dysfunction is comparable to that in patients without encephalopathy. The pathogenesis of encephalopathy is uncertain; changes in brain amino acids have been implicated, as have changes in CBF. CBF in patients with sepsis remains responsive to changes in arterial partial pressure of carbon dioxide ($PaCO_2$) (Fig. 10–4), although it is severely reduced in comparison with normal flow rates and in comparison with the elevated systemic blood flow typical in patients with sepsis.

Diagnosis. Septic encephalopathy is a diagnosis of exclusion. Lumbar puncture excludes nosocomial meningitis, a rare but treatable event in critically ill patients, and CT scanning excludes intracranial catastrophes.

Treatment. Septic encephalopathy has no specific treatment. Generally patients appear to recover neurologic function if the septic episode is successfully managed. However, no studies have characterized the neurologic and neuropsychologic sequelae of sepsis.

CENTRAL NERVOUS SYSTEM INFECTIONS

Meningitis

Background. Although meningitis occurs commonly, the clinical presentation, etiology, and treatment vary markedly based on the patient's age and immune status.

Diagnosis. The clinical presentation of meningitis typically includes fever, headache, meningismus, vomiting, and confusion. However, the frequency of each of these findings varies depending on the pathogen. Very young, elderly, and debilitated patients may show little evidence of central nervous system infection. When the diagnosis is suspected, the first critical determination is the presence of focal signs. If no focal findings are present, lumbar puncture should be performed immediately. If focal signs are present, antibiotics should be given empirically and a CT scan obtained before diagnostic lumbar puncture. Lumbar puncture

TABLE 10–7. Typical Cerebrospinal Fluid Changes in Viral and Bacterial Meningitis

TEST	NORMAL	VIRAL	BACTERIAL
WBC/mm³	0-5	10-500	>1000
Protein (mg/dl)	15-40	50-100	>150
Glucose (mg/dl)	50-75	normal	<30
Stain for pathogen			Positive in >80%

may precipitate herniation in patients with elevated ICP. Typical cerebrospinal fluid findings associated with bacterial and viral central nervous system infections are listed in Table 10–7. Latex agglutination is the most reliable method of rapidly establishing the diagnosis of common infections.

Treatment. The primary treatment for meningitis is empiric administration of bactericidal antibiotics (ideally within 1 hour of entertaining the diagnosis). Antibiotics are adjusted as necessary as more definitive culture results become available. In an immunocompetent adult the likely pathogens are *Neisseria meningitidis* (ages 10 to 50) and *Streptococcus pneumoniae* (age greater than 50). Both are adequately treated with penicillin G. In neonates ampicillin and a third-generation cephalosporin, such as cefotaxime, cover *Escherichia coli* and group B streptococci. In an older child (6 weeks to 10 years), cefuroxime or a combination of ampicillin and chloramphenicol provides coverage for both *N. meningitidis* and *Haemophilus influenzae*. Widespread resistance to ampicillin among *H. influenzae* strains precludes use of that drug alone until specific sensitivities are determined. Recent studies suggest that dexamethasone reduces the incidence of sensorineural hearing loss in infants and children with bacterial meningitis. Glucocorticoids may also be useful in patients with evidence of cerebral edema.

In the rare case of fulminating meningitis with signs of impending herniation, monitoring and aggressive control of ICP may improve outcome. Although the mechanisms of intracranial hypertension in meningitis are multifactorial, increased ICP does not imply irreversible injury.

Encephalitis

Herpes encephalitis is the most common fatal encephalitis in the United States. Adults have altered mental status, seizures, fever, and headache. Focal neurologic signs are present in at least 75% to 85% of cases.

Diagnosis. Lumbar puncture is the primary diagnostic test. EEG is sensitive but nonspecific, demonstrating periodic temporal spikes and slow waves. The technetium brain scan shows frontotemporal focal abnormalities in 50% of patients. Magnetic resonance imaging (MRI) may also demonstrate abnormalities. When the diagnosis is in doubt, brain biopsy usually proves definitive.

Treatment. The introduction of vidarabine greatly improved the outcome from herpes encephalitis. The more recently released acyclovir appears to be less toxic and more effective. Therapy should be initiated as soon as possible, even before brain biopsy if that cannot be performed immediately, because of the increased morbidity and mortality that accompany deterioration in the level of consciousness.

Brain Abscess

Brain abscesses typically spread from remote or contiguous sites of infection such as cranial injuries, cutaneous infection, pulmonary infections, and mastoiditis. Symptoms may be nonspecific and subacute. Fever, headache, and focal neurologic deficits occur in less than 50% of patients, less commonly accompanied by vomiting, seizures, meningismus, and changes in the level of consciousness. Although the initial course may be slowly progressive, sudden deterioration may occur if meningitis, ventriculitis, or cerebral edema with herniation occurs.

Diagnosis. If focal deficits are present, lumbar puncture should be delayed until a CT scan has been obtained. Early in the course of a brain abscess, a radionuclide brain scan may best detect abscesses; later the CT scan becomes more sensitive, especially in the detection of cerebral edema and mass effect. Cerebrospinal fluid resembles that seen in acute bacterial meningitis.

Treatment. The two central components of therapy are antibiotics and surgical drainage. Glucocorticoids are equivocally efficacious once appropriate antibiotics have been given. The microbes associated with brain abscess include *Staphylococcus aureus,* Enterobacteriaceae sp., *Bacteroides* sp., and, in immunocompromised hosts, a wide variety of opportunistic organisms. Pending definitive culture results, intravenous penicillin G 20 million units daily and metronidazole 30 mg/kg/d after a 7.5 mg/kg loading dose cover most organisms. Nafcillin or vancomycin may be appropriate if *S. aureus* is suspected. If possible, surgical drainage should accompany antibiotic treatment.

TRAUMATIC CENTRAL NERVOUS SYSTEM INJURY

Head Injury

Head injury is a major public health problem. Annually at least 50,000 patients in the United States die of acute head injury; another 50,000 survive with disabling sequelae. Because these patients tend to be young and free of chronic systemic disease, they and society may carry the economic burden of their disability for many years.

Pathophysiology. Head injury includes a heterogeneous group of injuries. Autopsy may show the brain to be focally or diffusely injured. Focal lesions include cerebral contusions, hematomas, infarctions, and infections. Diffuse injuries include diffuse axonal injury, hypoxic brain damage, diffuse brain swelling, and diffuse punctate brain hemorrhages. The lesions found at autopsy represent both primary and secondary brain injury. Primary injuries occur before medical attention; secondary injuries occur after initiation of medical management and therefore can potentially be modified.

The reduction of the long-term sequelae of brain injury occupies the research efforts of numerous investigators and clinicians. At present, clinical protocols designed to limit the sequelae of intracranial mass lesions, hypotension, hypoxia, and cerebral edema are well established and continuing to evolve. In contrast, no currently available treatment reduces the progression of harmful biochemical processes that occur after brain trauma.

The biochemical basis of secondary brain injury has been studied primarily in animal models of acceleration-deceleration injury. Those investigations have shown that prostaglandin metabolites, O_2 free radicals, Ca^{++}, excitotoxins (glutamate and aspartate), intracellular acidosis, and cholinergic receptors are integrally involved in the pathogenesis of head injury. Investigational drugs are available that reduce the production of thromboxane A_2, scavenge O_2 free radicals, block the effects of excess Ca^{++}, antagonize the effects of glutamate and aspartate, alkalinize brain tissue, and block cholinergic receptors. Despite remarkable progress in applying pharmacologic developments to experimental models of head injury, only a few of the potential interventions have progressed to clinical trials. Of those that have, none has yet proved sufficiently efficacious to be added to routine care.

TABLE 10–8. Causes of Intracranial Hypertension Following Head Trauma

CAUSE	MECHANISM
Mass lesions	Local expansion
Brain swelling	Vascular congestion, hyperemia
Brain edema	
Cytotoxic	Cellular swelling secondary to hypoxia or ischemia
Vasogenic	Breakdown of blood-brain barrier, interstitial accumulation of protein
Interstitial	Hydrocephalus
Secondary vasodilation	
Hypercarbia	Increased extracellular H^+ concentration
Hypoxia	Increased local metabolite concentration (adenosine?)
Hypertension	Impaired autoregulation

Clinical attempts to limit secondary injury continue to be directed at rapid evacuation of large intracranial hematomas, at the prompt recognition and treatment of hypoxia and hypotension, at medical stabilization of head-injured patients, and at control of intracranial hypertension. Space-occupying intracranial lesions reduce cerebral perfusion pressure (CPP) and CBF, particularly in the brain adjacent to an expanding lesion. Hypoxia and hypotension, common accompaniments of acute head injury, dramatically worsen neurologic function in animals with experimental injury. In fact, levels of hypoxia (40 mm Hg) and hypotension (equivalent to 90 mm Hg systolic) that alone produce no adverse sequelae alter the pathogenesis of mild head injury so that it more closely resembles severe head injury.

Medical complications following head injury may also increase morbidity and mortality. Because these patients often require extended intensive care, they are likely to acquire complications such as pneumonia, pulmonary emboli, nutritional depletion, stress gastritis, and maxillary sinusitis secondary to prolonged nasal intubation.

The most critical secondary event after head injury is severe intracranial hypertension. Intracranial hypertension may result not only from space-occupying lesions but also from brain swelling and cerebral edema (Table 10–8). Because the skull is a noncompliant container, increases in volume can be accommodated only to a limited extent. Once volume has expanded beyond the ability of the intracranial contents to compensate, ICP rises abruptly and may

TABLE 10–9. Glasgow Coma Scale Score

COMPONENT	RESPONSE	SCORE
Eye opening	Spontaneously	4
	To verbal command	3
	To pain	2
	None	1
	SUBTOTAL (1- 4)	
Motor response (best extremity)	Obeys verbal command	6
	Localizes pain	5
	Flexion-withdrawal	4
	Flexion (decortication)	3
	Extension (decerebration)	2
	No response (flaccid)	1
	SUBTOTAL (1- 6)	
Best verbal response	Oriented and converses	5
	Disoriented and converses	4
	Inappropriate words	3
	Incomprehensible sounds	2
	No verbal response	1
	SUBTOTAL (1- 5)	
	TOTAL (3-15)	

increase sufficiently to reduce cerebral perfusion pressure, according to the equation:

$$CPP = MAP - ICP \qquad (Eq.\ 2)$$

where

CPP = Cerebral perfusion pressure
MAP = Mean arterial pressure

Jugular venous pressure replaces ICP in the equation if it exceeds ICP, as is usually true in the absence of intracranial hypertension.

Diagnosis. The initial diagnostic maneuver after acute stabilization of the head-injured patient is to assess the extent of injury and to assign a Glasgow Coma Scale (GCS) score for prognostic purposes (Table 10–9). After assessment and initial stabilization of extracerebral injuries, CT scanning discloses the presence or absence of subdural or epidural hematomas and provides a preliminary assessment of ICP. Abnormally small ventricles at the time of initial CT scanning correlate with the later development of intracranial hypertension.

Treatment. The treatment of acute head injury consists of general supportive care, stabilization of associated injuries, surgical interventions for intracranial lesions that exert a mass effect, and control of ICP. To accomplish the last, most clinicians recommend placing an intracranial monitoring device in any patient brought to the emergency department with a GCS score of 8 or less.

General supportive care is directed at preventing pneumonia, pulmonary emboli, maxillary sinusitis, nutritional depletion, and stress gastritis. Pneumonia prevention, a challenge in patients who require prolonged mechanical ventilation, necessitates frequent turning to prevent pooling of secretions in dependent lung regions. Electrically operated beds that turn in a wide arc at frequent intervals are an expensive means of ensuring turning but may be cost effective to the extent that they limit the incidence of nosocomial pneumonias. In patients with head injury, ventilation-perfusion mismatch develops despite initially clear chest roentgenograms; consequently, most require supplemental inspired O_2 and some require positive end-expiratory pressure (PEEP). In a few patients severe respiratory failure develops, sometimes secondary to central neurogenic pulmonary edema, in which case greater levels of PEEP and higher minute ventilation may be necessary to maintain adequate gas exchange. In general, if lung dysfunction is sufficiently severe to require PEEP, the effects on ICP are negligible.

Antibiotics should be administered cautiously to patients with head injury. Because fever is common in these patients, they are often given broad-spectrum antibiotics almost from the outset of their hospitalization. If antibiotics can be prescribed specifically for demonstrated infections rather than for nonspecific signs, the rate at which resistant nosocomial infections develop may be slowed.

Prevention of pulmonary emboli is more controversial in head-injured patients than in patients less likely to be harmed in the rare instance of bleeding complications from prophylactic doses of heparin. Pneumatic stockings appear to offer comparable protection against deep venous thrombosis and do not increase the risk of hemorrhagic complications.

Prolonged artificial airway support in head-injured patients necessitates a choice among oral endotracheal intubation, nasal intubation, and tracheostomy. Although nasal intubation is associated with a 15% to 20% incidence of maxillary sinusitis, nasal tubes can be used if care is taken to diagnose and treat sinusitis.

Because of accelerated catabolism in the first days to weeks after head injury, nutritional depletion occurs rapidly and contributes to morbidity and mortality. Although controversy continues regarding the choice between enteral

TABLE 10–10.   Strategies for Controlling ICP Following Severe Head Injury

STRATEGY	MECHANISM
Endotracheal intubation	Prevention of hypoxia and hypercarbia
Neuromuscular blockade*	Prevention of coughing and straining
Passive hyperventilation*	Reduction of CBF and cerebral blood volume
Fluid restriction*	Limitation of cerebral edema
Head positioning*	Facilitation of cerebral venous drainage
Osmotic diuresis	Reduction of brain water
Sedation/narcosis*	Reduction of $CMRo_2$, limitation of CBF response to noxious stimuli
Fever control	Limitation of $CMRo_2$
Barbiturates†	Reduction of $CRMo_2$, CBF, ICP
Glucocorticoids†	Limitation of cerebral edema
Decompressive craniectomy*	Increase space for brain expansion

ICP = Intracranial pressure, CBF = cerebral blood flow, $CMRo_2$ = cerebral metabolic rate for oxygen.
*Controversial.
†Little or no demonstrable benefit.

and parenteral nutritional support, most investigators agree that aggressive nutritional support, starting within 48 hours of admission to the ICU, maximizes survival.

Prevention of stress gastritis is a fundamental aspect of care of a patient with head trauma. Originally called Cushing's ulcer in patients with intracranial pathologic conditions, stress gastritis has been a common source of morbidity throughout the history of neurologic and neurosurgical intensive care. Surgery for refractory bleeding is rarely necessary. Aggressive use of antacids, a practice that has been supplanted in many medical centers by the use of H_2 antagonists, has virtually eliminated life-threatening hemorrhage. However, gastric alkalinization permits overgrowth of bacteria, providing a reservoir of bacteria that may be passively regurgitated and aspirated to precipitate nosocomial pulmonary infection. Sucralfate appears to offer stress ulcer prophylaxis comparable to that provided by antacid therapy and may become the preventive measure of choice.

The control of ICP, usually defined as maintenance below 15 to 20 mm Hg, is the cornerstone of management of severe head trauma. Although understanding of the pathophysiology of head injury has progressed rapidly over the last decade, the basic strategies for controlling ICP have changed little (Table 10–10). Surprisingly little information is available to confirm the efficacy of most individual components of commonly practiced protocols. Maintenance of a patent airway is universally accepted as the central element because of the potentially disastrous effects of hypoxia and hypercarbia on brain oxygenation and ICP. Passive hyperventilation is also a routine part of therapy, even in patients who have normal ICP. The rationale is that reducing $Paco_2$ reduces CBF, cerebral blood volume, and ICP. However, few convincing data support the clinical practice of routinely restricting CBF in head-injured patients. For the 50% of patients with hyperemia, attempts to produce cerebral vasoconstriction may be warranted; for the other half who have both reduced flow and lowered metabolism, unnecessary hyperventilation may result in inadequate cerebral O_2 delivery. Data concerning head positioning are also limited. In many patients the modest ICP reduction produced by the common practice of keeping the head elevated 15 to 30 degrees is more than offset by the reduction in mean arterial pressure associated with the semisitting position. Another standard practice, fluid restriction to approximately two thirds of calculated maintenance, probably exerts negligible influence on ICP.

Conclusive data now demonstrate that routine administration of glucocorticoids and barbiturates is unwarranted. Although certain patients might benefit from either or both modalities, neither offers anything to the majority of patients with head injury.

Much remains to be learned about the proper care of patients with head injury. Evaluation of generally accepted but unproven concepts and of the ability of new pharmacologic agents to limit secondary injury must continue.

Spinal Cord Injury

Approximately 200,000 persons in the United States are quadriplegic. To that number are added an additional 7000 to 10,000 patients per year who become paraplegic or quadriplegic as a result of acute spinal trauma. About 5000 persons die before reaching the hospital or after admission because of spinal cord injury or associated injuries. Like the victims of head injury, those suffering spinal cord injury tend to be young and to carry their deficit and its personal and societal costs through several decades.

Pathophysiology. The spinal cord, encased in the spinal canal, may be compressed and deformed by forces sufficiently violent to disrupt the bony and ligamentous attachments of the canal. Forces that produce cord injury include flexion, extension, compression and rotation, and shear and tension. Spinal cord injury, like head injury, has both primary and secondary components. The primary injury includes shearing and disruption; the subsequent secondary injury includes the deleterious effects of hypoxia, hypotension, and inappropriate stabilization, as well as vascular and biochemical events that occur in the hours after the injury.

The characteristic lesion associated with acute spinal cord injury begins in the central gray matter and within hours extends into the white matter. This has prompted the assumption that early interventions interrupting the sequential course of the injury might preserve spinal cord function. Within minutes after experimental spinal cord compression, hyperemia and small hemorrhages appear in the central gray matter. These subsequently expand into large areas of hemorrhage. Concurrently, spinal cord blood flow becomes critically limited, as is evidenced by a decline in tissue O_2 saturation. Within 4 hours gray matter is infarcted; within 8 hours edema and infarction have spread through the white matter.

The mechanisms of the progressive ischemia and infarction in the spinal cord after compressive injury have not been completely elucidated. However, many of the factors implicated in head injury have also been implicated in cord injury. Among these, endogenous opioids, vasoconstrictive amines, and O_2 free radicals have received considerable attention.

Diagnosis. Two rules are critical in the diagnosis of spinal cord injury. The first is that the emergency care team must consider the possibility of spinal cord injury in comatose, head-injured patients. Severe head injury is commonly accompanied by spinal cord compression, which must be excluded by appropriate radiographic studies before efforts to stabilize the spinal canal are terminated. The second rule is that other injuries accompanying a spinal cord injury must not be missed. Spinal cord injury is accompanied not only by head injury but also by severe injuries to the thorax, extremities, and abdomen. Because of the lack of sensation below the level of the lesion, a patient with spinal cord disruption may not report pain. Consequently, a comprehensive physical examination is required in addition to a thorough neurologic examination.

The two most useful individual diagnostic tests are cervical spine roentgenograms (anterior and lateral) and cervical CT scans. Approximately 10% to 15% of patients with cervical spine injuries have lesions evident on CT scan but not on plain films of the neck. Myelography is a controversial diagnostic test. The potential value of more precise anatomic diagnosis must be weighed against the difficulty of the procedure, the possibility of precipitating seizures, and the risk of arachnoiditis induced by contrast media in patients with bloody cerebrospinal fluid.

Treatment. The primary approach to treatment is to avoid inadvertently aggravating the spinal injury and to control the cardiovascular, pulmonary, and gastrointestinal complications of acute paraplegia or quadriplegia (Table 10–11). The immediate responses to acute spinal cord injury are hypertension and tachycardia secondary to sympathetic discharge. However, if the lesion is located at or above T1, neurogenic shock quickly follows. Although neurogenic shock is manifested as hypotension and bradycardia, systemic perfusion is usually adequate. Hypotension responds to fluid infusion; in fact, worsening of hypotension or failure to respond to volume expansion suggests bleeding from an associated injury. In the later recovery phase after cervical or high thoracic spinal cord transection, autonomic hyperreflexia often becomes a problem. This syndrome, characterized by severe hypertension and tachycardia in response to noxious stimulation below the level of the lesion, is often precipitated by distention of a hollow viscus.

Pulmonary complications of cervical spine injury include paralysis of the respiratory musculature and respiratory failure secondary to associated injuries. Nosocomial infection and pulmonary emboli are delayed complications. A lesion at C5 paralyzes the intercostal musculature but is usually compatible with spontaneous ventilation. However, higher lesions often compromise diaphragmatic function sufficiently to limit forced vital capacity (FVC) to a level that precludes adequate clearing of secretions. Such patients should be carefully monitored to detect impending hypoxic or hypercarbic respiratory failure. Measurement of FVC at intervals allows timely intubation and support of ventilation and secretion clearance. Mechanical ventilation and weaning in patients with spinal cord injury is managed as in other patients with acute respiratory failure. Prevention of nosocomial pulmonary infection requires the same attention to turning, chest physiotherapy, and suctioning that are necessary in the head-injured patient. The most scrupulous care must be provided to patients who have a postinjury FVC that equals or barely exceeds the criterion for intubation, that is, 15 ml/kg.

In these immobile patients, prevention of pulmonary embolism necessitates prevention of

TABLE 10–11. Systemic Complications of Spinal Cord Injury

ORGAN SYSTEM	MECHANISM	MANAGEMENT
Cardiovascular		
Hypotension	Loss of sympathetic tone (early)	Volume expansion
		Rarely pressors
Bradycardia	Same as above	Rarely atropine
		Same as above
Autonomic hyperreflexia	Loss of supraspinal inhibition of sympathetic discharge	Antihypertensives
		Avoid noxious stimulation
Pulmonary		
Respiratory insufficiency	Reduced forced vital capacity, reduced tidal volume if severe	Intubation
		Ventilatory support
Posttraumatic pulmonary failure	Same as adult respiratory distress syndrome (see Chapter 1)	Intubation
		PEEP
		Mechanical ventilation
Nosocomial infection	Inadequate clearance of secretions; prolonged tracheal intubation	Turning
		Suctioning
		Careful use of antibiotics
Gastrointestinal		
Gastric atony	Reflex ileus	Nasogastric intubation
Genitourinary		
Urinary retention	Neurogenic bladder	Continuous or intermittent bladder catheterization

deep venous thrombosis with pneumatic compression stockings or minidose heparin (usually 5000 IU subcutaneously every 12 hours). Air swallowing, in association with gastric atony and generalized paralytic ileus, frequently produces abdominal distention. Nasogastric intubation should be performed before or immediately after admission to the ICU. Since rapid catabolism accompanies spinal injury, nutritional support is essential. Some patients tolerate jejunal feedings through a small-lumen nasoenteric tube. Those who do not may require intravenous hyperalimentation. Urinary retention occurs acutely. Continuous bladder catheterization is usually required while the patient is in the ICU, although intermittent catheterization may be appropriate in institutions where that technique has been extensively practiced.

The specific management of spinal column injury is limited to traction stabilization or surgical stabilization. Gardner-Wells tongs or a halo is commonly used with 5 to 10 pounds of traction. Because a patient in cervical traction is difficult to turn, an electrically operated, rotating bed facilitates care and may limit subsequent problems with pulmonary infection, decubitus formation, and deep venous thrombosis.

High doses of methylprednisolone in the first 24 hours after spinal cord trauma slightly but significantly improve neurologic outcome. Other pharmacologic treatments that address

the biochemical sequelae of spinal compression have been unsuccessful. Naloxone, remarkably effective in animals, is ineffective in humans. Free radical scavengers have yet to be subjected to adequate clinical trials, although preliminary data in experimental cord injury appear promising. Aggressive surgical approaches, such as decompression laminectomy and cervical cord cooling, have attempted to limit the progression of cord edema and infarction, but the results have not been encouraging.

Postoperative Neurosurgical Intensive Care

After elective and emergency neurosurgical procedures, most patients are admitted to an ICU for observation or continued intensive monitoring and therapy. Although the necessity for routine admission of neurologically intact patients has been questioned, the practice appears justifiable because of the potential for prompt recognition and treatment of complications that otherwise would result in severe morbidity and mortality. Adverse occurrences in the postoperative period include intracranial hemorrhage, cerebral edema, diabetes insipidus (DI), and SIADH. Intracranial hypertension secondary to bleeding or cerebral edema may produce rapid deterioration of neurologic status. If neurologic deterioration is promptly recognized, CT scanning facilitates diagnosis, after which temporizing medical therapy or definitive surgical therapy may be undertaken. The management of intracranial hypertension is discussed elsewhere in this chapter. The management of DI and SIADH is reviewed briefly here.

Diabetes Insipidus

Hypernatremia is a consequence of free water depletion, combined water and sodium depletion (water depletion greater than sodium depletion), or sodium gain. The differential diagnosis begins with an assessment of intravascular volume followed by analysis of possible contributing causes (Fig. 10–5).

DI, a pharmacologically correctable cause of hypernatremia, is a consequence of injury to the posterior pituitary gland or the pituitary stalk. It is an infrequent complication of closed head trauma, skull fractures, and neurosurgical procedures, especially those involving the pituitary gland. Decreased secretion of antidiuretic hormone (ADH) from the posterior pituitary gland results in water diuresis, progressive dehydration, and hypernatremia. Urinary output may exceed 700 ml/h; despite serum hyperosmolality the urine remains dilute.

DI must be distinguished from solute diuresis induced by vigorous intravenous fluid administration or radiographic contrast media and from diuretic-induced polyuria. The diagnosis depends on demonstrating inability to concentrate urine or reduce urinary volume despite hypovolemia or hypernatremia induced by dilute polyuria. Characteristically, the excessive urinary output is associated with urinary osmolality that is inappropriately low (60 to 200 mOsm) relative to serum osmolality, and with urinary specific gravity less than 1.005.

The management of DI is both supportive and pharmacologic. Input and output must be

carefully monitored because hypovolemia and hypernatremia develop rapidly. Other valuable monitors include serum and urinary electrolytes and osmolality, urinary specific gravity, BUN, creatinine, and frequent weight determinations. An awake, alert patient who can tolerate oral hydration usually ingests sufficient water to maintain electrolyte balance and euvolemia. If fluid must be replaced in a patient who cannot regulate fluid intake, solutions containing low sodium concentrations should be given to replace water losses. If total losses are modest, 5% dextrose in 0.2% saline plus supplemental potassium can replace the hourly urinary output plus estimated insensible losses. However, intravenous administration of large quantities of 5% dextrose may produce hyperglycemia, superimposing glycosuria-induced polyuria on DI. If the urine output remains excessive (greater than 200 to 250 ml/h) or if maintaining fluid balance is difficult, 1-desamino-8-D-arginine vasopressin (DDAVP) or aqueous vasopressin reduces urinary output. DDAVP, considered the drug of choice because of its limited systemic effects, is given in a dose of 1 to 2 mg subcutaneously or intravenously twice a day. The dose of vasopressin is 5 to 10 IU intramuscularly or subcutaneously to control excessive urinary output. As output decreases, intravenous or oral fluid intake can be tapered. Since the duration of DI is variable, further pharmacologic treatment is dictated by the recurrence of polyuria. If long-term therapy is required, DDAVP can be administered intranasally as needed to control urinary output.

DI also develops commonly as a manifestation of brain death. If the brain-dead patient is a potential organ donor, careful management of the DI is essential to preserve the viability of the transplantable organs. In combination with vasodilation, hypovolemia may result in grossly inadequate perfusion of potentially lifesaving organs.

Syndrome of Inappropriate Antidiuretic Hormone Secretion

SIADH is an essential consideration in the differential diagnosis of hyponatremia (Fig. 10–6). The measurement of serum osmolality helps to distinguish among causes of SIADH. When osmolality is high, serum sodium levels are depressed as a result of the accumulation of other osmoles, such as glucose, mannitol, or alcohols. When osmolality is low, estimation of intravascular volume helps to separate the various causes.

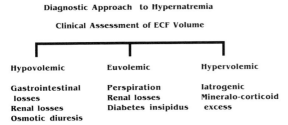

Diagnostic Approach to Hypernatremia

Clinical Assessment of ECF Volume

Hypovolemic	Euvolemic	Hypervolemic
Gastrointestinal losses	Perspiration	Iatrogenic
Renal losses	Renal losses	Mineralo-corticoid excess
Osmotic diuresis	Diabetes insipidus	

Figure 10–5. Diagnostic approach to hypernatremia. In hypernatremic patients, clinical assessment begins with the adequacy of extracellular fluid volume. Based on the subsequent classification into hypovolemic, euvolemic, and hypervolemic status, potential etiologic sequences can be assessed.

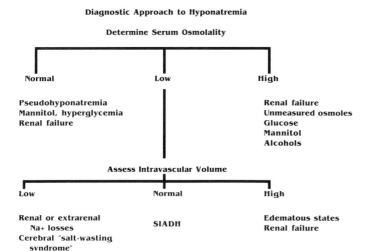

Diagnostic Approach to Hyponatremia

Determine Serum Osmolality

Normal — Low — High

Normal:
Pseudohyponatremia
Mannitol, hyperglycemia
Renal failure

High:
Renal failure
Unmeasured osmoles
Glucose
Mannitol
Alcohols

Assess Intravascular Volume

Low — Normal — High

Low:
Renal or extrarenal
Na+ losses
Cerebral "salt-wasting syndrome"

Normal:
SIADH

High:
Edematous states
Renal failure

Figure 10-6. Diagnostic approach to hyponatremia. The evaluation of hyponatremia depends on the sequential assessment of serum osmolality and intravascular volume. This permits determination of a likely etiologic sequence.

A wide variety of central nervous system disorders, including head trauma, tumor, subarachnoid hemorrhage, and brain abscess, are associated with inappropriate secretion of ADH. Usually self-limited, SIADH most commonly develops 3 to 15 days after trauma or surgery and usually resolves within 7 days. The excessive ADH secretion causes continued renal excretion of sodium despite hyponatremia and associated hypoosmolality. Urinary osmolality is therefore high relative to serum osmolality. A patient with SIADH has no clinical evidence of dehydration; renal and adrenal function are normal.

The clinical manifestations of hyponatremia depend on the severity of the hyponatremia and the rapidity with which it develops. If the serum sodium level falls slowly, even to 120 mEq/L, symptoms are frequently mild. If the hyponatremia occurs more quickly, symptoms usually include anorexia, nausea, vomiting, irritability, and hyperreflexia, which may progress to seizures, stupor, and coma.

The mainstay of treatment for these water-overloaded, euvolemic patients is water restriction (500 ml/d). In the absence of severe neurologic complications of hyponatremia, the serum sodium level should be gradually corrected. Recently the syndrome of central pontine myelinolysis was described in patients who had undergone excessively rapid correction of hyponatremia. If the hyponatremia is severe (serum sodium less than 110 mEq/L), hypertonic (3% to 5%) saline solution can return the serum sodium level toward normal. Because of the rapid increase in extracellular and intravascular volume produced by hypertonic saline solution, it must be used with caution and patients must be carefully monitored to prevent

acute pulmonary edema. An alternative treatment regimen for rapid correction of hyponatremia is the administration of 0.9% saline solution in combination with a loop diuretic. Because the sodium concentration of diuretic-induced urinary losses is usually less than that of 0.9% saline solution, serum sodium levels increase. That approach is sound in patients who have limited cardiac reserve and require rapid partial correction of hyponatremia. When pharmacologic treatment is desirable for persistent SIADH, demeclocycline is effective.

NEUROMUSCULAR DISEASES

Diseases that cause acute neuromuscular compromise result in a small percentage of ICU admissions. However, the scrupulous application of sound principles of critical care medicine permits many of these patients to return to their previous level of activity.

Guillain-Barré Syndrome

The Guillain-Barré syndrome (GBS), an acute inflammatory polyradiculopathy, is the most common cause of rapidly progressive weakness in the United States, affecting 20 to 80 persons per million population per year. Because respiratory failure develops in 25% to 30% of patients, many patients with GBS are admitted to ICUs for close observation and monitoring or for mechanical ventilation, often for prolonged periods.

Pathophysiology. GBS is an immunologically mediated disease, apparently including features of both cell-mediated and humoral immune injury. Demyelination of peripheral

TABLE 10–12. Differential Diagnosis of Acute Weakness

DIAGNOSIS	CLINICAL FEATURES
Guillain-Barré syndrome	Dysesthesias of the distal extremities Usually progresses from distal to proximal Increases CSF protein levels (delayed)
Myasthenia gravis	Decremental response to repetitive nerve stimulation Preserved reflexes No sensory abnormalities
Amyotrophic lateral sclerosis	Increased reflexes Normal CSF Normal sensation
Multiple sclerosis	Long tract signs (e.g., hyperreflexia)
Polymyositis	Muscle pain and tenderness Preserved deep tendon reflexes
Diphtheritic neuropathy	Paralysis of pharyngeal and laryngeal muscles Numbness of lips Lower CSF protein
Botulism	Normal CSF Prominent bulbar systems
Tick paralysis	Normal CSF Improvement after tick removal
Poliomyelitis	Increased cells and protein in CSF Preserved sensation
Acute intermittent porphyria	Prominent abdominal pain CSF protein normal Increased serum delta-aminolevulinic acid
Shellfish poisoning	Facial and distal extremity numbness Descending paralysis

CSF = cerebrospinal fluid.

nerves and nerve root ganglia is the most prominent feature; axonal injury is less consistently identified. The disease resembles the laboratory model of experimental allergic neuritis, a characteristic injury produced by immunizing rabbits against peripheral nerve antigen. In this model, myelinolysis is associated with acute weakness similar in distribution and onset to GBS. Experimental allergic neuritis can be transferred passively by inoculation of uninfected animals with lymphocytes or intraneural injection of cell-free serum. The specific initiating sequence in the clinical syndrome remains unknown. Although the disease is preceded by viral illness, mycoplasmal infection immunization, or other factors in about 50% of patients, in some no precipitating event can be identified.

Diagnosis. GBS must be differentiated from other causes of acute weakness (Table 10–12). However, the clinical features of GBS are usually sufficiently distinctive to prompt the correct diagnosis. GBS begins with dysesthesias of the distal extremities. Weakness follows after a variable interval of hours to days. Classically, the weakness begins distally and extends proximally, although it may initially be diffuse. Facial and cranial nerve paresis is common. The rate and extent of progression of the disease are variable. Rarely progressive for more than 1 month, weakness reaches its maximum within 2 weeks in half of patients. Occasionally the onset is explosive, with ventilatory failure occurring within a few hours. In other patients the weakness progresses little. Autonomic dysfunction, present in many patients, is often most severe in those with the most profound weakness. Hypotension, hypertension, tachyarrhythmias, and bradyarrhythmias are common and may be life threatening.

Physical examination generally shows symmetric weakness with depression or loss of deep tendon reflexes. The cranial nerves are usually symmetrically involved. Sensory loss varies from mild in most cases to profound in rare cases. Intellectual function is preserved.

The laboratory examination is generally unremarkable. Hyponatremia secondary to SIADH occurs occasionally. The cerebrospinal fluid is normal in the first few days, but then elevated protein levels, sometimes as high as 1 to 2 g/dl, develop. Nerve conduction studies typically demonstrate profound slowing of conduction, primarily in proximal nerves.

Treatment.   If good supportive care is provided, recovery is likely. Most patients with GBS recover to nearly their premorbid level of function. The mortality rate is approximately 5%, primarily occurring in those who require prolonged ventilator support or who have severe autonomic dysfunction. Less than 10% remain seriously handicapped. Poor prognosis appears to correlate with advanced age, severity of paralysis, and prolonged progression of disease.

Management of the respiratory and cardiovascular consequences of the disease is the essential aspect of nursing and medical care. Respiratory care begins with close observation and monitoring of respiratory muscle function. Frequent documentation of FVC and peak negative inspiratory pressure (PNIP) should provide early warning of impending respiratory failure. Most clinicians recommend intubation when FVC falls below 20 ml/kg or PNIP becomes less negative than 25 cm H_2O. Patients should be intubated before respiratory function deteriorates sufficiently to produce hypoxia and hypercarbia.

Cardiovascular management consists of prompt treatment of arrhythmias and hemodynamic disturbances. When possible, rapidly reversible interventions are preferable to long-acting agents. For instance, esmolol may terminate tachyarrhythmias but can be rapidly withdrawn if bradyarrhythmias develop. Sodium nitroprusside controls episodic hypertension but can be eliminated immediately if hypotension develops.

Specific treatment for GBS does not exist. Corticosteroids are probably not useful and may increase the risk of infectious complications. Despite intense controversy the role of plasmapheresis in the acute phase now appears well established. Plasmapheresis consists of blood removal, centrifugation to separate plasma from cellular elements, resuspension of the cellular elements in 5% albumin in saline solution, and reinfusion. Patients particularly likely to benefit from plasmapheresis are those who have had symptoms for less than 7 days and who require mechanical ventilation. In such patients the severity and duration of symptoms may be reduced.

Myasthenia Gravis

Myasthenia gravis (MG) is characterized by weakness and rapid muscular fatigue. The incidence of MG is approximately 5 per 100,000 population, with two distinct peaks, the first at about age 20 and the second in the fifth decade. Women predominate in the younger group and men in the older. Patients who have MG may require admission to an ICU for myasthenic or cholinergic crises or for management after thymectomy. Myasthenic patients are classified

TABLE 10–13.   Clinical Classification of Myasthenic Patients

GROUP	FEATURES
1	Isolated ocular involvement
	Rarely progresses to generalized disease
2-A	Mild generalized MG
	Benign course
	Good response to treatment
2-B	Moderately severe generalized MG
	Usually progresses from ocular through other muscles
3	Acute fulminating MG
	Common respiratory involvement
	Poor response to drug treatment
	High mortality
4	Late, severe MG
	Usually starts as group 2-B or 3
5	Neonatal MG (transient)
6	Congenital MG

MG = myasthenia gravis.

according to the distribution and course of their disease (Table 10–13).

Pathophysiology.   MG is a disease of neuromuscular transmission. The acetylcholine (ACh) receptors at the postsynaptic myoneural junction are reduced in number and are morphologically abnormal. Because of the reduced number of ACh receptors, the amplitude of spontaneous miniature end-plate potentials is diminished.

The cause of MG is autoimmune. Both cell-mediated and humoral immunity contribute to the disease manifestations. More than 80% of patients have a circulating antibody to the ACh receptor. Considerable evidence suggests that the thymus is centrally involved in the initiation and progression of the disease. Eighty percent of patients under 50 years of age have microscopic thymic lymphoid hyperplasia. Thymomas occur in 10% of patients.

Diagnosis.   The diagnosis is usually apparent from the clinical presentation. Because of weakness of the extraocular muscles, most patients have ocular symptoms. Bulbar symptoms, including difficulties with chewing and swallowing, commonly occur before limb weakness becomes prominent. Severe weakness of the respiratory musculature is a rare early symptom.

The diagnosis is confirmed by demonstrating improvement following the administration of a cholinesterase inhibitor or by eliciting an exaggerated response to a competitive neuromuscular blocker. The edrophonium (Tensilon) test is the most commonly employed diagnostic maneuver. If a 2 mg test dose produces no untoward reaction, an additional 8 mg is injected. Muscle strength is then evaluated. As an alternative, neostigmine can be used, especially in small children. A placebo control may be helpful when testing anticholinesterase response.

Curare, a nondepolarizing neuromuscular blocker, is occasionally used to confirm the diagnosis in equivocal cases. Because of the extreme sensitivity of myasthenic patients to curariform drugs, a small systemic dose often elicits profound symptoms. Because of the risk of sudden ventilatory failure, curare is also occasionally given as a regional test, in which the circulation to one arm is occluded by a tourniquet and a small dose of curare is injected intravenously distal to the tourniquet. This test can demonstrate weakness with minimal risk of respiratory compromise. However, a few patients with disproportionately severe ventilatory muscle failure may demonstrate an equivocal response to regional injection but definitive deterioration of ventilatory function with systemic injection. The only commonly employed blood test assesses the presence of the anti-ACh receptor antibody.

Treatment. The mainstay of therapy for MG is the administration of anticholinesterase agents, such as pyridostigmine or neostigmine, to increase the availability of ACh at the myoneural junction. Pyridostigmine, approximately one fourth as potent per milligram as neostigmine, produces fewer gastrointestinal side effects. Typical intravenous doses of pyridostigmine and neostigmine are 0.5 mg and 2 mg, respectively.

Corticosteroids are used in more severe generalized disease. After steroids are initiated, weakness often worsens before improving. Other immunosuppressive agents have occasionally been used in refractory cases. Azathioprine, used with caution because of its sometimes unacceptable depression of immune function, is effective with or without concurrent corticosteroid therapy. Thymectomy is currently recommended for patients who have thymic hyperplasia and moderate to severe disease. The response, often delayed for weeks to months, is most striking in younger patients. Plasmapheresis is commonly employed for acute exacerbations of the disease or in preparation for surgery.

In patients receiving long-term treatment for MG, myasthenic crisis (a severe exacerbation) or toxic effects of excessive anticholinesterase medications may develop. In either case it is customary to withhold anticholinesterase medication, provide ventilatory support if needed, and reinstitute medication several days later. Compulsive attention to respiratory care is essential. Measurement of FVC and PNIP provides early warning of impending respiratory failure. Intubation is indicated when FVC falls below 15 to 20 ml/kg or PNIP becomes less negative than 25 to 30 cm H_2O. Intubation should be performed before the onset of hypoxia and hypercarbia.

In myasthenic crisis patients are generally resistant to anticholinesterase therapy; in patients who are in cholinergic crisis, pyridostigmine or neostigmine aggravates weakness and autonomic symptoms.

Other Chronic Neurologic Diseases

Occasionally, patients with other chronic neurologic diseases require intensive care. Amyotrophic lateral sclerosis (ALS), a chronic, inexorably progressive disease, usually causes death by interfering with ventilatory function and airway protection. Rarely a patient with ALS recovers sufficiently from respiratory failure caused by an episode of pneumonia to permit weaning from mechanical ventilation and discharge from the hospital.

The management of multiple sclerosis (MS) has gradually improved during the past few decades. Baclofen and to a lesser extent dantrolene have become valuable agents for the control of spasticity caused by the upper motor neuron syndrome. Carbamazepine is useful for the control of dystonic spasms. Amitriptyline controls episodic pain in approximately half of patients and is also frequently effective in controlling the pseudobulbar symptoms of pathologic laughing and weeping.

No treatment is clearly effective in delaying the progression of the more severe cases of MS. MRI has demonstrated frequent discrepancies between the clinical manifestations of the disease and anatomic lesions. Corticosteroids and adrenocorticotropic hormone appear to shorten the duration of acute episodes but do not arrest the disease. Azathioprine possibly slows the downhill progression of some patients. Cyclophosphamide also seems to slow the course of the disease, especially in younger patients who are still ambulatory. The role of cyclosporine is undergoing investigation. Copolymer 1, a synthetic peptide, produces improvement in mild cases. Elective intubation or ventilation is rarely used in patients whose MS has advanced to the point of ventilatory failure.

Although effective immunization has reduced paralytic polio to the status of a rare disease, many patients who suffered infection in the epidemics of 40 to 50 years ago now have late complications of their disease. Ventilatory insufficiency is the most life threatening of these late complications. Patients with late postpolio respiratory insufficiency have usually been free of mechanical ventilatory assistance for many years but begin to decompensate as aging reduces muscle strength and lung elasticity. Management varies among medical centers but includes such modalities as tracheostomy with continuous or nocturnal home mechanical ventilation, mouth positive-pressure ventilation, and cuirass ventilation with the Emerson wrap negative-pressure ventilator. Improvement of symptoms is common with long-term support of ventilation, but the effect on outcome is unclear.

SEIZURES

Seizures, a common complication of critical illness, result from numerous traumatic and metabolic insults. However, all are characterized by paroxysmal uncontrolled neuronal discharge with or without spread to normal brain tissue. Epileptic patients, about 1% of the population, also require intensive care for episodes unrelated to their seizure diagnosis. Status epilepticus (SE), a life-threatening form of primary and secondary seizure, is a medical emergency that often must be managed in the ICU after initial stabilization in the emergency department or elsewhere in the hospital.

Classification System. Seizures are classified by their clinical and EEG characteristics (Table 10–14). Epileptic syndromes are categorized as partial, generalized, undetermined (fitting into neither of the first two categories), or special (such as febrile seizures). Individual seizures are classified as partial seizures, generalized seizures, or unclassified seizures. Tonic-clonic convulsions constitute the majority of seizures that require urgent attention in the ICU.

Diagnosis. Accurate diagnosis of the type of seizure is essential for the selection of appropriate antiseizure medication. *Partial seizures* usually accompany a single, discrete area of structural brain abnormality, from which clinical and EEG changes originate. The majority of partial seizures originate in the temporal lobe. Partial seizures that produce no impairment of consciousness are called *simple* partial seizures. Simple partial seizures may have motor, sensory, autonomic, or psychic manifestations. Although the EEG commonly demonstrates focal epileptiform activity over the appropriate cortical area, it may be normal.

TABLE 10–14.   International Classification of Epileptic Syndromes and Seizures

I. Classification of epileptic syndromes
    A. Localization-related epilepsies and syndromes
    B. Generalized epilepsies and syndromes
    C. Undetermined epilepsies and syndromes
    D. Special syndromes
II. Classification of epileptic seizures
    A. Partial seizures
        1. Simple partial seizures (consciousness not impaired)
        2. Complex partial seizures (consciousness impaired)
        3. Secondarily generalized seizures
    B. Generalized seizures
        1. Absence seizures
        2. Myoclonic seizures
        3. Clonic seizures
        4. Tonic seizures
        5. Tonic-clonic seizures
        6. Atonic seizures
    C. Unclassified seizures

Modified from Riela AR: Management of seizures. Crit Care Clin 1989;5:863–879. With permission.

Auras, which are sensory, autonomic, or psychic phenomena, such as unpleasant odors or tastes, that frequently accompany complex partial seizures, are examples of simple partial seizures.

Complex partial seizures are accompanied by alteration of consciousness. Complex partial seizures are often accompanied by automatisms, involuntary although coordinated behaviors occurring during impaired consciousness. Typical automatisms include eating behaviors, such as chewing or swallowing; motor activity, such as walking; and speech, often unintelligible. The typical EEG demonstrates unilateral or bilateral discharge most frequently from the temporal or frontal lobes. When partial seizures become *secondarily generalized,* they often have tonic, clonic, or tonic-clonic clinical manifestations, accompanied on EEG by bilateral abnormal epileptiform activity. Although the archaic term "grand mal" is commonly applied to both secondarily generalized seizures and primary generalized seizures, the distinction between the two is important because the treatment may differ.

Generalized seizures involve both cerebral hemispheres simultaneously, as is evident from both the clinical findings and the EEG. Consciousness is typically impaired. Generalized seizures include absence, myoclonic, atonic, clonic, and tonic-clonic seizures. *Absence seizures,* typically occurring in patients less than 20 years of age, are brief episodes, occasionally of simple impairment of consciousness but more commonly incorporating clonic, tonic, or automatic behaviors. Originally termed petit mal seizures, they are associated with EEG findings of a generalized 3 Hz spike and wave discharge. Hyperventilation for 3 minutes frequently precipitates absence seizures. *Myoclonic seizures* are sudden muscle contractions that symmetrically involve the extremities or facial musculature. The EEG reveals a generalized "fast" 4 to 6 Hz spike and wave discharge. *Atonic seizures,* also called drop attacks, are characterized clinically by a sudden loss of muscle tone, usually without impairment of consciousness. The EEG displays generalized polyspikes, flattening, or low-voltage fast activity. *Clonic seizures* are usually generalized jerking movements, accompanied by impairment of consciousness. The EEG demonstrates fast activity with generalized spike or polyspike and wave discharge. *Tonic seizures* consist of muscle stiffening or rigidity, impairment of consciousness, and EEG findings similar to those associated with clonic seizures. *Tonic-clonic seizures,* also called grand mal convulsions, combine features of clonic and tonic seizures and are universally associated with impairment of consciousness. The EEG resembles that associated with tonic and clonic seizures.

The World Health Organization defines *status epilepticus* as "a condition characterized by an epileptic seizure that is sufficiently prolonged or repeated at sufficiently brief intervals so as to produce an unvarying and enduring epileptic condition." Most clinicians define SE as seizures exceeding 30 minutes in duration. The mortality rate is approximately 10%.

SE is classified into two general categories, nonconvulsive and convulsive. Nonconvulsive SE primarily refers to absence or partial SE. Convulsive SE consists of tonic, clonic, tonic-clonic, or myoclonic seizures.

Absence SE (spike-wave stupor or petit mal status) produces a continuous mild impairment of function. Most patients appear dull and confused. The EEG shows a generalized epileptiform or a paroxysmal change from baseline. This condition should also be treated vigorously, although it is not a medical emergency. *Complex partial SE* resembles absence SE with long episodes of confusion or psychotic behavior with or without automatisms. Although not as urgent as convulsive SE, this condition should be treated vigorously. *Convulsive SE* usually is tonic-clonic. Tonic or clonic SE occurs primarily in children. *Myoclonic SE* consists of impairment of consciousness with rapid muscle jerks occurring irregularly in a generalized but asymmetric fashion. A specific form of myoclonic SE occurs after global hypoxic and ischemic events. These seizures are refractory to treatment and portend a poor outcome. *Tonic-clonic SE* represents a medical emergency because of the associated morbidity and mortality. Idiopathic tonic-clonic SE most often results from alcohol withdrawal or noncompliance with antiepileptic therapy and generally responds well to treatment. More commonly, generalized tonic-clonic SE implies acute cerebral disease such as tumors, cerebrovascular disease, or severe hypoxic brain injury. These seizures are frequently difficult to control.

Treatment. Antiepileptic medications have improved steadily over the past three decades; they exert more specific effects on individual seizure types and cause fewer side effects. Antiepileptic therapy should be based on an accurate diagnosis. A single medication is used until seizure control is attained or unacceptable side effects occur. Only then should a second antiepileptic medication be started. Polypharmacy increases the incidence of side effects and may complicate the maintenance of therapeutic serum levels.

Many neurologists believe that isolated, first seizures require no treatment. If possible, treatment should be deferred until a full evaluation of the patient is completed. Epileptic patients with breakthrough seizures frequently require no medical intervention. When breakthrough seizures occur, possible causes should be evaluated. Noncompliance is the most common reason.

If treatment appears necessary in patients with isolated or breakthrough seizures, clinicians should avoid the tendency to treat all seizures as if they represented SE. Unduly aggressive management may lead to unnecessary complications. For example, intravenous administration of diazepam *following* a seizure is unnecessary, ineffective, and potentially life threatening.

Tables 10–15 and 10–16 list the characteristics of several antiepileptic drugs.

Phenobarbital is most often used in the pediatric population. Indications include all forms of neonatal seizures, generalized and partial seizures of childhood, febrile convulsions (when treatment is required), and SE. Phenobarbital may aggravate absence seizures. In adults phenobarbital is used primarily in generalized tonic-clonic seizures and in secondarily generalized seizures. It can be given orally, intramuscularly, or intravenously. Dose reduction may be necessary in both renal and

TABLE 10–15.   Pharmacologic Characteristics of Antiepileptic Drugs

DRUG	PREPARATIONS	HALF-LIFE (AVERAGE)	PROTEIN BOUND (%)
Phenobarbital	PO, IM, IV	96 h	40-50
Phenytoin	PO, IV	24 h	90
Primidone	PO	12 h	0-50
Ethosuximide	PO	30 h	0
Carbamazepine	PO, PR	18 h	70
Valproic acid	PO, PR	12 h	90

PO = oral, IM = intramuscular, IV = intravenous, PR = rectal.

hepatic disease. Therapeutic levels range between 10 and 30 μg/ml. The side effects of phenobarbital include dose-related drowsiness, mental clouding, and decreased cognitive performance.

Phenytoin is primarily indicated for partial seizures, including secondarily generalized tonic-clonic seizures. Important in the treatment of SE, phenytoin is also used in many of the primary generalized seizures including tonic, clonic, tonic-clonic, atonic, and possibly myoclonic seizures. It is ineffective against absence seizures and does not prevent febrile convulsions. Phenytoin can be given orally and intravenously; absorption from intramuscular injection is erratic. The therapeutic range is 10 to 20 μg/ml. It is 90% protein bound, metabolized by the liver through parahydroxylation, and excreted in the urine. Because this compound is metabolized in the liver by a saturable enzyme system, small increments in dose may result in dramatic increases in serum concentration once a critical serum level is attained. The side effects of phenytoin include dose-related complications such as nystagmus, diplopia, ataxia, mental dulling, sedation, dyskinesias, and, at toxic levels, increased seizure frequency. Side effects unrelated to dose include many cosmetic effects, such as hirsutism, worsening acne, coarsening of facial features, and gingival hyperplasia. Severe reactions such as Stevens-Johnson syndrome, aplastic anemia, and hepatic failure occur more frequently with phenytoin than phenobarbital.

Primidone has a phenytoin-like action and is transformed by hepatic metabolism into phenobarbital. It is primarily indicated for the treatment of partial seizures in adults and has been effective in refractory myoclonic seizures. Therapeutic levels range from 5 to 12 μg/ml. Phenobarbital levels should also be monitored in patients who receive primidone because phenobarbital toxic effects may occur despite therapeutic levels of primidone. The side effects closely resemble those associated with phenobarbital, although primidone may produce less sedation.

Ethosuximide is used mainly for absence seizures in children. It is metabolized primarily by the liver. Therapeutic levels range between 40 and 100 μg/ml. Side effects consist primarily of gastrointestinal dysfunction, including abdominal pain, nausea, vomiting, and anorexia. Headache, hiccups, and a lupuslike reaction have been described.

Carbamazepine, highly effective against all types of partial seizures, has been used in both primary and secondarily generalized tonic-clonic seizures. Carbamazepine typically induces its own metabolism, resulting in an increasing dose requirement with long-term use. The therapeutic range is 4 to 12 μg/ml. Dose-related side effects include nystagmus, diplopia, ataxia, dizziness, and sedation. Mild nausea and abdominal discomfort can occur with initiation of this medication or with toxic levels. Cognitive impairment may occur at higher concentrations but is less frequent than with phenobarbital or

TABLE 10–16.   Common Antiepileptic Medications

DRUG	THERAPEUTIC LEVEL (μg/ml)	METABOLISM	SIDE EFFECTS
Phenobarbital	10-30	Hepatic	Drowsiness; decreased cognition
Phenytoin	10-20	Hepatic	Sedation; ataxia
Primidone	5-20	Hepatic	Sedation
Ethosuximide	40-100	Hepatic	Gastrointestinal distress
Carbamazepine	4-12	Hepatic	Ataxia; nausea; cognitive impairment
Valproic acid	50-100	Hepatic	Sedation; nausea; hepatic failure

phenytoin. Very rarely, hepatic or renal failure occurs.

Valproic acid is used in all forms of primary generalized seizures, including absence, tonic, clonic, tonic-clonic, myoclonic, and atonic seizures. This medication has usually been employed in combination with other medications to control refractory partial seizures, although recently it has been used alone. Therapeutic levels vary from 50 to 100 μg/ml. Dose-related side effects, often milder than those accompanying other antiepileptic medications, include sedation, tremor, nausea, vomiting, and abdominal pain. The most significant side effect, hepatic failure, occurs most frequently in children less than 2 years of age who are neurologically impaired and receiving multiple antiepileptic drugs.

SE requires an aggressive, systematic approach to treatment. Once generalized tonic-clonic SE is diagnosed, the goal should be to control seizures within 60 minutes. The first 10 to 15 minutes is used for evaluation and provision of basic cardiopulmonary support. After evaluation and stabilization, antiepileptic medications are introduced for continuing seizures. Because no ideal drug for SE is available, a benzodiazepine and phenytoin are used together. Many physicians prefer intravenous diazepam, starting with a dose of 10 mg at a rate no faster than 2 mg/min. The most significant side effects are respiratory depression and hypotension. Recently lorazepam has been successfully used in SE. The usual dose is 2 to 4 mg given intravenously. The advantages of lorazepam over diazepam include a longer duration of antiseizure activity and possibly fewer side effects. Phenytoin is mixed in normal saline solution at 20 mg/kg and normally infused intravenously at a rate of less than 50 mg/min. Hypotension and cardiac arrhythmias may necessitate reducing the infusion rate.

Errors in the control of SE are common. If diazepam is given alone, SE typically recurs within 20 to 30 minutes. Excessive administration of diazepam may produce respiratory depression. Recurrence of SE may also occur if an inadequate loading dose (20 mg/kg) of phenytoin is given. In this emergency situation, full loading doses should be given rapidly. Inadequate dosage of medications is the most common reason for failure to control seizures. If SE remains refractory to treatment, an underlying cerebral disorder is usually present. An EEG should be obtained to more accurately characterize the seizure. A second antiepileptic

TABLE 10–17. Treatment of Status Epilepticus

Phase 1: Stabilization and Evaluation (0 to 15 Minutes)

a. Assess cardiorespiratory status
b. Oral airway; O_2 as needed
c. Observe clinical seizure (diagnosis); obtain brief history and perform brief physical and neurologic examination
d. Start intravenous lines (two preferable)
e. Perform tests: complete blood count, electrolytes, blood urea nitrogen, creatinine, antiepileptic drug levels, drug screen, and metabolic screen
f. Glucose 25 g and vitamin complex intravenously

Phase 2: Seizure Control (Next 20 to 30 Minutes)

a. Diazepam intravenously not faster than 2 mg/min up to 40 mg or lorazepam up to 10 mg
b. As giving benzodiazepines, infuse phenytoin 20 mg/kg in normal saline at rate no faster than 50 mg/min while monitoring electrocardiogram and blood pressure
c. In young children, may start with phenobarbital 20 mg/kg either intravenously or mixed intravenously and intramuscularly

Phase 3: Refractory Seizure Treatment Options (Next 30 Minutes)

a. Intubate, obtain electroencephalogram, and consider general anesthesia
Meanwhile:
b. Infuse more phenytoin (10 mg/kg) *or*
c. Infuse phenobarbital 20 mg/kg not faster than 100 mg/min watching for hypotension *or*
d. Infuse diazepam 100 mg in 500 ml of 5% glucose at 40 ml/h *or*
e. Administer paraldehyde intravenously (if available) as a 4% solution in normal saline or give 0.3 ml/kg up to 15 ml mixed with an equal volume of mineral oil as an enema *or*
f. Administer valproic acid 20 mg/kg with an equal volume of water and give as a retention enema *or*
g. Give a bolus of lidocaine 2 mg/kg intravenously followed by an infusion of 3 to 10 mg/kg/h

Phase 4: General Anesthesia for Totally Refractory Seizures

Phase 5: Maintenance Care

Modified from Riela AR: Management of seizures. Crit Care Clin 1989;5:863-879. With permission.

medication should be introduced while general anesthesia is considered. General anesthesia may occasionally be indicated if seizures remain refractory to multiple antiepileptic medications (Table 10–17). Once SE is terminated, a maintenance plan for chronic care is instituted.

PSYCHOLOGIC AND PSYCHIATRIC DYSFUNCTION

Agitated or delirious patients are a constant source of frustration for ICU personnel and a potential source of danger to the patients themselves. Although no single diagnostic or-therapeutic approach can be applied to the en-tire range of psychologic and psychiatric distur-bances, several general principles appear valid.

Since the development of the first ICUs, psychologic problems have plagued both pa-tients and personnel. Patients admitted to ICUs have life- or function-threatening disease pro-cesses. They temporarily lose control over their environment. Intubation or tracheostomy pre-vents effective communication. Day-night cycles are disrupted, with bright lighting, noise, and activity continuing around the clock. Sleep is difficult, and prolonged rest may be impossible. Even such elementary orienting information as the time and date becomes obscure. Pain and discomfort are common but may be inade-quately appreciated by caregivers. Painful pro-cedures occur frequently, often with insufficient explanation. The patients most vulnerable to psychologic dysfunction in this environment are those who are elderly, have a history of mental illness or substance abuse, have had extensive surgery or a complicated intraoperative course, or are receiving multiple medications.

The response of individual patients to inten-sive care varies but commonly takes the form of anger, depression, agitation, disorientation, or frank psychosis. Unfortunately, the differentia-tion of reactive psychologic disturbances from organic causes is imprecise. Life-threatening or-ganic causes of psychologic deterioration, that is, hypoxemia and sepsis, must be considered and either excluded or treated. The careful in-terview, a critical part of the diagnosis of psy-chologic disorders, is impractical with most pa-tients, especially those unable to talk. In most other patients, symptomatic interventions are sufficient pending recovery from the primary illness.

Diagnosis.   Patients who become acutely dis-oriented should be presumed to have hypoxia or sepsis until evidence demonstrates otherwise. Consequently, an arterial blood gas determina-tion or placement of a pulse oximeter may prove invaluable in excluding or proving a treatable diagnosis. Sepsis often cannot be disproven immediately; however, blood cultures should be obtained and a search begun for signs of infection. Withdrawal syndromes can be sus-pected from the history. An acute central nervous system disorder, such as infection or intracranial hemorrhage, should be suspected in patients at risk for those complications. Lumbar puncture or CT scanning is often necessary to exclude potentially remediable causes of acute

delirium or aberrant behavior. In the majority of instances, a thorough diagnostic evaluation, although essential, does not disclose a specific cause.

Treatment.   Attention to the details of the critically ill patient's environment does much to limit psychologic dysfunction. Bedside person-nel should attempt to orient patients frequently to date and time. Calendars and clocks are useful reference points. Mealtimes can be treated as specific events, even if "breakfast" consists only of changing to a new bag of enteral feeding solution. Radio or television may pro-vide stimulation, especially for an alert patient who is confined to the ICU for a protracted period. Windows are essential in distinguishing day from night. Reducing nocturnal illumina-tion and commotion facilitates sleep. Conversa-tions among caregivers about the patient's condition should take place away from the bedside, particularly if the subject matter im-plies poor prognosis. Physical restraints, popu-lar with personnel, should be used only if they prevent risk to the patient (for example, are used to control repeated attempts at self-extubation). Passive restraints tend to reinforce a patient's misperception of being held against his or her will by unsympathetic or dangerous persons and may actually worsen delirium.

For patients who have no specific organic cause for agitation, a variety of pharmacologic agents are available, although none is entirely satisfactory. Use of sedatives should be avoided unless the risk/benefit ratio is clearly positive. Diazepam has several drawbacks. Its terminal elimination half-life may be extremely pro-longed, particularly in elderly patients or those with liver disease. Diazepam often produces only transient hypnotic effects; therefore a patient may doze after a 5 to 10 mg intravenous dose of diazepam but promptly awaken with only enough sedative effect remaining to reduce behavioral inhibitions. Lorazepam 1 to 4 mg intravenously produces more stable, sustained sedation, even though its pharmacologic half-life is shorter than that of diazepam. Lorazepam exerts profound amnesic effects. Midazolam has recently been used extensively for sedation. In the ICU its advantages include a short duration of action, excellent amnesic effects, and suit-ability for continuous infusion. However, it is expensive. Haloperidol is commonly employed to reduce agitation in the ICU. The dose usually employed, 1 to 2 mg intravenously, is far lower than the doses commonly used to control a psychiatric patient during a severe schizo-phrenic episode. Higher bolus doses create the risk of hemodynamic depression in fragile patients. However, large doses can be administered in small increments.

The treatment of ethanol withdrawal merits special attention. Typically observed within 48 hours after cessation of ethanol ingestion, withdrawal commonly is manifest as anxiety, tremors, tachycardia, mild fever, and seizures. An occasional patient manifests symptoms only after 4 days or more in the hospital. The treatment is administration of sufficient benzodiazepine to control the manifestations. Diazepam is often given in 5 mg increments until a total loading dose of 50 to 100 mg has been given. Usually, approximately half of the dose given in the preceding 24 hours is required on each successive day. The drug must be carefully titrated to achieve adequate suppression of symptoms without ventilatory or cardiovascular depression. Lorazepam is a satisfactory alternative. Recently the centrally acting alpha$_2$-receptor agonist clonidine has been employed to reduce both the psychic disturbances associated with ethanol withdrawal and the hyperadrenergic state, a manifestation that also responds to beta blockade. In the future, clonidine or a related compound may be routinely employed in patients withdrawing from ethanol abuse.

BRAIN DEATH

Brain death must be accurately diagnosed for two reasons. First, the ability to state unequivocally that survival is impossible provides ICU personnel with a legally and ethically sound rationale for withdrawing life support. Second, in some patients accurate diagnosis of brain death permits harvesting of transplantable organs. Although brain death criteria must be met before organ donation, they have never been intended as the sole criteria for a decision to withhold or withdraw care when donation is not a consideration. In an era when transplantation techniques are well advanced but transplantable organs are in critically short supply, all potential donors must be identified and their families counseled regarding organ donation.

Because of the possibility of organ donation, the medical management of the brain-dead patient has become a vital topic. Paradoxically, sound intensive care of one deceased patient may preserve life or improve the quality of life for several people: the recipients of transplanted kidney, heart, liver, pancreas, and lung.

Diagnosis. The impetus for defining the criteria for brain death originated from the legal necessity of stating without doubt that a potential donor could not survive. Consequently a multicenter study was performed to determine criteria by which brain death could be distinguished from irreversible coma. Patients were entered if they exceeded 1 year of age and had been cerebrally unresponsive for at least 15 minutes. Clinical, neurologic, and EEG examinations were performed on admission and subsequently at 6, 12, and 24 hours, at 2 and 3 days, and weekly thereafter until death or recovery. Because the confirmatory test in this study was sustained EEG silence, patients were excluded if they were unresponsive in association with drug intoxication or hypothermia. Three criteria for cerebral death, including cerebral unresponsivity, apnea, and electrocerebral silence, were met by 187 patients, of whom 185 died. Although pupillary dilation and complete lack of cephalic reflexes added little diagnostic specificity, they were considered worthwhile indicators by the investigators; spinal reflexes were not. They concluded that the chances of even temporary survival were slight if the five criteria were met for at least 30 minutes occurring at least 6 hours after hospital admission. Determination of absent brain blood flow was mentioned as a confirmatory test.

The criteria for brain death just outlined are time consuming to confirm, and they exclude patients with intercurrent sedative intoxication or hypothermia from consideration. Four-vessel cerebral angiography, a potential confirmatory test in such situations, is expensive and time consuming. Therefore the early "flow phase" of radionuclide brain scanning has emerged as a valuable technique that can be easily performed in most ICUs. Unlike EEG diagnosis, a single negative study is adequate to make an unequivocal diagnosis. The primary limitation of the technique is lack of evaluation of the posterior circulation. Its greatest advantage is rapid assessment of cerebral perfusion.

Supplementary techniques have been applied recently as early harbingers of brain death, although in most cases radionuclide scanning continues to be the definitive test, with or without EEG. Those techniques include brainstem auditory evoked potentials and transcranial Doppler ultrasonography. The former shows absence of all waves or all but the first (medullary) wave in brain-dead patients. Transcranial Doppler ultrasonography of the middle cerebral artery (Fig. 10–7) characteristically shows a progressive fall in cerebral perfusion pressure, with initial loss of diastolic flow followed by oscillating flow as cerebral blood

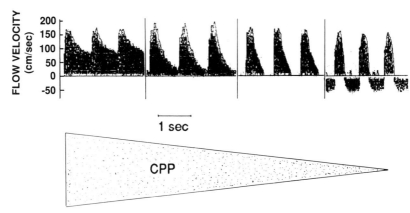

Figure 10–7. Changes in flow velocity in the middle cerebral artery as cerebral perfusion pressure (CPP) declines because of increasing intracranial pressure. As CPP declines, flow velocity in the middle cerebral artery initially demonstrates progressive loss of the diastolic flow component. Then, as intracranial pressure approaches critical values, flow velocity becomes bidirectional. Ultimately, if intracranial pressure exceeds mean arterial pressure, flow ceases in the middle cerebral artery (not shown). (Modified from Hassler W, Steinmetz H, Gawlowski J: J Neurosurg 1988;68:745-751. With permission.)

flow ceases. Because these tests can be performed repeatedly, they can be used to determine when a radionuclide study should be performed. Table 10–18 summarizes the tests commonly used to diagnose brain death.

Management. Management of the brain-dead patient requires application of all the principles of sound cardiovascular, pulmonary, and renal intensive care. Care directed at these organ systems frequently follows an interval during which aggressive neurologic intensive care, including osmotic diuresis and fluid restriction, has produced moderate to severe hypovolemia. In addition, the occurrence of cerebral death is typically accompanied by profound systemic vasodilation and DI, both of which complicate volume replacement. Finally, resuscitation is constrained by the concern of some transplantation teams that pulmonary artery catheterization may damage the donor heart and that pharmacologic control of DI may damage the donor kidney.

TABLE 10–18. Criteria for Brain Death

Clinical

1. Coma with cerebral unresponsivity
2. Apnea
3. Pupillary dilation
4. Absent cephalic reflexes

Monitoring

1. Evoked potentials
2. Processed electroencephalogram
3. Doppler ultrasonography

Confirmatory

1. Electroencephalogram (maximal sensitivity)
2. Radionuclide brain scan

Management of the cardiovascular system is based on conventional criteria for providing adequate preload, afterload, and contractility. Inadequate maintenance of cardiac output compromises the kidneys and liver; prolonged beta-adrenergic stimulation may damage the heart. Systolic blood pressure declines to less than 90 mm Hg in approximately half of donor candidates. In young donors empiric volume expansion without invasive monitoring may be adequate. However, pulmonary artery catheterization should be considered if blood pressure cannot easily be restored. Inotropic agents should be used with caution. A low-dose infusion of dopamine (less than 3 μg/kg/min) tends to reverse venodilation, support blood pressure, and improve renal perfusion. Higher doses of dopamine (greater than 10 μg/kg/min) or administration of epinephrine or norepinephrine may reduce perfusion of the kidneys and liver and produce subclinical changes in myocardial contractility and compliance that persist into the posttransplant period.

Pulmonary management requires an assessment of the competing needs of multiple organ systems. If the lungs are to be transplanted, they ideally should be "dry." However, the necessity for timely fluid resuscitation may compromise that requirement. Adequate oxygenation of systemic tissues may require PEEP, but PEEP may further reduce cardiac output in patients with tenuous volume status and loss of vascular tone. A fraction of inspired oxygen exceeding 0.60, if maintained for prolonged periods, may damage the pulmonary parenchyma. If therapeutic hypocapnia has been employed to assist in ICP control, the $Paco_2$ should be permitted

TABLE 10–19.   Care of the Brain-Dead Organ Donor

ORGAN SYSTEM	MANAGEMENT STRATEGY
Cardiovascular	Replace intravascular volume Avoid alpha-adrenergic drugs Pulmonary artery catheter if empirical therapy fails
Pulmonary	$Paco_2 \approx 40$ mm Hg PEEP as necessary to limit $Fio_2 \leq .60$
Renal	Control diabetes insipidus Provide effective cardiovascular support Consider low-dose dopamine
Other	Control hypothermia Consider hydrocortisone Specific organ preservation before organ removal (still experimental)

to return to 40 mm Hg to prevent the systemic consequences of alkalemia.

Effective renal management is essential. After renal transplantation, acute renal failure commonly occurs. The kidneys may be damaged not only by poor preservation after removal from the donor, but by prolonged renal hypoperfusion before removal. Restoration of circulating blood volume and avoidance of exogenous vasoconstrictors are essential. Control of polyuria necessitates control of hyperglycemia and DI. Often water diuresis treated by replacement with saline solution or lactated Ringer's solution results in hypernatremia before declaration of brain death. Rapid correction of hyponatremia is difficult because the necessary quantities of free water, administered as 5% dextrose in water, produce hyperglycemia and perpetuate the urinary losses with osmotic diuresis. An appropriate fluid in that situation is 0.45% saline solution without dextrose. Vasopressin, given in the physiologic doses necessary to control water diuresis, produces little if any vasoconstriction. Therefore a continuous infusion of 1 to 3 units/h should be considered. Alternatively, subcutaneous vasopressin or DDAVP, considered by some to be the drug of choice because of its limited systemic effects, may be given in twice-daily doses of 1 to 2 μg subcutaneously or intravenously.

Other supportive care may be necessary. Hypothermia commonly develops in these poikilothermic patients and may necessitate warming. Hypopituitarism, a theoretical problem in brain-dead donors, is inconsistently documented and of questionable importance. However, if the delay from the initial determination of death to organ removal is prolonged,

hydrocortisone may be given in a dose of 50 to 100 mg. In the future, specific organ-preserving agents may be given as part of therapy before organ removal. Such agents include Ca^{++} entry blockers, adrenergic antagonists, and free radical scavengers. However, data are insufficient to routinely include such interventions in management. A summary of suggestions for the care of potential donors is listed in Table 10–19.

SUGGESTED READINGS

General Reviews

Grenvik A, Safer P (eds): Brain failure and resuscitation. New York, 1981, Churchill Livingstone

Prough DS (ed): Neurologic critical care (Critical Care Clinics). Philadelphia, 1989, WB Saunders

Rogers MC, Traystman RJ (eds): Neurologic intensive care (Critical Care Clinics). Philadelphia, 1985, WB Saunders

Ropper AH, Kennedy SF (eds): Neurological and neurosurgical intensive care. Rockville, Md, 1988, Aspen Publishing

Stroke

Consensus Conference: Treatment of stroke. Br Med J 1988;297:126-128

Gelmers HJ, Gorter K, del Weerdt CJ, Wiezer HJA: A controlled trial of nimodipine in acute ischemic stroke. N Engl J Med 1988;318:203-207

Grotta JC: Current medical and surgical therapy for cerebrovascular disease. N Engl J Med 1987;317: 1505-1516

Wechsler LR, Ropper AH: Management of stroke in the intensive care unit. Semin Neurol 1986;6:324-331

Subarachnoid Hemorrhage

Allen GS, Ahn HS, Preziosi TJ, et al: Cerebral arterial spasm — a controlled trial of nimodipine in patients with subarachnoid hemorrhage. N Engl J Med 1983;308: 619-624

Jan M, Buchheit F, Tremoulet M: Therapeutic trial of intravenous nimodipine in patients with established cerebral vasospasm after rupture of intracranial aneurysms. Neurosurgery 1988;23:154-157

Kirsch JR, Diringer MN, Borel CO, Hanley DF: Cerebral aneurysms: mechanisms of injury and critical care interventions. In Prough DS (ed): Neurologic critical care (Critical Care Clinics). Philadelphia, 1989, WB Saunders, pp 755-772

Petruk KC, West M, Mohr G, et al: Nimodipine treatment in poor-grade aneurysm patients: results of a multicenter double-blind placebo-controlled trial. J Neurosurg 1988; 68:505-517

Solomon RA, Fink ME, Lennihan L: Early aneurysm surgery and prophylactic hypervolemic hypertensive therapy for the treatment of aneurysmal subarachnoid hemorrhage. Neurosurgery 1988;23:699-704

Thie A, Spitzer K, Kunze K: Spontaneous subarachnoid hemorrhage: assessment of prognosis and initial management in the intensive care unit. J Intensive Care Med 1987;2:103-114

Intracerebral Hemorrhage

Godersky JC, Biller J: Diagnosis and treatment of spontaneous intracerebral hemorrhage. Compr Ther 1987;13: 22-30

Poungvarin N, Bhoopat W, Viruyavejakui A, et al: Effects of dexamethasone in primary supratentorial intracerebral hemorrhage. N Engl J Med 1987;20:1229-1233

Young WL, Prohovnik I, Ornstein E, et al: Monitoring of intraoperative cerebral hemodynamics before and after arteriovenous malformation resection. Anesth Analg 1988;3:1011-1014

Global Cerebral Ischemia

Brain Resuscitation Clinical Trial I Study Group: Randomized clinical study of thiopental loading in comatose survivors of cardiac arrest. N Engl J Med 1986;314: 397-403

Cohan SL, Mun SK, Petite J, et al: Cerebral blood flow in humans following resuscitation from cardiac arrest. Stroke 1989;20:761-765

Forsman M, Aarseth HP, Nordby HK, et al: Effects of nimodipine on cerebral blood flow and cerebrospinal fluid pressure after cardiac arrest: correlation with neurologic outcome. Anesth Analg 1989;68:436-443

Kirsch JR, Dean JM, Rogers MC: Current concepts in brain resuscitation. Arch Intern Med 1986;146:1413-1419

Levy DE, Caronna JJ, Singer BH, et al: Predicting outcome from hypoxic-ischemic coma. JAMA 1985;253: 1420-1426

Maiese K, Caronna JJ: Coma following cardiac arrest: a review of the clinical features, management, and prognosis. J Intensive Care Med 1988;3:153-163

Prough DS, Furberg CD: Nimodipine and the "no-reflow phenomenon" — experimental triumph, clinical failure? [editorial]. Anesth Analg 1989;68:431-435

Hypertension and Cerebral Blood Flow

Barry DI: Cerebrovascular aspects of antihypertensive treatment. Am J Cardiol 1989;63:14C-18C

Baumbach GL, Heistad DD: Cerebral circulation in chronic arterial hypertension. Hypertension 1988;12:89-95

Haas DC, Streeten DHP, Kim RC, et al: Death from cerebral hypoperfusion during nitroprusside treatment of acute angiotensin-dependent hypertension. Am J Med 1983;75:1071-1076

Paulson OB, Waldemar G, Schmidt JF, Strandgaard S: Cerebral circulation under normal and pathologic conditions. Am J Cardiol 1989;63:2C-5C

Encephalopathy

Diagnosis and treatment of Reye's syndrome. JAMA 1981;246:2441-2444

Isensee LM, Weiner LF, Hart RG: Neurologic disorders in a medical intensive care unit: a prospective survey. J Crit Care 1989;4:208-210

Mahoney CA, Arieff AL: Uremic encephalopathies: clinical, biochemical, and experimental features. Am J Kidney Dis 1982;2:324-336

Shaywitz BA, Rothstein P, Venes JL: Monitoring and management of increased intracranial pressure in Reye syndrome: results in 29 children. Pediatrics 1980;66: 198-204

Neurologic Infections

Benson CA, Harris AA: Acute neurologic infections. Med Clin North Am 1986;70:987-1011

Lebel MH, Freji BJ, Syrogiannopoulos GA, et al: Dexamethasone therapy for bacterial meningitis: results of two double-blind, placebo-controlled trials. N Engl J Med 1988;319:964-971

Mampalam TJ, Rosenblum ML: Trends in the management of bacterial brain abscesses: a review of 102 cases over 17 years. Neurosurgery 1988;23:451-458

Roos KL, Scheld WM: The management of fulminant meningitis in the intensive care unit. Crit Care Clin 1988;4:375-392

Sepsis

Bolton CF, Young GB: Sepsis and septic shock: central and peripheral nervous systems. In Sibbald WJ, Sprung CL (eds): Perspectives on sepsis and septic shock. Fullerton, Calif, 1986, Society of Critical Care Medicine, pp 157-171

Bowton DL: CNS effects of sepsis. In Prough DS (ed): Neurologic critical care (Critical Care Clinics). Philadelphia, 1989, WB Saunders, pp 785-792

Sprung CL, Peduzzi PN, Shatney CH, et al: The impact of encephalopathy on mortality and physiologic derangements in the sepsis syndrome. Crit Care Med 1988; 16:S398

Head Injury

Butterworth JF IV, DeWitt DS: Severe head trauma: pathophysiology and management. In Prough DS (ed): Neurologic critical care (Critical Care Clinics). Philadelphia, 1989, WB Saunders, pp 807-820.

Eisenberg HM, Frankowski RF, Contant CF, et al: High-dose barbiturate control of elevated intracranial pressure in patients with severe head injury. J Neurosurg 1988; 69:15-23

Jennett B: Treatment of severe head injuries. J Intensive Care Med 1988;3:284-286

Teasdale G, Jennett B: Assessment of coma and impaired consciousness: a practical scale. Lancet 1974;2:81-84

Ward JD: Intracranial pressure monitoring. In Critical care: state of the art. Fullerton, Calif, 1989, Society of Critical Care Medicine, pp 173-185

Ward JD, Choi S, Marmarou A, et al: Effect of prophylactic hyperventilation on outcome in patients with severe head injury. In Hoff JT, Betz AL (eds): Intracranial pressure VII. New York, 1989, Springer-Verlag, pp 630-633

Spinal Cord Trauma

Albin MS: Acute cervical spinal injury. In Rogers MC, Traystman RJ (eds): Neurologic intensive care (Critical Care Clinics). Philadelphia, 1985, WB Saunders, pp 267-284

Bracken MB, Shepard MJ, Collins WF, et al: A randomized, controlled trial of methylprednisolone or naloxone in the treatment of acute spinal-cord injury. N Engl J Med 1990;322:1405-1411

Ducker TB: Treatment of spinal-cord injury [editorial]. N Engl J Med 1990;322:1459-1460

Faden AI: Pharmacotherapy in spinal cord injury: a critical review of recent developments. Clin Neuropharmacol 1987;10:193-204

Luce JM: Medical management of spinal cord injury. Crit Care Med 1985;13:126-131

Epilepsy

Browne TR, Mikati M: Status epilepticus. In Ropper AH, Kennedy SF (eds): Neurological and neurosurgical intensive care, 2nd ed. Rockville, Md, 1988, Aspen Publishing

Commission on Classification and Terminology of the International League Against Epilepsy: Proposal for classification of epilepsies and epileptic syndromes. Epilepsia 1985;26:268-278

Riela AR: Management of seizures. In Prough DS (ed): Neurologic critical care (Critical Care Clinics). Philadelphia, 1989, WB Saunders, pp 863-880

Zaret BS: Status epilepticus. In Rippe JM, Irwin RS, Alpert JS, Dalen JE (eds): Intensive care medicine. Boston, 1985, Little, Brown, pp 1069-1078

Syndrome of Inappropriate Antidiuretic Hormone Secretion and Diabetes Insipidus

Al-Mufti H, Arieff AI: Hyponatremia due to cerebral salt-wasting syndrome: combined cerebral and distal tubular lesion. Am J Med 1984;77:740-746

Anderson RJ, Chung H-M, Kluge R, Schrier RW: Hyponatremia: a prospective analysis of its epidemiology and the pathogenetic role of vasopressin. Ann Intern Med 1985;102:164-168

Ayus JC, Krothapalli RK, Arieff AI: Changing concepts in treatment of severe symptomatic hyponatremia: rapid correction and possible relation to central pontine myelinolysis. Am J Med 1985;78:897-902

Forrest JN Jr, Cox M, Hong C, et al: Superiority of demeclocycline over lithium in the treatment of chronic syndrome of inappropriate secretion of antidiuretic hormone. N Engl J Med 1978;298:173-177

Brain Death

Fink MP: In vivo organ preservation in brain dead patients. J Intensive Care Med 1989;4:53-54

Goodman JM, Heck LL, Moore BD: Confirmation of brain death with portable isotope angiography: a review of 204 consecutive cases. Neurosurgery 1985;16:492-497

Hassler WL, Steinmetz H, Gawlowski J: Transcranial Doppler ultrasonography in raised intracranial pressure and in intracranial circulatory arrest. J Neurosurg 1988;68:745-751

Youngner SJ, Landefeld CS, Coulton CJ, et al: "Brain death" and organ retrieval: a cross-sectional survey of knowledge and concepts among health professionals. JAMA 1989;261:2205-2210

Guillain-Barré Syndrome

Chad D: Guillain-Barré syndrome. In Rippe JM, Irwin RS, Alpert JS, Dalen JE (eds): Intensive care medicine. Boston, 1985, Little, Brown, pp 1083-1087

Kleyweg RP, van der Meche FGA, Meulstee J: Treatment of Guillain-Barré syndrome with high-dose gammaglobulin. Neurology 1988;38:1639-1641

McKhann GM, Griffin JW, Cornblath DR, et al: Plasmapheresis and Guillain-Barré syndrome: analysis of prognostic factors and the effect of plasmapheresis. Ann Neurol 1988;23:347-353

Ropper AH: ICU management of acute inflammatory-postinfectious polyneuropathy (Landry-Guillain-Barré-Strohl syndrome). In Ropper AH, Kennedy SF (eds): Neurological and neurosurgical intensive care, 2nd ed. Rockville, Md, 1988, Aspen Publishing, pp 253-268

Myasthenia Gravis

Levin KH: Critical care of myasthenia gravis. In Rippe JM, Irwin RS, Alpert JS, Dalen JE (eds): Intensive care medicine. Boston, 1985, Little, Brown, pp 1088-1090

Mier-Jedrzejowicz AK, Brophy C, Green M: Respiratory muscle function in myasthenia gravis. Am Rev Respir Dis 1988;138:867-873

Perlo VP: Treatment of the critically ill patient with myasthenia. In Ropper AH, Kennedy SF (eds): Neurological and neurosurgical intensive care, 2nd ed. Rockville, Md, 1988, Aspen Publishing, pp 247-252

Chronic Progressive Neurologic Disease

Davison AN: The need for a new strategy for the treatment of multiple sclerosis. J Neurol 1988;235:327-329

Jubelt B, Cashman NR: Neurological manifestations of the postpolio syndrome. Crit Rev Neurobiol 1987;3:199-220

Killian JM, Bressler RB, Armstrong RM, Huston DP: Controlled pilot trial of monthly intravenous cyclophosphamide in multiple sclerosis. Arch Neurol 1988;45:27-30

Rodriguez M: Multiple sclerosis: basic concepts and hypothesis. Mayo Clin Proc 1989;64:570-575

Swanson JW: Multiple sclerosis: update in diagnosis and review of prognostic factors. Mayo Clin Proc 1989;64:577-586

Ethanol Withdrawal

Baumgartner GR, Rowen RC: Clonidine vs. chlordiazepoxide in the management of acute alcohol withdrawal syndrome. Arch Intern Med 1987;147:1223-1226

Morris JC, Victor M: Alcohol withdrawal seizures. Emerg Med Clin North Am 1987;5:827-839

Rosenbloom A: Emerging treatment options in the alcohol withdrawal syndrome. J Clin Psychiatry 1988;49:28-32

Sebastian P: Delirium. In Rippe JM, Irwin RS, Alpert JS, Dalen JE (eds): Intensive care medicine. Boston, 1985, Little, Brown, pp 1079-1083

Psychiatric Disturbances

Lumb PD: Sedatives and muscle relaxants in the intensive care unit. In Furhman BP, Shoemaker WC (eds): Critical care: state of the art. Fullerton, Calif, 1989, Society of Critical Care Medicine, pp 145-171

11

ACUTE RENAL FAILURE

ALAN S. TONNESEN, MD

Acute renal failure (ARF) is a disastrous complication in critically ill patients. Acute tubular necrosis (ATN) is the most common form of ARF in the ICU. ATN is most commonly due to ischemia or nephrotoxins.

Most current concepts of the pathogenesis of ATN have been derived from animal models, which are poor analogs of ATN as seen in the ICU population. The most popular model of ARF is clamping of the renal artery for 40 to 180 minutes with various interacting, prophylactic or therapeutic modalities applied. Although no one doubts that total cessation of renal circulation causes renal damage, the extrapolation of conclusions from this model to the nonhypotensive patient with an intact renal circulation in whom ARF develops over a few hours to a few days is open to question. Until more realistic models are developed, significant progress in reducing the incidence of ARF or shortening its course is unlikely.

In the first section of this chapter, renal physiology is outlined to clarify the pathogenesis of ATN and of the fluid and electrolyte abnormalities seen in critically ill patients. Subsequent sections discuss the pathogenesis of ATN and its complications and their management.

RENAL PHYSIOLOGY
Renal Blood Flow

Renal blood flow (RBF) is the sine qua non of renal function, and its maintenance should be high on the intensivist's list of priorities. RBF is determined by renal perfusion pressure (RPP) and renal vascular resistance (RVR):

$$RBF = \frac{RPP}{RVR} \qquad (Eq. 1)$$

$$RPP = MAP - RVP \qquad (Eq. 2)$$

where
MAP = mean systemic arterial pressure
RVP = renal venous pressure

Factors that elevate either the central venous pressure or intraabdominal pressure elevate RVP and thus diminish RPP. The control of RVR is multifactorial, as shown in Table 11–1.

Autoregulation

Both RBF and glomerular filtration rate (GFR) exhibit autoregulatory phenomena over RPP ranging from about 50 to 60 mm Hg up to about 150 mm Hg (Fig. 11–1, *A*). Patients with prior ischemic insults may have markedly impaired autoregulation (Fig. 11–1, *B*) over the entire range of pressures, while the autoregulatory range of chronically hypertensive subjects shifts to a higher minimal MAP before RBF falls.

Autoregulation is an intrinsic property of the preglomerular arterioles and can be enhanced by the other factors that influence RVR. Increased stretch (as in hypertension) of the afferent arteriole increases intracellular

TABLE 11–1. Control of Renal Arteriolar Resistance

	AFFERENT ARTERIOLE	EFFERENT ARTERIOLE
Autoregulation	+ or −	+ or −
Angiotensin II	+ +	+ + +
Arginine vasopressin	+	+
Sympathetic tone		
Alpha	+ +	+ +
Beta	−	−
Dopamine	− −	− −
Atrial natriuretic peptide	− −	+ or −
Prostaglandins	−	−

Plus signs indicate an increase in tone, and minus signs, a decrease. The number of signs is intended to show only directional changes and not a ratio of potencies of the different agents.

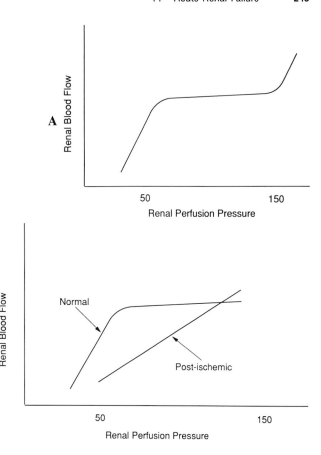

Figure 11–1. **A,** Autoregulation is due predominantly to the intrinsic properties of the renal arterioles, in which stretch of the vessel caused by elevated transmural pressure increases the vessel's tone. Although intact renin-angiotensin and sympathetic systems may enhance the effectiveness of the reflex, they are not necessary for its action. **B,** Autoregulation is impaired after ischemic insults in animal models of acute tubular necrosis. The curve is shifted downward and to the right. As a result, renal blood flow is diminished at any, even normal, renal perfusion pressure. The clinical implication is that mild depressions in renal perfusion pressure may result in additional ischemic injury to the kidneys and should be aggressively prevented or treated.

calcium, which causes vasoconstriction, whereas decreased stretch (as in hypotension) is associated with the opposite response.

Sympathetic Tone

Alpha receptors mediate significant vasoconstriction; dopamine receptors, significant vasodilation; and beta receptors, unimportant dilation. Beta receptors also stimulate renin release. Changes in sympathetic tone rapidly modulate vascular resistance and mediate many of the effects of anesthesia, hemodynamic abnormalities, mechanical ventilation, and positive end-expiratory pressure (PEEP) on renal function.

Angiotensin II

Angiotensin II is the biologically active end product of the actions of renin on angiotensinogen, which produces angiotensin I, and of angiotensin converting enzyme on angiotensin I. Angiotensin II can be generated entirely within the kidney or in the systemic vasculature. The rate-limiting step is the generation of renin. Renin release is stimulated and suppressed in a feedback loop (Table 11–2).

Systemic administration of angiotensin II causes greater constriction of the efferent arteriole than of the afferent arteriole. When generated via the intrarenal mechanism, the constriction is isolated to the efferent arteriole. The predominant constrictor effect on the efferent arteriole sustains glomerular capillary pressure and increases filtration fraction, thus maintaining GFR as RBF begins to decline.

Arginine Vasopressin

Arginine vasopressin (AVP) release is normally regulated by extracellular fluid osmolality,

TABLE 11–2.   Regulation of Renin Release

INCREASED RENIN	DECREASED RENIN
Decreased arteriolar stretch	Increased arteriolar stretch
Beta-adrenergic stimulation	Increased angiotensin level
Decreased chloride transport by macula densa	Increased chloride transport by macula densa
Prostaglandins	Increased atrial natriuretic peptide

which is sensed at the level of the hypothalamus. After rising above a threshold characteristic for each individual, between 275 and 285 mOsm/kg H_2O, osmolality elevations of as little as 1% to 2% stimulate AVP release. Hypovolemia resulting from loss of more than 10% to 15% of blood volume also causes AVP release even in the presence of an osmolality below the subject's threshold. Hypotension is an even more potent stimulus for AVP release. Finally, a variety of stressful stimuli, such as pain and nausea, cause AVP release by neurogenic mechanisms involving central dopaminergic receptors.

AVP causes vasoconstriction, especially in the superficial cortical nephrons, and increases the collecting duct's permeability to water. The latter action is potentiated by prostaglandins and, in the presence of a hypertonic medullary interstitium, favors the reabsorption of water from the collecting duct. This results in production of hypertonic urine. Vasopressin has a variety of extrarenal actions in addition to vasoconstriction, but these have minimal relevance to critically ill patients.

Atrial Natriuretic Peptide

Atrial natriuretic peptide (ANP, or atriopeptin) is a 28–amino acid peptide synthesized and stored within granules of cells of the atrial walls. It is released in response to distention of either the right or the left atrium.

In usual concentrations ANP has little effect on renal blood flow, but with higher levels or when the renal vasculature is constricted, especially by angiotensin II, it is a potent renal vasodilator. The vasodilator effect primarily affects the afferent arteriole and may even have some constrictor effect on the efferent arteriole. These attributes help to sustain glomerular capillary pressure and thus GFR. ANP also promotes translocation of water from the vascular to the interstitial space.

Prostaglandins

All the eicosanoid series can be produced by the kidney, but the cyclooxygenase pathway predominates. Under normal circumstances prostaglandins play no role in regulating renal vascular resistance. When the kidney is under the influence of vasoconstrictors, however, the production of vasodilator prostaglandins is stimulated and the vasoconstrictor response is significantly blunted. Blockade of prostaglandin production by nonsteroidal antiinflammatory drugs under such circumstances leads to increased vascular resistance and decreased blood flow.

Miscellaneous Factors

Thromboxanes are renal vasoconstrictors. They may participate in the pathogenesis of certain forms of acute renal failure but seem to have little effect under normal circumstances. Adenosine is a renal vasoconstrictor after ischemic injury and it has been hypothesized that it may be an important mediator of renal vascular tone in renal failure. Acetylcholine is a potent renal vasodilator but probably does not participate in normal regulation of arterial tone.

Glomerular Filtration Rate

The rate of filtration is described by the Starling equation:

$$GFR = Kf[(Pgc - Pt) - r(COPgc - COPt)] \quad (Eq. 3)$$

where
Kf = Ultrafiltration coefficient
Pgc = Hydrostatic pressure in the glomerular capillary
Pt = Hydrostatic pressure in the proximal tubule
r = Reflection coefficient
COPgc = Colloid osmotic pressure in the glomerular capillary
COPt = Colloid osmotic pressure in the proximal tubule

Ultrafiltration Coefficient

The ultrafiltration coefficient (Kf) is a reflection of both permeability and surface area available for filtration. Permeability may change because of alterations in the capillary endothelial cell, in the basement membrane, and in the slits between the foot processes, each of which presents a progressively more restrictive filtration barrier. Changes in endothelial structure that limit filtration are believed to be rare and transient. Foot process fusion is an important factor in several forms of glomerulonephritis and nephrotic syndrome but is not seen in human ATN. The surface area of the glomerular capillary apparatus is variable. Contractile elements in the glomerular mesangium respond to several vasoactive hormones (such as AVP and angiotensin II). When these constrict, the surface area available for filtration decreases in a reversible fashion. The importance of this action is unclear and has not been clearly implicated in any human form of ARF. The glomeruli are structurally normal in ATN.

Hydrostatic Pressure Gradient

The hydrostatic pressure in the glomerular capillary bed (Pgc) is determined by the mean arterial pressure (MAP), the absolute resistance of the arterioles, and the balance between preglomerular and postglomerular vascular resistance. The conducting interlobar, arcuate, and interlobular arteries cause some pressure reduction to below systemic levels, but the major reduction occurs at the afferent arteriole. The higher the mean arterial pressure, the lower the afferent arteriolar resistance, and the greater the efferent arteriolar resistance, the greater the capillary pressure favoring filtration. Pgc can never exceed systemic pressure. The Pgc in humans is estimated to be between 40 and 60 mm Hg.

The Pgc is opposed by the intratubular pressure (Pt), which is approximately 10 mm Hg. The latter pressure is elevated when filtration occurs in the presence of obstruction at any downstream point in the nephron.

Reflection Coefficient

The reflection coefficient is approximately 1.0, indicating that it nearly completely prevents filtration of macromolecules such as albumin.

Oncotic Pressure Gradient

The oncotic pressure is 20 to 25 mm Hg in normal human plasma, largely because of albumin. The reflection coefficient in the normal glomerulus is close to 1.0, so the oncotic pressure in the filtrate approaches zero. On initial inspection, it appears that the oncotic pressure gradient opposing filtration is 20 to 25 mm Hg. However, as formation of protein-free filtrate occurs, the glomerular capillary plasma oncotic pressure is raised progressively as the nonfiltered macromolecules are concentrated in the glomerular capillary plasma (Fig. 11–2, *A*). If plasma flow is sluggish, oncotic pressure in the plasma rises until it equals the hydrostatic pressure gradient, at which time filtration ceases. This state is termed filtration equilibrium (Fig. 11–2, *B*). When plasma flow is rapid, the plasma oncotic pressure does not equal the hydrostatic pressure gradient at the point where blood exits via the efferent arteriole. This state is termed filtration disequilibrium (Fig. 11–2, *C*).

GFR is inversely and linearly related to the oncotic pressure in plasma. At any hydrostatic pressure gradient, GFR rises as oncotic pressure is lowered. Thus crystalloid regimens, which significantly reduce plasma oncotic pressure, sustain GFR despite significantly lower arterial pressures, higher renal arteriolar resistances, and lower blood flow. This may be viewed as either an advantage (sustained GFR) or a disadvantage (GFR and urine flow are maintained even at relatively low values of RBF, thus masking marginal renal perfusion).

Net Ultrafiltration Pressure Gradient

The net ultrafiltration pressure gradient is proportional to the area between the curves describing the hydrostatic pressure gradient and the oncotic pressure gradient (Fig. 11–2). The net ultrafiltration pressure gradient is the mean difference between the hydrostatic pressure gradient and the rising oncotic pressure gradient. The greater the net ultrafiltration gradient, the higher the GFR. Although renal blood flow does not appear explicitly in the Starling equation, glomerular plasma flow is an important determinant of the rate of rise of the oncotic pressure gradient and thus the net ultrafiltration pressure gradient.

Practical Application of the Principles of Filtration

In critically ill patients it is crucial to avoid activating the neurohumoral systems that cause glomerular constriction (Table 11–1; see sections on arginine vasopressin and the renin-angiotensin system). The hydrostatic pressure favoring filtration is supported by sustaining an adequate blood pressure and avoiding arteriolar constriction as discussed in the section on renal blood flow. Fluid regimens that use crystalloid, thus depressing the plasma oncotic pressure, favor filtration at any given hydrostatic pressure. To the extent that hemodynamics can be sustained with crystalloid solutions alone, they favor maintenance of glomerular filtration. A note of caution is that the kidney's oxygen consumption is directly proportional to the amount of sodium filtered at the glomerulus. If the crystalloid fluid replacement results in severe anemia, marginal blood pressure, and vasoconstriction because of marginal plasma volume, the balance between renal oxygen supply and demand could theoretically become unfavorable.

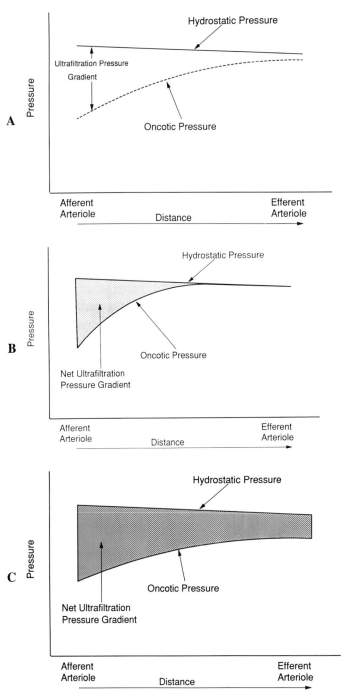

Figure 11–2. **A,** Oncotic pressure rises as glomerular capillary plasma passes from the afferent to the efferent arteriole because water is filtered from the plasma. As a result, the ultrafiltration pressure gradient becomes progressively smaller. **B,** Filtration equilibrium occurs when the plasma flow rate is low in relation to the balance between glomerular capillary and oncotic pressure. The blackened area between the oncotic and hydrostatic pressure curves represents the net ultrafiltration pressure gradient. **C,** Filtration disequilibrium occurs when the plasma flow rate is high in relation to the balance between glomerular capillary pressure and oncotic pressure. The cross-hatched area represents the net ultrafiltration pressure gradient. The cross-hatched area should be compared to the blackened area in **C,** which represents the smaller net ultrafiltration pressure gradient during states of low plasma flow. Thus plasma flow rate through the glomerular capillary bed is a major determinant of oncotic pressure. (Reproduced with permission from Maddox DA, Brenner BM: *Annual Review of Medicine,* vol 28, © 1977 by Annual Reviews Inc.)

Tubular Transport

Membrane-bound pumps, most notably the sodium–potassium–adenosine triphosphatase (Na-K-ATPase) pump, are responsible for the reabsorption out of, and secretion of substances into, the glomerular filtrate. There are several varieties of pumps, including primary active transport, secondary active transport, and carrier-mediated transport. Nearly all transport processes are in some way coupled to the transport of sodium.

Primary active transport requires direct hydrolysis of high-energy compounds, for example, the Na-K-ATPase pump on the basal membrane (interstitial side) of the tubule (Fig. 11–3). Secondary active transport occurs when the electrical or chemical gradients generated by the primary pump are coupled to movement of other substances. Transport proteins for

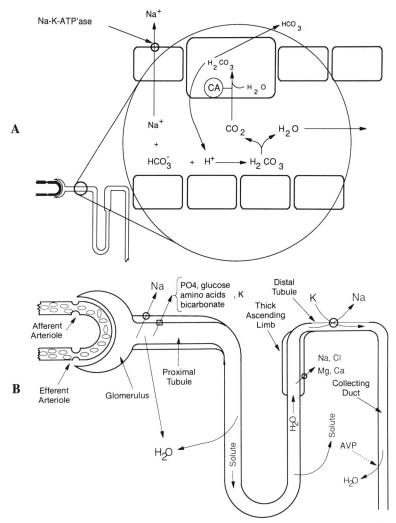

Figure 11–3. **A,** Metabolic pumps on the basal membrane of the tubular cells remove sodium from the cell interior, favoring diffusion of sodium from the filtrate into the cell. This activity is coupled to the transport of many substances, as described in the text. Sodium and bicarbonate (HCO_3^-) are filtered by the glomerulus. The process of HCO_3^- reabsorption is described in the text. CA = carbonic anhydrase. **B,** Both the active transport processes and the passive permeability properties of the nephron are sharply localized to individual segments of the nephron (axial heterogeneity). Active processes are represented by arrows passing through the tubular wall via the circles, and passive movements of water and ions are represented by arrows passing through the tubular walls without circles. For example, sodium, cloride, magnesium, and calcium are actively pumped from the filtrate in the thick ascending limb.

glucose are located in the luminal membrane. When both a sodium and a glucose molecule combine with the transport protein and the concentration gradient for sodium exists, the glucose and sodium are transported into the cell. Phosphate and amino acids are transported in a similar fashion. When sodium and the other substance are transported in the same direction, the process is termed cotransport. When the sodium and another substance move in opposite directions, it is termed countertransport. Hydrogen and calcium ions are countertransported with sodium. A primary

hydrogen ion ATPase pump also is present in the distal nephron.

Proximal Tubule

Sodium. Between 60% and 70% of the filtered sodium is reabsorbed by the proximal tubule (Fig. 11–3). The Na-K-ATPase pump in the basal membrane removes three sodium ions from the cell in exchange for two potassium ions. Potassium then diffuses out of the cell across the basal membrane down its concentration gradient. This segment is permeable to water, which passively follows the sodium, balancing the osmotic pressure across the tubule. Most of the water passes via the intercellular (paracellular) pathway.

Potassium. Nearly all filtered potassium is reabsorbed in the proximal tubule. The potassium pumped into the cell in exchange for sodium across the basal membrane diffuses down its concentration gradient into the interstitium because the permeability of the basal membrane to potassium is high. The net effect of the sodium and potassium fluxes is that the pump creates a negative charge inside the cell, favoring uptake of potassium across the luminal membrane.

Glucose. Nearly all of the filtered glucose is absorbed proximally by a sodium-glucose cotransport carrier. The maximal rate of glucose transport is approximately 300 mg/min. When the filtered load of glucose (plasma glucose × GFR) exceeds the maximal rate of transport, glucose is excreted in the urine, causing an osmotic diuresis. Glucosuria may result from one or more of three abnormalities: high plasma glucose, elevated GFR, or impaired transport.

Amino Acids. Virtually all the amino acids are reabsorbed by the proximal tubule in a system analogous to glucose transport. Damage to this segment produces aminoaciduria.

Phosphate. Phosphate is reabsorbed primarily by the proximal tubule under the influence of parathyroid hormone (PTH) by a sodium-dependent cotransport mechanism. There is also a distal PTH-sensitive transport system. PTH inhibits the reabsorption of phosphate, reducing its plasma level. Calcium is partially complexed with phosphate. If the phosphate level rises, the ionized calcium level falls, stimulating PTH release. After PTH exerts its effect, the calcium concentration rises. Glucagon, corticosteroids, and insulin may also regulate phosphate reabsorption.

Bicarbonate. Bicarbonate filtered into the proximal tubular fluid reacts with secreted hydrogen ions (Fig. 11–3, *A*) to form carbonic acid and sodium chloride. Carbonic acid dissociates into carbon dioxide and water. Carbon dioxide diffuses into the tubular epithelial cell, where it is hydrated, under the influence of carbonic anhydrase, to release hydrogen ions and bicarbonate. Hydrogen ions are secreted in exchange for sodium by a hydrogen-sodium countertransport mechanism. The bicarbonate diffuses down its electrochemical gradient across the basal membrane, into the interstitium. Bicarbonate reabsorption parallels sodium reabsorption.

Organic Acids and Bases. Organic acids in plasma, such as ketones, are actively secreted into the tubular lumen. Specific sodium cotransport proteins in the basal membrane combine with the acid and in the presence of sodium are transferred into the cell. The acid then diffuses into the filtrate through the luminal membrane, down its concentration gradient.

The proximal tubules produce ammonia from glutamine when metabolic acidosis is present. Ammonia diffuses into the filtrate and combines with hydrogen ions to form ammonium. The membrane is not permeable to the charged ammonium ion, which therefore becomes "trapped" in the filtrate.

Hydrogen Ion. Hydrogen ions secreted into the proximal tubular fluid combine with bicarbonate as discussed earlier and also react with phosphate and sulfate salts to form titratable acid. Other hydrogen ions combine with ammonia as described previously. These mechanisms account for excretion of "fixed" (that is, noncarbonic) acid, about 1 mEq/kg/d.

Calcium and Magnesium. Much of the filtered calcium and some magnesium are reabsorbed proximally and are probably both influenced by PTH.

Loop of Henle

THICK ASCENDING LIMB

Sodium and Chloride. Sodium and chloride are transported actively out of the thick ascending limb (Fig. 11–3, *B*). This lowers the osmolality of the tubular fluid because this segment of the nephron is impermeable to water.

Magnesium. The thick ascending limb is the major site for magnesium reabsorption (Fig. 11–3, *B*). Loop diuretics or disease of this segment causes magnesium wasting.

Distal Tubule

Sodium. Sodium can be reabsorbed against large concentration gradients by the distal tubule (Fig. 11–3, *B*). This transport is stimulated by aldosterone.

Potassium. Potassium is excreted in proportion to sodium reabsorption (Fig. 11–3, *B*) and is markedly increased by long-term aldosterone stimulation. The increase caused by aldosterone is associated with structural alterations of the luminal membrane that increase its surface area. Aldosterone increases the permeability of the luminal membrane to potassium and increases sodium reabsorption, which renders the lumen more electronegative. Potassium diffuses from the cell into the lumen down its electrical and chemical gradient. The faster fluid flows past the distal tubular cells, the more efficiently the gradients are maintained and the greater is the potassium loss. Thus any diuretic state tends to cause potassium loss.

Collecting Duct

The collecting duct has the capacity to reabsorb sodium. This segment may be sensitive to atrial natriuretic peptide, which inhibits sodium reabsorption. Permeability to water is regulated by AVP (Fig. 11-3, B), but water movement is a passive process, with water moving from areas of low to high osmolality.

Concentration

Final urinary concentration depends on a highly integrated series of functions involving every segment of the nephron (Fig. 11–3, B) plus the distribution of renal blood flow. Some of the intrinsic properties of more proximal nephron segments set the basis for regulation of final urinary osmolality by vasopressin. Concentrating and diluting ability is adversely affected by many diseases because integrity of all nephron segments is necessary for generation of maximal urinary osmolality.

Proximal Reabsorption

The proximal tubule (Fig. 11–3, B) normally reabsorbs 60% to 70% of the filtrate in an isotonic fashion. The proportion reabsorbed depends to some extent on filtration fraction, which is the proportion of plasma flow filtered. The higher the filtration fraction, the higher the oncotic pressure in the peritubular capillary and the greater the ability to reabsorb water. As GFR falls, the proportion of the filtrate reabsorbed by the proximal tubule rises somewhat, leaving less for more distal reabsorption. If proximal reabsorption is impaired by ischemia or toxins, the distal mechanisms are overwhelmed and the maximal urinary osmolality diminishes.

Descending Limb

The filtrate entering the descending limb is isotonic, but osmolality increases progressively during descent because the epithelium of the descending limb is water permeable but solute impermeable (Fig. 11-3, B). Thus water is passively extracted into the more hypertonic interstitium by passive forces. About half of the filtrate entering the descending limb is removed during descent.

Ascending Thin Limb

Progressively decreasing osmolality is observed in the ascending limb because it is impermeable to water and permeable to solute (Fig. 11–3, B). Thus solute passively leaves the filtrate, but volume changes little. The fluid entering the thick ascending limb is approximately isotonic.

Ascending Thick Limb

The thick ascending limb actively removes solute from the filtrate but is impermeable to water (Fig. 11–3, B). The filtrate becomes progressively more hypotonic. It is the active reabsorption of solute in this segment that provides the energy for production of the concentrated medullary interstitium. The active pumping in this segment is associated with a high level of oxygen consumption. In addition, the blood supply of the thick ascending limbs is tenuous. Thus they are commonly damaged during renal ischemia.

Collecting Duct

The collecting duct has variable permeability, which is regulated by AVP (Fig. 11–3, B). The final concentration of the urine cannot be higher than the osmolality of the medullary interstitium at the tip of the loops of Henle, nor significantly more dilute than the filtrate entering the collecting duct. Arginine-vasopressin increases the water and urea permeability of the collecting duct, allowing water to move passively from the duct into the interstitium, from which it is removed by the capillary blood flow. Prostaglandins modulate the effect of AVP on the collecting duct.

Peritubular Capillary and Vasa Recta Flow

The ratio of the rate of filtration of water and solute into the interstitium to the rate of blood flow through the interstitium is critical. A high ratio of water entry to blood flow dilutes the medullary concentration because the plasma does not carry the water away rapidly enough. A low ratio allows the blood to remove an excessive amount of solute, which overwhelms the countercurrent exchange mechanism and washes out the medullary concentration gradient.

The passive countercurrent exchange of water and solute between the ascending and descending vasa recta helps prevent medullary washout. Drugs (perhaps anesthetics) and diseases (sickle cell disease and possibly sepsis) that disturb the distribution of blood flow through the medulla prevent the development of a high medullary osmolality and limit maximal urinary concentration.

DIAGNOSIS OF ACUTE RENAL FAILURE

Acute renal failure is defined as a reduction in GFR occurring over hours to days in a patient with previously stable function. The previous level of function may or may not have been normal. A common clinical categorization consists of prerenal, intrinsic or parenchymal renal, and postrenal causes. Detection of postrenal causes is critical because therapy is radically different from that for intrinsic disease. Discrimination between prerenal and intrinsic renal causes is more difficult and less useful.

The pathogenesis of ARF should be considered in the framework of normal renal physiology outlined previously. Although renal function is classically discussed in terms of filtration, reabsorption, and secretion, all three components are critically dependent on adequate renal blood flow. Of these, filtration is the sine qua non of renal function and is the most important functional loss in ARF. Tubular dysfunction is an important component of ARF when ATN is present, and tubular damage is probably intimately related to the sustained suppression of glomerular filtration in ATN.

Estimation of Filtration Rate

Creatinine is considered the best available physiologic substrate for estimating GFR. Estimation of GFR from plasma creatinine concentration is associated with several problems:

1. Creatinine is filtered and secreted, and the degree of secretion increases as the plasma level rises. Thus the measurement of serum creatinine or creatinine clearance (Ccr) overestimates GFR by as much as 30% in renal failure.

2. The rate of creatinine production is proportional to muscle mass ($15 \text{ mg} \cdot \text{kg}^{-1} \cdot \text{day}^{-1}$ for women and $20 \text{ mg} \cdot \text{kg}^{-1} \cdot \text{day}^{-1}$ for men) and gradually falls with age. Not only does muscle mass vary with age, sex, and physical conditioning, it falls rapidly in critically ill patients. Thus the normal range of production is wide

and production is variable in critically ill patients.

3. Because the plasma level varies inversely with GFR and volume of distribution and directly with muscle mass, abrupt changes in GFR are not reflected immediately in the plasma creatinine level. Thus, if the plasma level is used to monitor GFR, the recognition of declining or improving renal function is delayed.

4. Creatinine concentration is falsely elevated by the presence of noncreatinine chromogens, such as ketones, flucytosine, and some cephalosporins (for example, cephalothin, cefoxitin, and ceforanide) when measured by spectrophotometric methods.

5. Creatinine secretion is impaired by some drugs (for example, cimetidine and trimethoprim-sulfamethoxazole), leading to increases in creatinine concentration, although GFR is unchanged.

6. The plasma creatinine concentration is geometrically related to the GFR after reaching steady state. Thus a halving of GFR leads to a doubling of plasma creatinine. A patient with a normal GFR of 100 ml/min and normal plasma creatinine level of 0.7 mg/dl needs to lose 50% of the GFR and wait 2 to 3 days for equilibrium to occur before the plasma creatinine level exceeds the upper limit of normal plasma creatinine (1.5 mg/dl). The resulting broad range of normal and abnormal values seriously limits the diagnostic utility of the plasma creatinine level and argues strongly for monitoring of creatinine clearance as an estimate of GFR.

Creatinine clearance is an imperfect measure of GFR, but it is far superior to measurement of plasma creatinine concentrations alone. Measurement of urine flow rate is associated with errors in volume because of unequal bladder emptying at the beginning and end of the collection period. These errors can be reduced by collecting large volumes of urine. For example, a 10 ml error represents a 20% error in a 50 ml collection and a 5% error in a 200 ml collection. Unfortunately, the longer the collection time, the less relevant the data for acute decision making in patients with declining renal function. In general, clearances calculated from collections of 2 hours' duration are representative of values calculated from longer collections.

Renal Dysfunction and Renal Failure

A reduction in GFR that requires modification of diet or drug dosage can be termed renal dysfunction. A loss sufficient to result in acidosis, hyperkalemia, or fluid overload despite a normal intake is termed renal failure. When the creatinine clearance falls below 40 ml/min (approximately $25 \; \text{ml} \cdot \text{m}^{-2} \cdot \text{min}^{-1}$, or 40% of normal), several drugs require dosage reduction. This level of dysfunction also narrows the range of compensation for variations in catabolism and intake of protein and electrolytes. When GFR is less than 15 ml/min (approximately $10 \; \text{ml} \cdot \text{m}^{-2} \cdot \text{min}^{-1}$, or 15% of normal), the ability to compensate for changes in intake or production is exhausted, which results in abnormalities of extracellular fluid volume or composition. Deviation from normal fluid volume status and hemodynamic parameters causes transient reductions in GFR. Thus filtration failure should be diagnosed when Ccr is $< 10 \; \text{ml} \cdot \text{m}^{-2} \cdot \text{min}^{-1}$ for 2 days or longer after adequate fluid and hemodynamic resuscitation.

Tubular Abnormalities

Evidence of tubular dysfunction and damage is required for a diagnosis of ATN (Fig. 11–4 and Table 11–3). Tubular dysfunction is manifest as abnormalities in reabsorption and secretion. A number of tests based on abnormalities of tubular function aid in differentiating between oliguria caused by prerenal factors and that caused by intrinsic renal damage. Reabsorption of water causes the concentration of (the nonreabsorbable) creatinine in the tubular fluid to rise. When tubular reabsorption is depressed by tubular dysfunction or cell death, urinary creatinine concentration fails to increase normally and the ratio of urine to plasma concentration falls. The tubules' ability to produce a concentrated medullary interstitium is impaired, resulting in inability to concentrate or dilute the final urine. Impairment of sodium reabsorption causes the proportion of filtered sodium that is excreted to increase. Thus the fractional excretion of sodium (FeNa) rises (Table 11–3). The excretion of glucose, bicarbonate, and amino acids increases because of damage to the proximal tubule where these substances are normally completely reabsorbed. Beta$_2$ microglobulin is a small protein that is filtered and then removed from the filtrate by the proximal tubules. Patients with ATN excrete increased amounts.

Thus tubular dysfunction can be defined as inability to appropriately concentrate or dilute the urine, concentrate creatinine or urea, and reabsorb sodium. Typical values for urinary findings in ATN are shown in Table 11–3.

Elevation of FeNa in the stressed or oliguric patient reflects tubular dysfunction or death.

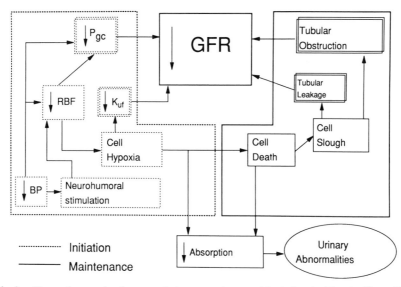

Figure 11–4. The pathogenesis of acute tubular necrosis caused by ischemia. The double outlined boxes represent the four major hypotheses regarding the cause of filtration failure. The areas outlined by dashed lines represent factors operative during the initiation phase of ATN, and those outlined with solid lines represent factors active in and responsible for the maintenance phase after correction of the initiating factors. Nephrotoxins may operate during the initiation phase to produce the same overall results as cellular hypoxia. Cellular dysfunction or cellular death results in impaired reabsorption and secretion, thus producing the chemical abnormalities shown in Table 11–3. The sloughing of dead cells and formation of casts produce characteristic signs in the urinary sediment (Table 11-4).

TABLE 11–3. Urinary Indices in Oliguria

	PRERENAL	TUBULAR DYSFUNCTION
UNa (mEq/L)	<20	>40
FeNa (%)	<1	>2
RFI	<1	>2
Urine/plasma creatinine ratio	>40	<20
Urine/plasma urea ratio	>8	<3
Plasma urea/creatinine	>20	10
UOsm (% of plasma)	>120	80-120
TCH$_2$O (ml/h)	<−15 >+15	−15 to +15
Urine chloride	<20	>20

UNa = sodium concentration in the urine. FeNa = fractional excretion of sodium. RFI = renal failure index. UOsm = osmolality of urine in milliosmoles per kilogram of water. FeNa is calculated by dividing the clearance of Na by the clearance of creatinine (Cr) and converted to a percent by multiplying by 100: FeNa (%) = 100 × (UNa/PNa)/(UCr/PCr). PNa = concentration of sodium in plasma. UCr = concentration of creatinine in urine. The renal failure index is similar: RFI = UNa/(Ucr/Pcr). Total water clearance (TCH$_2$O): TCH$_2$O = V/t − { (UOsm/POsm) × V/t}. V = urine flow rate in milliliters. t = time in minutes.

Unfortunately, the FeNa test does not reliably identify individual patients whose GFR improves after correction of fluid and hemodynamic abnormalities, even though it correctly classifies most groups of patients. FeNa remains elevated during the first 1 to 2 weeks of the diuretic phase, indicating persistent tubular dysfunction.

Tubular damage may be detected by finding abnormal cellular enzymes in the urine. These include lactic dehydrogenase, L-alanine aminopeptidase, ligandin, beta-glucuronidase, N-acetylbeta-D-glucosaminidase, gamma-glutamyltranspeptidase, leucine aminopeptidase, and alkaline phosphatase. Adenosine deaminase–binding protein is a basement membrane antigen whose levels are elevated in acute pyelonephritis, renal allograft rejection, prerenal oliguria, and ATN. These tests are mostly of research interest.

The urinary sediment should always be examined when renal dysfunction is suspected (Table 11–4). In ATN, tubular epithelial cells slough and form epithelial cellular and granular casts. Excretion of epithelial cells and cellular casts indicates structural tubular injury. White blood cells and white blood cell casts may be present in ATN but are more commonly associated with inflammatory conditions, such as pyelonephritis or allergic interstitial nephritis. Hematuria, red blood cell casts, and heavy proteinuria are associated with acute glomerular injury, not ATN. The presence of crystals of sulfonamide drugs or uric acid may give clues regarding the etiology of ARF.

Urine Flow Rate

ARF is subclassified as anuric (urine flow rate <100 ml/d), oliguric (100 to 400 ml/d), nonoliguric (400 to 2000 ml/d), or polyuric (>2000 ml/d). For many years, ATN was recognized only in association with oliguria. However, most patients with ATN are not oliguric. The classi-

TABLE 11–4. Abnormalities Observed in Urinary Sediment in Acute Kidney Disease

FINDING	ACUTE TUBULAR NECROSIS	GLOMERULONEPHRITIS	INTERSTITIAL NEPHRITIS	PYELONEPHRITIS
Red blood cells	0	+ + +	0	
Red cell casts	0	+ + +	0	0
White cells	0	0	+	+ + + +
White cell casts	0	+	+	+ + + +
Eosinophiluria	0	0	+	0
Epithelial cells	+		+	
Cellular casts	+ +	0	+ +	
Pigmented casts	+ +	+	0	0
Granular casts	+ + +	0	0	+
Protein	+	+ + +	+	+ +
Lipid	0	+ +	+	0
Crystals	0	0	0	0

0 indicates that the finding is generally absent. The plus signs indicate a semiquantitative estimate of the degree of abnormality likely to be seen. Blanks indicate an absence of good information.

fication is useful because nonoliguric patients have sustained a lesser insult and have a better prognosis for recovery of renal function and survival. In any category of patients with ATN the presence of oliguria or anuria doubles the mortality rate.

Oliguria

The minimal urine output consistent with normal renal function is related to osmolar balance. Electrolytes and urea account for most of the urinary osmoles. A normal diet produces approximately 12 mOsm $\cdot$ kg^{-1} $\cdot$ day^{-1}, or 0.5 mOsm $\cdot$ kg^{-1} $\cdot$ hour^{-1}. Maximally concentrated urine contains approximately 1 mOsm/ml. Thus a urine output of at least 0.5 ml $\cdot$ kg^{-1} $\cdot$ hour^{-1} is required to maintain osmolar balance. If the urine osmolality is lower, a higher urine output is needed to maintain osmolar balance. Patients can produce less urine than this with a normal GFR if the proportion of filtrate reabsorbed proximally increases because of reduction in renal blood flow. Critically ill patients may excrete 1½ to 3 times the normal osmolar load, necessitating a significantly higher urine output. Most patients with a urine flow rate less than 0.5 to 0.7 ml $\cdot$ kg^{-1} $\cdot$ hour^{-1} have a depressed GFR and are at risk of ARF. Most clinical studies of patients with ARF have defined oliguria as 400 ml/d or less, equivalent to only 0.24 ml $\cdot$ kg^{-1} $\cdot$ hour^{-1}. Thus the definition of oliguric renal failure should not be confused with the definition of oliguria per se.

Classification

ARF secondary to ATN can be classified according to three components: filtration failure, tubular dysfunction or damage, and urine output. For early recognition, monitoring of filtration by frequent, repetitive measurements of creatinine clearance should be routine in high-risk, critically ill patients. When creatinine clearance falls, evidence for tubular and glomerular injury should be sought by measurement of FeNa and water clearance and examination of the urinary sediment.

Other Diagnostic Procedures

Renal uptake of technetium-99m dimercaptosuccinic acid, intravenous urography, computed tomography scans, and retrograde pyelography have limited value in evaluating ARF patients. Radionuclide flow scans are useful for documenting vascular patency when major arterial or venous occlusion is suspected. Angiography is used when vascular repair is contemplated, recognizing the risk of further damage secondary to injection of a radiocontrast agent.

Ultrasonography is highly useful for eliminating urinary tract obstruction and assessing kidney size, which is reduced in chronic renal disease and may be increased by edema during ATN.

Biopsy is rarely performed in critically ill patients because ATN is by far the most likely diagnosis. Biopsy may be indicated in patients with evidence of glomerular injury or interstitial nephritis because some of these patients respond to antiinflammatory therapy. Biopsy is occasionally performed during prolonged anuria to clarify the prognosis for recovery of function. If cortical necrosis is found, long-term dialysis is usually required.

PATHOGENESIS OF ACUTE TUBULAR NECROSIS

The events initiating ARF are different from those maintaining it (Fig. 11–4). A variety of physiologic disturbances can alter glomerular hemodynamics, causing the acute phase of filtration failure. The sustained reduction in GFR during ATN probably results from tubular damage.

Initiation Phase of Ischemic Acute Tubular Necrosis

Reduced Renal Blood Flow

During the initiation phase of ischemic ATN, renal blood flow is believed to be reduced to a level that does not support GFR. Ischemic damage occurs to the tubules, particularly the proximal tubule and thick ascending limb of Henle's loop (Fig. 11–4). RBF is about 60% of control values in patients in shock. Most of the reduction is due to hypotension, but RVR is elevated rather than reduced.

Research has failed to demonstrate a primary role for the renin-angiotensin system in the vasoconstriction seen in ARF. Inhibition of prostaglandin synthesis potentiates a variety of renal insults but is not an initiating factor by itself. Vasopressin is a potent vasoconstrictor, but its role in inducing ARF is unclear. Blockade of alpha-adrenergic receptors improves renal perfusion after ischemic insults. In theory, blockade of these receptors coupled with maintenance of MAP could improve maintenance of RBF. Calcium channel blockers provide some protection against norepinephrine-induced ATN in animals but not against ARF caused by renal arterial clamping. Thus the protective effect appears to result from vasodilation, not prevention of cell death by calcium entry.

Atrial natriuretic peptide has provided excellent protection against ischemic ATN in animal models. Stimulation of endogenous release by aggressive volume expansion may explain some of the protective value of fluid loading in patients at risk for ATN, as well as in animal models. The mechanism of this protection may involve vasodilation, but this is unproven.

Tubular Dysfunction and Damage

The ischemic damage during ischemic ATN is maximal in the pars recta of the proximal tubule and thick ascending limbs of the deeper, juxtamedullary nephrons. This probably relates to the high rates of sodium transport and their location in an area with a tenuous blood supply.

The blood supply to the juxtamedullary region of the kidney is much less than to the superficial cortex. The outer medullary vasculature is congested with erythrocytes during ATN. It has been hypothesized that cellular swelling during ischemia extracts fluid from the extracellular and vascular spaces, leaving behind the erythrocyte-rich blood congesting the vasculature. Thus blood flow to this region may be more impaired for a longer time than elsewhere in the cortex.

During the initiation phase of ATN, proximal tubular dysfunction results in delivery of increased amounts of solute to the loop of Henle, increasing pumping activity by the thick ascending limb. Two findings support the importance of increased metabolic activity in damaging this nephron segment. First, ischemic damage to the thick ascending limb is worse when renal perfusion is only impaired, thus permitting some filtration, rather than totally occluded. Second, inhibition of electrolyte transport by furosemide can protect against ischemic injury to the thick ascending limb when the drug is given before the insult. Defective reabsorption of sodium and chloride at this site and in the proximal tubule releases renin, activates the tubuloglomerular feedback loop, and results in a reduced glomerular plasma flow and GFR, tending to perpetuate the ischemia. The relatively greater loss of deeper nephrons and of the thick ascending limb might also explain the early

and nearly universal loss of concentrating ability in ischemic acute renal failure.

Mechanisms of Ischemic Damage

LOSS OF ADENOSINE TRIPHOSPHATE

The rate at which the energy stores are depleted is determined by the balance between the rate of sodium transport and the delivery of oxygen and substrate. Sodium transport is determined primarily by the filtered load of sodium. When this balance is upset, ATP levels fall, followed by inhibition of pumping by the Na-K-ATPase membrane pump. If ATP–magnesium chloride is infused, or renal blood flow is improved, cellular energy stores are restored and ATN is prevented.

CALCIUM ACCUMULATION

Intracellular calcium concentration rises after reperfusion because of increased membrane permeability produced by oxygen radicals. However, calcium channel blockers do not protect animals against renal failure by preventing intracellular calcium accumulation. This failure to protect may be due to the presence of abundant intracellular calcium stores or alternate calcium channels.

REDUCED ULTRAFILTRATION COEFFICIENT

The epithelial cell bodies and podocytes may flatten and increase the degree of coverage of the glomerular capillary bed during the initiation phase of ischemic ARF, thus reducing Kf (Fig. 11–4). Reperfusion rapidly reverses this finding, which is not important during the maintenance phase of ARF. Angiotensin II can produce similar changes in glomerular ultrastructure. The reduction in Kf may be due to reduction in surface area available for filtration rather than a change in permeability. In addition, preferential shunting of blood through short capillary loops or contraction of the glomerular mesangium could cause such changes. Thus changes in Kf may acutely reduce filtration.

NET ULTRAFILTRATION PRESSURE GRADIENT

A reduction in MAP or RBF or an increase in the ratio of afferent to efferent arteriolar resistance decreases the net ultrafiltration pressure gradient. This is probably the major reason for the acute failure of filtration during the shock stage.

Maintenance Phase

Reduced Renal Blood Flow

RBF remains depressed in established ATN even after full hemodynamic resuscitation. However, restoration of total RBF to normal, by volume loading and vasodilators, does not restore filtration during the maintenance phase. In some animal models autoregulation is markedly impaired, with blood flow falling passively with blood pressure (Fig. 11–1, *B*). In addition, the renal vasculature of kidneys damaged by ischemia becomes hyperreactive to sympathetic nerve stimulation. Paradoxically, responsiveness to infused vasoconstrictors, such as angiotensin and norepinephrine, is reduced.

The accumulation of blood cells in the vasa recta may be due to endothelial damage during the initiation phase. In addition, tubules, dilated by obstruction and swelling, may impinge on the peritubular capillaries, increasing vascular congestion.

Reduced Ultrafiltration Coefficient

Glomerular structure is normal or minimally abnormal in ATN. A reduced Kf is not believed to be important during the maintenance phase (Fig. 11–4).

Reduced Net Ultrafiltration Pressure Gradient

The result of tubular obstruction is to raise tubular pressure, depressing the ultrafiltration pressure gradient.

Tubular Obstruction

Cellular anoxia or toxins cause dysfunction of membrane sodium pumps. Swelling and death of the tubular cells, especially of the proximal tubular and thick ascending limb segments, result. The processes resulting in cell death begin during the initiation phase. The cellular swelling and subsequent sloughing of necrotic debris obstruct the tubule (Fig. 11–4), elevating the proximal tubular pressure. This slows flow through the remaining portion of the nephron, allowing Tamm-Horsfall proteins to reach a concentration that causes precipitation into obstructive casts. Interstitial edema or extrinsic compression can also lead to tubular obstruction.

The preceding hypothesis is not universally accepted because histologic damage does not seem to correlate with the degree of dysfunction, especially in humans. However, some have argued that a strong correlation exists between the degree of tubular necrosis, the degree of tubular obstruction, and the degree of functional impairment.

Backleak of Glomerular Filtrate

The pathologic picture, especially in animal models, reveals extensive tubular necrosis with denudation of the basement membrane. This, coupled with the apparently normal glomeruli, suggests that filtrate may be formed and then leak back through the damaged tubules to be reabsorbed into the circulation (Fig. 11–4). This mechanism is applicable only during maintenance of ARF, not initiation. In human, nonoliguric renal failure as much as 44% of the filtrate may be reabsorbed. The GFR in these patients was depressed to an average of 5 $ml \cdot min^{-1} \cdot 1.73 \ m^{-2}$. Even if no backleak had occurred, GFR still would have been depressed by 90%. Thus the quantitative contribution of backleak to GFR reduction was minimal.

Therapeutic Implications

These hypotheses have therapeutic implications. The congested vessels can be flushed out by raising perfusion pressure and reducing vascular resistance. Increased renal perfusion pressure should decrease the medullary congestion and improve GFR. Volume loading should release atrial natriuretic peptide (ANP), which helps restore renal blood flow and favors filtration. The more rapidly substrate delivery to the cells is restored, the more rapidly cell swelling is reversed and vascular congestion is cleared, and the less necrosis occurs. Rapid establishment of osmotic diuresis during the initiation phase may flush out necrotic debris as it forms and prevent the formation of obstructing casts.

CAUSES OF ACUTE RENAL FAILURE

ARF is classified into prerenal, parenchymal, and postrenal. Parenchymal ARF may be caused by anoxia, toxins, metabolic abnormalities, immunologic disorders, infiltration of parenchyma, and acute infection (Table 11–5). In many cases the etiology is multifactorial and one abnormality potentiates the effects of another. Among the critically ill, however, the majority of cases are related to renal anoxia, toxic chemicals, and metabolic factors.

Postrenal causes (Table 11–5) must be diagnosed quickly because therapy is usually a

TABLE 11–5. Causes of Acute Renal Failure

Anoxic or Ischemic Causes

Shock
  Hypovolemic
  Cardiogenic
  Vasogenic
Vascular occlusion
  Venous thrombosis
  Arterial
  Thrombosis
  Embolism
  Stenosis
Drugs
  Radiocontrast agents (may decrease ultrafiltration coefficient)
  Nonsteroidal antiinflammatory drugs
  Angiotensin converting enzyme inhibitor drugs
  Vasoconstrictors
Systemic diseases
Sepsis
Sickle cell disease
Hemolytic-uremic syndrome
Vasculitis
Malignant hypertension
Chronic hypertension
Hepatorenal syndrome
Disseminated intravascular coagulation
Elevated intraabdominal pressure
Diabetes mellitus

Toxins
Environmental Agents

Heavy metals
  Mercury
  Arsenic
  Lead
  Bismuth
  Uranium
  Barium
  Gold
  Copper
  Iron
  Cadmium
Organic solvents
  Carbon tetrachloride
  Ethylene glycol
  Trichloroethylene
Mushroom poisoning
Paraquat
Chlordane
Elemental phosphorus

Drugs

Antibiotics
  Aminoglycosides
  Amphotericin
  Sulfonamides
  Colistin/polymixin
  Tetracycline
  Cephalosporins
  Rifampin
Anti-cancer agents
    Cisplatin
    Doxorubicin
    Interferon

Interleukin-2
Nitrosoureas
Methotrexate
Mitomycin C
Mithramycin
Streptozotocin
5-Azacitidine
Miscellaneous agents
  Acetaminophen
  Anesthetics (methoxyflurane)
  Cyclosporine
  EDTA
  Mannitol
  Nonsteroidal antiinflammatory drugs
  Radiocontrast agents
  Lithium

Metabolic Causes

Hyperuricemia (tumor lysis syndrome)
Hypercalcemia
Hypokalemia
Myoglobinuria
  Excessive muscle activity
    Seizure
    Malignant hyperthermia
    Vigorous exercise
  Muscle ischemia
    Crush injury
    Improper intraoperative positioning
    Carbon monoxide poisoning
  Hypokalemia
  Hypophosphatemia
  Drug overdose
    Alcohol
    Methanol
    Cocaine
    Narcotics
    Amphetamines
    Phencyclidine
  Head injury
  Hyperthermia
  Hypothermia
  Viral infection
  Snake bites
  Electrical burns
  Succinylcholine
  Genetic diseases
    Glycogen storage disease
    Muscular dystrophy
Hemoglobinuria
  Transfusion reaction
  Burn injury
  Congenital red cell diseases
  Heat stroke
  Cardiopulmonary bypass
  Malaria
  Snake venom
  Prosthetic heart valve
  Drugs
  Water intoxication
Multiple myeloma
Obstructive jaundice
Oxalate

TABLE 11–5. Causes of Acute Renal Failure—cont'd

Immune Causes	Infiltrative Causes
Allergic interstitial nephritis	Tumor
Penicillins	Amyloid
Cephalosporins	Sarcoid
Sulfonamides	
Rifampin	**Infectious Causes**
Phenytoin	Interstitial infection
Cimetidine	Systemic effect of sepsis elsewhere
Nonsteroidal antiinflammatory drugs	
Thiazides	**Postrenal Causes**
Furosemide	*Obstruction*
Triamterene	Intraluminal obstruction
Glomerulonephritis	Stones
Secondary to infection elsewhere	Clots
Abscesses	Extrinsic compression
Bacterial endocarditis	Tumor
Ventriculoperitoneal shunts	Iatrogenic (ligation)
Poststreptococcal	
Secondary to systemic autoimmune disorder	*Disruption*
Vasculitis	Traumatic
	Iatrogenic

surgical intervention and untreated obstruction may lead to permanent kidney damage. Ultrasound examination of the kidneys and collecting systems is the best single test for obstruction.

Ischemia and Anoxia

Hypotension by itself can reduce renal blood flow and glomerular capillary pressure sufficiently to halt filtration. However, it rarely results in ARF unless accompanied by significant systemic soft tissue damage or infection. Hypotension also stimulates the sympathetic nervous system, renin release, and vasopressin release, which further reduce renal blood flow. Hypotension is a potent contributor to ARF in conjunction with a variety of other renal insults.

Vascular Occlusion

Acute renal arterial or venous occlusion may result from thrombosis, trauma, generalized arteritis, or embolism of atheromatous material, especially during aortic surgery. Major vascular occlusion usually results in renal infarction rather than ATN. Early recognition and revascularization are critical to outcome but exceedingly difficult to achieve.

Sepsis

Sepsis is believed to be a major risk factor for ARF, but the mechanisms have not been fully clarified in clinical or experimental studies. RBF has been reported to fall in septic patients. Endotoxin causes variable changes in RBF and RVR, but GFR generally falls. Urine flow rate may increase or decrease, but urine osmolality falls. Endotoxin may cause sequestration of leukocytes in peritubular capillaries with stasis of erythrocytes. In addition, endothelial lesions appear, resulting in peritubular capillary disruption. Endotoxin greatly potentiates the effect of renal ischemia in rats. The latter conforms to the suspicions of many clinicians that even brief episodes of hypotension or low cardiac output in patients with toxic effects may result in rapid loss of renal function, whereas the kidneys of patients without sepsis often tolerate prolonged hypotension. Many of the effects of endotoxin can be reproduced by infusion of cachectin (TNFa), an endogenous mediator of inflammation. Cachectin promotes vasoconstriction of many vascular beds and damages the endothelium. Its role in ARF will undoubtedly receive attention in the future. Finally, bacteremia may potentiate the nephrotoxicity of aminoglycoside antibiotics.

Hepatorenal Syndrome

The hepatorenal syndrome (HRS) is defined as oliguria, rising serum creatinine level, low urine sodium and FeNa levels, and no significant abnormalities on urinalysis in a patient with established liver disease, most commonly cirrhosis. The prognosis is uniformly bad and depends primarily on the reversibility of the hepatic lesion. Most evidence suggests a functional lesion. Evidence for the presence of tubular damage exists. For example, enzymuria and elevated beta$_2$ microglobulin excretion are found in cirrhotic patients with HRS. Evidence for renal vasospasm is present in washout curves of radio-active xenon injected into the renal artery and on renal arteriograms.

Despite the apparent functional nature of the lesion, suggested management strategies have met with limited success. Relative hypovolemia may result from hypoalbuminemia and pooling of blood in the splanchnic and peripheral venous beds. Absorption of endotoxins may occur because of collaterals that bypass the reticuloendothelial system of the liver and because of the absence of bile salts. Aldosterone levels do not correlate with the sodium reten-tion. Correction of increased intraabdominal pressure by paracentesis or insertion of a peritoneovenous shunt has improved renal function in some cases.

Increased Intraabdominal Pressure

Increased intraabdominal pressure, caused by tense ascites or postoperative changes, may cause significant renal dysfunction or ARF. Elevation of renal venous pressure or direct renal compression seems the most likely mech-anism. Renal function responds to measures that reduce the tension. Intraabdominal pres-sure can be estimated by measuring bladder (greater than 25 mm Hg is abnormal) or intragastric pressure.

Toxicity

Many drugs and nontherapeutic chemicals are associated with ARF (Table 11–5). Readers are referred to more extensive reviews for details.

Aminoglycosides

The proximal tubules accumulate aminogly-cosides, causing tubular dysfunction and necro-sis. Dysfunction may appear or persist after drug administration has stopped, since renal tissue half-life is about 100 hours. Toxicity may be potentiated by hypokalemia, gram-negative bac-teremia, volume depletion, magnesium deple-tion, increased frequency of dosage, and male sex. Gentamicin causes interstitial nephritis in females.

Nonsteroidal Antiinflammatory Drugs

Nonsteroidal antiinflammatory drugs inhibit the production of renal vasodilator prostaglan-dins. Thus vasoconstriction is unopposed and the risk of ARF caused by other factors may be potentiated.

Angiotensin Converting Enzyme Inhibitors

Angiotensin converting enzyme inhibitors may cause ARF when arterial inflow is impeded by renal arterial stenosis. In such patients GFR is sustained by an increased filtration fraction caused by an increase in efferent tone secondary to angiotensin II stimulation. A reduction in efferent arteriolar tone caused by blockade of angiotensin II production reduces glomerular ultrafiltration pressure.

Radiocontrast Agents

Ionic radiocontrast agents cause renal failure. Risk factors include preexisting renal disease, diabetes mellitus, type of study, volume of contrast injected, heart disease, and perhaps dehydration. Although dehydration may in-crease the risk, intentional overhydration does not have a major protective effect. Replacement of the urine lost through the osmotic diuretic effect of the radiocontrast agent is critical.

Metabolic Causes

Myoglobinuria

Myoglobinuria caused by rhabdomyolysis has been associated with multiple causes (Table 11–5). Rhabdomyolysis has been suggested as a cause of ARF in sickle cell disease.

Myoglobinuria is associated with a rise in se-rum creatine phosphokinase (CPK) and lactic dehydrogenase (LDH) levels in a ratio of about 10:1, indicating severe muscle damage. Patients with myoglobinuria are at risk for ARF, al-though the exact mechanism is unclear because myoglobin itself is not a potent nephrotoxin. It seems likely that the combination of hypov-olemia and tissue destruction with activation of inflammatory mediators leads to reductions in RBF and GFR. The filtered myoglobin may then precipitate in the tubules, sustaining the reduction in GFR.

In animal models significant protection is afforded by saline loading or mannitol infusion. The injury is worsened by dehydration. Because myoglobin is more soluble in alkaline solutions, plasma pH should be kept normal or alkaline. A brisk solute diuresis should be induced with or without a diuretic with proximal tubular action, such as mannitol. Although these steps are rational, clinical studies demonstrating improved outcome after alkalinization and diuresis are not available.

Rhabdomyolysis-induced ARF is associated with hyperuricemia, hyperkalemia, hyperphosphatemia, hypocalcemia, and disproportionately elevated plasma creatinine levels. Hypocalcemia is due to tissue calcium deposition. Hypercalcemia commonly develops during the diuretic phase of rhabdomyolysis-induced ARF and is probably related to elevation of 1,25-$(OH)_2$-vitamin D.

Hemoglobinuria

Hemoglobinuria results when hemolysis outstrips the body's ability to bind and degrade hemoglobin. In an ICU this most commonly occurs when clerical error results in ABO or Rh transfusion incompatibility. Hemoglobin itself is not a significant nephrotoxin, but its presence combined with dehydration and hemodynamic instability commonly leads to ARF. Comments relative to the pathogenesis and management of myoglobinuric ARF are applicable in hemoglobinuria.

Jaundice

The risk of ARF after biliary surgery for obstructive jaundice is related to the bilirubin level. It has been suggested that renal dysfunction is related to absorption of excessive endotoxin because of a deficiency of bile acids in the gastrointestinal tract. Establishing diuresis before surgery by mannitol administration appears protective.

Immune Causes

Several drugs cause allergic interstitial nephritis (Table 11–5). About 50% of patients have a rash, 75% have fever, 80% have eosinophilia, and many have eosinophiluria.

RISK OF ACUTE RENAL FAILURE

The incidence of ARF is estimated to be between 0.1% and 4.9% of hospitalized patients. One might predict that the incidence of ARF would be higher in ICUs, but this has received little attention. In one study of all patients with ARF, 63% were in ICUs, but it is not entirely clear whether ARF or the critical illness occurred first. Identification of patients at high risk should lead to more intense monitoring of renal function, fluid balance, and hemodynamic

TABLE 11–6. Potential Risk Factors for Acute Renal Failure

Physiologic or Metabolic Abnormalities

Physiologic factors
  Advanced age
  Hemodynamic abnormalities
    Elevated or reduced central venous pressure
    Hypotension
    Reduced renal perfusion pressure
    Low or high cardiac index
    High or low oxygen extraction ratio
    High or low oxygen consumption
    High or low systemic vascular resistance
  Positive fluid balance
  Edema
  High protein intake
  Hypokalemia
  Low plasma fibronectin levels
Signs of sympathetic nervous system activation
  Tachycardia
  Sweating
  Cool skin
Signs of kidney stress
  Low fractional excretion of sodium
  High fractional excretion of potassium
  Oliguria or polyuria
  Negative free water clearance
  High urinary osmolality
  Urine/plasma osmolality
  Low osmolar excretion (urinary osmolality × volume)

Procedures

Major vascular procedures with
  Aortic clamping
  Renal artery clamp
  Renal vascular interruption
Cardiopulmonary bypass
Operations for obstructive jaundice
Blood transfusion
Major orthopedic procedures
  Pelvis
  Femur
  Lumbar spine
  Thoracic spine
Major trauma

---

function. Surprisingly little data are available to define risk factors. Potential and reported risk factors for ARF include the etiologic factors already presented in Table 11–5. Table 11–6 presents other factors that have identified high-risk patients or are related to one or more of the hypotheses regarding the pathogenesis of ATN.

Physiologic Abnormalities

Certain physiologic abnormalities (Table 11–6) may be related to ARF. The role of advanced age has been unclear. After correction for the effects of underlying diseases, age may not be an independent risk factor. Nevertheless, even a healthy elderly patient has decreased reserves in every organ system.

High or low central venous pressure (CVP) is a potential risk factor. An elevated CVP results in an even higher RVP, thus reducing RPP. Conversely, low filling pressures are associated with hypovolemia. Hypovolemia causes both direct depression of cardiac output and activation of protective neurohumoral systems.

Positive fluid balance is commonly seen before onset of ATN. Possible reasons include translocation of fluid out of the intravascular space resulting in hypovolemia, fluid and salt retention because of activation of the renal regulatory hormones, or even the onset of renal failure itself. The positive water and sodium balance results in edema.

Several medical procedures have been associated with a high risk of ARF (Table 11–6), the mechanisms of which have not been clarified.

Massive muscle injury, visceral trauma, shock, severe sepsis, and hypoxia have been associated with an increased risk of ATN. Although ARF developed in only 5.2% of severely injured patients, injuries of more than one site were associated with a significantly increased risk of ARF: 3.2% of patients with a single major injury, compared with 18% of those with more than one major injury. Isolated, noncritical injuries were associated with a less than 1% chance of ATN. In contrast, two critical injuries were associated with a 30% risk. Among patients in whom ATN developed, oliguria occurred in 25.9% of patients with multiple injuries and 13.8% of patients with isolated injuries. Injuries to the abdomen, thigh or leg, head, or cervical spine were directly correlated with the incidence of ARF.

Chronic Disease States

Hypertension (Table 11–5) is associated with chronic vascular disease and causes a shift of the autoregulatory range to higher values. Diabetes mellitus causes chronic renal insufficiency and generalized vascular disease.

Long-Term Drug Therapy

Long-term use of diuretics is associated with a variety of abnormalities that may predispose to ARF, including hypovolemia, activation of the renin-angiotensin axis, hypokalemia, reduced RBF, and hypertension. NSAIDs are discussed in a previous section.

Short-Term Drug Therapy

Certain drugs may cause tubular necrosis in uniquely susceptible patients or in toxic doses (Table 11–5). They may be considered risk factors because of the variable expression of their toxicity or because they may potentiate the effects of other injurious factors, such as sepsis or ischemia.

Mortality Rate

Several factors influence the mortality rates of patients with ARF. Outcome in patients with multiple organ failure correlates with the number of organs failing. The sicker the patient with renal failure, the worse the prognosis. ARF is a disease that complicates other frequently lethal diseases.

Surgical patients with ARF, especially after cardiovascular, trauma, general, and aortic surgery, usually have a poorer outcome than medical patients.

Hypovolemia, cardiogenic shock, cardiovascular complications, hypotension, heart failure, use of inotropic drugs, prior heart disease, tachycardia, hypervolemia, and preoperative hypotension are associated with an increased death rate in patients with ARF. Sepsis is frequently cited as the most common cause of death in ARF.

Central nervous system depression, underlying malignancy, burn injury, jaundice, pancreatitis, malnutrition, a requirement for parenteral nutrition, hypercatabolism, and disseminated intravascular coagulation correlate with mortality rate. Male sex and advanced age have sometimes been correlated with mortality rate. As discussed earlier, oliguric patients are at greater risk of dying than nonoliguric ones.

Patients who require hemodialysis may have a higher mortality rate than those who do not. However, mortality rate is unrelated to the dialysis intensity, duration, or number of times. The influence of prior renal disease on outcome is not clear.

Mortality rates have changed little since the introduction of hemodialysis. This may be due to a more elderly or sicker population of patients in more recent series and to elimination of ARF in many clinical situations associated with a better prognosis, such as obstetrics, because of better resuscitation skills. These hypotheses have not been critically tested.

MANAGEMENT OF ACUTE RENAL FAILURE

Prevention

Several maneuvers to ameliorate or prevent renal failure have been studied in animal models. These factors were chosen because they interfered with one or more of the hypothetic pathogenic mechanisms. Fluid loading, vasodilators, blockade of the renin-angiotensin system, adrenergic receptors, calcium channel blockers, vasopressin, thromboxane, adenosine, administration of ATP, prostacyclin, atrial natriuretic factor (ANF), and diuretics have been studied. Most of these have shown some protection but only when started before or immediately after the insult.

Volume Loading

Volume loading with saline solution before a renal insult has been one of the most consistently protective maneuvers in animal models and in perioperative fluid management in humans. The mechanism of its protective value has not been fully elucidated. Early studies suggested that suppression of the renin-angiotensin axis was responsible, but this probably plays little if any role. Protection seems to correlate best with solute excretion rate. Volume loading stimulates ANF release, and ANF infusions have been protective in a few studies of ischemic renal failure. Volume loading should always be attempted during the initiation phase of ARF.

Diuretics

Diuretics should not significantly affect damaged nephrons because their site of action is on the luminal side of the tubule and they interfere with reabsorption of solute. Tubules that are significantly hypoxic, poisoned, or dead or are distal to glomeruli that are not filtering are not functioning and should be unresponsive to diuretics. The diuresis occasionally seen must result from action on nephrons that have not yet been rendered nonfunctional. In fact, the few controlled trials available document no beneficial effect of diuretics on ARF. The specific effects of mannitol and furosemide are discussed in the section on diuretics.

Dopamine and Dobutamine

Dopamine is a renal vasodilator, inhibits sodium reabsorption, and supports cardiac output. It has been used alone or in conjunction with furosemide to support renal perfusion. Controlled clinical trials of dopamine for prevention of ARF are lacking. It increases urine output but not GFR in oliguric patients. To the extent that it improves cardiac output, it is a useful drug and secondarily improves renal function. Nevertheless, dobutamine usually causes a greater increase in cardiac output, reduction in filling pressure, and improvement in renal function than does dopamine. Thus, if cardiac performance is impaired, dobutamine alone or in combination with 3 to 5 $\mu g \cdot kg^{-1} \cdot min^{-1}$ of dopamine is the preferred agent.

Calcium Channel Blockade

Calcium channel blockers may protect against ARF because calcium accumulates in dying cells and these agents are vasodilators. However, supporting evidence is not available.

Metabolic Factors

High levels of protein intake are associated with progression of chronic renal disease and with more severe renal failure in animal models of ischemic renal failure. Hyperglycemia may also increase the risk of renal damage if an ischemic event occurs.

Intake, output, body weight, osmolality, and electrolyte concentrations must be monitored to prevent water and electrolyte overload. Water requirements are directly proportional to metabolic rate. Normally 1 ml of water is required for each kilocalorie (kcal) of energy expended, but about 70% of this water requirement is responsible for excretion of solute generated by metabolism. Thus oliguric patients with renal failure should need only 0.3 to 0.5 ml/kcal. Nonoliguric patients may require a much larger than normal volume of water to excrete solute because of inability to concentrate the urine. In addition, other body fluids are lost to varying degrees that may be difficult to measure, such as in diarrhea or insensible losses from wound surfaces and perspiration. Respiratory losses may be markedly elevated (for example, because of dyspnea, fever, or elevated respiratory dead space) or depressed (the ventilated patient may have no respiratory losses if the ventilator circuit provides effective humidification.)

These patients frequently require fluids for administration of multiple drugs and for intravenous nutrition, which are greater than the renal and extrarenal losses. Nutrition and drugs should be administered in concentrated form via the gut or parenterally. Water balance is then restored by ultrafiltration.

SODIUM

Hyponatremia usually results from water overload. Treatment generally is the limitation of water intake and removal of any excess via dialysis. Sodium replacement should be guided by serial measurements of plasma sodium concentration and measurement of the sodium concentration of other losses, such as gastric or fistula drainage, coupled with assessment of the extracellular fluid volume.

POTASSIUM

Hyperkalemia is prevented and treated by removal of potassium from all administered fluids, administration of potassium-binding resins via the gastrointestinal tract, and dialysis. Hyperkalemia is more common in patients who have catabolism, retained necrotic tissue, or anuria. Aqueous penicillin contains significant amounts of potassium. If hyperkalemia occurs with electrocardiographic changes, intravenous calcium can be given to antagonize the electrophysiologic effects of hyperkalemia on the heart. Respiratory or metabolic alkalosis and insulin administration cause redistribution of potassium to the intracellular space. Dialysis may cause hypokalemia, which can be treated by increasing the potassium concentration in the dialysate or administering potassium.

ACIDOSIS

The 1 mEq/kg body weight of nonvolatile acid produced each day, which is normally excreted by the kidney, accumulates, causing a metabolic acidosis. Acidosis blunts the actions of catecholamines and causes nausea, vomiting, central nervous system dysfunction, compensatory hyperventilation, and glucose intolerance. Administration of acetate or bicarbonate and removal of acids by dialysis are effective therapy. Most patients seem to tolerate a lower than normal pH (7.28 to 7.35).

CALCIUM

Hypocalcemia results from hyperphosphatemia, hypoalbuminemia, and abnormalities in levels of parathyroid hormone and vitamin D and from precipitation in tissue in rhabdomy-

olysis and pancreatitis. Ionized calcium levels must be measured because the relationship between total and ionized calcium is severely disturbed in critically ill patients. Hypercalcemia occurs during the diuretic phase, especially when rhabdomyolysis was the initiating event. This is related to reabsorption of calcium deposited during the acute phase. Hypercalcemia may also occur during the maintenance phase of ARF and may require calcitonin.

PHOSPHORUS

Hyperphosphatemia often accompanies hyperkalemia because both phosphorus and potassium are predominantly excreted by the kidney. In addition, both are intracellular ions and their concentrations rise rapidly when tissue damage is present. Phosphate administration should be limited , and removal should be enhanced with phosphate-binding agents in the gastrointestinal tract and by dialysis. Hypophosphatemia sometimes occurs after stabilization and institution of nutrition.

AZOTEMIA

Proteins are degraded to urea, which the kidney excretes. Nutrition requires administration of amino acids or protein, but utilization of essential amino acids with reduced total amounts of nitrogen may limit the rate of urea accumulation. After dialysis is initiated, essential amino acids are replaced with usual sources of protein and the increased urea is removed by dialysis.

Nucleotides are metabolized to uric acid, which is also excreted by the kidney. Excessive uric acid production occurs during lytic tumor therapy. Allopurinol limits uric acid production. Dialysis stops the progressive rise in uric acid level.

ENZYMES

Amylase and lipase levels rise during renal insufficiency because they are excreted in the urine. This causes diagnostic ambiguity when pancreatitis is suspected. However, patients with pancreatitis and ARF have extremely high levels of these enzymes.

HORMONE LEVELS

Production of parathyroid hormone and growth hormone is increased during ARF. Because the kidney degrades many polypeptide hormones, their levels rise during ARF. The physiologic impact of these elevations is not certain, and interpretation of the levels is difficult.

Cardiovascular Factors

Hypertension is uncommon during ARF unless a systemic disease has caused both or unless the hypertension itself is the cause of ARF. Hypervolemia commonly occurs during ARF, following attempts to reverse any hemodynamic contribution to the onset of acute renal failure.

Uremia is associated with pericarditis and tamponade, but both are rarely significant in dialyzed patients. When pericarditis occurs early in the course of ARF, a systemic disease, such as autoimmune disease or vasculitis, is probably the cause of both.

Potassium, calcium, magnesium, and acid-base abnormalities cause arrhythmias, as do pericarditis, toxic effects of drugs, and underlying heart disease. Correction of the metabolic disturbance must be coupled with antiarrhythmic agents for optimal response.

Hematologic Factors

Inadequate red blood cell production because of decreased erythropoietin, iatrogenic losses for laboratory testing, losses to dialysis circuits, shortened red cell life span, and hemorrhagic complications, such as gastrointestinal blood loss, cause anemia. Adequate nutrition, prophylaxis against gastrointestinal hemorrhage, and transfusion are indicated. Platelet dysfunction occurs even with a normal platelet count because of abnormalities in von Willebrand factor. It is best detected by measuring bleeding time. Correction can be effected by cryoprecipitate or desmopressin (DDAVP). DDAVP 0.3 µg/kg intravenously over 30 minutes or subcutaneously stimulates release of von Willebrand factor from the endothelium. Improvement in bleeding time begins within an hour and lasts for about 4 hours. Ten units of cryoprecipitate also improves bleeding time for about 4 hours. Unfortunately, both therapies are short lived and the response cannot be improved by increasing the dosage or by combining their use. However, sequential administration may be a useful strategy. Platelet transfusion is usually not effective because the defect lies in the abnormal environment of the uremic patient, not in the platelets themselves. Dialysis shortens bleeding time, as does transfu-sion of sufficient red blood cells to correct the anemia to a hematocrit value of 25% to 30%.

Gastrointestinal Factors

In the past, gastrointestinal hemorrhage occurred in one fourth to one third of patients and was often fatal. Its incidence has probably decreased since vigorous prophylaxis against gastrointestinal bleeding has become routine. Azotemia is accompanied by anorexia, nausea, and vomiting, which are best controlled by adequate dialysis.

Infections

Pneumonia, wound infections, and other infections are probably the most common direct cause of death during ARF. Infections may occur in arteriovenous fistulas or the peritoneum secondary to dialysis. Careful monitoring for infectious complications is mandatory.

Pharmacologic Factors

Many drugs or their metabolites are excreted by filtration, secretion, or both. Renal failure prolongs the elimination half-life and the duration of action, necessitating a longer dosage interval of many drugs used in critical care. The volume of distribution of many drugs may be increased because of an increase in extracellular fluid volume, resulting in a need for a larger dose than normal. Doses of toxic drugs, such as aminoglycosides, should be adjusted by individualized pharmacokinetic analysis. Nomograms relating dose schedules to plasma creatinine concentration or creatinine clearance are not useful.

Dialysis
Hemodialysis

The mortality rate of ARF was reduced by the introduction of hemodialysis, which nearly eliminated death caused by acidosis, fluid overload, and electrolyte abnormalities. Unfortunately, since its clinical introduction, there has been little further improvement in outcome.

INDICATIONS

Dialysis is indicated for hyperkalemia; acidosis; removal of drugs, metabolites, or toxins; fluid overload with pulmonary edema; and pericarditis. It is also used to maintain the BUN

TABLE 11–7. Outcome and Complications

	BUN < 60	BUN < 100
Number	17	17
Number of hemodialyses	16	8
Duration of hemodialysis	23 days	22 days
Mortality	58.8%	47.1%
Oliguric	71%	
Nonoliguric	20%	
Sepsis	8	11
Hemorrhage	4	10
Cardiovascular	6	6
Adult respiratory distress syndrome	3	2
Bowel infarct	1	1
Hepatic failure	2	1
Seizures	0	1

BUN < 60 = patients dialyzed to maintain BUN < 60. BUN < 100 = patients dialyzed to maintain BUN < 100. None of the differences were statistically significant.
From Gillum DM et al: Clin Nephrol 1986;25:249. With permission.

below a specified level, usually less than 100 mg/dl, although this has no demonstrable advantage (Table 11–7).

COMPLICATIONS

Hemodialysis in critically ill patients is often complicated by significant hypotension because of reduced cardiac output. The latter is caused by a reduction in stroke volume incompletely compensated by an increase in heart rate. Substitution of bicarbonate for acetate as the buffer may better preserve cardiac output. Meticulous attention to maintenance of pulmonary capillary wedge pressures in unstable patients helps to sustain cardiac output, but addition of or an increase in catecholamine support is frequently needed. Avoidance of hypotension is critical because animal models of ischemic renal failure exhibit an exaggerated vasoconstrictor response to sympathetic nerve stimulation. Paradoxically, sensitivity to exogenous catecholamines is diminished. Kidneys of patients with ARF demonstrate multiple lesions of different ages, implying that episodic insults occur during the maintenance phase.

Dialysis is also accompanied by sequestration of white blood cells in the lungs and by hypoxia. The latter is also due to carbon dioxide removal by the dialysis membrane with subsequent hypoventilation. White blood cell sequestration is transient and depends on the composition of the dialysis membrane.

Even if regional heparinization is used, heparin commonly is inadequately reversed, resulting in anticoagulation of the patient after hemodialysis is completed. Measurement of partial thromboplastin time is necessary to regulate protamine administration. A synthetic prostacyclin analog should soon be available, which may be used when heparin must be avoided. Patients with contraindications to heparinization, such as recent stroke or head injury, may not be candidates for dialysis.

Air embolization is a risk because blood is pumped through the circuit, necessitating air traps and alarms.

Continuous Arteriovenous Hemofiltration

Continuous arteriovenous hemofiltration (CAVH) is an attractive alternative to intermittent hemodialysis because the equipment is simpler and the rapid changes in volume status and substrate concentrations caused by hemodialysis are avoided. However, arterial access is required for CAVH and not for hemodialysis.

INDICATIONS

The ultimate role of CAVH in ARF will depend on the results of appropriately controlled clinical trials. The indications for CAVH with or without dialysis fluid are the same as for hemodialysis, but CAVH may sometimes be used in hemodynamically unstable patients who do not tolerate hemodialysis. As mentioned previously, avoidance of hypotension is probably critical to avoid repetitive renal insults. Removal of large volumes of fluid is more effective with CAVH because the removal can be effected over a longer period. This allows time for mobilization of fluid from the interstitial fluid space, thus maintaining a more stable blood volume. Consistent fluid removal enhances the ability to administer fluid for nutrition. CAVH has generally, but not uniformly, been associated with greater hemodynamic stability. If hypotension occurs, filtration slows, providing a negative feedback loop, which contributes to cardiovascular stability. Bleeding is more common with CAVH because heparin is administered continuously. Air embolism is not a significant problem because the blood flow through the circuit is driven by the patient's blood pressure. Clotting of the filter, problems maintaining vascular access, and low clearance rates of solute are the major problems in CAVH.

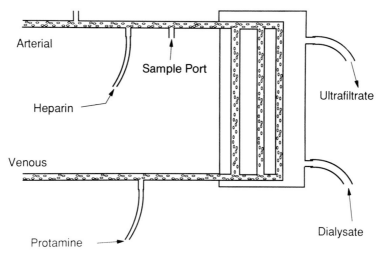

Figure 11–5. Continuous arteriovenous hemofiltration (CAVH). See text for full discussion. The stippled areas represent the blood pathway. Dialysate is perfused in the countercurrent direction to blood flow. T-shaped connectors are present on the arterial and venous limbs to allow fluid and drug infusion or blood sampling.

TECHNIQUE

Arterial and venous catheters are inserted and connected with short lengths of tubing to a filtration cartridge primed with heparinized saline according to the manufacturer's instructions. All air must be purged from the system. Heparin infusion is begun, and the arterial and venous lines are opened to begin blood flow. If systemic heparinization is not contraindicated, a bolus of heparin (approximately 70 units/kg) is administered, followed by an infusion into the arterial inflow line to the cartridge (Fig. 11–5). The infusion is adjusted to maintain the partial thromboplastin time of systemic blood at twice the upper limit of the normal value or the activated coagulation time (ACT) between 150 and 200 seconds. If regional heparinization is used, heparin is infused into the arterial inflow line at 300 to 500 units/h and an ACT is measured on a blood sample drawn from the sampling port on the venous return side of the cartridge. The heparin infusion is then adjusted to achieve an ACT of 150 to 200 seconds. A protamine infusion into the venous return line is begun at a rate of 1 mg of protamine per 100 units of heparin (Fig. 11-5). Subsequent protamine infusion rates are adjusted to keep the partial thromboplastin time, measured on a sample of systemic blood, near the upper range of normal.

REPLACEMENT FLUID

Filtration proceeds at a rate proportional to the surface area of the membrane, the mem-

brane permeability, the difference between hydrostatic pressure in the blood path of the cartridge and the pressure in the filtrate compartment of the cartridge, the plasma colloid osmotic pressure, and the blood flow. Filtration can reach high rates (15 to 20 ml/min) when pressure and flow are high, which leads to rapid reduction in plasma volume. Simply adjusting the vertical distance between the collection device and the filter changes the hydrostatic pressure gradient, changing the rate of filtration. Filtration usually falls to 5 to 10 ml/min during the first few hours, probably as a result of partial occlusion of the membrane.

Fluid replacement should include fluid required for nutrition (intravenous or enteral), drug administration, and the achievement of the desired net fluid balance. For example, filtration rate = 450 ml/h; parenteral nutrition fluid = 125 ml/h; drug administration (20 ml/h) = 480 ml/d; desired net negative fluid balance above insensible losses = 2400 ml/d (200 ml/h). The fluid administration rate should be 200 ml/h less than the filtration rate, or 250 ml/h. The total fluid input is 145 ml/h. Thus an additional 95 ml/h must be administered. The composition of this fluid is tailored to correct any electrolyte abnormalities.

HEMODIAFILTRATION

Solute removal can be enhanced significantly by passing peritoneal dialysis fluid through the ultrafiltration cartridge in a direction opposite to blood flow (Fig. 11–5). This overcomes the limited solute removal by CAVH alone. Solute removal is increased in proportion to the flow rate of the dialysate. Maximal solute removal is achieved at a dialysate flow rate of about 30 ml/min. A low concentration of dextrose is used in the dialysate to prevent hyperglycemia. Concentrations of sodium, potassium, phosphate, calcium, and other substances in the dialysate are adjusted to achieve the desired balance. However, severely catabolic patients may require supplemental conventional hemodialysis.

Peritoneal Dialysis

Peritoneal dialysis can be instituted rapidly to control acute hyperkalemia or acidosis, although it is less efficient than hemodialysis. The equipment and access techniques are simple, and the principles are straightforward. Peritoneal dialysis can be used when anticoagulation is contraindicated. Its use after abdominal surgery is controversial. If the peritoneum has not healed sufficiently, dialysate commonly leaks out of the abdomen into the abdominal wall or through the skin. When healing has progressed, adhesions may make distribution of the dialysate inadequate and increase the risk of bowel injury during catheter insertion. Peritoneal dialysis can be used in the presence of intraabdominal infection, and antibiotics may be delivered via the dialysate. Many regard the presence of an intraabdominal vascular prosthesis as an absolute contraindication to peritoneal dialysis. The rate of fluid removal is related to maintenance of an osmotic gradient between the dialysate and the extracellular fluid. The higher the dialysate osmolality and the more frequent the changes, the greater the rate of fluid removal. Electrolyte abnormalities are controlled by alteration of the electrolyte concentrations in the dialysate.

Complications include bowel perforation or bleeding as a result of catheter insertion, peritonitis, protein loss, and hyperglycemia, especially when concentrated dialysate solutions are used. Solutions with a dextrose concentration higher than 4.5% should rarely be used. The absorption of dextrose and other substances from the peritoneum is proportional to their concentration in the dialysate and can be used as a partial route of administration for nutritional purposes.

Nutrition

The role and particulars of nutrition in management of ARF remain controversial. Many believe that adequate nutrition is critical to survival, but animal studies suggest that intravenous amino acids may potentiate aminoglycoside nephrotoxicity and the effects of renal ischemia. At least 10 g of essential amino acids per day is required to maintain protein synthesis, but 30 to 40 g daily is generally recommended. Dialysis clears 10 to 20 g of amino acids per day, so patients aggressively dialyzed need increased amounts of amino acids during dialysis. Peritoneal dialysis removes 8 to 12 g of protein per day. Fluid restriction is often a difficult problem in critically ill patients with ARF. Intravenous nutritional fluid can be based on a 70% dextrose solution, which provides 40% more calories per milliliter of fluid than the traditional 50% dextrose base. Many clinicians prescribe standard nutritional fluids once dialysis has been established, reserving the expensive essential amino acid formulations for retarding BUN increase before dialysis. Intravenous lipid emulsions allow administration of 2 kcal/ml, which is helpful in restricting fluid. Hyperlipidemia must be monitored and the dosage adjusted accordingly.

Improved survival in patients receiving nutritional support has not been well documented. Use of a parenteral or enteral diet rich in essential and branched chain amino acids in conjunction with hemodialysis appeared to improve the negative nitrogen balance in a group of patients with posttraumatic ARF. Overall outcome was not affected, however.

Diuretics

Indications

Several of the suggested indications for diuretic administration are seen in critically ill patients (Table 11–8). Hypertension in a critically ill patient should rarely be treated with a diuretic except as a continuation of prior therapy. Vasodilators, alpha-adrenergic blockers, calcium channel blockers, angiotensin converting enzyme inhibitors, and beta blockade

TABLE 11–8.   Suggested Indications for Diuretic Therapy

Hypertension
Fluid overload
Therapeutic dehydration
Acceleration of excretion
Dilution of nephrotoxins
Acute oliguria
Renal failure

are generally more effective and safer during the acute, unstable phase of an illness.

Fluid overload should not be diagnosed on the basis of evidence of expanded extravascular fluid volume (that is, edema) but rather when circulatory overload with supramaximal filling pressures is present.

Therapeutic dehydration, most commonly with an osmotic diuretic, is often attempted in patients with intracranial hypertension. Meticulous attention to sustaining an adequate intravascular volume is necessary and requires monitoring of wedge pressures, vascular resistance, and cardiac index. As dehydration approaches a critical lowering of blood volume, blood pressure and heart rate are often well maintained. As blood volume falls, systemic vascular resistance rises and cardiac index falls, indicating the need for infusion of fluid that will remain in the vascular space.

Diuresis has been proposed as a means of speeding the elimination of drugs that are excreted by the kidney. This is generally ineffective because most drugs are excreted by filtration and secretion. Diuretics do not change GFR unless hypovolemia is produced, in which case GFR falls. Diuretics may actually compete with the target drug for secretory sites, further reducing its excretion.

The tubular epithelium is exposed to high concentrations of nephrotoxins that are excreted by the kidney. Some evidence suggests that mannitol may reduce toxicity of a few nephrotoxins, such as amphotericin B and cisplatin, but the evidence is far from convincing. Furosemide may actually potentiate the toxicity of aminoglycosides.

The use of diuretics in oliguric patients with critical illness is mentioned primarily to be condemned. Oliguria should be considered a sign of fluid deficit, electrolyte imbalance, or inadequate hemodynamic performance. The diuretic may induce urine flow, causing the physician to relax, inappropriately, further diagnostic and therapeutic efforts.

Diuretics have been evaluated for their usefulness in preventing, diagnosing, and treating ARF. Furosemide and mannitol have been tested for their ability to (1) aid in differentiating parenchymal from prerenal failure, (2) halt the progression to parenchymal renal failure, (3) convert oliguric to nonoliguric ARF and (4) shorten the course of established ARF. Generally, no clinical value for the suggested uses has been demonstrated. Uncontrolled trials have tended to show some benefit, and the few controlled trials have shown no effect other than establishing a higher urine flow rate in some patients. A response in urine flow rate is seen in patients with well-established ARF and does not occur in the presence of prerenal oliguria if filtration rate is low. Thus no diagnostic information is obtained. The only clinical situation that appears to benefit from prophylactic administration of mannitol is perioperative administration in patients with obstructive jaundice (see the discussion of jaundice as a cause of ARF). Diuretics have been suggested as a prophylactic measure during vascular surgery, but adequate volume resuscitation appears equally effective (see the discussion of vascular surgery as a cause of ARF).

Diuretics have a limited role in established ARF and have not been demonstrated to modify the outcome significantly. Some patients respond to diuretics, making administration of drugs and nutritional fluids easier.

Proximal Tubular Diuretics

Mannitol and acetazolamide have their maximal effect on the proximal tubule. Furosemide and metolazone have a minor action at this site (Table 11–9).

OSMOTIC DIURETICS

Mannitol is a nonmetabolizable alcohol that is filtered but not reabsorbed. Large quantities of sodium are reabsorbed in the proximal

TABLE 11–9. Diuretics

DRUG	ROUTE	ONSET (min)	DURATION (h)	EXCRETION
Metolazone	PO	60	24	Urine
Furosemide	PO	60	6-8	Filtration, secretion
	IV	5	2	
Mannitol	IV	5	1-2	Filtration
Acetazolamide	PO	30	12	Secretion, filtration

PO = oral; IV = intravenous.

tubule, followed by water, thus maintaining isotonicity of the fluid. When a nonreabsorbable solute is present in the filtrate, the water is retarded from following the sodium. This dilutes the sodium concentration in the filtrate. The proximal tubule is not capable of generating large sodium concentration gradients. Thus sodium reabsorption is decreased. This increases the total amount of sodium delivered to the distal tubule, which is capable of generating large gradients between the tubular fluid and the interstitium but which has limited capacity. The distal stimulation of sodium reabsorption increases potassium excretion. Thus the mannitol, water, and excess sodium and potassium are excreted. The rapid flow of tubular fluid prevents the development of the medullary interstitial concentration gradient. Therefore the urine tends to be isosmotic.

Although mannitol protects a variety of animal models against ARF, the exact mode of protection is not clear and lack of protection is sometimes reported. Several actions of mannitol might be protective. Mannitol is a renal vasodilator and a scavenger of oxygen free radicals, as well as a diuretic. The latter is important because most studies demonstrating protection have correlated the protection with an increase in solute excretion rate before the renal insult. Mannitol may prevent tubular obstruction by maintaining brisk flow through the proximal tubule and Henle's loop, thus flushing any precipitants out of the nephron before they can form obstructing casts. Mannitol elevates proximal tubular pressure and should facilitate flushing of partially obstructing debris from the nephron. The most severe damage occurs in the proximal tubules, the nephron segment where mannitol exerts its major effect. Hypertonic mannitol also aids in volume expansion, another potentially protective procedure. Cell swelling has been postulated to be an important pathogenic mechanism, and hypertonic agents may reduce cell swelling. If sludging of red and white blood cells in peritubular capillaries is important in pathogenesis, hemodilution provided by mannitol may be protective. Despite these rationalizations and the fact that mannitol has performed better than furosemide in most animal models, few well-controlled clinical studies of its use in preventing or treating ARF have been conducted. Mannitol may be protective in jaundiced patients perioperatively and during therapy with amphotericin B, radiocontrast agents, and cisplatin. Although experimental studies show significant effects, solid clinical documentation of benefit is lacking.

CARBONIC ANHYDRASE INHIBITORS

Acetazolamide interferes with the hydration of carbon dioxide, thus inhibiting bicarbonate reabsorption in the proximal tubule (Fig. 11–3). It also interferes with phosphate and calcium reabsorption, leading to increased urinary excretion. Although distal sites can reabsorb some of the increased bicarbonate, they are incapable of reabsorbing it all. The fractional excretion of bicarbonate can reach 45% of the filtered amount. Alkalinization of the tubular fluid inhibits the ammonium ion trapping, resulting in increased reabsorption of ammonia. This could be a problem in patients with hepatic decompensation. The primary reason for using acetazolamide in the ICU is for treatment of metabolic alkalosis. One to three doses of 250 mg each usually corrects the problem in 24 to 36 hours.

Loop Diuretics

Furosemide, bumetanide, and ethacrynic acid have their primary action in the thick ascending limb of Henle's loop, where they inhibit the secondary active reabsorption of chloride by inhibiting Na-K-ATPase. These agents have minor actions in the proximal and distal tubule. The inhibition of thick ascending limb transport impairs magnesium and calcium reabsorption (Fig. 11–3). Increased delivery of sodium to the distal tubule stimulates hydrogen ion and potassium secretion, leading to hypokalemia and alkalosis. Furosemide must reach the luminal surface of the thick ascending limb to exert its action. The drug is filtered and actively secreted by the proximal tubule. If filtration or secretion is impaired, the amount of drug reaching the site of action is reduced. This impairs the drug's effectiveness.

Metolazone is similar to the thiazide diuretics but acts on the proximal tubule and thick ascending limb, as well as the distal tubule. When it is administered in conjunction with a loop diuretic, a massive diuresis sometimes results. Thus the combination is used in attempts to stimulate urine flow in patients who have not responded to other diuretics.

FUROSEMIDE IN RENAL FAILURE

Furosemide is a weak renal vasodilator and increases solute excretion through the distal nephron because its major site of action is in the thick ascending limb of Henle's loop. Thus it seems unlikely to be highly protective because the proximal tubule is generally the most severely affected segment. Its protective effects seem to correlate with an increase in solute excretion. Furosemide has been mildly protective in ischemic models but is not useful or is even detrimental in nephrotoxic models. Controlled clinical trials have failed to demonstrate any benefit.

Distal Tubular Diuretics

Thiazides, triamterene, metolazone, and spironolactone act distally. The thiazides are of little interest in critical care other than the complications they induce in electrolyte and volume status in patients subsequently admitted to the ICU. Triamterene and other potassium-sparing diuretics are rarely used in critically ill patients. Spironolactone acts by inhibiting aldosterone action and is used to sustain diuresis in patients with significant activation of the renin-angiotensin-aldosterone system. Examples include cirrhotic patients with ascites and chronic congestive heart failure.

SUGGESTED READINGS

Beutler B, Cerami A: Cachectin: more than a tumor necrosis factor. N Engl J Med 1987;316:379-385

Brezis M, Rosen S, Silva P, Epstein FH: Renal ischemia: a new perspective. Kidney Int 1984;26:375-383

Broe M, Heyrman R, Backer W, et al: Pathogenesis of dialysis-induced hypoxemia: a short overview. Kidney Int 1988;33:S57-S61

Cade R, Wagemaker H, Vogel S, et al: Hepatorenal syndrome: studies of the effect of vascular volume and intraperitoneal pressure on renal and hepatic function. Am J Med 1987;82:427

Dixon BS, Anderson RJ: Nonoliguric acute renal failure. Am J Kidney Dis 1985;6:71-80

Fontanarosa P: Radiologic contrast-induced renal failure. Emerg Med Clin North Am 1988;6:601-616

Humes HD: Role of calcium in pathogenesis of acute renal failure. Am J Physiol 1986;250:F579-F589

Makhoul RG, Gewertz BL: Renal prostaglandins. J Surg Res 1986;40:181-192

Mason J: The pathophysiology of ischaemic acute renal failure. Renal Physiol 1986;9:129-147

Moran SM, Myers BD: Course of acute renal failure studied by a model of creatinine kinetics. Kidney Int 1985;27:928-937

Solez K: Pathogenesis of acute renal failure. Int Rev Exp Pathol 1983;24:277-333

Sondheimer JH, Migdal SD: Toxic nephropathies. Crit Care Clin 1987;5:883-907

Teschan PE: Nutrition in renal failure. Artif Organs 1986;10:301-305

Zarich S, Fang LST, Diamond JR: Fractional excretion of sodium: exceptions to its diagnostic value. Arch Intern Med 1985;145:108-112

12

INFECTIOUS DISEASE

MORRIS BROWN, MD, AND ANDREW JACKIW, MD

Sepsis is a leading cause of death in critically ill patients. Therefore signs and symptoms of infection must be routinely monitored and, when discovered, thoroughly investigated because early recognition and intervention are essential for successful management. The key factor in treating sepsis is identification of the source and type of offending organisms. A complete history and directed physical examination frequently provide the information needed for correct diagnosis based on clinical knowledge. Properly performed tests determine the susceptibility of the presumed organisms to antimicrobial agents. The location of the infection must be taken into consideration, since this may significantly influence the choice of antibiotics. Finally, other host factors may influence not only choice of drug, but also dosage and route of administration.

APPROACH TO THE INFECTED PATIENT

Clinical Manifestations

Fever is one of the most common clinical findings in sepsis. It may be related to tumor necrosis factor, interleukin-1, or various pyrogens elaborated as monokines from macrophages and peripheral monocytes. Although all infections can cause fever, elevated body temperature can accompany many other disease states, including mechanical trauma, neoplastic diseases, hemopoietic disorders, vascular accidents, diseases caused by immune mechanisms, and acute metabolic disorders. A chill or rigor commonly accompanies the fever. Fever with rigors may also occur with noninfectious diseases, such as lymphoma. Further, chills may be evoked or perpetuated by the intermittent administration of antipyretic agents, without infection being present.

Fever is frequently an early and only manifestation of underlying disease. Whether the fever is intermittent, remittent, sustained, or relapsing can aid immeasurably in formulating a diagnosis. An intermittent fever, in which wide variations exist between the peak and nadir, suggests pyogenic infections (particularly abscesses), lymphoma, and miliary tuberculosis. A remittent fever is characterized by an elevated temperature that falls to near normal every day. This is the most common type of fever and is not diagnostic or characteristic of any disease process. A sustained fever, one having a persistent elevation without significant variation, is typical of untreated typhoid or typhus. A relapsing fever has short febrile periods between prolonged periods of normothermia. Relapsing fevers are characteristic of malaria, rat-bite fever, and occasionally pyogenic infections. An increased mortality rate has been suggested in patients unable to generate a fever greater than 99.6° F in the first 24 hours of an infection or in hypothermic patients. Indeed, hypothermia is seen most commonly in patients who are at the extremes of age or have chronically debilitating or immunosuppressant conditions.

Tachypnea and tachycardia are also common clinical manifestations of sepsis. Azotemia, oliguria, and an active urinary sediment are common renal manifestations of infection. A mild nephropathy with an active urinary sediment may be the sole manifestation, or progression to acute tubular necrosis and renal failure may occur. Leukocytosis with a shift to immature neutrophils ("left shift") is one of the main hematologic findings in sepsis, although leukopenia may also be present. Thrombocytopenia, with or without coagulation abnormalities, is also common. When present, coagulation abnormalities may be manifest as prolonged prothrombin time (PT) or partial thromboplastin time (PTT) or as disseminated intravascular coagulation. The most common central nervous system manifestation of sepsis is altered mental status. The presentation may take the form of disorientation, confusion, lethargy, or obtundation, which may result from a decrease in cerebral blood flow. A recently described polyneuropathy in critically ill patients is manifest as impaired deep tendon reflexes and muscle weakness and wasting caused by primary axonal degeneration of the sensory and motor fibers. Hepatic dysfunction characterized by increased transaminase levels and cholestatic jaundice is common in patients with sepsis. Stress ulceration with gastrointestinal bleeding may be related to altered mucosal blood flow, hypoxia of the gastric mucosal cells, release of mucosal lysozyme, disruption of the gastric mucosal barrier, and the irritative effect of acid and bile on the hypoxic gastric epithelium.

HOSPITAL-ACQUIRED INFECTIONS

Urinary Tract Infections

The urinary tract is the most frequent site of infection in hospitalized patients, accounting for approximately 40% of hospital-acquired infections. Since most critically ill patients have an indwelling catheter, it is not surprising that the urinary tract is a common source of infection. The risk of infection in a patient with an indwelling Foley catheter is 5% per day. However, in critically ill patients the urinary tract is a less likely source of infection than other sites, such as the respiratory tract.

Bacteremia develops in one of six patients who have urinary tract infections. The urinary tract is the most common source of gram-negative bacteremia. The mortality rate of bacteremic urinary tract infections is approximately 30%. Many antibiotics are highly concentrated in the urine, which helps to eradicate the infection. Therefore, although urinary tract infections are potentially catastrophic, the majority are readily treated without significant sequelae. However, the urinary tract should be considered a possible source of infection if the patient has bacteriuria and a clinical picture consistent with infection.

Wound Infections

Most surgical wound infections are caused by the introduction of bacteria directly into the tissue during an operation. They account for 10% of all infections in postsurgical ICU patients. Wounds should be observed for any signs of infection, such as erythema and induration. Any purulent material should be sampled and sent for Gram stain and culture studies. Taking samples from the wound surface for culturing is not useful because surface organisms may be contaminants. Biopsy with microscopic examination for organisms invading live tissue and an inflammatory response is the most specific means of diagnosing a wound infection that does not produce pus. Most wound infections are evident 3 to 7 days after surgical intervention. Infections developing within 24 hours are generally fulminant infections by *Clostridium* or beta-hemolytic streptococci. Later surgical wound infections are generally caused by gram-negative bacilli, anaerobic bacteria, and staphylococci. The administration of prophylactic antibiotics has greatly reduced the postoperative wound infection rate.

Pneumonia

The most serious complication among hospital-acquired infections is lower respiratory tract infection. Hospital-acquired pneumonia occurs in up to 15% of ICU patients and is the leading cause of death in this population. The major organisms causing pneumonia in critically ill patients are gram-negative bacilli and *Staphylococcus aureus.* The diagnosis of pneumonia in critically ill patients who are maintained with mechanical ventilatory support can be difficult. Critically ill patients in whom nosocomial pneumonia develops frequently do not exhibit the classic signs (such as violent shaking chills, chest pain, cough producing rust-colored sputum, dullness to percussion over the affected lobe, and consolidation of lung parenchyma on chest roentgenogram) described for community-acquired pneumococcal pneumonia. Physical examination by itself cannot be used to make the diagnosis. Laboratory studies also have limitations. Normally, sputum obtained solely from below the vocal cords is sterile. However, in patients with an artificial airway (endotracheal tube or tracheostomy) the trachea is colonized within 24 to 48 hours. Thus Gram stain and culture of material aspirated through the artificial airway may be contaminated by the colonizing bacteria in the trachea. Antibody coating and quantitative cultures have not significantly improved diagnostic efficacy. Protected brush catheter bronchoscopy has recently been advocated as an effective adjunct to the diagnosis of pneumonia for patients maintained with mechanical ventilatory support. However, no sampling technique, other than open lung biopsy, has been found to prevent tracheal contamination completely. Semiquantitative culturing of the protected brush specimen may be the most specific diagnostic test except for lung biopsy. Specimens containing more than 10^3 colony-forming units/ml show a high correlation with infection diagnosed by other means. Diagnosis of nosocomial pneumonia is generally based on signs and symptoms of infection, bacteriologic verification, and finding a new pulmonary infiltrate on chest roentgenogram that is unchanged by physical therapy (that is, not atelectasis).

Pathogenesis. Most nosocomial pneumonias develop secondary to several contributing factors. First, normal oropharyngeal flora is suppressed by the use of antibiotics or by underlying illness. Next, hospital-acquired organisms colonize the oropharyngeal mucosa. Nosocomial bacteria are conveyed to patients by manifold means, such as hands of health care givers, nonsterile suctioning of the oropharynx, and contaminated bedside articles. Third, these organisms are delivered to the tracheobronchial tree by microaspiration (a normal phenomenon), contaminated humidifiers, and instrumentation such as endotracheal suctioning. The passage of organisms into the tracheobronchial tree is easier in patients with artificial airways because normal defense mechanisms, such as the turbinates, nasal mucosa, and gag and cough reflexes, are bypassed. Finally, impaired clearance of material from the tracheobronchial tree amplifies the insult. Clearance is impaired by many pathologic alterations found in critically ill patients, including decreased cough effectiveness and mucociliary dysfunction. These defense mechanisms are discussed in detail in Chapter 3.

Specific Etiologic Agents. *Pseudomonas* pneumonia is extraordinarily difficult to treat and causes a necrotizing pneumonia that is often rapidly progressive. Diagnosis by routine Gram stain and culture studies presents no unusual problems. When the disease is suspected, empiric treatment with at least two antibiotics must begin immediately. The current standard therapy consists of an aminoglycoside plus either a penicillin or a second- or third-generation cephalosporin. Aztreonam is a viable additional drug whose role is not yet fully defined. The organism often becomes resistant to cephalosporins during therapy, so it must be grown on culture repetitively and therapy adjusted accordingly.

Staphylococcus aureus pneumonia is a common pneumonia occurring early in critical illness. It produces lung necrosis and advances rapidly. No special diagnostic tests are required. Many medical centers start therapy with vancomycin because of the incidence of resistance to penicillins. First- and second-generation cephalosporins are often useful alternatives to penicillin or vancomycin.

Legionnaires' pneumonia is caused by a peculiar gram-negative organism that contaminates the water of some buildings and hospitals. The organism typically produces a pneumonia without a purulent sputum. Bronchoalveolar lavage specimens are tested with stains and antibody techniques. The disease must be treated with erythromycin or tetracycline.

Pneumocystis carinii is another organism that causes pneumonia without purulent sputum. *P. carinii* pneumonia is seen in immunosuppressed patients. Bronchoalveolar lavage with appropriate staining is necessary for rapid identification. Prognosis is poor, primarily because of the severely compromised hosts the disease attacks.

Viral pneumonia is recognized predominantly in immunocompromised hosts. The sputum is usually bland, containing few or no organisms. Serologic testing, examination of bronchoalveolar lavage fluid sediment, cytology, and tissue culturing are necessary to make the diagnosis. Cytomegalovirus, herpesvirus, influenza, and varicella should all be considered.

Mycobacteria may cause pneumonia in immunocompromised hosts and present diagnostic confusion.

Intravascular Device–Related Infections

With advances in technology and invasive monitoring, intravascular device–related bacteremia has become a common problem, accounting for more than 25,000 cases of bacteremia annually. Contamination of intravascular devices may occur anywhere along the line from the infusate bottle to the skin entry site. Predisposition to intravascular device–related bacteremia is determined by both patient factors and hospital factors. The patient-related factors generally reflect the severity of underlying disease. Hospital-related factors are more controllable and include the type of catheter, site of insertion, technique of placement, and duration of cannulation. Recommendations for prevention of intravascular device–related infections should be based on the Centers for Disease Control guidelines. The introduction of organisms into the infusate occurs whenever the integrity of the bag, line, or catheter is broken. The number of times an infusion line is opened for withdrawal of specimens or administration of medications is directly correlated with the incidence of infection. The proper role of changing catheters to new sites or over guidewires is still actively discussed. Recently a silver-impregnated collagen cuff was demonstrated to reduce the rate of infection at the insertion site and to prolong the time the catheter remains in the patient. Not only must catheters be inserted with meticulous sterile technique, the site must be inspected, cleaned, and covered every day and whenever it becomes contaminated.

Intraabdominal Infections

Abdominal infections generally occur in patients who have undergone intraabdominal procedures, especially if intraperitoneal hemorrhage occurred. Risk factors for infection include prolonged operative time, use of foreign substances, inadequate drainage, presence of devitalized tissue, hematoma formation, and fecal contamination at the time of surgery. Acalculous cholecystitis is another potential cause of abdominal infection in the postoperative period. Stress ulceration with significant gastrointestinal bleeding and perforation, or perforation of mechanical origin, such as nasogastric drainage, can result in intraabdominal infection in the absence of prior surgical intervention. Large bowel perforation because of massive dilation or because of ischemia during shock can produce intraabdominal infection in the absence of prior violation of the peritoneum or gastrointestinal tract. Pancreatitis is sometimes complicated by secondary infection. The diagnosis of intraabdominal infection depends primarily on physical examination with adjunctive radiologic evaluation, including computed tomography, ultrasonography, and abdominal roentgenography. Other findings associated with abdominal infection include ileus, diarrhea, distention, nausea, and vomiting. Diagnostic peritoneal lavage or aspiration of ascitic fluid sometimes establishes the presence of infection.

Sinusitis

One of the recognized complications of nasotracheal intubation is sinusitis. Sinusitis accounts for 5% of nosocomial infections in critically ill patients. However, this infection is frequently difficult to diagnose and often goes unrecognized. Patients may have fever and leukocytosis but few other signs or symptoms of overt infection. Less than half of patients have purulent nasal drainage. The diagnosis of sinusitis relies on roentgenograms of the paranasal sinuses. Unfortunately, these are frequently of suboptimal quality when taken in the critical care unit with a portable apparatus. However, if sinuses are opacified or an air-fluid level is noted and aspiration reveals purulent material, the endotracheal tube should be removed and replaced via the oral route and topical vasoconstrictor (such as phenylephrine) and antibiotic therapy should be initiated. Patients generally respond well and rarely require surgical drainage.

Central Nervous System Infections

Nosocomial central nervous system infections are uncommon in critically ill patients unless they have predisposing conditions, such as neurosurgical procedures or central nervous system trauma. All pyogenic infections of the cranial contents originate by either hematogenous spread or extension from contiguous sites. Acute meningitis is a medical emergency that requires high-level diagnostic and therapeutic skills because it has a significant mortality rate. Symptoms include headache, stiff neck, seizures, and altered mental status. Bacterial meningitis is differentiated from aseptic meningitis syndrome by analysis of the cerebrospinal fluid. All febrile patients with lethargy, headache, or confusion of sudden onset, even if only low-grade temperature is present, should be subjected to a lumbar puncture after assessment for signs of elevated intracranial pressure.

Incidence of brain abscess has remained constant even with the introduction of broad-spectrum antibiotic coverage. It is associated with high morbidity and mortality rates. The most common age for occurrence is between 30 and 40 years, and brain abscess is frequently associated with sinusitis or otitis. Streptococci are the most common etiologic organisms. Treatment has improved with the advent of better imaging techniques that allow guided drainage for diagnosis and therapy. Although the mortality rate has decreased, significant incidence of neurologic residual, primarily seizure disorders, remains.

Endocarditis

Infective endocarditis (IE) is associated with significant morbidity and mortality. It accounts for approximately 5 of every 1000 hospital admissions, with mortality rates from 10% to 60% reported. IE is a microbial infection of the heart valves or the endocardium in proximity to congenital or acquired cardiac defects. The infection may develop abruptly or insidiously and is fatal if left untreated. The foremost factor governing the development of IE is seeding of the blood with bacteria. The portal of entry of bacteria may be overt; intravenous drug use, a dental or surgical procedure, or a broken bone is more than sufficient. Seeding from transient covert bacteremia caused by trivial injuries of the gut or the oral cavity is equally capable of causing IE.

Hemodynamic events are important in development of IE. Before contamination with bacteria, sterile vegetations consisting of platelets and fibrin form at sites of high flow rates in areas of structural change or abnormalities that alter the endothelial surface. The vegetation becomes the nidus on which microorganisms are implanted. A subsequent bacteremia may seed these primed sterile vegetations. The adherent bacteria are protected from circulating phagocytic cells by a thin coating of circulating platelets and fibrin.

IE occurs most often in patients with preexisting heart disease, but virulent organisms can seed normal cardiac valves. Infection most commonly involves the left side of the heart, with the mitral, aortic, tricuspid, and pulmonary valves involved in decreasing order of frequency. Patients with IE require prolonged therapy with bactericidal rather than bacteriostatic antibiotics to eradicate infection.

Transient bacteremia is common, even in normal hosts. Normally this bacteremia is low grade, with fewer than 10 colony-forming units/ml of blood. The size of the bacteremia is proportional to the amount of trauma affecting the mucosal surface and to its microorganism infestation. The incidence of bacteremia also varies with the type of procedure. Symptoms of endocarditis usually begin insidiously and include weakness, fatigability, weight loss, feverishness, night sweats, anorexia, and arthralgias. Embolic phenomena may produce paralysis, chest pain, acute vascular insufficiency, hematuria, abdominal pain, or sudden blindness. Chills are uncommon.

Physical examination findings may be normal early in the course of infection. As the disease progresses, however, patients appear chronically ill and pale and have temperature elevation. The fever is most often remittent with afternoon or evening spikes. Cutaneous lesions are common and may include petechiae in the mucosa of the mouth, pharynx, or conjunctiva. Splinter hemorrhages, Osler's nodes, clubbing of the fingers, and mild jaundice may be noted. Cardiac findings are usually those of the underlying heart disease with major changes in cardiac murmurs, primarily development of a new diastolic murmur. Other findings may include splenomegaly without splenic tenderness, arthritis, and evidence of embolic phenomena.

Acute endocarditis often involves a normal heart, whereas the subacute infection almost invariably affects an abnormal heart. Acute endocarditis is particularly common in intravenous drug users. The infection is usually fulminant with high fever, leukocytosis, and systemic toxic effects. Chills, petechiae, and embolic phenomena are prominent. Metastatic abscesses frequently follow septic embolism. The organisms involved in acute endocarditis are more virulent. Death, if therapy fails, usually ensues in several days to 6 weeks.

Prosthetic valve infections develop in 2% to 3% of patients the first year after valve placement and 0.5% each year thereafter. Approximately one third of infections in the first year develop within 2 months of surgery and are probably due to colonization of the prosthesis or suture sites during surgery. Prosthetic valve infections that occur more than 2 months after surgery may result from implantation of organisms at surgery or colonization of the prosthesis or its attachment site during transient bacteremias. Therefore patients with prosthetic valves should receive prophylactic microbial agents when undergoing procedures known to produce bacteremia.

Before the antibiotic era, IE was uniformly fatal. With appropriate antibiotic therapy, however, more than 70% of patients with infection on endogenous valves and 50% with infection on prosthetic valves survive the infection. The prognosis is worse with gram-negative bacilli, fungal endocarditis, presence of congestive heart failure, extremes of age, polymicrobial bacteremia, and involvement of multiple heart valves. The most common cause of death in treated endocarditis is congestive heart failure caused by valve destruction or myocardial damage.

Antimicrobial therapy must be initiated early and in sufficient dosage to kill the offending organisms. Bacteriostatic drugs that only inhibit organisms are ineffective; bactericidal drugs are necessary for cure. Antibiotic therapy is generally required for 4 to 6 weeks. Prosthetic valve infections should be treated for 6 to 8 weeks, and patients should be monitored closely for signs of valve dysfunction and embolism. Mechanical valves are more likely to require replacement than bioprostheses.

Prophylaxis. The risk of IE is related to procedures associated with a high incidence of bacteremia and to the underlying cardiac condition. Procedures that increase risk include dental procedures, upper airway manipulations, and gastrointestinal or genitourinary procedures. Prophylaxis is recommended for all dental procedures, including routine professional cleaning, that are likely to cause gingival bleeding. Prophylaxis is required for all surgical procedures on the respiratory tract, including tonsillectomy with or without adenoidectomy; bronchoscopy, especially with a rigid bronchoscope; and other surgical procedures, including biopsy involving the respiratory mucosa. Gastrointestinal or genitourinary procedures that require prophylaxis include cystoscopy, urinary tract surgery, vaginal hysterectomy, gallbladder surgery, colon surgery, esophageal dilatation, colonoscopy, and gastrointestinal endoscopy with biopsy. Prophylaxis is not necessary for percutaneous liver biopsy, barium enema, gastrointestinal endoscopy without biopsy, or uncomplicated vaginal delivery. If infection is not suspected, prophylaxis is not required for dilatation and curettage, cesarean section, or sterilization procedures. However, some clinicians believe that prophylaxis is prudent for patients with prosthetic heart valves.

Cardiac conditions placing patients at risk for endocarditis can be divided into low-, intermediate-, and high-risk groups. Low-risk conditions do not require prophylaxis for endocarditis. The intermediate group generally warrants prophylactic therapy. In the high-risk group every precaution should be taken and patients should definitely receive antibiotic prophylaxis.

Fungal Infections

Broad-spectrum antibiotic therapy, organ transplantation, prosthetic cardiac valves, and immunosuppression from neoplasm, transplants, burns, and drugs have increased the incidence of fungal infections. Clinical manifestations range from thrush to disseminated candidiasis. Organs involved with systemic disease include the kidneys, brain, myocardium, and eyes. The pathologic hallmark is diffuse microabscess with a combined suppurative and granulomatous reaction. The diagnosis of candidemia may be difficult because the specificity and sensitivity of serum antibody tests have been uniformly disappointing and cultures are often negative. Although not all patients with candidemia require antifungal therapy, amphotericin B is the drug of choice if treatment is indicated. The recent availability of parenteral fluconazole, a much less toxic drug, has liberalized the indications for treatment. The prophylactic application of nystatin to the upper gastrointestinal tract mucosa and vagina during the course of broad-spectrum antibiotic treatment is common, although its efficacy is not clearly defined. When candidemia occurs in conjunction with intravascular devices, particularly when parenteral nutrition is administered, it usually responds to removal of the device.

Infections in Immunocompromised Hosts

Infections in immunocompromised hosts present special challenges because the incidence of infection is high, the spectrum of potential pathogens is much greater than in normal hosts, the unusual organisms are difficult to diagnose, and the therapeutic options are often marginally effective and significantly toxic. These patients often must be treated empirically for gram-positive, gram-negative, anaerobic, fungal, and viral infections. The signs of infection for the most part represent the body's response to infection; for example, pus contains copious white blood cells and may be absent or appear to be serosanguineous fluid in a leukopenic patient. Thus fever and cardiovascular instability may be the only presenting symptoms in a compromised patient with sepsis.

Septic Syndrome

The definition of the septic syndrome is based on easily acquired clinical data that can be applied to a broad population of patients. The clinical evidence is based on a high index of suspicion and does not require confirmation with positive cultures of blood or material from a closed space. Indeed, the septic syndrome can be defined in terms of the systemic response to infection, expressed as tachycardia, fever or hypothermia, tachypnea, and evidence of inadequate organ perfusion. That is, the systemic response is what differentiates sepsis from simple infection or bacteremia. The object of such a broad definition is to facilitate early recognition and prompt institution of therapeutic interventions.

Sepsis has been estimated to occur in 1 of 100 hospitalized patients in the United States. Although the precise incidence is unknown, it has been estimated, that up to 500,000 cases of sepsis occur each year in the United States. When the septic syndrome is accompanied by hypotension unresponsive to fluid therapy, it is often referred to as septic shock. Shock develops in approximately 40% of patients with sepsis. The increased survival of immunocompromised patients, those receiving organ transplants, and those with malignancy and inflammatory disease, as well as the use of invasive medical devices and procedures, has increased the incidence of sepsis.

The septic syndrome can be identified as a systemic manifestation of presumed sepsis. The definition of the septic syndrome includes many of the more common clinical manifestations of sepsis. In a recent study of patients with the septic syndrome, the mortality rate was nearly 30% of the 382 patients enrolled. Only 45% of these patients had positive blood cultures, and almost 64% had either shock on entry into the study or the development of shock after entry. The adult respiratory distress syndrome (ARDS) developed in 25% of these patients. Although the traditional definition of sepsis requiring positive blood or closed-space culture and shock was not met by the majority of patients, the overall mortality rate was significant and similar to those reported by several investigators in patients with sepsis. The incidence of ARDS was also similar to previously published reports. Clearly the septic syndrome has a clinically significant morbidity and mortality. Progression from the septic syndrome to the associated clinical sequelae of septic shock and ARDS can be prevented by intervention at the onset of the septic syndrome. Identification and clinical evaluation of the criteria for the septic syndrome may demonstrate an appropriate point for evaluating therapeutic interventions.

Septic Shock

Septic shock is one of the most common causes of death in ICUs. It is a form of circulatory shock that usually develops as a complication of an overwhelming infection. Like any other form of shock, it is a state in which oxygen consumption by the body tissues is inadequate to meet the body's metabolic demands. It has been estimated that more than 130,000 gram-negative bacteremias occur in the United States each year and that shock intervenes in up to 40% of these patients, resulting in a 50% to 90% mortality rate. *Escherichia coli* is the most common causative organism, followed by *Klebsiella, Enterobacter, Proteus,*

Pseudomonas, and *Serratia.* A recent increase in the incidence of gram-positive bacteremia and fungemia has important implications for the necessarily empiric treatment of these patients. As is evident from the causative agents, infection sites are usually the urinary, intestinal, biliary, and female genital tracts. The preponderance of infection occurs in elderly men and childbearing women. Nonspecific predisposing conditions are common and include diabetes mellitus, cirrhosis of the liver, burns, neoplasms, drug therapy, such as chemotherapy and steroids, and invasive therapeutic or monitoring devices.

Pathophysiology. Unfortunately, it has become common to label septic shock as gram-negative shock or endotoxin shock. Gram-negative bacillary endotoxin seems to be only one of the culprits in the pathogenesis of shock syndrome. Indeed, clinical differentiation between gram-positive and gram-negative infection is extremely difficult. The gram-negative bacilli have a complex, three-layered cell wall. The lipopolysaccharide component of the outermost layer has been particularly interesting because of its association with endotoxin properties. Endotoxin is a complex molecule consisting of an outer core of repetitive sugar moieties, an O antigen–specific side chain conferring serologic specificity, and an inner core linked to a structure termed lipid A. Endotoxin and other bacterial products activate cell membrane phospholipases to liberate arachidonic acid and release leukotrienes, prostaglandins, and thromboxanes. These inflammatory mediators primarily influence vasomotor tone, microvascular permeability, leukoagglutination, and the aggregation of platelets. Bacterial endotoxin can trigger a cascade of enzymatic processes, which leads to the release of vasoactive kinins, particularly kallikrein. The microorganisms activate the classic complement pathway, whereas endotoxin activates the alternate pathway. Complement activation, leukotriene generation, and the direct effects of endotoxin on neutrophils lead to the accumulation of inflammatory cells in the lung. This has been proposed as the underlying mechanism for initiation of ARDS, which is a common accompaniment of septic shock. Disseminated intravascular coagulation also occurs; the pathogenesis probably involves activation of the intrinsic clotting system by Hageman factor, leading to activation of kallikrein. This in turn activates the potent vasodilator bradykinin, which results in peripheral blood pooling and increases capillary permeability and localized tissue damage.

Presentation. The classic features of septic shock include fever, tachycardia, elevated white blood cell count, hypotension, and evidence of decreased organ perfusion, such as oliguria, mental status changes, and jaundice. Some patients have hypothermia. White blood cell count or platelet count may be decreased. Tachypnea with a resultant respiratory alkalosis is common early in septic shock. As shock progresses, metabolic acidosis with an elevated serum lactate level becomes evident. The clinical manifestations usually begin abruptly with chills, fever, nausea, vomiting, diarrhea, and prostration. Organ systems involved by septic shock include the cardiac, renal, respiratory, and hematologic systems. Cardiac failure may develop, primarily related to myocardial depressant factors. Disseminated intravascular coagulation is common with septic shock. Septic shock is an important cause of ARDS and severe respiratory failure. The kidneys are also target organs in septic shock, resulting in acute renal failure. Oliguria occurs early and probably results from inadequate renal perfusion.

Diagnosis. Unfortunately, many patients do not have typical symptoms and signs of sepsis. Therefore shock caused by sepsis is often difficult to diagnose, especially in elderly or immunocompromised patients. Of patients who have symptoms suggesting septic shock, approximately half have positive blood cultures. Of patients with positive blood cultures, 40% have a hemodynamic profile consistent with septic shock. Therefore a negative blood culture does not exclude the diagnosis of septic shock. Detection of bacteremia generally depends on recovery of microorganisms from blood cultures. Although blood cultures are a sensitive assay for bacteremia, their usefulness is limited by the ability to detect only viable bacteria and by the time required to grow the microorganisms in vitro. A minimum of 10 ml of blood for each culture should be obtained from adults. Two or three separate blood samples should be obtained for culture when bacteremia is suspected. When the total blood volume cultured is 30 ml from three independent punctures, 99% of bacteremias can be detected. During the initial assessment the patient must be thoroughly evaluated for potential sources of sepsis. The most common sources of bacteremia are the respiratory, genitourinary, and gastrointestinal tracts. Intravenous catheters are a frequently overlooked source of sepsis.

The hemodynamic abnormalities of septic shock have recently been extensively investigated. Using radionuclide gated pool scans with concomitant thermal dilution cardiac output measurements, systemic pressures, flows, and left ventricular volumes, several investigators have identified a significant decrease in left ventricular ejection fraction with the onset of hypotension. The decrease in ejection fraction is associated with left ventricular dilation and maintenance of stroke volume and cardiac output. Similarly, right ventricular ejection fraction is decreased with concomitant right ventricular dilation. These changes in ventricular function during sepsis are not evident when cardiac output is evaluated alone with thermal dilution pulmonary artery catheters. Recent evidence suggests that the cardiovascular abnormalities and the multiple organ system dysfunction found in septic shock are probably not caused directly by microorganisms but in part by release of harmful endogenous substances such as tumor necrosis factor and interleukin-1. In addition, endotoxin may serve as one of multiple mediators that produce septic shock and hemodynamic alterations. Other mediators of septic shock are alpha hemolysin, interleukin-2 as well as myocardial depressant substances, kinins, endorphins, eicosanoids, platelet-activating factor, superoxide radicals, and other lymphokines.

Treatment. Treatment of septic shock is directed at two primary therapeutic goals: rapid reversal of perfusion failure and identification and control of infection. The high mortality rate associated with septic shock reflects the inadequacy of therapeutic approaches. The basics of treatment are eradication of the microbial source of sepsis with appropriate antibiotics, surgical drainage of any focus of infection, improvement of cellular oxygen delivery, and maintenance of adequate tissue perfusion. To this end, aggressive intravascular volume replacement therapy is often needed. As soon as the diagnosis of septic shock is entertained, appropriate culture studies should be performed and the patient treated empirically with broad-spectrum antibiotics. If intravascular catheters are possible sites of infection, immediate replacement of these catheters should be considered. Once the source of infection is determined and the infecting agents are identified, the clinician can limit antibiotic treatment to the organisms involved.

Early aggressive intervention, including fluid resuscitation, vasoactive drug support, mechanical ventilatory support, and surgical drainage of any infected site, is essential for successful treatment. Fluid remains the mainstay in the treatment of septic shock. The fluid of choice for volume resuscitation is controversial. Regardless of the fluid infused, survival can be improved if stroke volume or cardiac output improves in response to fluid challenge. Drugs with predominantly alpha-adrenergic effects should generally be avoided because in the low-flow state of hypodynamic septic shock, peripheral vascular resistance increases. Dopamine and dobutamine have been used successfully to treat septic shock, since these drugs have predominantly beta-adrenergic effects and increase cardiac output because of increased contractility and heart rate. Maintaining urine flow is important to prevent renal failure. Urine output should ideally be kept between 30 and 40 ml/h with fluid resuscitation, inotropic agents, and if necessary drugs, such as dopamine and norepinephrine, to sustain adequate renal perfusion pressure.

Corticosteroids have been advocated in the past as adjunctive therapy for septic shock. However, more recent studies suggest that high-dose corticosteroids provide no benefit in the treatment of severe sepsis and septic shock and should no longer be recommended. Efforts are now being directed toward techniques for early diagnosis of the septic syndrome, identification of markers of causative organisms, and more promising pharmacologic or immunologic drugs to reduce the still unacceptably high mortality rate of systemic sepsis. The recent introduction of antibodies to the core antigens of bacteria shows promise in reducing complications of septic shock when the antibodies are given soon after recognition of the septic syndrome.

PREVENTION

The prevention of infection is crucial. Some principles should be followed: hands must be washed before and after any contact with a patient and between procedures on the same patient; invasive devices should be removed as soon as they stop contributing significant information or therapeutic potential; sterile technique is mandatory whenever normal anatomic barriers are breached; long-term prophylactic antibiotics should be avoided; prophylactic antibiotics are most effective when given before soiling of tissue and are generally ineffective if not administered within 2 to 6 hours after the contamination of tissue; and body fluids and exudates must not be allowed to accumulate. Multiple organisms and multiple sites of infection are the rule, not the exception, in patients who are critically ill.

DIAGNOSIS AND ASSESSMENT

Diagnosis

The diagnosis of an infectious disease requires demonstration of the infecting organism on or within the host's tissue. Techniques available to identify pathogenic microorganisms include direct microscopic examination by stain-enhanced microscopy, wet mount, immune microscopy, or electron microscopy. Direct microscopic examination of body fluids, exudates, and tissues is one of the simplest and most helpful laboratory procedures available for the diagnosis of infectious disease. In many situations the examination accurately and specifically identifies the causative agent. Wet mounts are used for the diagnosis of fungal and parasitic infections. Gram stain is the single best technique available for the rapid diagnosis of bacterial infection. It can be applied to virtually all clinical specimens and is of particular value in the examination of exudates, aspirates, and body fluids.

Immune microscopy combines the specificity of immunologic procedures with the speed and convenience of direct microscopy. In this technique specimens are stained with specific antibody preparations, labeled with fluorescent compounds, and examined with a fluorescence microscope. Viral, bacterial, fungal, or parasitic organisms may be identified. Enzyme-linked immunosorbent assay (ELISA) is similar to immunofluorescence except that antiserum is reacted with an enzyme-labeled, antispecies conjugate. Electron microscopy is a technique particularly valuable in the identification of virus particles. It identifies certain viruses that do not produce cytopathic effects in cell culture.

Because direct microscopy is relatively nonspecific, newer techniques are aimed at the rapid detection of microbial agents, byproducts, or genomes. Techniques available include counterimmunoelectrophoresis, particle agglutination, radioimmunoassay, DNA probes, and gas chromatography.

Respiratory Sources. When the suspected source of infection is the tracheobronchial tree, antimicrobial therapy is generally guided by sputum culture, despite its reported unreliability. Colonization of upper airways and endotracheal tubes is responsible for this inaccuracy. Bronchoscopic aspirates and bronchial washing have been reported inaccurate for the same reason. Transthoracic needle aspiration may be used to diagnose pneumonia, especially in immunocompromised patients. However, this procedure carries significant hazards in critically ill patients. The plugged telescopic catheter brush technique may also be used to improve diagnostic accuracy. However, false-positive results have been reported in as much as 41% of cases. Open lung biopsy, although obviating oropharyngeal contamination, has not been associated with an improved outcome.

Urinary Sources. Assessment of the urinary tract is generally by Gram stain and culture. A urine culture is necessary only if bacteriuria and at least 10 white blood cells per high-powered field are present. Urosepsis is the cause of more than 3000 deaths per year in the United States and is responsible for a significant increase in hospital costs. However, the urinary tract appears to be an infrequent source of systemic sepsis in critically ill patients unless obstruction or urinary tract instrumentation has occurred. Anaerobic urinary tract infections primarily caused by clostridia have been reported in critically ill patients. Anaerobes should be suspected if Gram stain of the urine shows gram-positive or gram-negative rods with subsequent negative aerobic cultures. Cystitis emphysematosa (gas in the bladder wall), a rare condition visible on roentgenograms of the kidney, ureter, and bladder, should raise the possibility of an anaerobic urinary tract infection. The diagnosis is confirmed by obtaining a urine specimen by suprapubic needle aspiration, since clean-catch midstream specimens generally cannot be obtained from critically ill patients.

Wound Source. The diagnosis of a wound infection depends on a thorough knowledge of the patient's history, physical examination, and bacteriologic information from Gram stain and culture studies. Most wound infections can be diagnosed by careful physical examination and confirmed with appropriate cultures. Swab specimens for culture taken from the surface of wounds that appear benign do not help confirm the source of sepsis, since almost all such cultures are positive. If a wound is suspected as the septic source, quantitative cultures should be used to confirm the diagnosis. Greater than 10^5 organisms per gram of tissue strongly suggests wound sepsis, and aggressive topical and systemic antibiotic therapy is indicated.

Neurologic Source. Assessment of a patient with neurologic injury generally requires Gram stain and culture of a sample of cerebrospinal fluid. However, meningitis associated with head or spinal cord injury is an uncommon problem. Indeed, gram-negative meningitis, although highly lethal, is an unusual cause of systemic sepsis and death in trauma patients. The incidence of meningitis may be higher in critically ill medical patients, but no specific data are available to confirm the incidence of meningitis as a cause of septic syndrome in this population.

Abdominal Source. The diagnosis of intraabdominal sepsis, especially in postoperative patients, may be difficult. Early diagnosis and drainage of an infected site are essential for improved survival. A clinical diagnosis of sepsis should logically include the abdomen if the patient has sustained blunt or penetrating trauma resulting in intraperitoneal soilage from damage to the colon or alimentary tract. Prolonged elective surgical procedures with enteric anastomoses may also predispose to abdominal abscesses. Chest roentgenograms and flat and upright abdominal films are frequently obtained but are usually nondiagnostic. Barium or Gastrografin studies may be hazardous and are usually not useful. Diagnostic ultrasonography has the advantage of being relatively inexpensive compared with other noninvasive imaging techniques. In addition, it can be performed at the bedside, which is a significant advantage for critically ill patients. Although ultrasonography has been reported accurate for diagnosis of abdominal abscess in the general population, the accuracy in critically ill postoperative patients is probably not as good. Nuclear studies, including gallium scans, are generally not helpful. Radioactive tagging of endogenous leukocytes has also been used but has limitations, since all inflamed areas concentrate leukocytes and since uptake in the liver and spleen compromises evaluation of these areas. Computed tomography (CT) has become the preferred method for the diagnosis of intraabdominal abscesses. Unfortunately, clinical criteria for ordering CT scans have not developed as rapidly as the technology. CT scanning should be done only if a reasonable probability exists that the information will direct clinical decisions. This probability should be based on a decision-making process in which negative and positive results actually direct therapy in different directions. Some authors believe that abdominal exploration is the only definitive test in some instances, especially when unexplained failure of a single organ system develops. Whether reoperation significantly affects outcome in larger populations of critically ill patients with multisystem organ failure is less clear. It appears that a properly timed reexploration may prevent multisystem organ failure and significantly improve survival. However, whether the course of established multisystem organ failure can be altered with reexploration remains unanswered.

TREATMENT

Susceptibility

Once the organisms have been identified by appropriate culture studies, susceptibility of the isolated pathogens to antimicrobial agents must be determined. Several tests may provide this information. Organisms are susceptible to an antimicrobial agent if they are inhibited in vitro by a concentration of the agent that is lower than the serum concentrations achievable with the usual drug dosage. The minimal inhibitory concentration (MIC) is the lowest concentration of antimicrobial agent that prevents visible growth after a 24-hour incubation period. The MIC of an antimicrobial agent defines the susceptibility and resistance of a defined population of organisms. All susceptibility tests are based directly or indirectly on MIC determinations. Minimum bactericidal concentration (MBC) is the lowest concentration of antimicrobial producing at least a 99.9% reduction in the original inoculum. The MBC can be determined by quantitative subculture. This same technique can be used to determine the minimal lethal concentration (MLC). The most commonly used method for determining antimicrobial susceptibility is the disk-diffusion test, which defines the zone of growth inhibition around an antimicrobial-containing disk. This growth is inversely proportional to the MIC of the antimicrobial. The disk-diffusion method most often used is the Kirby-Bauer procedure. Disk-diffusion testing, however, is not useful for slow-growing fastidious or anaerobic organisms. Its usefulness is also limited because it provides only semiquantitative data. Because MIC determination and disk-diffusion methods require overnight incubation, commercially available systems were developed that produce susceptibility results in 3 to 7 hours. These automated systems can rapidly determine susceptibilities of multiple drugs at one time.

Antibiotic Therapy

Antibiotic therapy often must be started before full organism identification and sensitiv-ity information is available. Thus empiric agents are frequently administered initially. Some factors that must be considered before selecting empiric antibiotic regimens are the likely focus of infection, the organisms endemic to a given hospital and ICU, and the pharmacology of the antimicrobials, including the spectrum of activity, especially based on results of testing of organisms isolated in the ICU, pharmacokinetics, appropriate dosage and dosage intervals, and toxicities.

During the first 48 hours of empiric antibiotic therapy the patient must be monitored closely for changes in clinical status. If no improvement is noted, the physician should consider the possibility of an undrained focus of infection, inappropriate antibiotic selection, inadequate dosage or dosage schedule, early antibiotic-induced toxicity, such as drug-related fever or hypersensitivity reaction, or inadequate time to manifest clinical improvement with appropriate therapy. When culture and sensitivity results become available, the least toxic and narrowest antibiotic regimen should be selected. The administration of antibiotics may change the predominant organism so that resistant bacteria arise. Further, nothing prevents a secondary infection at a different site in these frequently immunocompromised patients. This dynamic situation requires that the patient's condition be continually monitored and antibiotic therapy adjusted according to the most recent culture and sensitivity data.

Penicillins. Penicillins can be classified on the basis of antibacterial activity. They generally inhibit cell wall biosynthesis through penicillin-binding proteins and are bacteriostatic. All penicillins are excreted into urine via glomerular filtration and secretion by the renal tubular cells. In addition, most penicillins are actively secreted into the bile, resulting in significantly higher biliary than serum concentrations.

Hypersensitivity is the major adverse effect of the penicillins. Reactions range in severity from rash to immediate anaphylaxis. Indeed, allergic reaction to penicillin is the most common cause of anaphylaxis, a rare occurrence but potentially fatal. Patients with atopic dermatitis or allergic rhinitis do not appear to be at increased risk of anaphylaxis. Other adverse effects of penicillins are diarrhea, neutropenia, autoimmune hemolytic anemia, and impaired platelet aggregation, although bleeding is rare. Neurologic toxic manifestations include myoclonic seizures. Renal damage ranging from allergic angiitis to interstitial nephritis has been described. Electrolyte abnormalities are an important consideration with use of penicillins. Carbenicillin and ticarcillin may cause hypokalemia because they serve as nonreabsorbable anions. In addition, these two agents give a large sodium load to the patient because they are disodium salts and contain 5 mEq of sodium per gram of antibiotic. An alternative regimen includes a drug such as azlocillin, which is a monosodium salt with half the salt load. Hyperkalemia or hypernatremia can result from large doses of penicillin G because each million units has approximately 1.7 mEq of potassium or sodium, depending on the preparation.

Cephalosporins. Cephalosporins are the most frequently prescribed antimicrobials. These agents are divided into a well-accepted generation scheme. Their spectrum of activity varies with the generation. The first-generation agents are the most commonly used antibiotics for surgical prophylaxis.

Because the chemical structures of cephalosporins and penicillins are similar, cross-reactivity between the two drugs sometimes occurs. Immunologic studies indicate that as much as 20% of patients show cross-reactivity. Clinically, however, only 5% to 10% show cross-allergy with penicillin. Therefore, if the penicillin allergy is not an anaphylactic type, cephalosporins may be given.

Other side effects of cephalosporins include nephrotoxicity and hematologic abnormalities. Interstitial nephritis may result from cephalosporin therapy, especially in patients over the age of 60 years. Evidence suggests that the combination of a cephalosporin and an aminoglycoside potentiates nephrotoxicity. The Coombs test is positive in approximately 3% of patients receiving cephalosporins, although hemolytic anemia is rare. A serious bleeding diathesis with hypoprothrombinemia and qualitative or quantitative platelet abnormalities may be caused by cephalosporins, especially moxalactam.

Aminoglycosides. Aminoglycosides bind irreversibly to proteins in the ribosomes, so these agents are bactericidal. When therapy is initiated, a loading dose should be administered to achieve a therapeutic serum level rapidly. The clearance of aminoglycosides is linearly related to creatinine clearance. Although quantitative differences among individual agents may exist, all aminoglycosides share three toxicities; neuromuscular paralysis, ototoxicity, and nephrotoxicity.

NEUROMUSCULAR PARALYSIS. Aminoglycoside-induced neuromuscular paralysis is a rare but potentially lethal complication. It should be suspected if recovery from a nonde-polarizing neuromuscular blocking agent is delayed, the depth of neuromuscular blockade increases after antibiotic administration, or the neuromuscular block is difficult to reverse. The mechanisms whereby aminoglycosides potentiate neuromuscular blockade are inhibition of presynaptic release of acetylcholine and a blockade of postsynaptic receptor sites for acetylcholine. This block is enhanced by the presence of curare-like drugs, succinylcholine, magnesium, and myasthenia gravis. The block can be largely reversed with calcium administration and partially reversed with neostigmine.

OTOTOXICITY. All aminoglycosides may be ototoxic. Although individual agents are more likely to produce either auditory or vestibular toxic effects, all aminoglycosides are capable of producing both. Ototoxicity is potentiated by other agents, including ethacrynic acid, furosemide, and possibly other diuretics. The toxicity is correlated with the duration of aminoglycoside therapy, preexisting renal disease, and the patient's age. Ototoxic effects have been reported in approximately 5% of patients receiving aminoglycoside therapy.

NEPHROTOXICITY. All aminoglycosides may be nephrotoxic. Nephrotoxic effects as defined by a fall in glomerular filtration rate occur in 5% to 25% of patients receiving aminoglycosides. Monitoring of serum levels is important when patients are maintained with aminoglycoside therapy. Risk factors for nephrotoxicity include advanced age, prior aminoglycoside administration, preexisting renal dysfunction, concomitant administration of other nephrotoxic agents, hypotension, and prolonged administration of the drug.

Vancomycin. Vancomycin is a bactericidal glycopeptide that inhibits cell wall synthesis. It has a half-life of 6 hours and is eliminated via glomerular filtration. The most frequent side effects of vancomycin administration are fever, chills, and phlebitis at the infusion site. Ototoxicity manifest as eighth nerve damage is possible. A more serious complication is the red-neck syndrome following rapid infusion of the drug. This histamine-induced reaction is characterized by flushing and a maculopapular rash of the face, neck, and trunk. It is usually self-limited and abates with cessation of the drug, although occasionally antihistamines and fluid resuscitation are necessary. The reaction appears to be associated with rapid intravenous infusion of vancomycin. Therefore the drug must be infused slowly over 1 hour.

Vancomycin is most commonly used empirically for infections caused by gram-positive organisms — *Staphylococcus aureus,* non-*aureus* staphylococci, and *Enterococcus,* which are commonly resistant to penicillins and cephalosporins. It should be used sparingly for other infections when less toxic drugs are at least as effective. Staphylococci resistant to vancomycin are appearing.

Clindamycin. The major therapeutic use for clindamycin, a lincosamine antibiotic, is for anaerobic infections or in combination with an aminoglycoside or aztreonam. The most common and serious side effect of clindamycin is diarrhea with pseudomembranous colitis, which occurs in as much as 10% of clindamycin-treated patients. Drug-induced rashes occur in approximately 5% of patients. Itching, angioneurotic edema, urticaria, Stevens-Johnson syndrome, drug fever, and granulocytopenia have been reported. Abnormalities in liver function tests, particularly transaminase elevations, appear frequently. However, they are usually erratic, mild, and unassociated with other evidence of hepatotoxicity. Like aminoglycosides, clindamycin can potentiate neuromuscular blockade, although it does so much less frequently. Clindamycin is incompatible in solution with many commonly used drugs, such as ampicillin, barbiturates, aminophylline, calcium gluconate, magnesium sulfate, and phenytoin.

Metronidazole. Metronidazole is a nitroimidazole with potent bactericidal properties. It is most useful in the treatment of serious anaerobic infections, especially intraabdominal infections. Metronidazole has no activity against gram-positive or gram-negative aerobic organisms. The drug has little protein-binding activity and a half-life of 8 hours. Metronidazole is metabolized in the liver and eliminated in the urine and feces.

Side effects of metronidazole therapy include a reaction with disulfiram, potentiation of warfarin, and pseudomembranous colitis. However, colitis is a rare complication, and metronidazole is used as an alternative to vancomycin to treat pseudomembranous colitis. Neurologic manifestations, such as seizures, encephalopathy, and neuropathy, occur rarely.

Imipenem. Imipenem is a prototype of the thienamycin class of compounds, a carbapenem antibiotic. It offers broad-spectrum coverage with potent activity against most clinically important species of bacteria, including isolates resistant to other antibiotics. It is generally distributed to most tissues and body fluids following intravenous administration, although cerebrospinal fluid levels are modest. Most of the drug is eliminated in the urine where it is metabolized by an enzyme on the brush border of the renal tubular cells. Cilastatin is given simultaneously to inhibit this inactivation. Imipenem is generally well tolerated, although several adverse effects have been described. Approximately 3% of patients manifest allergic reactions, such as drug fever, pruritus, and urticaria. Nausea and vomiting, diarrhea, and abnormalities of liver function have been described, as have more serious adverse effects, such as seizures and superinfection.

Quinolones. The quinolones, such as norfloxacin, are broad-spectrum, orally administered antibiotics. The most common indications for fluorinated quinolones are urinary tract infections, prophylaxis for urosurgery, gonorrhea, and bacterial enteritis. Quinolones have also been used successfully to treat chronic osteomyelitis and soft tissue infections and have been useful both prophylactically and therapeutically in neutropenic patients. Although ciprofloxacin is active against *Pseudomonas,* drug resistance develops rapidly.

The side effects most often seen with quinolones involve the gastrointestinal tract, central nervous system, and urinary tract. The most frequent complaints are nausea, upper gastrointestinal discomfort, and dizziness. These reactions are usually mild and rarely necessitate changing to another antibacterial agent. Another phenomenon noted with quinolone therapy is the formation of quinolone crystals in the urine. The consequence of these crystals is uncertain, but no deleterious effects have been described.

Aztreonam. Aztreonam is the first of a new class of monocyclic beta lactams. The pharmacologic properties of this agent are not exceptionally different from those of other parenterally administered beta-lactam antibiotics that are not absorbed orally. Dosage must be adjusted in patients with renal failure or cirrhosis and during dialysis. The types of infection for which aztreonam should be considered as a single agent include urinary tract or biliary tract infections, gonorrhea, and gram-negative osteomyelitis. It should be considered in combination with other agents for abdominal sepsis, respiratory tract infections, septicemia in leukemia, and neonatal meningitis.

Hypersensitivity reactions are an important limitation of the use of beta-lactam antibiotics. However, several studies suggest that little cross-reactivity exists between aztreonam and other beta-lactam antibiotics. The most commonly reported side effects are local reactions, skin rash, nausea, and diarrhea. The overall incidence of side effects and abnormal laboratory results necessitating discontinuation of aztreonam is approximately 2.1%.

Although extensive work has been done on structure-activity relationships of monocyclic beta-lactams, aztreonam is the only agent currently available for patient use. Newer compounds are being developed, and further derivations will surely emerge. Aztreonam therapy for *Pseudomonas* infections appears to have results equivalent to those of aminoglycosides.

Beta-Lactamase Inhibitors

Beta lactamases are the major form of resistance to penicillins and cephalosporins. Because developing antibiotics with stability to a wide range of beta lactamases has been difficult, combinations of an antibiotic with beta-lactamase inhibitor have recently gained popularity. Clavulanate is a beta-lactamase inhibitor with little antibacterial activity of its own. It inhibits beta lactamases by destroying the enzyme. The combination of amoxicillin and clavulanate has been used successfully to treat skin infections, otitis, and upper respiratory infections. The combination does not significantly alter the pharmacologic properties of either drug. The combination of ticarcillin and clavulanate is effective in the treatment of intraabdominal infections, osteomyelitis, and urinary tract infections because of the increased activity of ticarcillin when used in conjunction with clavulanate. The combination has also been used for febrile neutropenic patients.

Sulbactam is a 6-desamino penicillin sulfone that also inhibits beta lactamases. Sulbactam has pharmacokinetics similar to those of ampicillin. Combined with ampicillin this agent has been used successfully to treat urinary, intraabdominal, and respiratory infections caused by beta lactamase–producing organisms.

Antifungal Agents

Amphotericin B is the most effective antifungal agent available. It must be administered in a large volume of fluid. It often causes fever and chills and occasionally hypotension or hypertension. The systemic reaction is blunted by antihistamines and steroids. Amphotericin B is a potent nephrotoxin and induces potassium wasting. Because it is cleared by the liver, the dose is not adjusted for the level of renal function. Administration usually begins with 1 to 5 mg slowly intravenously while the patient is observed for signs of cardiovascular instability. The dose is then increased so that the patient is receiving 0.5 to 1 mg/kg/d over 4 to 6 hours. The total dose administered ranges from 0.5 to 2 g, with the daily and total doses being greater for more serious infections.

Fluconazole is effective against *Candida* and a variety of other fungi. It can be administered intravenously, with few immediate reactions and minimal toxicity. Its role in the management of critically ill patients has not yet been defined.

Antiviral Agents

Awareness of viral pathogens in the ICU population is increasing. Patients in the ICU are often immunosuppressed, with defects in humoral or cell-mediated immunity. Underlying illness or procedures that alter immune mechanisms are common. Viruses are often secondary infectious agents in these patients. Viruses are etiologic agents in 10% to 30% of all cases of community-acquired pneumonias. In adults influenza virus is the most common cause of viral pneumonia. Approximately 10,000 to 15,000 cases of viral meningitis and encephalitis are reported each year in the United States. The most common cause of sporadic cases of encephalitis in the United States is herpes simplex virus type 1. More than half of viral meningitis cases are probably caused by enteroviruses. With the widespread use of polio vaccines, coxsackievirus and echoviruses are now responsible for the majority of viral meningitis epidemics during the early summer and fall. Primary infection with herpes simplex virus type 2 has been associated with meningitis in 0.5% to 5% of all infected patients. Other etiologic agents for viral infection include varicella zoster virus, Epstein-Barr virus, and cytomegalovirus.

Several antiviral agents with proven efficacy against infections caused by influenza A, herpes simplex virus, and varicella zoster virus are available. However, most antiviral agents have a restricted spectrum of activity because they inhibit specific events in viral replication. The development of viral resistance to antiviral agents may limit their effectiveness. Combinations of antiviral agents have been used successfully to increase their efficacy and decrease toxicity.

Pharmacokinetic studies of absorption, stability, tissue distribution, and metabolic fate of antiviral agents aid in selecting and determining the dose of antiviral agents. Unfortunately, no standardized or generally accepted correlations exist between in vitro inhibitory concentrations, achievable blood or body fluid concentrations of antiviral agents, and clinical response. The antiviral agents most commonly in use today are acyclovir, amantadine, vidarabine, idoxuridine, and trifluridine.

Acyclovir. Acyclovir is an antiviral agent with activity directed at herpes simplex virus types 1 and 2, varicella zoster virus, and Epstein-Barr virus. Approximately 70% of acyclovir is excreted unchanged in the urine, and less than 15% is excreted as minor metabolites. Intravenous administration is generally well tolerated. Irritation at the injection site, rash, nausea, central nervous system changes, and renal dysfunction have been described with acyclovir administration.

Amantadine. Amantadine is a symmetric amine with specific activity against influenza A viruses. Amantadine is available only in oral formulations. It is well absorbed, is not metabolized, and has a serum half-life of 14 hours. Following oral administration 95% of the dose appears in the urine unchanged. The major toxic effects of amantadine occur in the central nervous system and include anxiety, insomnia, and difficulty in concentration. The effects are probably related to the drug's dopamine-potentiating properties. Other potential toxic effects are nausea, edema, livedo reticularis, congestive heart failure, and urinary retention.

Vidarabine. Vidarabine is an analog of adenine deoxyriboside with activity against herpes simplex virus types 1 and 2, varicella zoster virus, and Epstein-Barr virus. The primary route of elimination is renal, with urinary excretion accounting for 50% of the dose. Gastrointestinal toxic effects are common and are manifest as anorexia, nausea, vomiting, and diarrhea. At higher doses vidarabine has been associated with hematopoietic abnormalities and neurotoxic effects, such as anemia, leukopenia, thrombocytopenia, tumors, seizures, and unusual pain syndromes in the extremities.

Interferons. Interferons are proteins or glycoproteins produced by cells in response to an inducer, including viruses. Numerous trials are under way to test the efficacy of various interferons against not only viruses but also malignancies. This work along with studies of newer antiviral agents will determine the future role of these agents.

Antibiotic Monitoring

The aminoglycosides and vancomycin are toxic drugs with a narrow difference between effective and toxic levels. The clinical response of infections correlates with the levels achieved.

The rate of response is improved when tobramycin or gentamicin peak levels are maintained above 7 µg/ml and when amikacin peak levels are sustained above 26µg/ml. The aminoglycosides are distributed in the extracellular fluid and excreted by the kidneys. Both of these variables change rapidly in critically ill patients, making careful and frequent drug level monitoring mandatory. Use of nomograms leads to major dosage errors for individual patients. The interpretation of the routinely obtained "peak and trough" levels is deceptively simple. Accurate interpretation requires knowledge of the dose administered (often not the dose intended because of variability of drug concentration in stock solutions and variability in the percentage of the dose that is actually infused). The exact relationship between the time of drug infusion and the time at which the plasma sample was obtained is crucial for these drugs, whose half-lives may be as short as 2 hours. The "peak" level sample must be obtained after the redistribution (alpha) phase, which is generally complete in about 30 minutes for the aminoglycosides and 60 minutes for vancomycin. The "trough" sample must be obtained immediately before administration of the dose. We advocate measurement of the trough level, a second sample taken after the redistribution phase is complete, a third sample taken about one third of the way through the dose interval, and a final sample taken at the end of the dose interval. The results are plotted with time on the horizontal axis and the log of the level on the vertical axis. It should be possible to draw a straight line through the three postdose levels and then extrapolate it to the end of the infusion to estimate the true "peak" level. When the three points do not fall on a straight line, inaccurate results must be suspected. The volume of distribution is calculated by knowing the change from the predose trough to the extrapolated peak level and the amount of drug administered. The half-life is estimated from the disappearance curve. This estimate can be made with the first dose of the drug, allowing for adjustment immediately after the last level is available, to significantly speed the time when effective concentrations are achieved.

SUGGESTED READINGS

Baigelman W, Bellin S, Cupples A, et al: Bacteriologic assessment of the lower respiratory tract in intubated patients. Crit Care Med 1986;14:864-868

Balk RA, Bone RD (eds): Septic shock. *Crit Care Clin* 1989;5:1

Bone RC, Fisher CJ, Clemmer TP, et al: The Methylprednisolone Severe Sepsis Study Group: a controlled clinical trial of high-dose methylprednisolone in the treatment of severe sepsis and septic shock. N Engl J Med 1987;317:653-658

Brown M: Antibiotic therapy: infection in anesthesia. Anesth Clin North Am 1989;7:923

Brown M: ICU-critical care. In Barash PG, Cullen BF, Stoelting RK (eds): Clinical Anesthesia. Philadelphia, 1989, JB Lippincott, pp 1455-1476

Centers for Disease Control Working Groups: Guidelines for prevention of intravascular infections. In Guidelines for the prevention and control of nosocomial infections. Atlanta, 1981, US Public Health Service

Craven DE, Kunches LM, Lictenberg DA, et al: Nosocomial infection and fatality in medical and surgical intensive care unit patients. Arch Intern Med 1988;148:1161-1168

Demling RH: Colloid or crystalloid resuscitation in sepsis. In Sibbald WJ, Sprung CL (eds): Perspectives on sepsis and septic shock. Fullerton, Calif, 1986, Society of Critical Care Medicine, p 275

Hessen MT, Kaye D: Nosocomial pneumonia. Crit Care Clin 1988;4:245-257

Karakusis PH: Considerations in the therapy of septic shock. Med Clin North Am 1986;70:933-944

Natanson C, Fink MP, Ballentyne HK, et al: Gram-negative bacteremia produces both severe systolic and diastolic cardiac dysfunction in a canine model that simulates human septic shock. J Clin Invest 1986;78:259-270

Natanson C, Parrillo JE: Septic shock. Anesthesiol Clin North Am 1988;6:73-85

Norwood MSH, Civetta JM: Evaluating sepsis in critically ill patients: ACCP Council on Critical Care. Chest 1987; 92:137

Ognibene FP, Parker MM, Natanson C, et al: Depressed left ventricular performance: response to volume infusion in patients with sepsis and septic shock. Chest 1988;93: 903-910

Tracy KJ, Lowry SF, Fahey TJ, et al: Cachectic/tumor necrosis factor induces lethal shock and stress hormone response in the dog. Surg Gynecol Obstet 1987;164: 415-422

Veterans Administration Systemic Sepsis Cooperative Study Group: Effect of high-dose glucocorticoid therapy on mortality in patients with clinical signs of systemic sepsis. N Engl J Med 1987;317:659-665

Zavitsky AL, Chernow B: Catecholamine sympathomimetics. In Chernow B, Lake CR (eds): The pharmacologic approach to the critically ill patient. Baltimore, 1983, Williams & Wilkins, pp 481-509

13

SELECTED RED AND WHITE BLOOD CELL DISORDERS

BRIAN D. OWENS, MD

ANEMIA

Anemia is a common abnormality among patients in the ICU, but many of these anemic patients are asymptomatic and do not need immediate treatment to increase their red blood cell (RBC) mass. On the other hand, some patients admitted to the ICU with a normal RBC mass have functional anemia. The common denominator among patients requiring therapy, that is, those with symptomatic anemia and those with functional anemia, when variables such as volume status are eliminated, is inadequate oxygen delivery to tissues.

Oxygen delivery is a function of cardiac output, oxygen-carrying capacity, and the affinity of hemoglobin for oxygen. In this chapter factors influencing oxygen-carrying capacity are discussed.

Reduction in tissue oxygen delivery as a result of decreased RBC mass is the classic form of anemia, which is recognized by a lower than normal hemoglobin level and hematocrit value. Anemia is the most common RBC abnormality seen in the ICU. Causes of decreased RBC mass can be divided into two categories: inadequate production and increased loss. Inadequate production of RBCs can be divided into three categories: inadequate stimulus, inadequate substrate, and failure of the production organ (marrow). Increased loss of RBCs results from hemorrhage or from destruction of cells in the organs or vascular compartment.

Evaluation of Anemic Patients

An initial evaluation of a patient with anemia is no different in the ICU than in any other

setting. After a thorough history and physical examination, assessment begins with information that is readily available: reticulocyte count, RBC indices, and peripheral blood smear. These tests and hemoglobin electrophoresis (in cases of suspected hemoglobinopathy) are the only tests needed before transfusion.

The reticulocyte count differentiates anemias caused by increased destruction from those attributable to decreased production. With special stains the percentage of immature RBCs can be determined. To correct the actual percentage of reticulocytes to an index, the clinician multiplies that percentage by the patient's hematocrit value divided by a normal hematocrit:

$$\text{Reticulocyte index} = \text{Reticulocyte \%} \times \frac{\text{Patient's Hct}}{\text{Normal Hct}} \qquad \text{(Eq. 1)}$$

This index must be corrected for the premature release of bone marrow reticulocytes into the peripheral blood under stimulated conditions. The prematurely released reticulocytes are present for more than 1 to 2 days; therefore the index is divided by 2 (range 1.5 to 3 depending on the severity of the anemia). Even without the special reticulocyte stain, the clinician can make the presumptive diagnosis of reticulocytosis when polychromasia (large, lavender-shaded RBCs) is seen on a routine smear of peripheral blood.

Significant reticulocytosis suggests a hemolytic problem, but it also occurs in patients responding to earlier hemorrhage, or to replacement for substrate deficiencies, such as iron, folate, or vitamin B_{12}, and in anemias caused by bone marrow destruction or replacement by tumor or fibrosis.

Automated RBC counters provide RBC indices with the patient's hemoglobin level, hematocrit value, and RBC number. The machines measure mean corpuscular volume (MCV), RBC number, and hemoglobin directly. Hematocrit, mean corpuscular hemoglobin, and mean corpuscular hemoglobin concentration (MCHC) are calculated. MCHC has little use clinically because it is unreliable. MCV is the most useful of the RBC indices because it allows classification of anemias caused by underproduction.

Finally, the peripheral blood smear enables the clinician to search for quantitative and qualitative changes in all cell lines and may indicate a specific reason for the anemia. Often special stains are used to reveal specific markers. In this chapter, however, changes seen on the readily available routine stain are emphasized.

Hemolytic Anemia

As previously mentioned, reticulocytosis is most commonly associated with hemolytic anemia. Hemolysis occurs intravascularly or, more commonly, extravascularly as a result of RBC ingestion by macrophages in the liver or spleen. Causes of hemolysis may be extrinsic, as in trauma from a prosthetic heart valve, or intrinsic, resulting from membrane or cytoplasmic malfunctions that cause the mononuclear-phagocyte system to eliminate cells.

The peripheral smear is helpful in diagnosis of hemolytic anemias. The most common morphologic abnormality in hemolytic anemias is spherocytes. Fragmented RBCs are the hallmark of traumatic RBC destruction, hypochromic target cells are common in thalassemia syndromes, and crescent-shaped cells are seen in sickle cell disorders.

Hemolytic anemias share a common laboratory profile. Levels of serum bilirubin, specifically the indirect or unconjugated fraction, are elevated as a result of transport of this hemoglobin breakdown product from the macrophages to the liver. In the absence of hepatic dysfunction, direct or conjugated bilirubin levels are normal. Rapid hemolysis may result in icterus or jaundice.

After RBC destruction hemoglobin attaches to a plasma globulin, haptoglobin, and the complex is rapidly removed from the serum by macrophages. The result is a low to absent haptoglobin level. With ongoing hemolysis, free hemoglobin remains in the serum. The hemoglobin is filtered in the kidney, reabsorbed in the proximal tubule, and metabolized. Iron from this metabolism appears in urine as hemosiderin.

Two additional markers, serum methemalbumin and urine hemoglobin, should be mentioned because they are found only in severe, intravascular hemolysis.

When anemia occurs in the hospital and is associated with reticulocytosis and spherocytes, an immunohemolytic anemia caused by an underlying disease or by drugs must be suspected. The diagnostic test in this situation is the Coombs test. In a direct Coombs test antibodies to immunoglobulin G (IgG) or C3 are incubated with the patient's RBCs. Agglutination indicates coating of RBCs with IgG or C3. The indirect Coombs test can be prognostic in this group of patients because it indicates quantities of IgG or C3 present. The patient's serum is incubated with normal RBCs. The direct Coombs test is then performed on the incubated RBCs, and a positive test indicates that the patient's serum contains additional IgG or C3.

Chronic Disease or Inflammation

Normocytic anemia or a normal MCV is associated with chronic inflammation or diseases, including osteomyelitis, connective tissue disorders, regional enteritis, renal or endocrine failure, or subacute bacterial endocarditis. The pathogenesis of anemia in these disorders is varied. In some cases evidence supports an abnormality in iron transport, which may result in a population of slightly hypochromic, microcytic cells. Anemias associated with endocrine failures may be the result of decreased stimulus to bone marrow by one or more of the endocrine hormones.

RBC production and maturation are influenced by numerous substances (catecholamines, thyroid hormone, anabolic and catabolic steroids, growth hormone, and cyclic nucleotides); however, production appears to be most responsive to erythropoietin, a glycoprotein produced by the kidney in response to hypoxic stimuli. Whether erythropoietin influences the differentiation of the marrow's pluripotent stem cell to an erythroid precursor is a matter for further elucidation. Clearly, erythropoietin is a potent stimulant to hemoglobin synthesis and to cells in the erythroid line at all levels of maturity.

The classic anemia caused by inadequate stimulus is seen in chronic renal failure, and the degree of anemia usually correlates with the level of azotemia. Erythropoietin levels are lower than in nonuremic patients with similar degrees of anemia. Although anemias associated with chronic diseases are usually mild, the anemia of uremia can be severe. Patients tolerate the anemia well because of physiologic compensation to a slowly developing chronic condition. They are at risk for acute decompensation when such complications as gastrointestinal blood loss intervene.

Bone Marrow Failure

Inadequate production of RBCs as a result of bone marrow failure occurs in primary and secondary marrow disorders and causes a normocytic anemia. In aplastic anemia the disorder is at the level of the pluripotent stem cell; therefore anemia, leukopenia, and thrombocytopenia are present. Half of cases of aplastic anemia in the United States are idiopathic. Fanconi's anemia is an uncommon, autosomal recessive, inherited disease often associated with multiple somatic defects. More commonly aplastic anemia follows exposure to drugs or toxins. Some agents, such as cancer chemotherapeutic drugs, ionizing radiation, benzenes, and chloramphenicol, predictably cause bone marrow depression in a dose-dependent manner. Interestingly, chloramphenicol is also included in a second group, along with phenylbutazone, insecticides, gold compounds, sulfa drugs, and organic arsenicals, that unpredictably results in an often irreversible aplastic anemia unrelated to dose or duration of administration. Aplastic anemia is associated with several viral illnesses, including hepatitis A, B, and non-A, non-B, Epstein-Barr virus, and viral respiratory illnesses.

Finally, bone marrow infiltration by tumor, fibrous tissue, or granulomas can result in significant anemia with or without reduction or increase in other cell lines. The peripheral smear may show a significantly elevated number of reticulocytes, but when correction is made for hematocrit as previously described, the index is normal. No definitive laboratory profile is available for these disorders, and a bone marrow biopsy and aspirate are indicated.

Substrate Deficiencies

Anemias commonly recognized as resulting from a lack of substrate are those caused by iron, vitamin B_{12}, and folic acid deficiency; however, sideroblastic anemias with failed porphyrin synthesis and the thalassemias resulting in inadequate globin synthesis must also be considered in this group. Because iron deficiency, sideroblastic anemias, and the thalassemias cause inadequate hemoglobin synthesis, they result in small RBCs with reduced hemoglobin (hypochromic, microcytic RBCs). Deficiencies of vitamin B_{12} and folate cause impaired DNA synthesis. Cell division is slowed while development of cytoplasmic components is unaffected, resulting in large or megaloblastic RBCs.

Iron deficiency is probably the most common cause of anemia among adults in the United States. Although iron deficiency can rarely result from inadequate intake (fad dieters, indigent or elderly people, clay ingesters) or poor gastrointestinal absorption (partial or total gastrectomy, malabsorption syndromes), by far the most common cause is blood loss. Blood loss may be natural as in menstruating females or abnormal as in gastrointestinal bleeding. With chronic blood loss the daily iron loss increases from the normal 1 to 1.5 mg. Depletion of iron stores increases the efficiency of the duodenal and jejunal mucosa by unknown mechanisms, so that 10% to 20% of ingested iron can be absorbed. An average adult in the United States ingests 10 to 20 mg of iron daily. When loss exceeds absorption, iron stores are depleted and iron deficiency ensues.

If iron deficiency is suspected, several laboratory tests should be performed. Serum iron levels are low, but this is also true in anemia of chronic disease. To differentiate between the two, the total iron binding capacity and serum ferritin concentration are useful. Total iron binding capacity decreases in chronic disease but usually increases in iron deficiency. On the other hand, serum ferritin commonly falls to very low levels in iron deficiency.

The sideroblastic anemias are a heterogeneous group of hypochromic, microcytic anemias characterized by markedly increased mitochondrial iron deposits in nucleated erythroid precursors in the bone marrow. Hemoporphyrin synthesis is disordered. Although a hereditary form exists, most sideroblastic anemias are acquired in association with ingestion of toxins and drugs (alcohol, isoniazid), neoplastic or inflammatory diseases, or aging.

Thalassemias are the final group of microcytic anemias. This group of genetic disorders covers a spectrum of disease from undetectable to incompatible with life. The underlying problem is inadequate or slow formation of one of the globin chains, alpha or beta. An in-depth discussion of these disorders is beyond the scope of this chapter. If thalassemia is the cause of a significant anemia, the patient's condition is probably already diagnosed. Otherwise, the diagnosis should be entertained in patients with unexplained microcytosis.

The only source of vitamin B_{12} for humans is dietary meat and dairy products. Obviously, strict vegetarians are at risk for vitamin B_{12} deficiency. Absorption of the vitamin is a complex process requiring several glycoproteins and a normal distal ileum. The most common cause of a vitamin B_{12} deficiency is pernicious anemia in which atrophy of the gastric mucosa (parietal cells) causes decreased secretion of intrinsic factor, a glycoprotein. Since intrinsic factor is not available to bind with vitamin B_{12}, and since absorption in the distal ileum is specific for that complex, vitamin B_{12} is not absorbed. Other causes of vitamin B_{12} deficiency are gastrectomy, disease of the terminal ileum, and intestinal organisms, including bacterial overgrowth after oral antibiotic therapy.

Vitamin B_{12} deficiency is not an acute process. A normal adult has 4 mg stored; the daily requirement is 2.5 µg. Symptoms of vitamin B_{12} deficiency are often gastrointestinal (glossitis, anorexia, diarrhea) and neurologic (peripheral paresthesia or dysesthesia, weakness, ataxia, diminished vibration sense, poor fine motor coordination, and disturbances of mentation).

Unlike vitamin B_{12} deficiency, folic acid deficiency commonly results from malnutrition. Body stores are between 5 and 20 mg, and the daily requirement is 50 µg. A deficiency takes only a few months to develop. Folic acid deficiency has the same hematologic and gastrointestinal manifestations as vitamin B_{12} deficiency. Folic acid deficiency has no neurologic manifestations; however, the clinician must be aware that deficiencies of vitamin B_{12} and folate may coexist. Large doses of folic acid reverse the hematologic manifestations of vitamin B_{12} deficiency while allowing neurologic dysfunction to progress.

Blood Transfusion

Therapy for anemia is based on diagnosis and treatment of the underlying disorder, but blood transfusion allows short-term correction of oxygen-carrying capacity. The decision to transfuse whole blood or packed RBCs is complicated. Factors to be considered include rapidity of onset of anemia, ongoing RBC loss, premorbid patient condition, adequacy of clinical compensation, and course and treatment of the underlying abnormality.

In an emergency patients can be transfused with type O, Rh-negative packed RBCs or with type-specific blood. Type O, Rh-negative packed RBCs have no A, B, or D antigens, so massive hemolysis as a result of recipient antibodies to these antigens is unlikely. The plasma does contain antibodies to both A and B antigens, but packed RBCs have most plasma and antibodies removed. If for some reason type O, Rh-negative whole blood is given to a non–type O recipient, the blood bank should ensure that low antibody titer units are used. If 2 or more units of type O whole blood is transfused, type-specific blood should not be used until the recipient's antibody titer is documented to be safe.

Type-specific blood requires that the recipient's blood be typed. No cross-matching is performed. The risk of finding an unexpected antibody during cross-matching is 1:1000 in recipients without prior transfusion and 1:100 in those with prior transfusion. Type-specific transfusions have proved safe in clinical use.

With the advent of acquired immunodeficiency syndrome (AIDS), infectious risks of blood transfusion have become the dominant force in changing physicians' practice patterns, even though other infectious and noninfectious complications are much more common. Complications of blood transfusions can most easily be classified as immunologically or nonimmunologically mediated.

Immunologically mediated transfusion reactions can be directed against RBCs, white blood cells, platelets, or serum proteins. The most dramatic of these is the intravascular hemolysis seen with the transfusion of ABO-incompatible blood. The antibody, most commonly a naturally occurring immunoglobulin M, attaches to the RBC antigen and activates the complement cascade, resulting in massive hemolysis, cardiovascular collapse, disseminated intravascular coagulation, and renal failure. Conscious patients are restless and complain of head, back, and chest pains. These episodes are better avoided than treated. If one occurs, the transfusion should be stopped immediately. The cardiovascular system must be supported by volume expansion and vasoactive drugs as necessary. Diuresis should be maintained with osmotic or loop diuretics. Dopamine may increase renal blood flow.

Extravascular hemolytic reactions are far less dramatic. The antibody immunoglobulin G does not fix complement. Antibody-coated RBCs are destroyed by reticuloendothelial cells, mostly in the spleen. Disseminated intravascular coagulation and renal failure are uncommon. This reaction may occur immediately or be delayed for up to 3 weeks.

Febrile responses to blood transfusion are usually immunologically mediated and directed against leukocyte or platelet antigens. They occur in 2% to 7% of blood product transfusions, produce variable patient discomfort, and cause alarm because an infectious origin must be considered. Since these reactions require sensitization, they occur in patients who have had prior transfusions and in women who have borne children. If the patient has a history of febrile reactions, leukocyte-poor blood prevents the problem. Pretreatment with antipyretics, antihistamines, and corticosteroids has variable efficacy.

Other important immunologically mediated reactions are allergic reactions, in which urticaria, pruritus, and angioedema result from an allergic reaction to plasma proteins, and anaphylactoid reactions seen in immunoglobulin A (IgA)-deficient patients whose anti-IgA is directed against donor IgA.

Nonimmunologic hazards of blood transfusion include hypervolemia, results of massive transfusion, and transmission of infectious agents. Hypervolemia is self-explanatory and is not discussed further.

Massive blood transfusions have predictable consequences. Most transfusions are of packed RBCs, which contain inadequate platelets and significantly reduced amounts of factors V and VIII. Transfusion of platelet concentrates or fresh-frozen plasma must be individualized. Rapid transfusion of 6 units of packed RBCs or transfusion of 10 units in a 24-hour period should be cause for consideration of platelet transfusion. Blood product therapy guided by appropriate laboratory results, such as platelet count and partial thromboplastin time is preferable, but a clinical coagulopathy in the face of massive transfusion suggests dilutional thrombocytopenia.

Metabolic accompaniments of massive transfusion are hypocalcemia caused by citrate binding of calcium, hyperkalemia, and acid-base abnormalities. Citrate toxicity, manifest as cardiac dysfunction, is important with rapid transfusion (1 unit/5 min). If volume has been adequately replaced but cardiac output is low in a patient receiving massive transfusion, calcium chloride supplementation must be considered.

Hyperkalemia is also a rare complication of transfusion. Despite serum potassium levels of 19 to 30 mmol/L in blood stored 21 days, clinically significant hyperkalemia is seen only at transfusion rates greater than 100 ml/min. Treatment of hyperkalemia with calcium should be based on serum levels or peaked T waves on electrocardiogram.

Metabolic acidosis is a theoretical, but rarely a clinical, problem in transfusion therapy. Although blood stored 21 days may have a pH of 6.9, much of that is a result of high partial pressure of carbon dioxide, which is rapidly corrected with ventilation. No good data are available to support bicarbonate prophylaxis during blood transfusion. Such therapy should be guided by arterial blood gases.

Finally, hypothermia can be induced by transfusion of blood that has been stored at 4° C. Consequences of hypothermia, including ventricular irritability and shivering with increased oxygen consumption and carbon dioxide formation, argue for warming transfused blood.

As previously mentioned, the fear of AIDS is the strongest influence in transfusion therapy today. The latest figures estimate the risk of exposure to human immunodeficiency virus(es) to be 1:40,000 to 1:1 million per unit transfused depending on geographic location. Although the risk is small, the devastating effects of this disease account for its unprecedented influence.

Hepatitis is a much more common viral complication of blood transfusion, occurring in approximately 3% to 10% of patients receiving transfusions. Less than 5% of cases of posttransfusion hepatitis are caused by the hepatitis B virus. Most cases are anicteric, non-A, non-B hepatitis for which no serologic marker exists. Risk of non-A, non-B hepatitis per unit transfused is 1:100. Unfortunately, chronic disease develops in 30% to 50% of patients infected with non-A, non-B hepatitis.

WHITE BLOOD CELL DISORDERS

White blood cells (WBCs) are separated into five types: neutrophils, lymphocytes, monocytes, eosinophils, and basophils. Functionally, they can be divided into those capable of phagocytosis and those whose primary activity is to modulate the immune response. WBCs have numerous metabolic activities. Obviously a discussion of WBC functions and abnormalities could fill an entire book (see suggested readings). This chapter focuses on neutrophil and lymphocyte functions, the importance of the WBC and differential counts, causes of neutrophilia, and importance of neutropenia.

Neutrophils

In healthy individuals neutrophils account for 50% to 60% of WBCs in peripheral blood; however, circulating neutrophils account for less than 5% of all the neutrophils in the body. Approximately 90% of these cells are stored as reserves in bone marrow. Another 7% to 8% are in tissues. Finally, of the 2% to 3% of neutrophils that form the blood pool, half exist in a marginated population that is attached to the vascular endothelium.

Neutrophils are phagocytes. They are the most important part of the immune response for microbial killing because of their numbers, motility, and efficiency. They are most active after moving out of the bloodstream and into the tissues.

Unstimulated neutrophils move out of the marrow and into the blood in response to several humoral factors that accompany activation of the complement system. Although phagocytosis occurs to a limited extent intravascularly, the function of blood in the neutrophil life cycle is to provide transportation. Circulating neutrophils respond to chemotactic stimuli, such as complement, leukotrienes, or bacterial products, by adhesion and aggregation. They become stimulated, which seems to involve activation of receptor sites that permit the cells to adhere to vascular endothelium near the stimulus site and to aggregate to other neutrophils. They then orient toward the stimulus and move through the vascular wall at junctions between endothelial cells. The passage through tissues is simplified by release of enzymes, such as collagenase and elastase. Neutrophils recognize material to be ingested because it is marked or opsonized by IgG antibodies or complement products. After ingestion, bacteria are destroyed by a system involving neutrophil myeloperoxidase and toxic oxygen products, such as hydrogen peroxide. Neutrophils are unable to reenter the vascular system after migrating out, and they survive 1 to 4 days after entering the tissue space. The WBCs, microorganisms, and damaged local tissues form pus.

Congenital and acquired diseases can affect any of the preceding neutrophil functions. It is unlikely that an adult with a congenital neutrophil dysfunction would be admitted to the ICU without a diagnosis, unless the patient had myeloperoxidase deficiency. Myeloperoxidase deficiency is the most common congenital neutrophil defect. It occurs in 1 in 2000 people and is inherited as an autosomal recessive trait. Fortunately, other microbicidal systems compensate for the deficiency, and unless additional defects are present in the immune system, the individual is not significantly compromised.

Acquired neutrophil dysfunction is seen in numerous diseases, some of which are associated with an increased incidence and severity of bacterial infections. Patients undergoing hemodialysis have impaired neutrophil adherence and aggregation. Diabetes mellitus, thermal injuries, sepsis, and malnutrition decrease neutrophil motility, response to chemotaxins, and microbicidal activity. Other diseases affecting neutrophil mobility are systemic lupus erythematosus, rheumatoid arthritis, some viral infections, and Down's syndrome. Malignancies, specifically leukemias, also suppress neutrophil function in multiple areas of the body.

Nonsteroidal antiinflammatory drugs, corticosteroids, and colchicine impair all aspects of neutrophil function.

Lymphocytes

Neutrophils are only one part of the body's defense system. The neutrophil is one of several effector cells that respond to stimulation of the immune system. The most important regulatory and effector cells of the immune system are the lymphocytes. They account for 25% to 33% of WBCs in peripheral blood and are further characterized as T cells, B cells, and large granular lymphocytes (LGLs).

Although T cells originate in bone marrow, their migration to the thymus is complete shortly after birth. In adults they are found mostly in lymph nodes, lymph, blood, and the spleen. A subset of T cells are the primary effectors of cell-mediated immunity and are capable of destroying foreign cells or cells infected by viruses. Equally important is their regulatory function. Helper and suppressor T cells activate or suppress immune responses involving cytotoxic T cells, B lymphocytes, and monocytes.

The primary function of B lymphocytes is to produce antibodies when appropriately stimulated. B cells are found in bone marrow, lymph nodes, the spleen, and peripheral blood. Although there are long-lived memory cells that recognize and respond to rechallenge by a previously recognized antigen, many B cells depend on T lymphocyte–derived factors for maturation and activation.

Understanding lymphocyte function and dysfunction requires an understanding of clinical immunology, which is not reviewed in this book. Although quantitative lymphocyte disorders do exist, qualitative disturbances of the immune system are a more common clinical problem. Efforts to solve the AIDS epidemic are rapidly increasing the understanding of lymphocyte function in health and disease.

Neutrophilic Leukocytosis

The most frequently encountered clinical problem involving WBCs is leukocytosis, specifically neutrophilic leukocytosis. The major concern is whether the increased neutrophil count is an indication of a bacterial infection. Although the clinician in the ICU can never ignore leukocytosis, he or she must realize that neutrophilia does occur with conditions other than infection and inflammation. Patient symptoms, physical examination, appropriate radiographic studies, and cultures support or detract from an infectious cause for leukocytosis.

Laboratory findings are helpful. Hemoglobin level, hematocrit, RBC indices, reticulocyte count, and platelet count can indicate problems with the erythroid cell line or the bone marrow or systemic diseases associated with neutrophilic leukocytosis. Vitamin B_{12} concentration and binding capacity are of no use, since both values are elevated in almost all cases of neutrophilia. Leukocyte alkaline phosphatase levels are markedly reduced in chronic myelogenous leukemia (and paroxysmal nocturnal hemoglobinuria). Unfortunately, this value moves toward normal with treatment, when concomitant infection is present, or with steroid administration.

The peripheral blood smear can provide important information. Neutrophilic leukocytosis caused by an infection often results in a "shift to the left." This means that more than 10% of the neutrophils are band forms or neutrophils with a nonsegmented nucleus. Band forms are not specific for infection, but they are a better indicator of an inflammatory process than total leukocyte count or fever. Other changes seen in infection are toxic granulation, vacuolated neutrophils, and Döhle bodies. Toxic granulation, like a nonsegmented nucleus, results when neutrophils experience a shortened marrow maturation time and are released into peripheral blood with primary azurophilic granules rather than their normal secondary granules. Vacuolated neutrophils represent neutrophils that have phagocytosed bacteria or antigen-antibody complexes in peripheral blood. They also are not specific for bacterial infection but do correlate with positive blood cultures. Döhle bodies are cytoplasmic inclusions, probably

fragmented endoplasmic reticulum, seen in infections, inflammation, pregnancy, and malignancy.

Several stimuli rapidly increase the neutrophil count in peripheral blood. Extreme emotional or physical stress, sudden temperature change, or administration of epinephrine or cryoprecipitate can cause intravascular neutrophils to demarginate. No immature forms are seen, and the neutrophilia lasts only minutes to hours unless the stimulus is repetitive or continuous.

Other stimuli cause neutrophilia in a matter of hours. Infection, inflammation, anesthesia and surgery, endotoxins, corticosteroids, and hydroxyethyl starch produce neutrophilia by stimulating release of the marrow reserve population.

Neutrophilia associated with corticosteroids deserves special mention. The neutrophil count increases significantly within 24 hours of initiation of therapy. Interestingly, the lymphocyte count decreases by as much as 50% over the same time period. With continued administration of corticosteroids the leukocyte count continues to increase in a dose-independent fashion for up to 2 weeks before it begins to decline. The count does not return to baseline until therapy is discontinued. No band forms, immature leukocytes, or toxic granulations are present on the peripheral smear in corticosteroid-induced neutrophilia.

Causes of more chronic neutrophilias include an autosomal dominant, benign, hereditary form, Down's syndrome, normal pregnancy, chronic myelogenous leukemia and other myeloproliferative diseases, chronic hemolysis or blood loss, lithium, asplenia, and of course bacterial infection and chronic inflammation. The leukocytosis occurring in these disorders is the result of increased proliferation from chronic stimulation or increased peripheral granulocyte survival.

Asplenia is important for two reasons. First, neutrophilia is always present with functional asplenia or surgical splenectomy. The degree decreases with time. More important, however, the asplenic patient is immunocompromised because of loss of the spleen's clearance of antibody-coated bacteria and because of decreased formation of IgG and IgM antibodies, which opsonize bacteria and allow neutrophils to identify and ingest them. Asplenia is associated with RBC abnormalities (nucleated RBCs, Heinz bodies, Howell-Jolly bodies) on peripheral smear.

Lithium causes a dose-dependent increase in neutrophils, usually to 1½ to 2 times normal levels. The neutrophilia does not resolve if therapy continues. It may be the result of direct lithium stimulation of the bone marrow.

Neutropenia

Although neutrophilia raises a concern of acute infection, neutropenia causes concern about susceptibility to overwhelming bacterial infection. In general, the likelihood of bacterial infection increases as the neutrophil count declines. The risk is slightly higher with absolute neutrophil counts between 500 and 1000/µl but increases markedly when counts fall below 200/µl.

Neutropenic patients are usually infected by endogenous bacteria or by strains with which they have been colonized. The most frequent isolates are *Staphylococcus aureus, Escherichia coli, Klebsiella,* or *Pseudomonas aeruginosa.* Common sites of infection are mucous membranes, skin and soft tissues, and lungs. Local infections are often complicated by septicemia. Symptoms of infection are malaise, chills, diaphoresis, and fever. Neutropenic patients become febrile because tissue macrophages and monocytes release pyrogens. Although erythema and tenderness occur in neutropenic patients, other signs of local infection (purulent exudates, fluctuant masses, and regional lymphadenopathy) may be absent.

Causes

Neutropenia may be either acute or chronic, and normal neutrophil counts differ significantly with age and race. In an ICU, neutropenia is most commonly drug induced. The diagnosis is one of exclusion. Unfortunately, the list of drugs capable of causing neutropenia includes cancer chemotherapeutic agents, numerous antibiotics, anticonvulsants, cardiac antidysrhythmic drugs, diuretics, sedatives, antithyroid agents, antiinflammatories, and others. Most ICU patients receive more than one possible causative drug, and if the neutropenia is thought to be drug induced, all possible causative agents must be stopped. The neutropenic patient remains at risk for an infection until the neutrophil count recovers.

Drug-induced neuropenia has certain characteristics, the most important of which is quantitative. Drug-induced neutropenias result in almost total disappearance of neutrophils (counts less than 100/µl are common). A second characteristic is temporal. Although immunologic effects of drug-induced neutropenia may appear shortly after exposure to the offending agent, the more classic interval is 2 to 3 weeks.

In addition to drugs, causes of neutropenia include congenital or hereditary disorders, hematologic diseases, viral infections, immunologic disorders, and systemic diseases (systemic lupus erythematosus, hypersplenism). Neutropenia developing in response to overwhelming sepsis carries a poor prognosis for recovery.

Therapy

A neutropenic patient in the ICU is at extreme risk for a life-threatening infection. Debilitation, inadequate nutrition, indwelling catheters, endotracheal tubes, and invasive procedures magnify the risk of neutropenia. Reverse isolation is of no benefit to these patients. Oral nonabsorbable antibiotics are protective, as is isolation in a laminar flow room, although such facilities are usually found only in large medical centers. In their absence, handwashing by the staff and a face mask for a patient who is not intubated are adequate.

Every febrile episode must be treated as life threatening. A careful physical examination with appropriate radiologic and laboratory studies and cultures must be performed. Indwelling catheters should be moved to new sites when possible. If the likely infecting organism is known, appropriate antibodies should be instituted. If the cause of the fever is obscure, empiric broad-spectrum antibiotics based on the most likely bacterial infections in the unit and their antibiotic sensitivities should be started immediately. Antibiotic coverage is then adjusted according to culture results. Febrile episodes in neutropenic patients have three outcomes:

1. If the patient responds to antibiotic therapy, it should be continued for at least 5 days after defervescence unless the infection requires prolonged treatment (as in bacterial endocarditis, pyelonephritis, and osteomyelitis).

2. If the fever persists but the patient remains stable and no cause for infection can be found, antibiotic therapy should be discontinued after 2 or 3 days. The patient must be closely monitored for signs of infection while other causes of fever are investigated.

3. The patient's clinical condition continues to deteriorate despite empiric or directed

antibiotic therapy. Attempts at diagnosis must continue. After 3 to 5 days, addition of amphotericin B should be considered. Antibiotic regimens are often adjusted to gain either broader coverage or more overlap for a suspected organism. Uncommon diseases such as tuberculosis deserve consideration.

The results of granulocyte transfusion for neutropenia remain controversial and difficult to evaluate. They are not beneficial prophylactically, nor are they of any benefit in nonbacterial infections. If granulocyte transfusions are being considered, the transfusion service that would supply the granulocytes should be consulted. They are not an option if marrow recovery is unlikely.

Two other therapies for neutropenia, lithium and splenectomy, deserve further mention. Although neither androgens nor glucocorticoids are used to treat neutropenia, lithium carbonate may be effective. Lithium directly stimulates marrow stem cells and causes neutrophilia as previously mentioned. It has been used to stimulate more rapid recovery in neutropenic patients but remains experimental. Splenectomy may benefit neutropenic patients with hypersplenism.

SUGGESTED READINGS

Acta Anaesthesiologica Scand 1988;32(Suppl 89)

Boxer LA, Stossel TP: Qualitative abnormalities of neutrophils. In: Hematology, ed 3. New York, 1983, McGraw-Hill Book Co, pp 802-815

Babior BM, Bunn HF: Megaloblastic anemias. In: Harrison's principles of internal medicine. New York, 1987, McGraw-Hill Book Co, pp 1498-1504

Bunn HF: Anemia. In: Harrison's principles of internal medicine. New York, 1987, McGraw-Hill Book Co, pp 262-266

Cline MJ: The white cell. Cambridge, Mass, 1975, Harvard University Press

Finch SC: Neutropenia. In: Hematology, ed 3. New York, 1983, McGraw-Hill Book Co, pp 773-793

Finch SC: Neutrophilia. In: Hematology, ed 3. New York, 1983, McGraw-Hill Book Co, pp 794-801

Gallin JI: Disorders of phagocytic cells. In: Harrison's principles of internal medicine. New York, 1987, McGraw-Hill Book Co, pp 278-283

Hardaway RM, Adams WH: Blood problems in critical care. I and II. In: Problems in critical care. Philadelphia, 1989, JB Lippincott, vol 3, nos. 1 and 2

Haynes BF: Enlargement of lymph nodes and spleen. In: Harrison's principles of internal medicine. New York, 1987, McGraw-Hill Book Co, p 278

Rappeport JM, Bunn HF: Bone marrow failure: aplastic anemia and other primary bone marrow disorders. In: Harrison's principles of internal medicine. New York, 1987, McGraw-Hill Book Co, pp 1533-1536

Schafer AI, Bunn HF: Anemias of iron deficiency and iron overload. In: Harrison's principles of internal medicine. New York, 1987, McGraw-Hill Book Co, pp 1493-1498

14

COAGULATION

NORIG ELLISON, MD

Blood is a body organ with specific functions just as the heart, kidney, and lungs are. One such function is to transport oxygen and nutrients to the other organs and to transport waste products, such as carbon dioxide and blood urea nitrogen, from other organs to the lungs and kidneys. The blood also has a clotting mechanism to seal off leaks in the blood vessels and prevent exsanguination when they are injured. The existence of such a mechanism is not without risk, since its initiation could lead to widespread or even complete clotting of blood. To prevent this catastrophe, a system of activators and inhibitors limits clot formation to the site of injury. A congenital or acquired imbalance in this system can lead to either excessive bleeding or thrombotic disorders.

NORMAL HEMOSTASIS

Abnormal bleeding occurs in many forms, varying from the purpura associated with platelet deficiency or the easy bruising in a patient taking coumarin to frank hemorrhage in a patient with a ruptured abdominal aneurysm. Hemostasis depends on vascular integrity, platelet function, and coagulation factors. No matter how meticulously a surgeon has secured hemostasis, a patient with hemophilia continues to bleed until factor VIII is increased to acceptable levels. Similarly, bleeding persists in the face of acceptable factor VIII levels and an adequate number of functioning platelets until vascular integrity is achieved in the case of a slipped ligature on an intercostal artery.

Although the spontaneous arrest of bleeding from ruptured vessels conveying blood under pressure involves complex physiologic principles, the physical principles are relatively simple. Blood escapes as long as the pressure within

the vessel exceeds the pressure at the orifice. Vasoconstriction of the blood vessel at the injury site, opening of anastomotic shunts, or sufficient blood loss reduces intravascular pressure and decreases blood flow. A rise in extravascular pressure (as with hematoma formation) also decreases the gradient.

The majority of blood vessels are less than 1 mm in diameter. In vessels of this caliber platelets and coagulation play the major role in securing hemostasis. Thus an efficient coagulation mechanism is essential to prevent bleeding. By common consent the suffix "a" is used to designate the activated form of a factor. Three factors (I, V, and VIII) do not exist in an enzymatically active form (Tables 14–1 and 14–2, Figure 14–1).

In response to vascular injury, platelets accumulate at the injury site where they come in contact with collagen-containing subendothelial basement membrane that has been exposed by the injury. Platelet aggregation (the affinity of platelets for one another) and platelet adhesion (the affinity of platelets for nonplatelet surfaces) develop simultaneously. In small injuries the resultant platelet plug may be sufficient to seal the defect. Platelet factor 3 (PF 3) is a phospholipid essential for activation of factor X by the complex of factors IXa and VIII and calcium ion, as well as for the conversion of prothrombin to thrombin. Platelet factor 4 (PF 4) is believed to play a role in preventing factor Xa inactivation by heparin. The final step in the formation of a clot, clot retraction, is probably due to a contractile mechanism found in platelets.

The final step is removal of the fibrin-platelet clot by the fibrinolytic system, which also has intrinsic and extrinsic pathways. The former is initiated by factor XII, and the latter by tissue activators. Both pathways convert plasminogen

TABLE 14—1. Coagulation Factors

FACTOR	SYNONYM	CLINICAL SYNDROME CAUSED BY DEFICIENCY
I	Fibrinogen	Yes
II	Prothrombin, prethrombin	Yes
III	Tissue factor, tissue thromboplastin	No
IV	Calcium	No
V	Labile factor, proaccelerin, plasma accelerator globulin (ac-G)	Yes
VI	No factor assigned to this numeral	
VII	Stable factor, proconvertin, autoprothrombin I, serum prothrombin conversion acceleration (SPCA)	Yes
VIII	Antihemophilic globulin (AHG), antihemophilic factor (AFG), thromboplastinogen, platelet cofactor I, antihemophilia factor A	Yes
IX	Plasma thromboplastin component (PTC), Christmas factor, auto thrombin II, antihemophilic factor B, platelet cofactor II	Yes
X	Stuart-Prower factor, autoprothrombin C (or III)	Yes
XI	Plasma thromboplastin antecedent (PTA), Rosenthal syndrome, antihemophilic factor C	Mild
XII	Hageman factor, glass factor	No
XIII	Fibrin stabilizing factor (FSF), Laki-Lorand factor, fibrinase serum factor, urea-insolubility factor	Yes

into plasmin, which cleaves both fibrinogen and fibrin. When plasmin cleaves fibrin into small pieces, they are called fibrin-split products. These products are removed normally by the reticuloendothelial system. If present in excessively high numbers, they are potent inhibitors of clot formation.

ROUTINE EVALUATION

History

The best means of detecting a hemorrhagic diathesis is a properly taken history, and one of the most important items to be checked is the hemostatic response to a prior surgical

TABLE 14—2. Minimum Levels of Coagulation Factors and Platelets Necessary for Effective Hemostasis, Distribution, and Fate of Clotting Factors After Transfusion Therapy, and Treatment Schedules

FACTOR	MINIMAL LEVEL FOR SURGICAL HEMOSTASIS (% OF NORMAL)	GENETIC PATTERN IN CONGENITAL DEFICIENCIES	IN VIVO HALF-LIFE (h)
I (fibrinogen)	50–100	Autosomal recessive	72–144
II	20–40	Autosomal recessive	72–120
V	5–20	Autosomal recessive	12–36
VII	10–20	Autosomal recessive	4–6
VIII	30	Males affected; females carriers	10–18
von Willebrand's	30	Autosomal dominant; variable penetrance	
IX	20–25	Males affected; females carriers	18–36
X	10–20	Autosomal recessive	24–60
XI	20–30	Autosomal recessive	40–80
XII	0	Autosomal recessive	50(?)–70
XIII	1–3	Autosomal recessive; some sex link possible	72(?)–120
Platelets	50,000–100,000/mm^3		

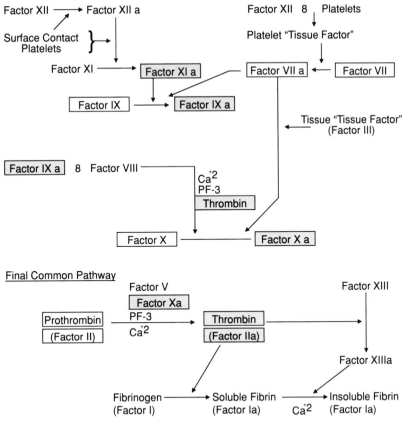

Figure 14–1. Coagulation cascade and its interrelationships. The four factors that constitute the prothrombin complex and are sensitive to coumarin administration — II (prothrombin), VII, IX, and X — are enclosed in boxes. The four activated factors that are inhibited by heparin — IIa (thrombin), IXa, Xa, and XIa — are shaded. This cascade demonstrates the interrelationships between extrinsic and intrinsic pathways in the first stage of coagulation. The concept of separate pathways is no longer valid. PF-3 = platelet factor 3.

THERAPEUTIC AGENT	DOSE (PER kg OF BODY WEIGHT)	
	INITIAL	MAINTENANCE
Cryoprecipitate	Precipitate from 100 ml	Precipitate from 14-20 ml/d
Plasma	10-15 ml	5-10 ml/d
Fresh or frozen plasma	10-15 ml	10 ml/d
Plasma	5-10 ml	5 ml/d
Cryoprecipitate	Precipitate from 70 ml	Precipitate from 35 ml twice daily
Plasma	10 ml	10 ml q 2-3 d
Plasma or II, VII, IX, X concentrate	60 ml; variable	7 ml/d
Plasma	15 ml	10 ml/d
Plasma	10 ml	5 ml/d
Plasma	5 ml	5 ml/d
Plasma	2-3 ml	None
Platelet concentrate	1-2 units per desired 10,000 increment in count	

experience. Equally important in the history is a detailed record of drug ingestion. Most patients taking anticoagulants volunteer that information, but they may neglect to mention that they are taking aspirin, which can have a coumarin-like effect in high doses and prolongs the bleeding time in low doses. Many other drugs impair platelet function. Drug history should include details about occupation and exposure to toxic agents or ionizing radiation. The age of onset is also an important clue; bleeding problems starting in infancy or early childhood suggest a congenital defect, and those starting in adulthood suggest an acquired defect.

Physical Examination

Discrete petechiae or prolonged bleeding after superficial trauma is usually due to vascular or platelet abnormalities. In contrast, the subcutaneous bleeding seen in coagulation factor deficiencies is usually an ecchymosis. Hemarthrosis or deep bleeding into muscles is more likely to occur with a coagulation factor deficiency.

Laboratory Tests

A screening hemostatic profile of any patient whose history suggests a hemorrhagic diathesis is essential. Such a profile might include prothrombin time (PT), activated partial thromboplastin time (aPTT), platelet count, fibrinogen level, and bleeding time. In the operating room an automated activated coagulation time (ACT) may be obtained. Especially in this era of cost containment, this profile cannot be obtained for every patient, nor should it be. However, in patients whose history or physical examination suggests the need for further evaluation, these tests are indicated. In addition, in procedures in which abnormal bleeding is a real possibility (such as cardiac surgery), a screening profile is recommended to rule out preexisting defects should abnormal bleeding later develop and to provide baseline values for comparison should repeat tests be ordered intraoperatively.

No one test or pair of tests is sufficient to make an accurate diagnosis of every bleeding disorder. For that reason a history of excessive bleeding must be given serious consideration, and quantitative assays of at least the three hemophilia factors (VIII, IX, and XI) should be performed in addition to the screening tests to rule out preexisting hemorrhagic diathesis.

CONGENITAL DEFICIENCIES

Congenital deficiencies are usually limited to one factor and are manifest in childhood. There may be a familial history of bleeding disorders. The incidence of the coagulation factor deficiencies varies greatly; the incidence of classic hemophilia A factor VIII deficiency is as high as 1:10,000 to 25,000 live births, whereas fewer than 100 cases of familial afibrinogenemia have been reported.

Table 14–3 lists the eight variables that must be considered whenever a coagulation factor is infused. Factor VIII replacement therapy, for which pharmacokinetics have been best worked out, is illustrated in Figure 14–2. The early rapid runoff reflects the redistribution from the vascular space, and the latter half reflects biodegradation. Although the shape of the curve varies depending on the apparent volume distribution and half-life for a given factor, each coagulation factor exhibits this characteristic double exponential curve (Fig. 14–2), with the exception of von Willebrand's disease. Patients with factor VIII deficiency are at risk for spontaneous bleeding if factor VIII levels fall below 10% (levels less than 1% are not uncommon), bleeding in response to minimal trauma if levels are less than 20%, and bleeding in response to major trauma or surgery if less than 30%. Throughout the perioperative and convalescent periods, therefore, factor VIII levels must be maintained above 30%. The treatment period varies with the procedure: 1 or 2 days may suffice for minor dental procedures, whereas 21 days or more may be necessary in cases of major orthopedic reconstruction.

Von Willebrand's disease (pseudohemophilia) may be the most common congenital deficiency of hemostasis. It is transmitted as an autosomal dominant gene with variable penetrance and is characterized by a deficiency of factor VIII and a prolonged bleeding time. Three areas of confusion exist with respect to von Willebrand's disease. First, the original report suggested the defect in platelets, but reevaluation of the same patient a generation later showed that factor VIII deficiency was part of the picture. Second, this entity is characterized by a cyclic variability and severity,

TABLE 14–3. Variables Influencing Coagulation Factor Replacement Therapy

Patient size	Extravascular distribution
Initial factor level	Half-life
Hemostatic level	Metabolic rate
Preoperative potency	Operations

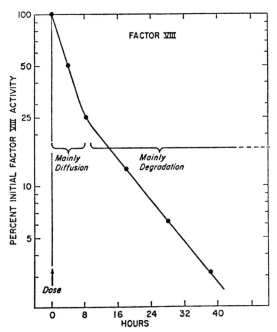

Figure 14–2. Response of factor VIII levels to one infusion. The graph shows the typical rapid rise and early rapid runoff, which reflects redistribution in the extravascular space. The slower decline subsequently represents degradation. Although the graph is a measure of factor VIII levels, all coagulation factors exhibit the same characteristic double exponential curve, the shape of which depends on the degree of extravascular distribution and the half-life of the factor.

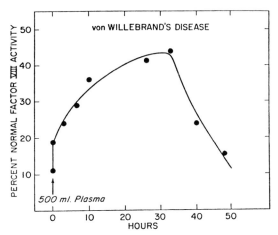

Figure 14–3. Response of factor VIII levels in patients with von Willebrand's disease. The initial rapid rise is followed by a progressive rise that reflects in vivo production of factor VIII. This contrasts with hemophilia A in which the peak level is achieved at the end of the infusion.

which are mirrored by a similar variability in laboratory tests. For this reason a patient with a strong history of bleeding problems may need further evaluation. Third, these patients seem to lack the stimulus to produce factor VIII rather than the ability to produce factor VIII. This is illustrated in Figure 14–3.

ACQUIRED DEFICIENCIES

In contrast to congenital deficiencies, which are usually limited to one factor, acquired deficiencies are usually multifactorial. In the critical care setting deficiencies of hemostasis in probable order of decreasing importance are disseminated intravascular coagulation (DIC), massive blood transfusion, inadequate surgical hemostasis, liver disease, thrombocytopenia, and anticoagulants.

Disseminated Intravascular Coagulation

DIC is a pathologic syndrome in which the formation of fibrin thrombi, the consumption of specific plasma proteins, the loss of platelets, and the activation of the fibrinolytic system suggest the presence of thrombin in the systemic circulation. Although coagulopathies associated with specific clinical entities have long been recognized, appreciation of a common denominator and the term "disseminated intravascular coagulation" are relatively recent developments. In 1972 DIC first appeared as a separate heading in *Index Medicus*. Although DIC may be looked on as a "disease of medical progress" that is now being diagnosed more frequently because larger numbers of critically ill patients are surviving longer, a more likely explanation is that the entity is now well accepted and being recognized more readily.

The clinical findings of DIC vary, with patients presenting thrombotic, hemorrhagic, or mixed pictures. Furthermore, some patients who present no clinical manifestation have a classic laboratory picture of DIC. No one pathognomonic laboratory test can be used to diagnose DIC. The following criteria can be used. In the absence of liver disease or blood transfusions, a screening triad of PT greater than 15 seconds, fibrinogen level less than 160 mg/dl, and platelet count of fewer than 150,000/mm^3. Abnormalities of all three indicate DIC. If two of three tests show abnormalities, either the thrombin time (more than 5 seconds greater than control values in the absence of heparin therapy) or levels of fibrin-split products must be abnormal to confirm the laboratory diagnosis.

The diagnosis of DIC is based on the finding of fibrin-split products in the bloodstream in conjunction with the decrease in levels of fibrinogen and platelets. As a practical matter in a typical clinical setting, the diagnosis of DIC can be presumed until proved otherwise when the fibrinogen level and platelet count are decreased.

DIC is never a primary disease state, nor does it develop in every patient who receives, for example, an incompatible blood transfusion. Diagnosis and treatment of the primary disease state are essential. The body has several defense mechanisms that eliminate any thrombin within the vascular tree. These include rapid blood flow, producing dilution of activated coagulation factors below threshold levels; liver and reticuloendothelial system clearance of activated coagulation factors; and inhibition of thrombin produced by naturally occurring plasma proteins, such as antithrombin III. In most cases of incompatible blood transfusion the combination of these three defense mechanisms prevents DIC. However, in cases of stagnant blood flow, such as shock; impairment of the liver and reticuloendothelial system, such as hypoxemia; or overwhelming insult, DIC may develop. In such cases fibrinolysis, a body defense mechanism in which plasminogen is activated to plasmin, which in turn destroys fibrinogen and factors V and VIII, is activated. The consumption of platelets and coagulation factors results in the hemorrhagic diathesis because no platelets or coagulation factors are available to seal off defects in vascular integrity. Furthermore, as previously mentioned, fibrin-split products possess anticoagulant properties that further aggravate the bleeding disorder.

The first treatment of DIC is always directed toward the primary cause. Stopping an incompatible blood transfusion or uterine evacuation of a dead fetus may be all that is required. In sepsis and other conditions in which the primary cause is not as readily removed, the treatment is supportive. Replacement of platelets and coagulation factors is required. The recognition that cryoprecipitate, which was originally developed for the treatment of hemophilia, contains one third of fibrinogen in the plasma from which it is derived has provided a specific therapeutic regimen for DIC. The risk of hepatitis is less with cryoprecipitate than with fibrinogen, which is a pooled product. The recognition that cryoprecipitate contains fibrinogen resulted in the discontinuation of fibrinogen concentrate preparation. The use of cryoprecipitate therefore increases levels of fibrinogen and factor VIII, both of which are depressed in DIC. Deficiencies of other coagulation factors, which may occur less commonly secondary to consumption, should be corrected with fresh-frozen plasma and platelet concentrates. The use of heparin remains controversial, especially for surgical patients who have fresh wounds. Heparin therapy in DIC is designed to stop clot formation and inhibit the continued consumption of coagulation factors and platelets so they can reach normal levels. Heparin doses of 40 to 80 units/kg are administered every 4 to 6 hours to prolong coagulation two to three times normal duration. The decision to employ heparin is not to be taken lightly. Some physicians believe that heparin therapy at best replaces one cause of bleeding with another and that theoretical reasons are insufficient to justify the use of such dangerous treatment. I have been extremely reluctant to use heparin therapy for surgical patients, especially those with a fibrinogen level less than 50 mg/dl, accompanying vasculitis, or local defects in the vascular system.

Massive Transfusion

Massive transfusion represents a paradox in that patients are bleeding actively and require blood, yet they are bleeding because they receive blood. Bank blood carries a hemostatic defect. Factors V and VIII in stored blood decrease after 21 days' storage to 20% to 50% of normal. However, this is still in excess of the minimal hemostatic level, so deficiency of these factors is rarely a primary cause of bleeding. In contrast, the hemostatic effectiveness of platelets decays within 48 to 72 hours, and a dilutional thrombocytopenia is believed to be the primary defect in massive transfusion. Whether deficiencies of factors V and VIII can aggravate or be aggravated by decreased platelet count is uncertain. Treatment with platelet concentrates is discussed later in the section on thrombocytopenia.

Inadequate Surgical Hemostasis

In a postoperative patient the possibility of inadequate surgical hemostasis must always be considered. Furthermore, some patients, who will ultimately stop bleeding because of effective clotting, may lose less blood if effective surgical hemostasis is achieved.

Liver Disease

Liver disease may produce bleeding because of defects in coagulation factors, thrombocytopenia related to hypersplenism, or excessive fibrinolysis, or on a mechanical basis as with esophageal varices. In addition to depressing the four vitamin K–dependent factors in the prothrombin complex, liver disease decreases production of factors V and XI. One iatrogenic cause of bleeding that may occur in critical care patients is the intestinal sterilization syndrome. The intestinal flora is a major source of vitamin K in humans. A patient whose gastrointestinal tract is sterilized with large doses of antibiotics preoperatively loses this source of vitamin K. If the patient is maintained with intravenous fluids or receives a restricted diet without vitamin K–containing foods, vitamin K stores become depleted in approximately 1 week. This syndrome is easily diagnosed on the basis of history, the finding of an isolated prolonged PT, and the prompt response to vitamin K administration. The treatment of bleeding caused by liver disease depends on the nature of the bleeding.

Thrombocytopenia

Although disorders of platelet function are more readily appreciated and diagnosed today, the most common cause of platelet-related bleeding is a reduction in platelet count. Therefore a platelet count is the first step in evaluation. Reduced platelet count may be due to decreased production, as with patients receiving cancer chemotherapy; increased utilization, as with DIC; increased destruction, as with idiopathic thrombocytopenic purpura or hypersplenism; or massive transfusion with bank blood containing no viable platelets. Both DIC and massive blood transfusion decrease the platelet count, which must be treated with platelet concentrate. In addition, decreased platelet count can occur on an immune basis. Platelet concentrates have little effect in such a case. Normal counts are 240,000 $\pm$ 100,000/mm^3. Although it is impossible to specify an absolute platelet count below which the risk of hemorrhage contraindicates surgery, a range of 50,000 to 75,000 is generally accepted, with an upper minimum level of 100,000. The template bleeding time of Ivy is now a well-accepted measure of platelet function and has been called the only test of platelet function capable of predicting excessive bleeding.

Platelets should not be transfused until sufficient surgical hemostasis has been achieved to avoid "transfusing the suction bottle." In a 70 kg adult, platelets from 1 unit of blood administered as a concentrate increase the platelet count by 5000 to 10,000/µl. Based on the patient's platelet count and the desired increase, the number of units of platelet concentrate needed can be calculated. Alternatively, the administration of 0.1 unit/kg is a commonly cited figure. The effectiveness of platelet transfusion therapy should be assessed by repeat platelet counts 1 and 24 hours after transfusion, as well as, ideally, bleeding times determined with both counts.

Anticoagulants

Two types of anticoagulants produce multiple hemostatic defects. Coumarin-like drugs inhibit production of factors II, VII, IX, and X, which together are known as the prothrombin complex or vitamin K–dependent factors. Heparin inhibits factors IXa, Xa, XIa, and IIa (thrombin). Small doses of coumarin inhibit factor VII, prolonging the PT while the aPTT remains normal. Larger coumarin doses depress factors X and II while prolonging PT. Small heparin doses inhibit factor IXa initially, resulting in a prolonged aPTT and a normal PT. Larger heparin doses affect factors Xa and IIa, prolonging both PT and aPTT.

APPROACH TO THE BLEEDING PATIENT

When the clinician is presented with unexpected bleeding in a critically ill patient, the tests outlined in Table 14–4 facilitate a rapid evaluation and guide to therapy. These tests can all be performed quickly and reliably. The ACT can be readily performed in the operating room or ICU while blood is being transported to the laboratory for other tests. Minimal equipment is required for an automated ACT. The clot can then be observed for retraction, a rough measure of platelet function, or lysis. Care must be taken not to confuse true fibrinolysis with the dissolution after vigorous shaking of a weak, friable clot caused by hypofibrinogenemia. Determining a fibrinogen level can obviously assist in making that distinction. As previously mentioned, no one test or pair of tests is sufficient as the basis for an accurate diagnosis in all cases, and often necessary secondary tests are suggested by the screening profile.

TREATMENT

The modes of treatment most frequently used to produce perioperative hemostasis are listed

TABLE 14—4. Primary (Screening) and Secondary Tests of Hemostasis

TEST	COMMENTS
Primary Tests*	
Activated coagulation time (ACT)	Can be done in operating room; observe for clot retraction and lysis
Fibrinogen level	Depressed in disseminated intravascular coagulation (DIC)
Prothrombin time (PT)	Prolonged in liver disease, vitamin K deficiency, coumarin anticoagulation, DIC.
Partial thromboplastin time (aPTT)	Prolonged in factors V and VIII deficiency (massive transfusion), hemophilias, or presence of heparin
Platelet count	
Secondary Tests	
Bleeding time	Widely accepted clinical test of platelet function
Platelet aggregation	More refined test of platelet function using various agents to determine the responsiveness of the platelets
Protamine titration	Definitive test used to confirm or disprove presence of heparin

*These are the initial tests used to confirm the presence of a disorder of hemostasis.

in a possible order of decreasing importance for use:

1. *Suture material* restores vascular integrity.

2. *Platelets* correct deficiencies in quantity or quality of platelets. Surgical bleeding has been shown to occur frequently with platelet counts less than 100,000/mm³ and especially below 50,000/mm³. Each unit of platelets increases the count by approximately 7500 to 10,000/mm³.

3. *Fresh-frozen plasma* (FFP) is the acellular portion of a single unit that is frozen at $-18°$ C within 6 hours of separation. FFP contains all coagulation factors as recommended for treatment of deficiencies of blood coagulation factors V, X, and XI and in the treatment of deficiencies of factors VII, VIII, IX, and XIII when cryoprecipitate or other specific concentrates are not available. When only packed red blood cells (RBCs) are used, 2 to 3 units of FFP might be required for every 10 units of RBCs to prevent deficiencies of clotting factors. Ideally, whole blood is used for such large-volume trans-

fusions, obviating the need for FFP. FFP is also used as an antidote for coumarin when an immediate effect is required. There is no formula for FFP administration in cases of coumarin administration because the level of clotting factors in the patient for a given PT varies greatly, as does the level of the clotting factors in the donor FFP. Two units of FFP should be administered and the PT checked.

4. *Specific antidotes* for heparin and coumarin are available. Protamine is the antidote for heparin and can be administered on the basis of the amount of heparin administered or, preferably, by means of protamine titration, which measures the amount of protamine required to neutralize the heparin in 1 ml of blood. For coumarin the specific antidote is vitamin K. However, unlike protamine, which acts instantly, vitamin K requires more than 4 hours to produce an effect. For that reason, in urgent cases the antidote to coumarin is FFP, which has an immediate effect (see paragraph 3 for dosage).

5. *Cryoprecipitate* is a fraction of plasma that contains in less than 3% of the original volume approximately 30% to 60% of factor VIII and is useful in the treatment of hemophilia A. Therapy during the operative period should be guided by the fact that individuals with factor VIII levels of less than 10% are at risk for bleeding with minimal trauma and those with levels of 10% to 20% are at risk with moderate trauma. Levels less than 30% should be raised immediately in cases of severe trauma or surgery. This fraction, which also contains factors I (fibrinogen) and XIII, is the only available source of fibrinogen since the preparation of fibrinogen concentrates was discontinued because of the high risk of hepatitis.

6. *Factor IX concentrate* contains factors II, VII, IX, and X and is used to treat patients with congenital deficiencies of these factors. This concentrate is a pooled product and carries a high risk of hepatitis. Therefore it is not used in other circumstances such as coumarin administration, where it would otherwise be the specific antidote.

THROMBOSIS

The other end of the hemostatic spectrum from bleeding is thrombosis. Considerable attention has been paid to the related issues of hypercoagulability and thrombosis in recent years.

Attempts to use a decreased time for a coagulation test as evidence of hypercoagulable state have proved unsuccessful. Hypercoagulability has been defined as a state in which objective evidence exists for in vivo activation of platelets or the coagulation mechanism with or without evidence of clinical thrombosis. In addition, deficiencies in any of the several coagulation inhibitors referred to previously may produce a hypercoagulable state. Measurement of PF 4 or beta thromboglobulin, which are released when platelets aggregate, or the peptides released when coagulation factors are activated is used as evidence of ongoing coagulation. Fibrinopeptide A, formed during the activation of fibrinogen, is the coagulation factor peptide that has been measured most extensively in the laboratory.

As mentioned in the discussion of DIC, among the several defense mechanisms that eliminate thrombin within the vascular tree are several naturally occurring proteins. Antithrombin III, probably the most important of these proteins, is normally a weak inhibitor of coagulation. However, as a cofactor for heparin, antithrombin III is a fast, highly effective inhibitor. Minidose heparin, which produces no change in coagulation that can be measured in the laboratory, is believed to work via antithrombin. Patients with congenital deficiency of antithrombin III are at great risk for recurrent venous thromboembolism.

Proteins C and S are vitamin K–dependent inhibitors of coagulation. Thrombomodulin complexes with thrombin and totally eliminates the latter's coagulation activation properties. Rather, the complex activates protein C, which utilizes protein S as a cofactor and degrades factors Va and VIIIa to decrease the generation of thrombin. Both congenital and acquired deficiencies of protein C and S have been reported. Patients who are homozygous for protein C deficiency typically have a fulminant lethal course marked by recurrent evidence of thrombotic disorders. Heterozygotes for protein C deficiency have a less lethal course but nevertheless have recurrent deep venous thrombosis, as do patients who are heterozygotes for protein S deficiency. An association between protein C deficiencies and DIC, major trauma and surgery, and cancer has been reported. Similarly, protein S deficiencies have been noted in several disease states ranging from lupus to nephrotic syndrome, as well as in women taking oral contraceptives.

Heparin is the mainstay in the treatment of active thrombotic disorders and should be administered in doses sufficient to prolong the aPTT. Although prolongation to 2 to 2½ times normal is commonly recommended, it has recently been suggested that heparin resistance makes achieving that goal difficult and unnecessary, since a prolongation to 1½ to 2 times normal is sufficient. Although the recognized causes of heparin resistance are multiplying, the argument that increased levels of factor VIII commonly seen in seriously ill patients blunt the effect of heparin on the aPTT and create the impression of serious underheparinization is persuasive.

The only major complication of heparin therapy, other than increased bleeding in cases of overdose, or with therapeutic doses when occult illnesses such as a gastrointestinal tract malignancy or ulcer are discovered, is heparin-induced thrombocytopenia. A slight decrease in the platelet count is often seen with the start of heparin therapy. In some patients, 7 to 14 days after the institution of heparin therapy new thrombocytopenia with a platelet count less than $100,000/cu^3$ occurs. In cases of reexposure to heparin therapy a shorter interval may ensue. In association with this new thrombocytopenia thromboembolic events in either the arterial or venous system are usually seen, with overall morbidity and mortality rates of 80% and 20%, respectively, reported. The mechanism for heparin-induced thrombocytopenia is believed to be a heparin-dependent platelet-aggregating factor in the IgG or IgM fractions of patients' sera. Platelet-inhibiting drugs, such as aspirin and dipyridamole, have been used in the treatment of these patients. However, the long half-life of these drugs makes them less desirable than iloprost, a synthetic analog of prostacyclin (PGI_2), which has been used effectively as an infusion in patients who require open heart surgery.

Long-term management of thrombotic disorders is usually with coumarin because it canbe taken orally. Heparin therapy should be maintained on the basis of aPTT determination until the PT has been adequately prolonged in response to coumarin therapy.

SUGGESTED READINGS

Bang NU: Diagnosis in management of thrombosis. In Shoemaker WC, Ayres S, Grenvik A, et al (eds): Textbook of critical care, ed 2. Philadelphia, 1988, WB Saunders, pp 886-896

Cartun SM, Snider EL: Thrombotic disorders: A clinical review. In Menitove JE, McCarthy LJ (eds): Hemostatic disorders and the blood bank. Arlington, Va, 1984, American Association of Blood Banks, pp 63-90

Colman RW, Robboy SS: Postoperative disseminated intravascular coagulation and fibrinolysis. Urol Clin North Am 1976;3:379-392

Consensus conference: platelet transfusion therapy. JAMA 1987;257:1777-1780

Consensus conference: fresh frozen plasma, indications and risks. JAMA 1985;253:551-553

Ellison N: Hemostasis in the trauma patient. Semin Anesthiol 1985;4:163-176

Ellison N: Coagulation evaluation and management. In Ream AK, Fogdal RP (eds): Acute cardiovascular management: anesthesia and intensive care. Philadelphia, 1982, JB Lippincott, pp 771-805

Ellison N, Jobes DR, Schwartz AJ: Heparin therapy during cardiac surgery. In Effective hemostasis in cardiac surgery. Philadelphia, 1988, WB Saunders, pp 1-14

Ellison N, Silberstein LE: Hemostasis in the perioperative period. In Stoelting RK, Barash PG, Gallagher TJ (eds): Adv Anesthesia 1986;3:67-102

Snyder EL (ed): Blood transfusion therapy, a physician's handbook, ed 2. Arlington, Va, 1987, American Association of Blood Banks

Tomasulo PA, Lenes DA: Platelet transfusion therapy. In Menitove JE, McCarthy LJ (eds): Hemostatic disorders and the blood bank. Arlington, Va, 1984, American Association of Blood Banks, pp 63-90

15

GASTROINTESTINAL TRACT FUNCTION AND DYSFUNCTION IN CRITICALLY ILL PATIENTS

KEITH L. STEIN, MD

Virtually any illness or injury necessitating admission to an ICU is accompanied by systemic perturbations. The consequences of these disturbances may contribute to morbidity or death of the patient.

The progression from single-system to multiple-organ failure is often insidious but nonetheless deadly. With advances in therapy aimed at preservation of organ perfusion, the final common pathway (often leading to death) evolved from hypovolemic shock during World War II to renal failure in the 1950s. During the conflict in Vietnam, respiratory failure and hypoxia came to the fore, prompting close attention to the effects of volume resuscitation and techniques for respiratory support. Recently hepatic dysfunction as a consequence of prolonged stress and illness (sometimes with associated sepsis) has been recognized.

Even in the modern era the gastrointestinal (GI) tract has often been characterized as a passive witness to the other systemic manifestations of disease. This myth is dissipating as evidence to the contrary mounts.

This chapter examines the importance of the GI tract from several perspectives. First, general aspects of assessment of its function and dysfunction are reviewed. Then aspects of GI dysfunction, including some particularly common or critical secondary diseases, are considered.

ASSESSMENT

Regardless of the rationale for admitting a patient to an ICU, a thorough examination of all organ systems is essential. An organized approach ensures rapid and complete evaluation of all essential elements. A rational plan for assessing the GI tract can be illustrated by the evaluation of acute abdominal pain or signs of peritoneal inflammation.

In the review of the patient's history, attention should be directed to past hospitalizations, particularly when surgery was required. Previously diagnosed systemic disorders (such as diabetes, lipid and metabolic disorders, and cardiac disease) must be cataloged. Specific abdominal visceral diseases, such as cholelithiasis, pancreatitis, gastric or duodenal ulcers, esophageal varices, diverticulosis, or oncologic processes, may also be present. A list of current medications, including the duration of their use and most recent ingestion, is essential. A review of family history should also be included.

The review of systems for the GI tract should include the occurrence of nausea, vomiting, diarrhea, constipation, hematemesis, hematochezia, melena, or jaundice; history of ethanol abuse; menstrual and sexual activity history; and a thorough description of the pain. Included in the last are pain's presentation at onset with attention to where and when it began, exacerbating or ameliorating responses (such as change in position, food or antacid intake), associated symptoms, and character of the pain (continuous or intermittent, sharp or dull, local or diffuse). Obviously a patient admitted to the ICU in unstable condition may not be able to provide any of this information. In this circumstance an effort should be made to harvest as much information as possible from family members.

When abdominal symptoms develop in a patient already resident in an ICU, the history must be tailored to this environment. In addition to the historical aspects just described, attention must be directed to evidence of other system failure. This includes respiratory failure with ventilatory support, episodic hypoperfusion with or without hypotension, exposure to broad-spectrum antimicrobial therapy, the use of prolonged intravenous hyperalimentation, the use of narcotic analgesics, frequency of blood and blood product transfusions, and evidence of septicemia. Metabolic derangements, such as abnormal serum sodium, potassium, phosphate, glucose, or magnesium levels or unexplained metabolic acidosis, must also be noted.

Initial assessment of the vital signs is essential. This should include a check for orthostatic hypotension and abnormal temperature. Physical examination of the abdomen begins with observation. Inspection may reveal distention, abdominal wall discoloration (such as Grey Turner's or Collins' sign), or scars from previous operations or trauma. Auscultation is appropriate to assess quality of bowel sounds. Their absence may suggest peritoneal inflammation or ileus. Unfortunately, the presence of apparently normal bowel sounds does not preclude intraabdominal disease. Hyperactive bowel sounds may suggest bowel obstruction.

Palpation of the abdomen helps to localize the point of maximum discomfort. Percussion may provide further evidence of distended air-filled loops of bowel or free intraperitoneal fluid. Elicitation of rebound tenderness is a particularly sensitive indicator of localized inflammation of the parietal peritoneum. For this finding to be significant, however, the point of greatest discomfort on palpation should be in close proximity to that noted on rebound. Under some circumstances a patient's anxiety may mask the usefulness of this finding. Appreciation of mass lesions and evaluation of the abdominal aorta and distal circulation are important to this part of the evaluation. Rectal and pelvic examinations are mandatory, with special attention to elicited tenderness, masses, and stool guaiac tests for blood.

Additional aspects of the physical examination include evaluation of the iliopsoas and obturator signs associated with change in lower extremity position. Complaints of pain during these maneuvers suggest inflammation in the vicinity of the psoas muscle or in the deep pelvis.

A thorough history and physical examination including all organ systems are critical for appropriate diagnosis of coincident or confounding medical illness.

Laboratory Evaluation

Although the diagnosis of an acute abdomen is based predominantly on the results of the history and physical examination, ancillary laboratory tests may help to confirm the diagnosis. The white blood cell count is often elevated and shows a predominance of immature neutrophils, a so-called left shift. However, overwhelming systemic infection may be associated with profound leukopenia and the identical left shift. In addition, the left shift may be associated with other conditions, such as pregnancy, exercise, hemorrhage, oncologic processes, and even myocardial infarction. Therefore the white blood cell and differential counts do not predict the need for surgical intervention in an acute abdomen independent of the physical examination.

The hematocrit and hemoglobin values may be depressed by occult or overt bleeding. Care in interpreting these results is essential because hemoconcentration in response to early stress may yield a misleadingly normal value. Blood samples for the purpose of typing and crossmatching should be sent to the blood bank, particularly if a patient is bleeding. Urinalysis is important because the hypovolemic state is often heralded by concentration of the urine, yielding a high specific gravity. Urinary tract infection is suggested in a patient with bacteria and white blood cells in the urine, although asymptomatic bacteria in a patient with an indwelling urinary drainage catheter may be a false lead.

Measurement of the serum amylase level is routine. This test is nonspecific because elevated amylase levels may have a wide variety of causes, including pancreatitis, parotitis, facial trauma, perforated peptic ulcer, ischemic bowel disease, and even head injury without other pathologic problems. Serum lipase level, when elevated, may aid in the diagnosis of pancreatitis. Ionized calcium and serum phosphate levels are routinely measured and corrected as needed.

Tests of hepatocellular function and bile transit are also important. These include serum lactate dehydrogenase, glutamate oxaloacetic transaminase, glutamic pyruvate transaminase, alkaline phosphatase, and direct and indirect measurement of bilirubin. Stress-induced hyperglycemia is identified by the measurement of blood glucose and a check of urine glucose and ketones.

Measurement of arterial pH, when coupled with assessment of the anion gap in serum electrolytes, reveals acidosis related to hypoperfusion (regional or generalized) with lactate accumulation. Hypoxemia may result from or exacerbate underlying ischemia. Therefore determination of arterial blood gases is essential to therapy for these critically ill patients.

A 12-lead electrocardiogram is required in all patients to evaluate precedent or current myocardial injury (a potential masquerader of abdominal distress).

Radiologic Evaluation

An admission chest roentgenogram is important for evaluation of the placement of invasive devices, assessment of cardiopulmonary dimensions and appearance, and search for the presence of free intraabdominal or intrathoracic air.

Plain films of the abdomen, including the kidney-ureters-bladder (KUB) view, are routine (although of low yield) for delineation of intraluminal and extraluminal gas patterns and recognition of abnormal masses or ascites. An abdominal film including the diaphragms, taken with the patient upright, or alternatively a lateral decubitus film is essential in the search for extraluminal gas consistent with a perforated viscus. The lateral decubitus film may also reveal aortic calcification consistent with atherosclerosis. Biliary stones are visualized by this examination in only 15% to 20% of patients who have them.

Ancillary radiologic evaluations include ultrasonography (helpful for biliary, pancreatic, renal, and pelvic viscera), computed tomography (useful for solid abdominal viscera), arteriography and red blood cell scanning (sometimes helpful in localizing bleeding), and white blood cell scanning (which occasionally reveals undiagnosed infectious loci). Also intermittently applied are imaging techniques involving the instillation of Gastrografin or barium, as well as liver and spleen scanning. The specific application of all of these techniques is guided by clinical suspicion based on the history and current physical examination. The indiscriminant use of these diagnostic tools is of relatively low yield.

Other Diagnostic Interventions

Under certain circumstances, invasive diagnostic procedures may be indicated. These include endoscopy (to detect GI bleeding), abdominal paracentesis, thoracentesis, and even diagnostic peritoneal lavage. The last may be of some value in discriminating the presence of intraabdominal sepsis but is not without complications, including false-positive results.

STABILIZATION

Initial resuscitation is aimed at producing cardiopulmonary stabilization and adequate cellular perfusion. This requires the prompt establishment of an adequate airway and ensurance of ventilation. Supplemental oxygen is required for all patients with compromised perfusion as evidenced by altered mentation, cardiovascular instability, or oliguria. Intravenous access is essential with large-bore, short-length (and therefore high-flow) intravenous catheters. Central venous access is a luxury unnecessary in the earliest phases of resuscitation. As time progresses, however, central access for infusion of vasopressors may become essential. In addition, repletion of intravascular volume and assessment of myocardial performance may be facilitated by the placement of a pulmonary artery catheter with measurement of cardiac output by thermodilution and mixed venous oxygen saturation.

Transfusion of red blood cells is begun to maintain hemoglobin at a level consistent with adequate cellular oxygen delivery. Though there is no absolute threshold, a hemoglobin level of 8 to 10 g/dl is generally considered the minimum acceptable. Arterial catheterization facilitates the frequent sampling of blood and assessment of arterial blood pressure. An indwelling urinary drainage catheter is an essential method of assessing adequacy of resuscitation, which is considered the return of an hourly output of at least 0.5 ml/kg body weight (in the absence of diuretics or glycosuria).

A nasogastric or orogastric tube is placed to decompress the stomach and simultaneously assess its content for the presence of bleeding. Appropriate therapy for prophylaxis or treatment of GI bleeding is applied as described in the sections that follow.

Antibiotic therapy is not automatically initiated unless the index of suspicion for a specific infectious process is sufficiently high. Antimicrobial therapy is then tailored to the most likely pathogens, including gram-negative bacilli and anaerobes. Special consideration of opportunistic infections, such as cytomegalovirus and *Candida,* as the primary pathogen must occur in patients who are immunocompromised or therapeutically immunosuppressed. If surgical intervention is anticipated, prophylactic antibiotics may include a bowel preparation as guided by surgical consultation.

Early consultation with the surgical specialist is essential for thorough evaluation of all intraabdominal crises. Therapy, including an operation, can then be coordinated with other diagnostic and therapeutic interventions.

In the sections that follow, specific disease entities are described in further detail. This includes attention to historical and physical findings, evaluation, and specific interventions required.

CHOLECYSTITIS

When evaluating a patient with an acute abdomen, particularly when right upper quadrant pain is noted, the clinician must seriously consider the diagnosis of acute cholecystitis. The latter entity is common in the United States, accounting for approximately one fifth of the 500,000 cholecystectomies performed each year.

The most common cause of acute cholecystitis is obstruction of the cystic duct by an impacted gallstone, although the precise mechanism by which this occurs is uncertain. The intense contractions of the gallbladder that result from cystic duct obstruction induce the pain of biliary colic and sometimes dislodge the stone. However, if the stone remains resident, a phase of edema formation, mucosal damage, and inflammation follows. Once the integrity of the gallbladder mucosa is compromised, the opportunity exists for bacterial invasion with subsequent sepsis, gangrene of the gallbladder wall, and perforation with peritoneal soilage.

The usual clinical presentation of acute cholecystitis is that of a 40- to 50-year-old overweight patient, more commonly a woman with several offspring, with a history including previous symptoms of biliary colic. This episode of right upper quadrant pain will have persisted for more than 6 hours. It may be associated with pain radiating to the epigastrium or back near the scapula. Frequently the patient complains of nausea and severe vomiting. A low-grade fever, usually less than 101° F, and mild tachycardia are usually noted. Physical examination reveals a nontoxic condition, anxiety, right upper quadrant rebound tenderness, guarding, and spasm. A mass is found in this area in approximately 20% of cases and is probably a result of

overlying omentum. Generalized peritonitis is rare, except after perforation.

The differential diagnosis must include peptic ulcer perforation or posterior penetration, appendicitis, hepatitis, myocardial ischemia, pneumonia, and pleuritic inflammation.

Laboratory evaluation reveals leukocytosis to 12,000 to 15,000/mm^3, with an increase in nonsegmented neutrophils, a so called left shift. Mild hyperbilirubinemia may be present, with the total bilirubin concentration usually less than 4 mg/dl. The serum amylase level is often elevated but nonspecific. Levels of liver enzymes, including serum transaminases and alkaline phosphatase, are typically elevated but rarely exceed two to three times the normal levels. A plain film of the abdomen may be useful in excluding other parts of the differential diagnosis but is rarely helpful in diagnosing cholecystitis.

An initial assessment specific to the biliary tree can be made through real-time ultrasonography. Its absolute value in diagnosing this acute cholecystitis is unclear. However, with the recent definition of diagnostic criteria, the sensitivity and specificity of this test have improved. Major criteria include the presence of gallstones or a completely nonvisualized gallbladder. The minor criteria include thickening of the gallbladder wall, tenderness of the gallbladder when palpated during the examination (sonographic Murphy's sign), gallbladder enlargement, and pericholecystic fluid. Cholescintigraphy with 99m-Tc-disopropyl iminodiacetic acid (DISIDA), when interpreted as nonvisualization of the gallbladder after 4 hours, implies cystic duct obstruction associated with acute cholecystitis. This latter test is considered strong supportive evidence when other evaluations are indeterminate. Which of these two radiographic techniques should be applied first remains a matter of debate. Abdominal computed tomography adds little to the diagnostic precision.

Acute acalculous cholecystitis occurs in 4% to 8% of cases of cholecystitis. This entity, as implied by its name, occurs in the absence of gallstones. As first described in casualties of the Vietnam conflict, acalculous cholecystitis is much more prevalent in the postoperative, post–burn injury, and posttraumatic period. Under these circumstances it accounts for 33% to 50% of acute cholecystitis. In contrast to the latter, acalculous cholecystitis is predominantly a disease of men with an incidence 1½ to 3½ times higher than in women.

The cause of acalculous cholecystitis is unknown. However, several factors are believed to contribute. A state of biliary stasis may result from prolonged fasting, fever, dehydration, parenteral hyperalimentation, anesthesia, and the use of narcotics for postoperative pain control. Transfusions or resorption of large hematomas may contribute to the pigment load and aggravate the problem. Ischemia as a result of episodic hypotension or hypoperfusion probably promotes mucosal injury and facilitates bacterial or fungal invasion. Even the application of positive-pressure ventilation with positive end-expiratory pressure may contribute, presumably by decreasing portal and choledochoduodenal blood flow.

As in calculous cholecystitis, the onset of right upper quadrant pain or tenderness is suggestive of the acalculous form. Clinical signs and symptoms are often more subtle in the acalculous variety, since they are typically more difficult to evaluate in critically ill patients with this disorder. The appropriate clinical scenario, when accompanied by fever and sepsis of undiagnosed origin, requires rapid radiologic evaluation of the gallbladder, as described previously. Ultrasonography usually reveals the sludge of inspissated bile accompanied by several of the aforementioned minor criteria. Cholescintigraphy usually does not visualize the gallbladder.

Treatment of critically ill patients with cholecystitis involves appropriately aggressive repletion of intravascular volume by rehydration, systemic antibiotic therapy, and prompt medical stabilization in preparation for surgical intervention. The antibiotic therapy must provide coverage for the most likely bacterial pathogens: *Escherichia coli,* other gram-negative organisms, *Streptococcus faecalis,* and anaerobes. Ampicillin and tobramycin with the addition of clindamycin or metronidazole is a reliable choice for non-penicillin-allergic patients. Maintenance of satisfactory organ perfusion, as evidenced by adequate urine output and clearing of the sensorium, may necessitate aggressive intravascular monitoring and pharmacologic intervention with vasopressors.

Controversy exists over the optimal timing and type of surgical intervention. Most authors have favored early cholecystectomy. Cholecystostomy has been suggested as an alternative only in patients deemed too ill to survive the more definitive procedure. Mortality rates in this population exceed 25%. As a result, cholecystectomy is indicated, even in this circumstance, as soon as medical stabilization occurs. Early diagnosis and prompt intervention are crucial in acalculous cholecystitis. Because of its insidious development and subtle presentation in critically ill patients, it is typically far advanced at the time of recognition. It is also more commonly complicated at the time of diagnosis by gangrene, necrosis, and perforation (in up to 40% of patients). Thus a chance at survival requires a high index of suspicion and precise aggressive therapy.

Morbidity and mortality rates associated with cholecystitis are clearly higher when this entity occurs in already debilitated critically ill patients. Complications include hemodynamic instability, pelvic or subphrenic abscess formation, pneumonia, and death. Ongoing sepsis leading to multiple–organ system failure is a frequent final pathway. Mortality rates with calculous cholecystitis approximate 5%. With acalculous cholecystitis, reported mortality rates range from 6.5% to 67% but usually are at least twice those with the calculous variety. A positive effect on prognosis occurs when operation is performed within 48 hours of the onset of symptoms.

PANCREATITIS

Acute inflammation of the pancreas may be mild or may become life threatening, particularly in patients with complicating medical problems. In the United States acute pancreatitis is caused by chronic alcohol ingestion or biliary tract disease, specifically cholelithiasis, in 80% of the cases. In the remaining 20% other factors may be implicated. Mechanical insult may result through direct pancreatic injury from trauma, surgery, or endoscopic retrograde cholangiopancreatography (ERCP) or through obstruction by tumor. Metabolic factors, including hypercalcemia, medications such as corticosteroids, azathioprine, thiazide diuretics, estrogens, L-asparaginase, and furosemide, or hyperlipidemia, may irritate the pancreas. Ischemia related to hypothermia, hypoperfusion, sepsis, or other shock states or following cardiopulmonary bypass (and even heart and heart-lung transplantation) can induce pancreatic dysfunction and injury. Infectious agents such as mumps and coxsackievirus have occasionally been implicated as the etiologic agent of pancreatitis.

Whatever the inciting agent or insult, inflammation of the pancreas may be difficult to diagnose even with a careful clinical evaluation. The initial features vary widely and may mimic other intraabdominal disease processes. Even when accumulated evidence strongly implicates pancreatitis, the possibility of concomitant perforated gastric or duodenal ulcer, severe or gangrenous cholecystitis, or even mesenteric infarction still exists.

Responsive patients note upper midabdominal pain, often severe and radiating to the back. The patients are nauseated and repeatedly vomit small amounts of normal gastroduodenal contents. Physical examination usually reveals local epigastric tenderness without true rigidity of the abdominal wall musculature. Patients are often anxious, restless, tachypneic, and tachycardic and may have orthostatic hypotension early in the course of the disease.

Laboratory evaluation to enhance the accuracy of the diagnosis begins with serum amylase determination. These levels are elevated in 95% of patients with acute pancreatitis. Unfortunately, such elevation lacks specificity because comparable elevations occur in a variety of other intraabdominal problems, such as acute biliary tract disease, tuboovarian disease, perforated peptic ulcer, intestinal obstruction, inflammation, and ischemia. Amylase levels may even be elevated by concomitant (or isolated) inflammation of the parotid gland. Isoamylase fractionation helps to identify patients with coincident salivary hyperamylasemia but is of no value in clarifying the origin of the amylase in at least 55% of the cases. Serum lipase levels are less sensitive (elevated in only 60% to 75% of those with pancreatitis) but may be more specific for pancreatic inflammation. Although comparison of the urinary clearances of amylase and creatinine has been used by some clinicians, it is currently considered of little additional value.

Other laboratory findings are often abnormal in pancreatitis but have limited diagnostic value. Included are leukocytosis with a shift to immature neutrophils, hyperglycemia, elevated serum lactic dehydrogenase and glutamic oxaloacetic transaminase levels, hypophosphatemia, ionized hypocalcemia, and metabolic acidosis. Elevated fibrinogen levels and methemalbuminemia have also been described.

Radiography is the next step in evaluation. Simple abdominal roentgenograms may suggest alternative diagnoses (such as through the presence of free intraperitoneal air with a perforated viscus) or even support the diagnosis of pancreatitis. The findings most frequently noted for the latter are the "sentinel loop" of localized small bowel ileus isolated in the left upper quadrant, distention of the transverse colon, and obscuration of the psoas muscle shadow. Occasionally, pancreatic calcification is evident, particularly in patients with a history of repeated bouts of pancreatitis.

Ultrasonography is useful in observation of the gallbladder (see section on cholelithiasis) but is of limited value in assessing the pancreas because of technical limitations (such as overlying gas-filled loops of bowel and adipose tissue). Computed tomography appears to be an excellent adjunctive technique for diagnosing pancreatitis and following its course. Abnormalities have been noted in at least 90% of cases of pancreatitis. Notable among these are localized or diffuse enlargement, loss of pancreatic outline with peripancreatic edema and blurring of the fat planes, thickening of the perirenal fascia, mesenteric edema, and inflammatory exudate.

The utility of diagnostic peritoneal lavage is a controversial issue. Advocates of this technique cite elevated amylase levels in free ascitic or lavage fluid in the absence of microorganisms as indicative of pancreatitis. When the diagnosis remains elusive in a patient with abdominal tenderness, peritoneal tap or lavage may be considered before exploratory celiotomy.

Acute pancreatitis sometimes has severe systemic manifestations. Admission to the ICU with frequent monitoring of vital signs, laboratory values, and fluid balance is essential under these circumstances. Recognition of these associated perturbations is essential to patient management. Intravascular volume rapidly moves into the retroperitoneal space. Concomitant diffuse capillary leak syndrome with interstitial fluid sequestration leads to profound hypovolemia. This in turn results in hypotension, tachycardia, tachypnea, depressed cardiac output, and organ hypoperfusion. Aggressive volume repletion is required, with particular attention to maintenance of adequate red blood cell mass and to the coagulopathic complications of marked rehydration. Following fluid therapy, patients may remain hypotensive, in a hyperdynamic state with low systemic vascular resistance characteristic of the inflammatory or septic state. (In fact, some authors attribute these systemic hemodynamic manifestations, at least in part, to pancreas-derived factors.) Despite apparently adequate volume resuscitation, hypovolemia may recur with ongoing fluid loss secondary to the diffuse "peritoneal burn." Many clinicians consider invasive hemodynamic monitoring for the measurement of pulmonary capillary wedge pressure and cardiac output to be essential for assessing response to the titration of fluid and vasopressor therapy.

Pancreatitis can be excruciatingly painful. However, agents used to control the discomfort must be chosen carefully. Opiate analgesics, particularly morphine, induce spasm of the sphincter of Oddi and, therefore, have the potential to exacerbate obstruction and bile stasis. Nausea and vomiting may worsen as a result of narcotic-induced stimulation of the medullary chemoreceptor zone. Meperidine has been used as an alternative to morphine, but its use may be complicated by myocardial depression or accumulation of the metabolite normeperidine (an analeptic). As a result, recent attention has been focused on the titration of intravenous synthetic narcotics, particularly fentanyl, or the use of epidural analgesia. Both techniques have been applied successfully, without the complications previously described.

Supportive therapy is aimed at preserving visceral perfusion and function, particularly of the renal and pulmonary systems. Noncardiogenic pulmonary edema with profound hypoxemia may occur, requiring ventilatory support to minimize the work of breathing resulting from decreased pulmonary compliance. Despite the lack of supporting scientific evidence, dopamine is often administered in low intravenous doses (1 to 2 μg/kg/min) to enhance renal perfusion and protection.

Nasogastric drainage is indicated if vomiting is a prominent problem. It appears to have no other value, in terms of disease progression or outcome. Oral food intake is prohibited until several days after resolution of the symptoms (particularly abdominal pain), since early feeding may precipitate a recurrence. Total parenteral nutrition does not specifically influence the course of the pancreatitis but is appropriate in severely ill, malnourished, and long-fasted patients.

No specific role has been defined for antimicrobial therapy in acute pancreatitis. Some clinicians administer antibiotics to patients with gallstone pancreatitis in anticipation of a bacterial component to the inflammatory process. In this circumstance second-generation cephalosporins or ampicillin with chloramphenicol have been applied. In general, antibiotic therapy should be applied to specifically documented infection and not to prophylaxis in pancreatitis.

If the cause of the pancreatitis involves an impacted gallstone, invasive intervention is usually indicated. Recently, ERCP has been advocated as both a diagnostic and a therapeutic tool, with sphincterotomy for relief of obstructive symptoms. Definitive biliary tract surgery, including cholecystectomy, operative cholangiography, and common bile duct exploration,

has been applied safely and successfully both early in the course and if delayed until stabilization occurs. Rarely is the operation followed by a recurrence of pancreatitis.

Several other pharmacologic interventions have been applied in both animal models and humans. These include glucagon, heparin, dextran, cimetidine, aprotinin, 5-fluorouracil, and somatostatin. To date, the therapeutic benefits have not been forthcoming. Studies continue, with recent evidence of improved cardiac performance in an *animal* model of pancreatitis as a result of methylprednisolone therapy. None of these interventions is currently advocated for clinical application.

Pancreatitis is a potentially lethal disease with mortality rates of 5% to 10%, and up to 20% in patients over 70 years of age. The best assessment of severity of pancreatitis and outcome prediction was developed by Ranson. Several modifications have been made since, but the essence remains the same. Evidence of shock, including massive fluid loss, declining hematocrit value, low serum albumin level, and metabolic acidosis, is a harbinger of a bad outcome. Concurrent hypocalcemia, renal insufficiency, elevated hepatic enzyme levels, altered blood glucose, hypoxemia, and respiratory insufficiency point to multisystem injury and are associated with a poor prognosis. Peritoneal lavage may be valuable in gauging the severity of pancreatitis soon after admission. The presence of greater than 20 ml of free intraperitoneal fluid and dark color of this or instilled lavage fluid may indicate a particularly severe attack. Postoperative pancreatitis carries a grave prognosis with a mortality rate of up to 60%. This may be attributed to difficulty and delay in diagnosis and the synergistic stress of recent operation. Hemorrhagic and necrotizing pancreatitis are generally the most severe varieties of pancreatitis and carry the highest mortality rate.

Despite successful fluid resuscitation, organ system support, nutritional therapy, and GI tract rest, complications may follow a bout of acute pancreatitis. Pseudocyst formation, particularly in patients with alcohol-induced pancreatitis, is the most common complication, occurring in up to 8% of patients. Pseudocysts may be suspected in patients in whom a peripancreatic fluid collection, as followed by abdominal computed tomography, persists more than 6 weeks. These pseudocysts usually are in continuity with the pancreatic ductal system and contain potent proteolytic enzymes. They may erode into surrounding vascular structures with lethal consequences. Drainage, either percutaneously or with formal surgical cystenterostomy, is indicated.

Pancreatic abscess is a potential late complication, occurring in 4% of acute pancreatic attacks. The usual onset is 2 to 4 weeks into the course of the disease. The demonstration of pancreatic or peripancreatic gas bubbles by abdominal computed tomography is the most specific diagnostic criterion. The more severe the initial attack as judged by Ranson's criteria, the more likely the development of an abscess. Treatment of the abscess involves drainage. Attention has been directed at comparison between closed drainage (laparotomy with pancreatic debridement and irrigation followed by closure with drains) and open drainage (placement of packs into the lesser sac changed periodically through the open abdominal wound) with some enthusiasm for the latter. Percutaneous catheter drainage has also shown some promise but is not popular at present. Monomicrobial gram-positive infection may be the cause of abscess in up to one third of the cases. Polymicrobial gram-negative abscesses account for most of the remainder and are associated with a particularly poor outcome. Without surgical intervention, pancreatic abscess has a 100% mortality rate. Even with aggressive management, including frequent re-operation for drainage of recurrent abscesses, the mortality rate remains at greater than 50%.

Other complications may occur, including rupture or thrombosis of the splenic, portal, or mesenteric vessels, perforation of the common bile duct, stomach, or colon, or even mesenteric ischemia.

Pancreatitis is a potentially lethal disease that may either be a primary problem or follow other systemic stresses. Prompt diagnosis and aggressive supportive therapy are essential. Even when these occur, morbidity and mortality rates are significant.

STRESS ULCERATION AND PROPHYLAXIS

GI integrity may be interrupted during the critically ill patient's stay in the ICU. Morbidity and mortality rates are frequently doubled or tripled with the onset of GI tract bleeding. Mortality rates as high as 40% to 65% have been reported. Stress-related ulceration of the upper GI tract is a generally avoidable complication, and preventive therapy is essential.

Stress ulceration has been described under a wide variety of circumstances. Curling in 1842 noted its association with severe burn injuries. In 1932 Cushing described a similar syndrome in patients with cranial trauma or tumors. Selye in 1950 commented that the common denominator for individuals at risk was activation of the neuroendocrine stress response. Identified risk factors include extensive thermal injury, head injury, coma, multiple trauma (particularly intraabdominal, thoracoabdominal, and spinal cord injuries), major or multiple surgeries, hypotension, sepsis, renal failure, pulmonary failure, hepatic failure, and mixed acid-base disorders. These factors are at least additive, if not synergistic.

The clinical presentation is the acute onset of painless upper GI tract bleeding in the setting of multisystem stress. Bleeding may be occult or may be overt with hematemesis or melena. Less than 10% of these patients have massive hemorrhage. The onset typically occurs within 7 to 14 days of admission to the ICU. Overt stress ulcer bleeding occurs in at least 20% of patients at risk who do not receive prophylactic therapy. Occult bleeding is more common and is found by nasogastric aspiration in over 50% of these patients.

Stress ulceration as the cause of upper GI tract bleeding is most efficiently and effectively diagnosed by upper GI tract endoscopy. The first endoscopy appropriately identifies the lesion in more than 80% of cases. The characteristic lesions are small, generally 1 to 2 mm in diameter, and red based early in their evolution. After 48 hours they become black based, 2 to 25 mm in diameter, and multiple. The ulcers are well circumscribed with little induration or edema and are usually distributed in the gastric fundus or proximal stomach. Radiographic techniques are of little value, since they detect these small lesions in only 20% of the cases.

Stress ulceration probably results from an imbalance between the destructive properties of gastric acid and pepsin and the protection by normal defense mechanisms. Splanchnic vasoconstriction with diminished gastric mucosal blood flow, ischemia, and tissue acidosis may be the common pathway for injury. When patients believed to be at highest risk and specific patient-related risk factors have been identified, prophylactic therapy can be applied with some scientific basis.

Preventive therapy currently involves the use of antacids, H_2 receptor antagonists, and sucralfate. Other interventions, such as topical prostaglandin E_2, are undergoing evaluation and may be of future use.

Antacids are given via the nasogastric tube.

Their titration is based on adequate neutralization of gastric acid, generally to a pH greater than 5. Intragastric pH is measured at least once per hour or even continuously with a pH electrode. Hourly antacid requirements may vary from 30 to 120 ml to achieve neutralization. This approach controls pH in almost all circumstances. Complications of this therapy include diarrhea or constipation, electrolyte shifts, and alkalosis. Nursing care must be intensified.

Antihistamine therapy with H_2 blockers may be applied with cimetidine, ranitidine, or famotidine delivered intravenously. The resulting decline in basal gastric acid secretion allows the intraluminal pH to rise above 5. This goal is most effectively achieved by continuous infusion, although intermittent bolus is frequently used. Several problems may be attributed to antihistamine therapy, including potential alteration in mental status, suppression of hepatic cytochrome P-450, producing altered drug levels (for example, of theophylline or phenytoin), and thrombocytopenia. The pharmacokinetic complications have been most notable with cimetidine and may not occur with ranitidine.

Studies comparing the efficacy and safety of antacids and H_2 blockers have failed to show clear superiority, though antacids may provide earlier and more complete control of pH. Antacids and H_2 blockers are often used effectively in combination.

Sucralfate, a polyanionic surface-active agent, does not change the intragastric pH but provides mucosal protection through its ability to bind to surface proteins and adsorb bile and pepsin. It can be given as a 1 g slurry via the nasogastric tube every 4 to 6 hours. Early reports suggest that, when used alone, it prevents gastric stress ulceration.

A currently acceptable prophylactic regimen is as follows:

- Identify and provide prophylaxis for all high-risk patients.

- Minimize the risk of aspiration of gastric contents by patient positioning and nasogastric suctioning.

- Combine H_2 receptor antagonists with antacids to diminish the volume and time needed for preventive therapy. Monitor gastric pH hourly when using this therapy.

- Consider using H_2 antagonists or sucralfate alone or in combination as an alternative to the preceding.

Recent studies have confirmed the safety and efficacy of these recommendations.

In the future the use of antacids in high volume for stress ulcer prophylaxis will probably be replaced by other methods. Sucralfate may become the preferred method of prophylaxis because it does not impair the acidic barrier to upper GI tract bacterial colonization and may thus diminish the incidence of aspiration-related bacterial pneumonitis. Bacterial aspiration pneumonitis is also prevented by keeping the stomach empty, and H_2 antagonists are particularly effective in this regard.

Some believe that enteral alimentation protects the upper GI tract. Indisputably, nutritional supplementation is beneficial for the recovery of critically ill patients and use of enteral alimentation is the preferred method in patients with adequate peristalsis and absorptive function. However, whether early enteral feeding truly prevents stress ulceration is unclear, and further study is warranted.

Most patients with stress ulcer–induced upper GI bleeding respond to nonoperative therapy. Although there is no evidence for the efficacy of saline lavage or antacid titration following the onset of bleeding, these therapies are routinely applied. The histamine receptor antagonists are ineffective in arresting bleeding. For patients who do not spontaneously stop bleeding after the aforementioned treatment, bleeding sites can often be controlled by endoscopic electrocoagulation techniques. Intraarterial vasopressin is rarely applied (and not favored because it may exacerbate mucosal ischemia), and angioembolic treatment is ineffective.

Operative intervention is unpopular because of the high incidence of morbidity, rebleeding, and mortality in this patient population. Comparative studies have suggested that, when surgery is necessitated by uncontrollable hemorrhage, the preferred technique may be vagotomy and pyloroplasty with directed oversewing of specific bleeding sites. Even this technique is associated with a 10% rebleeding rate and a mortality rate of approximately 25%. Clearly prevention is preferable to attempted cure.

In summary, a population at risk for stress-related gastric mucosal ulceration can be identified. These patients should receive prophylactic therapy that clearly prevents ulcer formation or progression to bleeding, such as titrated antacids or H_2 blockers. Future evaluation of other prophylactic interventions, such as sucralfate and prostaglandin E_2, is needed to advance understanding of, and ability to prevent, stress ulceration. Prevention is much easier than cure, and attention must be focused on the eradication of underlying contributory disease.

GASTROINTESTINAL BLEEDING

Hemorrhage from the GI tract may be present at patients' admission to the ICU or develop during their care. Bleeding from the GI tract results in more than 50 hospital admissions per 100,000 population per year in the United States. Up to 15% of these individuals have been estimated to require intensive care. Despite apparent advances in diagnosis and therapy, the overall mortality rate remains at approximately 10%. This may be due in part to the shifting patient population, in which almost half of affected individuals are over 60 years of age. Of patients with acute gastrointestinal hemorrhage, 85% have a source in the upper tract and the remainder have a lower tract site.

Upper Gastrointestinal Tract Bleeding

Upper gastrointestinal tract bleeding may be manifest as hematemesis, hematochezia, abdominal distention and epigastric discomfort, or syncope. It may initially be subtle, as the underlying cause of unexplained tachycardia and orthostatic hypotension. Historical data, such as the presence of peptic ulcer disease, hepatic dysfunction, history of GI bleeding, previous surgery, protracted or severe retching, heartburn, dysphagia, history of alcohol abuse, salicylate ingestion, or history of a bleeding diathesis, help to elucidate the situation.

Diagnosis is important, but stabilization is the first priority. Resuscitative efforts involve placement of large-bore peripheral intravenous access lines with the infusion of isotonic fluids pending completion of blood typing and cross-matching. Frequent vital sign measurement and assessment of orthostasis are essential for the titration of fluid resuscitation. In profound hypovolemic shock, emergency transfusion of type O, Rh-negative blood is initiated until type-specific blood becomes available. With this therapy in progress, laboratory studies, including blood cell counts, clotting studies, and blood chemistries, are performed urgently. In the case of massive transfusion, attention to secondary coagulopathies may necessitate repletion of platelets and clotting factors through transfusion of platelets and plasma. If blood is being transfused at greater than 100 ml/min, ionized hypocalcemia with hypotension and poor cardiac performance may result. Titration of supplemental calcium chloride may be empiric or guided by measured plasma levels of ionized calcium. Hypothermia must be avoided by warming of transfused products. Ventilatory support may be necessary to ensure adequate oxygenation, provide airway protection from aspiration of upper GI tract blood, facilitate patient rewarming by heating of inspired gases, and minimize the work and oxygen cost of breathing. Under any circumstance, supplemental oxygen is necessary for patients with acute anemia. Monitoring must routinely include bladder catheterization and temperature probe.

With restoration of acceptable perfusion as assessed by improved cardiovascular stability, mentation, and urine output, attention is redirected toward diagnosis. Bleeding stops spontaneously in approximately 80% of patients with acute GI hemorrhage when therapy is limited to cardiopulmonary stabilization.

Physical examination should include continuous assessment of hemodynamic status. Specific findings, such as cutaneous spider angiomas and palmar erythema, may suggest a diagnosis, in this case chronic liver disease and perhaps portal hypertension. Characteristic mucocutaneous changes associated with such syndromes as Peutz-Jeghers, Ehlers-Danlos, or hereditary hemorrhagic telangiectasia may also be apparent. The physical examination must be thorough and specifically include digital rectal examination and stool guaiac tests for the presence of blood. The next diagnostic evaluation is performed through placement of a nasogastric or orogastric tube with aspiration of stomach contents. Identification of the upper GI tract as the site of bleeding is rapidly confirmed by the presence of a bloody aspirate. Rarely is blood absent from the aspirate if the source of bleeding is the upper GI tract. This is most frequently related to duodenal ulceration and bleeding and can be diagnosed by passage of the gastric tube into the proximal small bowel. Upper tract GI bleeding can be virtually excluded if bilious aspirate free of blood (consistent with passage of the gastric tube into the proximal duodenum) is obtained.

In the case of upper GI hemorrhage the gastric tube is also used as the route of gastric lavage. Much attention has been directed at the use of iced saline solution or the addition of topical vasoconstrictors or topical thrombin to the lavage fluid. At present there is little scientific evidence to suggest that these have any more benefit than thorough lavage with room-temperature saline solution. Nonetheless, cold solutions are frequently used and may rapidly precipitate hypothermia with its arrhythmias and anticoagulant sequelae unless careful attention is paid to maintaining normal body temperature. During lavage the patient must be protected from aspiration of orogastric contents. This is best accomplished by positioning the patient in a head-down lateral decubitus position with continuous suctioning of the oropharynx.

Fiberoptic endoscopy is the next diagnostic step. This technique is far superior to radiographic methods in locating bleeding sites in the upper GI tract, particularly when applied early in the course of the disease. If it is performed within 12 hours of the onset of bleeding, an active site is identified in more than 40% of patients. This frequency declines progressively with time. Endoscopy is critical in patients with lesions of an unknown nature. For example, 60% of patients with known liver disease and esophageal varices who are examined for upper GI bleeding have a nonvariceal source of bleeding. In the 10% to 15% of patients in whom endoscopy fails to identify the source of upper GI tract bleeding, radiologic evaluation including air contrast studies is indicated. The highly invasive technique of vascular radiology may be applied in otherwise difficult to diagnose disease. A site may be identified when the rate of blood loss exceeds 0.5 to 1.5 ml/min. Therapy has occasionally been applied through these catheters, including localized regional vasoconstriction by vasopressin infusion, as well as embolization with clot or an inert substance, such as Gelfoam.

The most common cause of acute upper GI tract bleeding, accounting for up to 50% of cases, is peptic ulcer disease of the stomach or duodenum. These ulcers may result from repeated contact of the mucosa with acid and pepsin. They most commonly occur in the duodenal bulb or gastric antrum but can also be found in the esophagus and Meckel's diverticulum. Purported etiologic factors include altered acid and pepsin production, impaired mucosal bicarbonate secretion, altered feedback inhibition of the gastrin-acid pathway, increased parietal cell density, steroid therapy, and genetic factors. Endoscopy not only reveals these lesions but may also forewarn of propensity for continued bleeding or rebleeding. As summarized in an excellent recent review, the latter is suggested by any of the following: active arterial bleeding, a densely adherent clot attached to the lesion, an exposed or visible vessel, and an elevated red dot within a mucosal lesion.

Therapy initially consists of administration of parenteral H_2 receptor antagonists, such as ranitidine, and antacids via the gastric tube. Titration of this therapy must be guided by renal function (in terms of dosage of H_2 blockers and

avoidance of magnesium retention from antacids). Gastric pH is often difficult to monitor because of the persistence of blood in the gastric aspirate. As stated previously, most patients respond to this conservative management and require no further therapy. However, continued bleeding or rebleeding may necessitate more aggressive interventions, such as surgery. The determination is based on red blood cell transfusion requirements, with more than 6 units as the accepted threshold for additional intervention. The clinician must exercise caution in interpreting blood requirements, however, since redistribution of crystalloid rapidly infused during resuscitation requires 6 to 8 hours and may result in hemodilution. Ancillary therapy includes Nd:YAG laser endoscopic coagulation (although debate about its efficacy continues) or surgery, such as vagotomy with antrectomy or pyloroplasty. Continuous intravenous infusion of vasopressin is of uncertain benefit in this circumstance.

Upper GI tract bleeding from esophageal or gastric varices is another large etiologic category, accounting for 20% of these cases. Bleeding from these sites typically occurs in advanced hepatic cirrhosis and carries a particularly poor prognosis. It is the major cause of death in patients with hepatic failure. These patients cannot be discriminated from those with other types of upper GI tract hemorrhage on the basis of clinical findings. Indeed, as many as half of patients with a documented history of esophageal varices have bleeding from a *different* upper GI tract site, such as ulcer disease. Gastric tube insertion is not precluded by a history of varices, but prompt endoscopy is the preferred diagnostic procedure. The risk of bleeding from varices is high if endoscopy shows large varices with surface longitudinal venules that resemble whip marks.

Therapy is initially supportive as for all hypovolemic states. Once the diagnosis is made, specific interventions are applied. Despite the lack of scientific evidence substantiating its efficacy, intravenous infusion of vasopressin (begun at 0.2 to 0.4 unit/min and titrated as high as 0.9 unit/min) is routinely administered. This pharmacotherapy is fraught with complications. Vasopressin, as a profound vasoconstrictor, may result in severe systemic hypertension with diminished cardiac output or frank myocardial infarction, renal hypoperfusion and oliguria, or bowel infarction. Close monitoring of cardiac function, frequently including the use of a pulmonary artery catheter and simultaneous titration of vasodilators, such as nitroprusside, is essential. Other reported complications are arrhythmias and metabolic disturbances, such as hyponatremia from antidiuresis.

A Sengstaken-Blakemore (SB) tube is often used concomitantly or when vasopressin fails. Because of the large diameter of this triple-lumen tube, airway protection (to some extent from secretions and more effectively to prevent tracheal occlusion by the SB balloons) with elective endotracheal intubation usually precedes its insertion. The SB tube is placed via the orogastric route. Distal tip placement in the stomach is ensured by air insufflation with simultaneous auscultation over the upper abdomen. After the obligatory insertion of a conventional nasogastric tube into the esophagus, the gastric balloon is inflated with 250 cc of air. Acute onset of chest pain with balloon inflation suggests that the SB tube is too high, with the gastric balloon in the esophagus, and requires immediate deflation followed by repositioning. Approximately 2 pounds of traction is applied, typically by attachment of the SB tube to a football helmet. Continuous suction is applied to the esophageal nasogastric tube and intermittent suction to the gastric port of the SB tube. If bleeding does not promptly resolve, the esophageal balloon is inflated with the lowest volume that arrests bleeding, typically to a pressure of between 25 and 40 mm Hg. Some authors believe that deflation of the esophageal balloon for 30 to 60 minutes every 8 hours is advantageous. After 24 hours with no bleeding, the balloons are sequentially deflated, beginning with the esophageal balloon. The gastric balloon is later released, as long as no rebleeding occurs. Twelve to 24 hours later the entire SB tube is withdrawn. Although initial success in control of bleeding occurs in up to 90% of patients, rebleeding is frequent, occurring in up to 75% of patients. This is particularly true in cirrhotic patients with jaundice, ascites, or hepatic encephalopathy. Complications with the SB tube include rupture of the esophagus, pressure necrosis of the gastric mucosa, airway obstruction by improper positioning, and aspiration pneumonitis.

Endoscopic sclerotherapy is being evaluated as a method for immediate control and long-term therapy to prevent rebleeding from esophageal varices. Injection of such solutions as tetradecyl sulfate, sodium morrhuate, or thrombin has produced success rates of up to 90% for control of acute bleeding. Other techniques, such as endoscopic laser or electrocautery coagulation and transhepatic selective embolization of varices, seem to be of limited use.

Emergency surgical decompression of the portal vein through bypass techniques is generally reserved for patients with unrelenting hemorrhage and has been associated with a mortality rate of at least 50%. However, portasystemic shunting has attracted recent interest as a more effective and definitive therapy with fewer recurrences and a lower mortality rate (36%) than sclerotherapy for the control of variceal bleeding.

Bleeding from the upper GI tract may result from a variety of other, less common sources. The erosive gastritis that accompanies the profound stress state of the critically ill is discussed separately in the section on stress ulcer prophylaxis. Mallory-Weiss mucosal tears of the gastroesophageal junction infrequently require treatment other than antacids and parenteral H_2 blockers but should prompt removal of the nasogastric tube. An aortoenteric fistula must be considered if the patient has a history of abdominal aortic aneurysm or graft surgery. Any suspicion of this diagnosis should prompt urgent consultation with a vascular surgeon.

Lower Gastrointestinal Tract Bleeding

Typically the elderly patient who passes bright red blood (hematochezia) or dark red blood (melena) rectally is bleeding from the lower GI tract. However, since upper GI tract bleeding may have these same signs, the diagnoses already discussed must be considered simultaneously. When the nasogastric aspirate contains bile pigment but is free of blood, the bleeding is from the distal small bowel, colon, rectum, or anal canal. Brisk bleeding may result in hypovolemia and requires the same aggressive intervention as described for upper GI tract bleeding. Historical information, particularly of similar past episodes and workup, should be reviewed. Once again, careful digital rectal examination with evaluation of the contents of the rectal vault is essential.

Evaluation continues with the assistance of surgeons and gastroenterologists. Lower GI endoscopy with anoscopy, sigmoidoscopy, and then flexible colonoscopy is the most appropriate diagnostic course. Three fourths of these massive lower GI hemorrhages cease spontaneously, but treatment depends on the diagnosis. Therefore aggressive attempts at diagnosis are made. Barium studies of the lower GI tract are of little value and are probably contraindicated because they render endoscopy impossible. Red blood cell scanning with tagged red blood cells or technetium sulfur colloid may help to localize the bleeding site (although it does not determine the cause) and can detect bleeding at a rate of approximately 0.1 ml/min. In the case of persistent massive bleeding, arteriography frequently (80% of episodes) reveals the site, allowing specific surgical intervention.

The two most common causes of massive lower GI tract bleeding requiring intensive care are diverticular disease and arteriovenous malformations known as angiodysplasia. Colonic diverticula are typically a disease of the elderly. They are evidenced by episodic, painless, gross bleeding that resolves spontaneously. If a bleeding site is identified angiographically, selective arterial infusion of vasopressin may effect control. Embolization has been applied only anecdotally. If bleeding persists or recurs, emergency surgical intervention with hemicolectomy may be indicated once the bleeding site has been identified. If the source is uncertain, subtotal colectomy may be required for definitive control.

Angiodysplasia, typically of the right colon, also gives rise to episodic massive lower GI tract bleeding and is frequently recurrent. Diagnosis may be made angiographically when the site of the arteriovenous connection is suggested, although a specific bleeding site is rarely identified (in contrast to diverticular disease). Definitive therapy is through surgical resection.

Although an infrequent cause of lower GI tract bleeding, intestinal ischemia is worthy of mention, particularly as a sequela of acute superior mesenteric artery occlusion in a patient with vascular disease. Manifest as severe acute abdominal pain out of proportion to physical examination findings, mesenteric ischemia may occur along with global hypoperfusion after cardiogenic or hemorrhagic shock, atrial fibrillation, or major aortic surgery or in septicemia. Evaluation, performed along with aggressive resuscitative therapy as guided by invasive monitoring, should include a flat plate roentgenogram of the abdomen and colonoscopy. Colonoscopy confirms the dusky edematous pattern characteristic of intestinal ischemia. Prompt consultation with surgical specialists concerning revascularization or resection is required. Despite decisive management, the mortality rate remains high (at least 25%).

Other, less frequent causes of lower GI tract bleeding that must be considered are ulcerative colitis, Crohn's disease, radiation colitis, Meckel's diverticulum, and neoplastic disease.

In all cases of GI bleeding, attention is first paid to aggressive resuscitation followed promptly by diagnosis and consultation with surgeons and gastroenterologists. Despite advances in diagnosis and therapy, morbidity and mortality rates have remained at between 10% and 33%, the latter in patients whose onset of bleeding occurs in the hospital or who have a recurrence of bleeding, particularly elderly patients or those with concomitant systemic illness.

JAUNDICE AND HEPATIC DYSFUNCTION

The liver performs several essential functions in the maintenance of homeostasis: reticuloendothelial system function by the Kupffer cells; synthetic activity including glucose, albumin and other visceral proteins, and blood clotting factors; clearance of bile acids and bilirubin; and detoxification of some drugs, free fatty acids, ammonia, phenols, mercaptans, and amino acids.

Erythrocyte destruction by the reticuloendothelial system liberates hemoglobin, which is converted to bilirubin. This pigment is carried bound to protein, predominantly albumin, in this unconjugated and poorly water-soluble form to the hepatocytes. There conjugation occurs in the endoplasmic reticulum to form water-soluble conjugated bilirubin. This is followed by secretion onto the bile canaliculi, usually the rate-limiting step. The bile flows down the biliary tree into the duodenum where peristalsis delivers it for elimination in the feces. A small portion of the bile pigments undergoes enterohepatic recirculation.

Jaundice, or icterus, is the yellowish discoloration of skin, sclerae, and mucous membranes resulting from the accumulation of bilirubin or its conjugates. It becomes clinically detectable only when the total serum bilirubin level rises to three to four times normal. This accumulation of bilirubin may result from a wide variety of disorders affecting any portion of the clearance pathway. The most frequently applied discriminant is the relative proportions of unconjugated bilirubin (UB) and conjugated bilirubin.

Unconjugated hyperbilirubinemia may result from the following:

- Profoundly increased production of bilirubin related to hemolysis
- Impaired delivery of UB as a result of impaired myocardial function (particularly congestive heart failure) or portosystemic shunting (with cirrhosis or decompressive surgery)

- Limitation in hepatic uptake of UB as a result of drugs or metabolic derangements (including hyperthyroidism and Gilbert's syndrome type III)
- Insufficient conversion of UB to its conjugated form as is sometimes encountered in end-stage cirrhosis, chronic hepatitis, Wilson's disease, or hereditary disorders

Conjugated hyperbilirubinemia may result through the following pathways:

- Impaired biliary secretion as seen with hepatocellular dysfunction (viral or toxic hepatitis, Laennec's cirrhosis)
- Restriction of flow through the biliary tree resulting from cholestasis (intrahepatic: drugs, tumors, primary biliary cirrhosis; extrahepatic, or obstructive: ampullary or common duct obstruction, choledocholithiasis, acute cholecystitis, pancreatitis, pancreatic pseudocyst)

In the evaluation of hyperbilirubinemia, several diagnostic tests supplement the history and physical examination. Blood samples are analyzed for total bilirubin content, as well as indirect (UB) and direct (conjugated) fractions. Conjugated hyperbilirubinemia, the more common type encountered in the surgical arena, is further assessed by evaluation of hepatocellular enzyme, cholesterol, and serum alkaline phosphatase levels. Hepatocellular jaundice is characterized by mildly elevated bile acid levels and an alkaline phosphatase level usually less than three times normal. The serum cholesterol concentration is frequently decreased, and the serum aminotransferase levels (aspartate [AST or SGOT] and alanine [ALT or SGPT]) are usually markedly elevated. Patients with an abnormal prothrombin time do not generally respond to administered vitamin K. Virology studies and tests for specific antigens and antibodies to hepatitis viruses may then be indicated.

Unlike patients with direct cellular injury, those with cholestatic jaundice have sharply elevated bile acid levels, alkaline phosphatase levels greater than three times normal, increased serum cholesterol levels, and only mildly elevated AST and ALT concentrations. In these individuals the coagulopathy associated with an elevated prothrombin time normalizes after parenteral administration of vitamin K. Discrimination of specific mechanical causes of extrahepatic cholestasis is essential for appropriate treatment. Specific diagnostic interventions, such as ultrasonography and biliary scanning, and therapeutic interventions are discussed in the sections on assessment and on cholecystitis.

Since jaundice is a common symptom of underlying disease, therapy is directed at this problem and not at the elevated bilirubin level. Specific attention is given to avoiding factors known to exacerbate hyperbilirubinemia. These include acute hemolysis, impaired hepatic perfusion, and hypoxemia. Renal failure may also contribute to direct hyperbilirubinemia through impairment of renal excretion of conjugated bilirubin.

A particular type of jaundice worthy of note is that caused by postoperative cholestasis. After prolonged operations in which moderately severe blood loss requires a large transfusion of packed red blood cells, typically more than 20 units, jaundice may develop within 24 to 96 hours. This conjugated hyperbilirubinemia is believed to result from the combination of increased pigment load and impaired hepatic perfusion and thus clearance. In more severe forms conjugated bilirubin levels may exceed 40 times normal with an alkaline phosphatase level greater than five times normal. In the absence of multiple organ system failure these changes usually resolve within 2 to 4 weeks without permanent sequelae.

Although jaundice is generally a symptom rather than a discrete disease process, it may have a direct effect on other organs, as in the left ventricular dysfunction known as jaundiced heart. Jaundice alone carries a 1-year mortality rate of approximately 40%.

HEPATIC FAILURE

The liver's regenerative capabilities are impressive: normal hepatic function has been reported after resection of nearly 80% of the liver mass. Nonetheless, cellular injury resulting in massive hepatic necrosis can overwhelm this regenerative capability, resulting in acute fulminant hepatic failure or precipitous deterioration of chronic liver disease. Acute hepatic failure in the United States is most frequently a consequence of hepatitis B. Other causes are medications and toxins (acetaminophen, alpha methyldopa, ethanol, halothane, isoniazid, nonsteroidal antiinflammatory drugs, *Amanita phalloides* mushrooms, and carbon tetrachloride); ischemia (cardiovascular insufficiency, Budd-Chiari syndrome of hepatic vein occlusion); metabolic diseases (acute fatty liver of pregnancy, Wilson's disease, Reye's syndrome); or other viral hepatitides (A; non-A, non-B; D; herpes simplex; cytomegalovirus). Whatever the cause, the mortality rate is reportedly 80% to 90%, usually as a consequence of cerebral edema, hemorrhage, or septicemia. Cirrhosis, most commonly as a consequence of chronic alcohol abuse, predisposes the patient to hepatic failure.

Definitive diagnosis may be difficult. Presumptive diagnosis may be based on the history with special attention to viral syndromes, travel, medication and toxin exposure, transfusion, drug or alcohol abuse, and family history. This may be supplemented by other tests, including serum transaminase and lactate dehydrogenase levels as a reflection of hepatocellular injury; serologic tests including IgM anti-HBc for hepatitis B; coagulation parameters as evidence of diminished hepatic production of factors II, V, VII, IX, and X; renal function; and occasionally percutaneous liver biopsy for patients without severe coagulopathies. Evidence of the marked disturbance in metabolic pathways includes elevated serum ammonia levels and altered (often low) glucose levels. Physical examination is directed at assessment of neurologic impairment, cardiovascular status, pulmonary sufficiency and ability to protect the airway from aspiration, and evidence of specific predisposing disease such as herpetic vesicles. Circulatory status is assessed by invasive hemodynamic monitoring of cardiac output with the simultaneous assessment of perfusion by measurement of urine output. However, marked tissue hypoxia may be masked by the typical pattern encountered in hepatic failure: low systemic vascular resistance, elevated cardiac output, and normal arterial and venous oxygen saturation with peripheral shunting. Lactic acidosis may be the only indicator of altered perfusion, but the clinical utility of even this test is compromised by altered metabolic clearance.

Care of patients with hepatic failure is generally supportive in the hope of hepatic regeneration (or hepatic transplantation) and requires attention to detail. Specific aspects of management are best described in terms of the six major complications of hepatic failure: altered mental status, hypoglycemia, respiratory failure, bleeding, renal failure, and infection.

Probably because of metabolic derangements, mental status decompensation is common and may be rapidly progressive. Hepatic encephalopathy is described in stages: stage I — subtle intellectual impairment, mild personality changes, no asterixis; stage II — drowsy, capability of simple behavior on command, asterixis, diffuse slowing on electroencephalogram; stage III — stupor, response to painful stimuli, profound confusion, inarticulate speech, electroencephalographic abnormalities; stage IV — no response to pain, coma. Cerebral edema may exacerbate these mental status changes and be resistant to conventional therapies such as osmotic diuretics. Management of hepatic coma begins with minimization of complicating factors, such as the presence of gastrointestinal bleeding, infection, hypoglycemia, acid-base disturbances (notably hypokalemic metabolic alkalosis), excessive protein intake, and sedative medications. Particular attention must be paid to the use of drugs that depend on hepatic clearance for inactivation, such as benzodiazepines and narcotics. A gastric tube is placed for evacuation of upper GI tract blood, and magnesium citrate and enemas are used to purge the GI tract. GI tract bacteria (a source of free nitrogen) are suppressed through the oral administration of neomycin. The disaccharide lactulose is administered orally or rectally. Its mechanism of action is uncertain but may relate to its property as an osmotic laxative. It also provides an alternate carbohydrate nutrient source to gut bacteria, decreasing their elaboration of free nitrogen and simultaneously acidifying the gut lumen, which reduces ammonia absorption. Some investigators have suggested the use of parenteral branched chain amino acids as therapy for encephalopathy, but this remains controversial.

Hypoglycemia, as a consequence of impaired gluconeogenesis and glycogen depletion, is readily treated with intravenous glucose administration. Hypertonic dextrose may be required and is titrated to maintenance of normal serum glucose levels. Typically this requires 20 to 25 calories per kilogram of body weight per day administered as 20% to 25% dextrose via central vein infusion.

An important result of impaired mental status is respiratory insufficiency and failure. In patients with stage III or IV encephalopathy, protective airway reflexes are depressed or absent. Endotracheal intubation for airway protection and institution of mechanical ventilation are often required. Respiratory sufficiency is further compromised by aspiration pneumonitis, pulmonary edema, pleural effusions, intrapulmonary and portopulmonary shunting, and tense ascites. The development of acute respiratory failure, also known as adult respiratory distress syndrome, may necessitate the application of high inspired oxygen content and positive end-expiratory pressure. A Swan-Ganz pulmonary artery catheter may help these patients maintain appropriate intravascular volume and hemodynamic stability.

Bleeding is a common consequence of hepatic failure and a major cause of death in these patients. The cause of bleeding may be multifactorial and includes diminished synthesis of vitamin K–dependent factors by the liver, platelet sequestration by the spleen, and disseminated intravascular coagulation. Upper GI bleeding from gastroesophageal varices, peptic ulceration, and erosive gastritis may also occur (see discussion on upper gastrointestinal tract bleeding for further information on diagnosis and treatment). Specific therapy includes transfusion of red blood cells (generally to maintain a hematocrit value greater than 30 ml/dl) and fresh-frozen plasma if bleeding is significant or an invasive procedure is being performed. Hypothermia, a reported consequence of liver failure, may be exacerbated by rapid transfusion of cool blood products and should be avoided. Stress ulcer prophylaxis is essential and is described in detail in the section with that heading.

Infection and sepsis are frequently terminal complications in patients with hepatic failure. Careful attention to asepsis during all invasive procedures is critical. The occurrence of fever or an elevated or severely depressed white blood cell count with a shift to immature forms should precipitate a thorough culture evaluation of all body secretions and fluids, including blood. Antimicrobial therapy is directed at identified pathogens and rarely requires alterations in dosage (although dosage should always be checked).

Renal failure may result from altered perfusion during hemorrhage or from aggressive diuresis. In addition, some patients have the hepatorenal syndrome characterized by oliguria progressing to anuria with exquisitely low urinary sodium levels. Therapy is supportive with prevention of episodic hypoperfusion and with hemodialysis when appropriate. The combination of hepatic and renal failure carries a poor prognosis.

Liver transplantation for treatment of acute hepatic failure remains controversial. In selected patients without multiple–organ system failure, this procedure may be lifesaving. Early consultation with regional or national hepatic transplantation specialists is essential for identification of appropriate transplant recipients.

Hepatic function is essential to life. Despite advances in care of these critically ill patients, the mortality rate remains high. For those who survive, however, complete recovery of hepatic function to baseline levels is the most common outcome.

SUGGESTED READINGS

General

Alverdy JC, Saunders J, Chamberlin WH, et al: Diagnostic peritoneal lavage in intra-abdominal sepsis. Am Surg 1988;54:456-459

Bouwman DL, Altshuler J, Weaver DW: Hyperamylasemia: a result of intracranial bleeding. Surgery 1983;94:318-323

Shaff MI, Tarr RW, Partain CL, et al: Computerized tomography and magnetic resonance imaging of the acute abdomen. Surg Clin North Am 1988;68:233-254

Cholecystitis

Devine RM, Farnell MB, Mucha P: Acute cholecystitis as a complication in surgical patients. Arch Surg 1984;119:1389-1393

Johnson LB: The importance of early diagnosis of acute acalculus cholecystitis. Surg Gynecol Obstet 1987;164:197-203

Klimberg S, Hawkins I, Vogel SB: Percutaneous cholecystostomy for acute cholecystitis in high-risk patients. Am J Surg 1987;153:125-129

Peterson SR, Sheldon GF: Acute acalculous cholecystitis: a complication of hyperalimentation. Am J Surg 1979;138:814-817

Savino JA, Scalea TM, Del Guercio LRM: Factors encouraging laparotomy in acalculous cholecystitis. Crit Care Med 1985;13:377-380

Zewan RK, Burrell MI, Cahow CE, et al: Diagnostic utility of cholescintigraphy and ultrasonography in acute cholecystitis. Am J Surg 1981;141:446-451

Pancreatitis

Aziz S, Bergdahl L, Baldwin JC, et al: Pancreatitis after cardiac and cardiopulmonary transplantation. Surgery 1985;97:653-661

Barnett JL, Wilson JAP: Alcoholic pancreatitis and parotitis: utility of lipase and urinary amylase clearance determinations. South Med J 1986;79:832-935

Clavien PA, Hauser H, Meyer P, et al: Value of contrast-enhanced computerized tomography in the early diagnosis and prognosis of acute pancreatitis. Am J Surg 1988;155:457-466

Freeny PC, Lewis GP, Traverson LW, et al: Infected pancreatic fluid collections: percutaneous catheter drainage. Radiology 1988;167:435-441

Haas GS, Warshaw AL, Daggett WM, et al: Acute pancreatitis after cardiopulmonary bypass. Am J Surg 1985;149:508-515

Mayer AD, McMahon MJ: The diagnostic and prognostic value of peritoneal lavage in patients with acute pancreatitis. Surg Gynecol Obstet 1985;160:507-512

Pemberton JH, Nagorney DM, Becker JM, et al: Controlled open lesser sac drainage for pancreatic abscess. Ann Surg 1986;203:600-604

Ranson JHC, Rifkind KM, Roses DF, et al: Prognostic signs and the role of operative management in acute pancreatitis. Surg Gynecol Obstet 1974;139:69-81

Stress Ulceration and Prophylaxis

Borrero E, Margolis I, Banks S, et al: Antacid versus sucralfate in preventing acute gastrointestinal bleeding: a randomized trial in 100 critically ill patients. Am J Surg 1984;148:809-812

Bumaschny E, Doglio G, Pusajo J, et al: Postoperative acute gastrointestinal tract hemorrhage and multiple-organ failure. Arch Surg 1988;123:722-726

Driks MR, Craven DE, Celli BR, et al: Nosocomial pneumonia in intubated patients given sucralfate as compared with antacids or histamine type 2 blockers: the role of gastric colonization. N Engl J Med 1987; 317:1376-1382

Noseworthy TW, Shustack A, Johnston RG, et al: A randomized clinical trial comparing ranitidine and antacids in critically ill patients. Crit Care Med 1987; 15:817-819

Pingleton SK, Hadzima K: Enteral alimentation and gastrointestinal bleeding in mechanically ventilated patients. Crit Care Med 1983;11:13-16

Tryba M, Zevounou F, Torok M, et al: Prevention of acute stress bleeding with sucralfate, antacids, or cimetidine. Am J Med 1985;79:55-61

van Essen H, van Blankenstein M, Wilson JHP, et al: Intragastric prostaglandin E$_2$ and the prevention of gastrointestinal hemorrhage in ICU patients. Crit Care Med 1985;13:957-960

Gastrointestinal Bleeding

Cello JP: Diagnosis and management of lower gastrointestinal tract hemorrhage. West J Med 1985;143:80-87

Cello JP, Crass RA, Grendell JH, et al: Management of the patient with hemorrhagic esophageal varices. JAMA 1986;256:1480-1484

Gostout CJ: Acute gastrointestinal bleeding – a common problem revisited. Mayo Clin Proc 1988;63:595-604

Greenburg AG, Saik RP, Bell RH, et al: Changing patterns of gastrointestinal bleeding. Arch Surg 1985; 120:341-344

Hussey KP: Vasopressin therapy for upper gastrointestinal hemorrhage: has its efficacy been proven? Arch Intern Med 1985;145:1263-1267

Isenberg JI, Selling JA, Hogan DL, et al: Impaired proximal duodenal mucosal bicarbonate secretion in patients with duodenal ulcer. N Engl J Med 1987; 316:374-379

Krejs GJ, Little KH, Westergaard H, et al: Laser photocoagulation for the treatment of acute peptic-ulcer bleeding. N Engl J Med 1987;316:1618-1621

Provenzale D, Sandler RS, Wood DR, et al: Development of a scoring system to predict mortality from upper gastrointestinal bleeding. Am J Med Sci 1987; 294:26-32

Jaundice and Hepatic Dysfunction

Bismuth H, Samuel D, Gugenheim J, et al: Emergency liver transplantation for fulminant hepatitis. Ann Intern Med 1987;107:337-341

Corall I, Williams R: Management of liver failure. Br J Anaesth 1986;58:234-245

Matzen P: Diagnosis in jaundice: a contemporary approach. Dig Dis 1986;4:220-230

O'Connor M: Mechanical biliary obstruction: a review of the multisystemic consequences of obstructive jaundice and their impact on perioperative morbidity and mortality. Am Surg 1985;51:245-251

Peleman RP, Gavaler JS, Van Thiel DH, et al: Orthotopic liver transplantation for acute and subacute hepatic failure in adults. Hepatology 1987;7:484-489

Van Hootegem P, Fevery J, Blanckaert N: Serum bilirubin in hepatobiliary disease: comparison with other liver function tests and changes in the postobstructive period. Hepatology 1985;5:112-117

16

ENDOCRINOLOGY IN CRITICAL CARE

SIDNEY DEVINS, MD, KENNETH HASPEL, MD, AND BART CHERNOW, MD

HYPOTHALAMIC-PITUITARY AXIS

Critical illness affects the secretion of hormones from the hypothalamic-pituitary axis. Altered hormone release occurs rapidly in response to the physiologic changes induced by the stress of surgery and acute illness. Clinically relevant modifications of hypothalamic-pituitary release include the excessive or diminished secretion of adrenocorticotropin (ACTH), antidiuretic hormone (ADH), and thyrotropin (TSH).

Normal Physiology

The hypothalamic-pituitary axis epitomizes the intricacy of endocrinology. Various releasing and inhibiting factors produced in the hypothalamus help to regulate the secretion of pituitary hormones, which in turn stimulate target organs. The hormones released into the circulation from target organs then exert negative feedback on the hypothalamic-pituitary axis until homeostasis is achieved. The hypothalamus produces six well-described hormones with predictable actions on the pituitary gland (Table 16–1).

The pituitary gland has anterior and posterior components. The anterior pituitary gland (adenohypophysis) contains cells that synthesize and secrete TSH, ACTH, growth hormone (GH), leutinizing hormone (LH), follicle-stimulating hormone (FSH), prolactin, beta-lipotropin, and endorphins. The posterior pituitary gland (neurohypophysis) secretes ADH and oxytocin.

The anterior pituitary gland receives input from the hypothalamus via a portal system of capillaries. The posterior pituitary gland receives neuronal input from the supraoptic and paraventricular nuclei in the hypothalamus. ADH and oxytocin originate in these hypothalamic nuclei as prohormones, are packaged into vesicles, and are then transported along neurons (where they mature) to the posterior pituitary gland for storage.

TABLE 16–1. Relationship of Hypothalamic and Pituitary Hormones and Target Organs

HYPOTHALAMIC HORMONE	ANTERIOR PITUITARY HORMONE	TARGET ORGAN RESPONSE
Thyrotropin-releasing hormone (TRH)	↑ Thyroid-stimulating hormone (TSH), ↑ prolactin	↑ Thyroid hormone secretion, ↑ lactation
Growth hormone–releasing factor (GRF)	↑ Growth hormone (GH)	↑ Anabolism, ↑ free fatty acids, ↑ glucose (from GH), ↑ growth
Growth hormone–inhibiting factor (somatostatin)	↓ GH and TSH	Opposite of GH actions
Corticotropin-releasing hormone (CRH)	↑ Adrenocorticotropic hormone (ACTH) and beta lipoprotein	↑ Cortisol, ↑ aldosterone, ↑ adrenal synthesis of sex hormones
Gonadotropin-releasing hormone (GRH)	↑ Follicle-stimulating hormone (FSH)	↑ Testosterone/estrogen, ↑ sexual development, ↑ ovulation
Prolactin-inhibiting factor (dopamine)	↓ Prolactin	↓ Lactation, ? immune suppression

↑ = stimulates, ↓ = inhibits.

TABLE 16–2.   Antidiuretic Hormone Stimulation, Secretion, and Effect

	STIMULUS	SENSORS	RESPONSE	EFFECT
Osmolar:	↑ serum osmolality to 295 mOsm/kg H_2O or 1%-2% above baseline	Osmoreceptors in hypothalamus	↑ ADH secretion	Maintain serum osmolality between 275-285 mOsm/kg
Volume:	↓ blood volume by 10% or more	Baroreceptors of left atrium, carotid sinus, and ? left ventricle	↑ ADH secretion	Vasoconstriction and water retention to achieve normal plasma volume and pressure
Neural:	↑ sympathetic tone (secondary to baroreceptor activation of sympathetic nervous system)	Adrenergic pathways to supraoptic and paraventricular nuclei of hypothalamus	↑ ADH secretion	Additive and synergistic effects on vasoconstriction with catecholamines, fluid retention

↑ = increase, ↓ = decrease, ADH = antidiuretic hormone.

The products of target organs eventually exert negative feedback on the hypothalamic-pituitary axis to limit further hormonal outflow from the anterior pituitary gland. The release of posterior pituitary hormones depends on osmotic, volumetric, hormonal, and neural stimuli (Table 16–2). All of these stimuli may be altered in a critically ill patient and can be tested with provocative and inhibitory maneuvers (Table 16–3).

TABLE 16–3.   Hypopituitarism

DEFICIENT HORMONE	PROVOCATIVE TEST	RESPONSE EXPECTED
Luteinizing hormone (LH) follicle-stimulating hormone (FSH)	Gonadotropin-releasing hormone 100 μg IV	Response varies widely; FSH ↑ to >8-12LH ↑ to >3
Growth hormone (GH)	Insulin-induced hypoglycemia	Normal: GH >5 ng/ml above baseline or to a total >10 ng/ml
	L-Dopa 500 mg PO after overnight fast	Normal as above; measure GH at time 0 and q1h × 3
	Arginine 0.5 g/kg IV infused over 30 min	Normal as above; measure GH at time 0 and q30 min for 2 h
Thyroid-stimulating hormone (TSH)	Thyroid-releasing hormone (TRH) stimulation (500 μg IV bolus after overnight fast)	Normal, peak values ↑ to at least 2 × baseline (measure at time 0, then at 30 and 60 min)
Adrenocorticotropic hormone	Insulin-induced hypoglycemia	Normal: cortisol ↑ of 10 μg/dl or to maximum of >20 μg/dl suggests intact hypothalamic-pituitary axis
	Metyrapone (11-beta-hyroxylase blocker) 500 mg PO q4h × 6 (measure 24-h urine before and after)	17-Ketogenic steroids or 17-hydroxysteroids in urine 2-4 × baseline for a 24-h sample; serum 11-deoxycortisol ↑ to >7.5 μg/dl
	Overnight metyrapone test (single PM oral dose of 2-3 g)	Serum 11-deoxycortisol ↑ to >7.5 μg/dl
	Corticotropin-releasing hormone stimulation test	
Prolactin	TRH stimulation test	Normal: serum prolactin level should double (in general)
	Chlorpromazine 25 mg IM after overnight fast	Normal: prolactin ↑ to 2 × baseline. Measure at time 0 and q30 min to 2 h
Antidiuretic hormone (diabetes insipidus [DI])	Water deprivation to serum osmolality >295 mOsm/kg (measure urine osmolality)	Normal: 800-1220 mOsm/kg Partial DI: 400 mOsm/kg Complete DI: 200 mOsm/kg Nephrogenic DI: <150 mOsm/kg
	Administration of vasopressin after water deprivation	Normal: no ↑ in urine osmolality DI: >50% ↑ in urine osmolality Nephrogenic DI: <50% ↑ in urine osmolality

↑ = increase.

Alterations in Hypothalamic-Pituitary Hormone Secretion

Antidiuretic Hormone

The release of ADH into the circulation may be impaired or increased in critically ill patients. Impaired ADH release (diabetes insipidus) is commonly encountered in the ICU. It results from a variety of disorders but occurs most frequently after craniotomy. Intensivists use vasopressin (DDAVP) therapeutically to treat not only central diabetes insipidus, but also the bleeding disorder of uremic platelet dysfunction.

ANTIDIURETIC HORMONE HYPERSECRETION

ADH secretion by the posterior pituitary gland is sensitive to changes in osmolality, volume, and sympathetic nervous system tone. Although ADH secretion is more sensitive to osmolar changes, volume depletion leads to a more vigorous ADH response. ADH secretion is stimulated by a blood pressure reduction sensed at the baroreceptors of the left atrium and carotid sinus. This type of stimulus, however, is observed only after at least a 10% reduction in plasma volume. ADH secretion may also be increased by enhanced sympathetic nervous system tone. Sympathetic pathways travel from the baroreceptors to the tractus solitarius of the midbrain to settle on the supraoptic and paraventricular nuclei in the hypothalamus.

In congestive heart failure (CHF), ADH secretion is thought to be stimulated by a decreased "effective" circulating plasma volume, which produces a drop in mean arterial pressure, thus enhancing the baroreceptor reflex. This explanation, however, is inadequate to explain ADH release in low-output cardiac failure. Experimental and clinical data have shown stroke volume (or pulse pressure) to be an important determinant of ADH secretion. The left ventricle may contain receptors that sense a drop in stroke volume and subsequently stimulate ADH release. This notion is supported by the results of a clinical trial of afterload-reducing agents in patients with class III CHF. In that trial vasodilators produced little change in mean arterial pressure (mean drop of 5 mm Hg), yet water excretion was increased, ADH release was diminished, and cardiac output rose concomitantly. Whatever the mechanism for release may be, the antidiuretic action of ADH is intact in patients with CHF. Fluid accumulation results from enhanced water reabsorption in the distal tubule and collecting ducts of the medullary nephrons. Interestingly, the vasoconstrictive property of ADH is lost in patients with CHF, perhaps owing to down-regulation of ADH receptors. This phenomenon is fortunate, since increased afterload, secondary to vasoconstriction, is poorly tolerated by patients with low-output CHF.

ADH secretion is augmented in cirrhosis and nephrosis. The cause of fluid retention in these patients is multifactorial (elevated renin-angiotensin, aldosterone, and ADH levels), but ADH certainly plays a major role.

SYNDROME OF INAPPROPRIATE ANTIDIURETIC HORMONE SECRETION

The syndrome of inappropriate ADH secretion (SIADH) produces hyponatremia, serum hypoosmolality, natriuresis, and excessive urinary concentration. In the ICU, pulmonary disease, central nervous system disease, and malignancies account for the majority of cases (Table 16–4).

Diagnosis. The diagnosis of SIADH should be suspected in euvolemic patients with hyponatremia. Edematous disorders (such as CHF), hypovolemia, hypothyroidism, adrenal insufficiency, renal failure, and factitious hyponatremia (secondary to increased levels of circulating proteins, triglycerides, or glucose) must be excluded from the diagnosis. The finding of a urine sodium concentration greater than 40 mEq/L and urine osmolality greater than 100 mOsm/kg despite a low serum sodium level and osmolality supports the diagnosis.

The natriuresis occurring in SIADH is thought to result from elevated circulating levels of atrial natriuretic factor (ANF) released from the atria in response to SIADH-induced mild hypervolemia. ANF inhibits proximal tubule sodium reabsorption, which partially corrects this augmented plasma volume. Despite the patient's inability to dilute urine maximally, the urine sodium concentration may fall to very low levels (1 mEq/L). This situation occurs in patients who are being fluid restricted before surgery or are being treated for SIADH. In these patients ANF levels are likely to be low and plasma aldosterone concentrations are increased. Therefore a reduction of natriuresis may occur.

Clinical Manifestations. In the ICU, signs and symptoms of SIADH are related to hyponatremia. The preponderance of findings is neurologic. Lethargy, apathy, disorientation, agitation, anorexia, and nausea are common findings. The physical examination may demonstrate

TABLE 16–4. Causes of SIADH

Pulmonary disorders

Pneumonia
Tuberculosis
Abscess
Aspergillosis
Cancer

Malignancies

Lung
Duodenum
Pancreas
Lymphoma
Bladder
Prostate
Thymus

Central Nervous System Disorders

Encephalitis
Meningitis
Thrombosis
Hemorrhage
Abscess
Hematoma
Trauma

Drugs

Nicotine
Chlorpropamide
Tolbutamide
Carbamazepine
Morphine
Barbiturates
Clofibrate
Acetaminophen
Indocin
Cyclophosphamide
Vincristine
Isoproterenol

abnormal sensorium, diminished reflexes, Cheyne-Stokes respirations, and occasionally seizure activity. The severity of symptoms relates not only to the degree of hyponatremia, but also to the rate of fall of the serum sodium concentration (rapid decreases in serum sodium more frequently lead to neurologic sequelae). Although no clear, predictable association exists between the degree of hyponatremia and the extent of neurologic changes, most patients in whom seizures or coma develops have serum sodium levels less than 120 mEq/L.

Treatment. The most effective therapy for SIADH is elimination of the causative disorder. Immediate therapy, aimed at increasing the serum sodium to an acceptable level, consists of water restriction and in emergencies the infusion of hypertonic saline solution. In the ICU, water restriction is usually sufficient for correcting hyponatremia.

Sodium and water balance can be manipulated pharmacologically. Phenytoin and narcotic antagonists inhibit ADH release, and lithium carbonate and demeclocycline (an antibiotic) impair the renal tubular response to ADH. In the ICU and after surgery the necessity for pain control usually eliminates narcotic antagonists as therapeutic agents. Likewise, use of lithium carbonate, because of its effects on neuromuscular blockade (enhanced block) and the heart (arrhythmias), is usually avoided.

Water restriction is the treatment of choice in patients with SIADH. Demeclocycline, combined with water restriction, is an effective form of therapy when water restriction alone fails to resolve the hyponatremia. Demeclocycline 900 to 1200 mg/d is usually effective in increasing the serum sodium concentration. Its use should be avoided in patients with cirrhosis because a reversible demeclocycline-induced renal toxic effect is common. Superinfection is the only other serious side effect of demeclocycline therapy.

ICU Setting. ADH hypersecretion is common in the ICU. The consequence, hyponatremia, may lead to serious neurologic sequelae. A search for the cause of hyponatremia begins with an assessment of the patient's volume status and serum osmolality. In the ICU the hyponatremia usually results from free water excess (intravenous fluids), diuretic use, CHF, renal insufficiency, cirrhosis, vomiting, diarrhea, or osmotic diuresis (mannitol, glucose). Adrenal insufficiency and hypothyroidism are also important etiologic considerations. In the absence of these conditions, SIADH should be considered. A careful inspection of the patient's medications, pulmonary status, and central nervous system condition often reveals the cause of SIADH.

The goal of the ICU physician treating patients with hyponatremia is to prevent (or abolish) neurologic sequelae. Correction of the serum sodium level to at least 125 mEq/L is sufficient in nearly all patients. The rate at which the sodium can be safely corrected, however, is frequently debated. In patients with hyponatremia and no neurologic sequelae, a slow increase in sodium level should be attempted through water restriction. If, however, neurologic complications mandate the use of hypertonic saline solution, a more rapid increase in the serum sodium concentration is justified. Although some authors have suggested an increased frequency of central pontine myelinolysis after a rapid correction of serum sodium, others have not substantiated this claim. In the first 48 hours of therapy the physician probably should avoid correcting the serum sodium to normal or hypernatremic levels and avoid increasing the serum sodium by an absolute value of 25 mEq/L above baseline. When these parameters were followed in one retrospective study, central pontine myelinolysis did not occur. Of additional concern to the ICU physician is the possibility of precipitating CHF with hypertonic saline infusion. We therefore recommend that if hypertonic saline solution is used, a very slow rate of infusion (0.01 ml/kg/min) be tried at first to provide safe yet effective therapy for symptomatic hyponatremia.

ANTIDIURETIC HORMONE HYPOSECRETION (DIABETES INSIPIDUS)

Diabetes insipidus (DI) may be central or nephrogenic. Central DI is characterized by failure of the neurohypophysis to synthesize or secrete ADH. It may result from a variety of central nervous system disorders (Table 16–5). Depending on the extent of damage, varying degrees of polyuria and hypernatremia ensue as the kidney loses its ability to conserve water.

Nephrogenic DI (Table 16–5) is a disease of renal tubular resistance to the action of ADH and is characteristically less severe than central DI. Mild to moderate polyuria and hypernatremia occur because the kidney retains some of its ability to concentrate urine.

Clinical Manifestations. Central DI may be permanent or temporary depending on the location and severity of the damage to the neurohypophysis. The onset of DI is frequently abrupt. When DI occurs in the ICU, polyuria (urine output between 200 and 800 ml/h) and hypernatremia are the early manifestations. ICU patients who are not alert do not have free access to water and must rely on meticulous repletion of body fluids and electrolytes.

A distinctive course is observed in patients with central DI: (1) an initial diuretic phase of variable duration (hours to 5 days); (2) an antidiuretic phase, perhaps a result of ADH release from injured axons (hours to days); and (3) a final period of diuresis that may be permanent or resolve in time. This triphasic course makes appropriate fluid resuscitation a challenge for the ICU physician, since vigorous fluid replacement in the second phase can lead to volume overload and occasionally even hyponatremia.

Expected laboratory findings in DI include hypernatremia, serum hyperosmolality, and a dilute urine. The urine specific gravity is often less than 1.005, the maximum concentration is often only 100 to 200 mOsm/kg H_2O, and the urine dipstick test is usually negative for glucose and protein.

Diagnosis. The acute onset of polyuria in the ICU suggests glucosuria, the excretion of resuscitation fluids, or DI. The single most important laboratory finding suggesting DI is hypernatremia. Acute polyuria with hypernatremia helps the ICU clinician to distinguish DI from the other causes of polyuria. If a condition known to cause DI is present, polyuria with hypotonic urine develops, and hypernatremia is found, the physician need go no further to establish the diagnosis of DI. If uncertainty exists, a water deprivation test (Table 16–3) can be done. The diagnosis is made when patients demonstrate an inability to concentrate their urine despite serum hyperosmolality (295 to 300 mOsm/kg H_2O). If they then respond to exogenous vasopressin, central DI is the diagnosis. If the urine remains dilute despite the administration of vasopressin, the diagnosis of nephrogenic DI is made (Table 16–5).

Treatment. The treatment goal for DI is to normalize the serum sodium concentration, decrease polyuria, and avoid water intoxication. The currently recommended agent for hormone replacement therapy is DDAVP. DDAVP 5 to 20 µg twice a day administered intranasally or to

TABLE 16–5. Causes of Diabetes Insipidus

Central Diabetes Insipidus

Idiopathic	75% of outpatients
Acquired	Head trauma
	CNS surgery (postcraniotomy, majority of ICU patients)
	CNS infections (encephalitis, meningitis)
	CNS neoplasia (craniopharyngioma)
	Metastatic neoplasm (lung, breast)
	Granulomatous disease (tuberculosis, sarcoid, histiocytosis)
	Vascular abnormalities (aneurysm, thrombosis, Sheehan's syndrome)

Nephrogenic Diabetes Insipidus

Congenital	Rare
Acquired	Renal disease: chronic renal insufficiency, polycystic kidney disease, medullary cystic disease, pyelonephritis, acute tubular necrosis, postobstructive
	Electrolyte disorders: hypercalcemia, hypokalemia
	Drugs: amphotericin B, demeclocycline, lithium carbonate, alcohol, methoxyflurane
	Hematologic disease: sickle cell disease, multiple myeloma
	Nutritional: hypoproteinemia, excessive water intake
	Amyloidosis
	Sjogren's syndrome

CNS = central nervous system.

the buccal mucosa is usually sufficient to reduce polyuria. Alternatively, DDAVP may be given in doses of 50 μg/d perorally, an important route in patients with nasogastric tubes. Aqueous vasopressin may be administered subcutaneously or by intramuscular injection (in doses of 2 to 4 units repeated when polyuria recurs). Although intranasal DDAVP application provides an 8- to 24-hour duration of action, activity with parenteral administration lasts only 1 to 2 hours. In an emergency with profound polyuria, the aqueous preparation is preferable, since its short half-life allows titration. Resistance to vasopressin is seen in nephrogenic DI and with long-term DDAVP therapy (antibodies to vasopressin develop only after long-term therapy). If nephrogenic DI is suspected, pharmacologic manipulation may be necessary.

Pharmacologic agents with antidiuretic properties are considered effective for treating partial central DI and nephrogenic DI only. These agents include thiazide diuretics (salt depletion leads to decreased urine volume), chlorpropamide (250 to 500 mg/d), carbamazepine (700 to 1000 mg/d in divided doses), clofibrate (1 to 2 g/d in divided doses), and indomethacin (effective only for lithium-induced and congenital nephrogenic DI). In the ICU these compounds are of limited value.

Treatment with DDAVP should be continued for 7 to 10 days. If polyuria develops after withdrawal of DDAVP, the disease is likely to be permanent. Patients with confirmed DI should have an evaluation of anterior pituitary function, since the anterior pituitary gland commonly stops secreting hormones in these patients.

Adrenocorticotropic Hormone

Hypersecretion of Cortisol

Inappropriate hypercortisolism may result from Cushing's disease (pituitary hypersecretion of ACTH), or Cushing's syndrome (ectopic production of ACTH, adrenal tumors, adrenal nodular hyperplasia, and exogenous steroid use).

Pituitary ACTH hypersecretion causes bilateral adrenal hyperplasia (overstimulation) and hypercortisolemia. Cushing's disease, accounting for nearly 70% of all adult cases of hypercortisolemia, is a disorder of young women (20 to 40 years of age) with an 8:1 female to male ratio. Pituitary adenomas are responsible for ACTH hypersecretion in 70% to 90% of the cases; of these, 90% are microadenomas.

Macroadenomas can develop, and if so, local compression of tissues surrounding the pituitary gland leads to bitemporal hemianopsia and headache. Controversy exists concerning the cause of Cushing's disease. Some think the disorder is caused by excessive stimulation of the pituitary gland by corticotropin-releasing factor (CRF), whereas others believe the pituitary adenomas develop spontaneously.

Clinical Manifestations. Hypercortisolemia causes several signs and symptoms (Table 16–6). The increased frequency of opportunistic infections, the propensity for development of rib fractures (osteopenia), the muscular weakness, and the cardiovascular consequences of Cushing's disease challenge the ICU physician.

Glucocorticoids impair body defenses against infection in a variety of ways. They inhibit lymphokine release, chemotaxis, macrophage function, T and B cell function, and antibody production. Fungal, viral, parasitic, and bacterial infections may ensue. Even *Pneumocystis carinii* pneumonia is seen in patients with hypercortisolism.

Glucocorticoid-induced hypercalciuria and decreased intestinal calcium absorption may lead to secondary hyperparathyroidism. The result is normalization of the serum calcium concentration at the expense of bone mass. Osteopenia develops, causing fractures. In the ICU, rib fractures are particularly problems because atelectasis, pain, and pneumonia follow.

Endotracheal intubation of patients with the characteristic fat redistribution (central obesity)

TABLE 16–6. Clinical Manifestations of Cushing's Syndrome

> 75% of Patients
Central obesity
Hypertension
Hirsutism
Gonadal dysfunction
Neuropsychiatric disorders
Osteopenia
Back pain
Glucose intolerance
35% to 50% of Patients
Superficial fungal infections
Striae
Proximal muscle weakness
Acne
Bruising
20% of Patients or Less
Headache and visual field cuts
Hyperpigmentation
Renal stones (calcium)
Polyuria
Frank diabetes

is challenging. The head and neck are difficult to position because of the buffalo hump and moon facies seen in these patients. Patients with Cushing's syndrome may be difficult to wean from mechanical ventilation. They often have neuropsychiatric disorders, pulmonary disease, weakened bellows, cardiovascular abnormalities (atherosclerosis, CHF, stroke), and nutritional instability (glucose intolerance, ketogenesis). The ICU physician must address each of these disease manifestations before attempting extubation.

Wound healing is impaired by vascular disease, abnormal connective tissue, impaired cellular function, and nutritional alterations. Dehiscence therefore is a common occurrence in these patients.

The laboratory findings in Cushing's disease are nonspecific. Mild hyperglycemia (without frank diabetes) and modestly elevated red blood cell count, leukocyte count, and hematocrit value are seen. Serum calcium, blood urea nitrogen (BUN), and creatinine levels are usually normal. The mineralocorticoid effects of excessive pituitary ACTH stimulation are usually minimal, so hypokalemia and metabolic alkalosis are uncommon in Cushing's disease. Cushing's syndrome, however, often includes hypokalemia and alkalosis, and some argue that these findings strongly suggest ectopic ACTH production, exogenous steroid administration, or adrenal carcinoma as the source of hypercortisolism. In addition, the abrupt onset of hypercortisolism, although occasionally observed in Cushing's disease, implies ectopic ACTH production. The source, usually lung cancer (oat cell and bronchial carcinoma), may be unidentified before the development of this paraneoplastic syndrome. Tumor resection leads to resolution of the hypercortisolism. In some patients hypercortisolism results not from ectopic ACTH secretion, but from ectopic CRF secretion.

Diagnosis. The diagnosis of Cushing's disease (or syndrome) is based on the demonstration of hypercortisolism. Increased cortisol production can be detected by an elevated morning cortisol level, loss of the normal diurnal variation of cortisol secretion, and elevated 24-hour urinary concentrations of free cortisol, 17-hydroxycorticosteroids, and 17-ketosteroids. Unfortunately, the diagnosis in ICU patients is extremely difficult because stress enhances the secretion of ACTH and cortisol in critically ill patients. (Normal values for morning cortisol in these patients exceed 20 μg/ml.)

A common algorithm for the diagnosis of hypercortisolemia is presented in Figure 16–1. The overnight dexamethasone suppression test can be used in "stable" (nonstressed) patients to aid in the diagnosis. "Normal" patients respond with a decrease in the morning cortisol level to less than 5 μg/dl. Failure to do so signifies hypercortisolism. In addition, basal measurements (usually three separate levels) of ACTH can help to identify the source of hypercortisolism: (1) Cushing's disease is associated with "normal" ACTH levels of 50 to 200 pg/ml (inappropriately high in the presence of elevated circulating cortisol levels); (2) adrenal tumors are associated with low levels of ACTH (less than 30 pg/ml); and (3) ectopic ACTH production is associated with very high ACTH levels (greater than 200 pg/ml) (Fig. 16–1).

None of these tests produces reliable results in the ICU, however, because high circulating nonsuppressible cortisol and ACTH levels develop in critically ill patients. Therefore testing these patients before the resolution of their critical illness is fruitless.

Treatment. The therapy for Cushing's disease is designed to eliminate the source of ACTH secretion. Although ectopic ACTH production is eliminated by resection of the secreting mass, and adrenal carcinoma and hyperplasia are managed with surgical or medical adrenalectomy, patients with pituitary adenomas undergo transsphenoidal resection. Selective, transsphenoidal microadenomectomy is extremely successful (80% overall remission rate) and relatively safe and promptly reverses hypercortisolism. Although permanent damage to the remaining pituitary gland is rare, transient secondary adrenal insufficiency commonly necessitates glucocorticoid support for 6 to 18 months after the procedure. In addition, DI, requiring temporary DDAVP therapy, develops in a few patients postoperatively.

Additional surgery or radiation therapy may then be considered. Glucocorticoids should be given preoperatively while infections, hypertension, and hyperglycemia are controlled. Response to surgery should be documented by demonstration of resolution of the hypercortisol state. Secondary adrenal insufficiency may develop, necessitating postoperative glucocorticoid replacement.

Alternative therapy for hypercortisolism includes irradiation of the pituitary adenoma and surgical or medical adrenalectomy. Because adrenal insufficiency and Nelson's syndrome

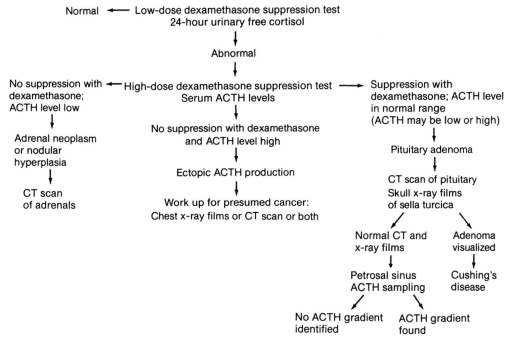

Figure 16–1. Diagnostic evaluation of hypercortisolemia for suspected Cushing's syndrome.

(diffuse hyperpigmentation with adrenal insufficiency) result from bilateral adrenalectomy, this technique, although effective, has been replaced by pituitary surgery and irradiation. Pituitary irradiation results in an 80% response rate in children but only 15% to 25% in adults. Radiation is useful in children who fail to improve with surgical resection and in those who cannot safely undergo resection.

Pharmacologic treatment for hypercortisolemia is used before surgery to control the hypercortisol state, in patients unable to undergo resection, and in patients with an unidentified source of ACTH secretion. Metyrapone, aminoglutethimide, mitotane, and ketoconazole all decrease adrenal cortisol production.

Hyposecretion of Adrenocorticotropic Hormone

ACTH regulation is under the direct influence of CRF from the hypothalamus, which is released in response to central nervous system stimulation. Cortisol released into the circulation provides negative feedback to inhibit further CRF and ACTH release. The normal, nonstressed adrenal gland secretes 25 to 30 mg of cortisol per day. Under stressful conditions the secretion of cortisol increases to 75 to 100 mg/d. The failure to increase cortisol release under those conditions may be the first indica-

tion of adrenal insufficiency. In patients being treated with glucocorticoid preparations, symptoms of secondary adrenal insufficiency develop under stressful conditions, not only from prolonged hypothalamic-pituitary suppression, but also from inadequate exogenous steroid replacement during the vulnerable period. Secondary adrenal insufficiency occurs in many ICU and postoperative patients.

SECONDARY ADRENAL INSUFFICIENCY

Secondary adrenal insufficiency results from either pharmacologic suppression of ACTH secretion or structural disruption of the hypothalamic-pituitary axis. Diseases that produce hypopituitarism, and thus adrenal insufficiency, include neoplasms, infarction, granulomatous disease (tuberculosis or sarcoidosis), infections, and surgery (hypophysectomy).

Adrenal insufficiency caused by exogenous glucocorticoid administration usually takes 1 to 4 weeks to develop depending on the agent used, the dosage, and the dose interval. Administered steroids suppress the nocturnal surge of ACTH that follows the decline in the evening cortisol level. This nightly ACTH release is responsible not only for the increased morning cortisol level, but also for the functional integrity of the adrenal cortex. Therefore agents that are given frequently, have a long half-life

(Table 16–7), or are administered in extremely high doses cause adrenal insufficiency quickly (5 to 7 days) by suppressing the nighttime ACTH surge. On the other hand, agents with a short half-life (Table 16–7) given once daily may not cause secondary adrenal insufficiency even after a prolonged course. In addition, the administration of steroids every other day appears to greatly reduce the incidence of adrenal suppression by allowing a late night ACTH surge on the nontreatment days. In general, steroid administration for more than 1 to 2 weeks should be tapered, since abrupt withdrawal may lead to acute adrenal insufficiency—the addisonian crisis.

Adrenal insufficiency or reduced adrenal reserve may be unmasked in critically ill patients at times when cortisol secretion should increase. The most vulnerable time for perioperative patients appears to be during anesthetic reversal and early recovery from surgery. In one study the plasma cortisol and ACTH responses to surgery and anesthesia in patients undergoing neck exploration were measured. All patients received identical anesthetic technique. Blood samples were collected every 10 minutes from start to completion of treatment. Neither plasma cortisol nor ACTH levels increased significantly during the surgical procedures; however, reversal of anesthesia and endotracheal extubation produced marked increases of both hormones. By the end of the first postoperative day all concentrations had returned to baseline.

Another study demonstrated significant increases of plasma cortisol in patients undergoing moderate (cholecystectomy) or severe (colectomy) surgical stress. The increases occurred 1 hour postoperatively, persisted for 24 hours in severe stress but not moderate stress, and returned to baseline levels in all patients by the fifth postoperative day. This information suggests that in the immediate period after surgical stress patients with suppressed adrenal function are the most vulnerable.

Other conditions that provoke hypersecretion of cortisol from the adrenal glands include infections, head injury, hemorrhage, and strenuous exercise. These conditions impair the normal inhibitory action of cortisol on ACTH release, causing maximal 24-hour cortisol output to be as high as 100 mg. The hypersecretion of cortisol may be an attempt to temper the body's physiologic response to stress. Whatever the mechanisms for increased cortisol secretion, cortisol levels increase in relation to degree of stress or severity of illness. Some have suggested that shifting from the production of other steroids, such as dehydroepiandrosterone (DHEAS), to cortisol may account for the increased cortisol secretion.

Clinical Manifestations. In contrast to primary adrenal insufficiency (Addison's disease), secondary adrenal insufficiency is not characterized by mineralocorticoid deficiency and its electrolyte abnormalities, since aldosterone secretion depends more on the renin-angiotensin system than on ACTH stimulation. The fluid and electrolyte imbalances (hyperkalemia, hyponatremia) and hyperpigmentation of primary adrenal insufficiency usually do not develop because ACTH and melanocyte-stimulating hormone (MSH) levels are suppressed in patients with secondary adrenal insufficiency. Additional clues differentiating primary from secondary adrenal insufficiency are the presence, in primary adrenal disease, of hyperpigmentation, electrolyte abnormalities, and eosinophilia (total cell count greater than 300/mm^3). It is instead the glucocorticoid deficiency that leads to the clinical manifestations of secondary adrenal insufficiency. These signs and symptoms (Table 16–8) may appear within 12 to 36 hours of steroid withdrawal or may be precipitated by stress, such as trauma, surgery, hemorrhage, or

TABLE 16–7. Properties of Commonly Prescribed Corticosteroids

AGENT	EQUIVALENT DOSE (mg)	MINERALOCORTICOID POTENCY*	GLUCOCORTICOID POTENCY†	DURATION OF ACTION (h)
Dexamethasone	0.75	0.00	25.0	72
Methylprednisolone	4.00	0.25	5.0	26
Prednisolone	5.00	0.80	4.0	24
Prednisone	5.00	1.00	4.0	24
Cortisol	20.00	1.00	1.0	8
Hydrocortisone	25.00	1.00	0.8	8
Cortisone	25.00	1.00	0.8	8

*The higher the number in this column, the more likely that the agent's use will cause metabolic alkalosis.
†The higher the number in this column, the more likely that the agent will suppress hypothalamic and pituitary adrenocorticotropic hormone.

infection. Postoperatively and in the ICU, gastrointestinal symptoms, cardiovascular complications, muscular weakness, and neuropsychiatric changes commonly develop.

The laboratory findings of secondary adrenal insufficiency include relatively normal electrolyte levels, normal aldosterone level, and

TABLE 16–8. Clinical Manifestations of Adrenal Insufficiency

Glucocorticoid Deficiency
Gastrointestinal

Anorexia
Nausea, vomiting
Abdominal pain
Diarrhea, constipation
Weight loss

Respiratory

Asthma

Skin

Hyperpigmentation (especially extensor surfaces, palmar creases, areolae, scars, mucous membranes, gingiva)

Cardiovascular

Impaired pressor response to catecholamines
Hypotension
Orthostatic hypotension

Muscular

Weakness, fatigue
Myalgias
Arthralgias

Renal

Impaired free water excretion

Neurologic

Personality change
Confusion
Psychosis
Increased sensations (hearing, taste, smell)
Apathy
Lethargy

Metabolic

Impaired gluconeogenesis (hypoglycemia)
Impaired lipogenesis
Hyponatremia

Miscellaneous

Lymphocytosis
Eosinophilia
Anemia
Fever

Mineralocorticoid Deficiency

Hypovolemia, hypotension, shock
Decreased cardiac output
Azotemia, hyponatremia
Hyperkalemia, acidosis, hyperchloremia
Salt craving
Impaired pressor responses to catecholamines

fasting hypoglycemia. The plasma cortisol and ACTH concentrations are low, and the cortisol response to the rapid ACTH stimulation test is suppressed because of adrenal gland atrophy. Interestingly, the degree of hypocortisolism may provide prognostic information. In one series of ICU patients, serum cortisol levels of less than 350 μmol/L were associated with a 100% mortality, whereas levels greater than 350 μmol/ L were associated with a 27% mortality rate. A study measuring cortisol levels and adrenal response to rapid ACTH stimulation testing found the highest mortality rate in patients with randomly measured cortisol levels greater than 60 μg/dl (regardless of their response to ACTH). The mortality rate was reduced in patients with lower random cortisol levels that increased to more than 18 μg/dl in response to ACTH stimulation. This study supports the concept that the degree of cortisol release reflects the severity of illness.

Diagnosis. Every ICU physician should include adrenal insufficiency in the differential diagnosis of shock unresponsive to the usual therapeutic interventions (volume expansion and vasopressors). The diagnosis hinges on the demonstration of reduced cortisol production. We believe that in a critically ill patient a morning serum cortisol level of less than 15 μg/dl suggests but does not confirm the diagnosis. A morning cortisol level greater than 15 μg/dl, however, virtually excludes the diagnosis of adrenal insufficiency in such a patient. In the preoperative evaluation the morning serum cortisol level is not an adequate test to exclude adrenal insufficiency because people vary in their circadian rhythms. A preoperative patient suspected of having adrenal insufficiency and a postoperative or critically ill patient with a morning cortisol level less than 15 μg/dl should undergo an ACTH stimulation test (250 μg cosyntropin intravenously). Measuring the basal plasma cortisol level just before injection, then again at 30 and 60 minutes after cosyntropin administration, establishes the functional integrity of the adrenal cortex. A normal response (an increase of at least 7 μg/dl above the baseline and an absolute value of at least 20 μg/dl after 30 or 60 minutes) excludes primary adrenal insufficiency. The rapid ACTH stimulation test is an excellent screening test, but an abnormal response does not differentiate primary from secondary adrenal insufficiency. Further testing may be warranted.

The plasma ACTH level, insulin hypoglycemia test, or long (3-day) ACTH infusion test all differentiate pituitary from adrenal failure. In primary adrenal insufficiency the plasma ACTH level is high (greater than 250 pg/ml) and the plasma cortisol response to a prolonged ACTH infusion is low (less than 20 μg/dl). In contrast, secondary adrenal insufficiency is characterized by a low circulating ACTH level (less than 50 pg/ml) and a normal response to the long ACTH infusion test (greater than 20 μg/dl) (Fig. 16–2). The availability of these tests and the relative hazards of performing the metyrapone test on critically ill patients makes the latter test inadvisable in the ICU.

Treatment. The mainstay of therapy for a critically ill patient with secondary adrenal insufficiency is glucocorticoid supplementation and intravenous fluid and glucose administration. Since aldosterone secretion is intact, mineralocorticoids need not be given. Therapy should be started immediately when adrenal insufficiency is suspected in a critically ill patient. If dexamethasone is used as the initial glucocorticoid replacement, reliable testing for adrenal insufficiency can be carried out, since no radioimmunoassay cross-reactivity exists between dexamethasone and serum cortisol determinations. If the diagnosis is established, or further testing is unlikely, hydrocortisone in intravenous doses of 50 to 100 mg every 8 hours or methylprednisolone in equivalent doses

(Table 16–7) may be used. After stabilization of the patient's condition, glucocorticoids are tapered to replacement levels. Hydrocortisone is given twice a day, 20 mg in the morning and 10 mg in the evening. Alternatively, prednisone may be administered orally, 5 mg in the morning and 2.5 mg in the evening.

RECOMMENDATIONS FOR PERIOPERATIVE STEROID COVERAGE.   Steroid coverage for the perioperative patient is indicated in the following conditions:

- Patients with known adrenal insufficiency
- Patients receiving long-term glucocorticoid therapy
- Patients with abnormal results of an ACTH stimulation test
- Patients who received steroid therapy for longer than 1 week in the previous 6 months
- Patients about to undergo hypophysectomy or adrenalectomy

Patients with vague medical histories should receive ACTH stimulation testing before elective procedures if adrenal insufficiency is suspected (Fig. 16–2). If adrenal insufficiency is confirmed, appropriate replacement therapy with hydrocortisone is instituted. When the diagnosis has not yet been established but

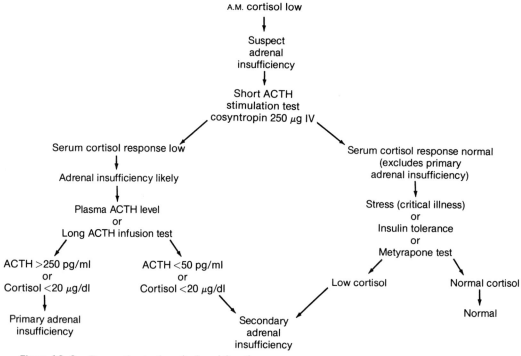

Figure 16–2. Provocative testing of adrenal function.

emergency surgical intervention necessitates steroid coverage, dexamethasone should be used so that postoperative adrenal testing can be accurately performed. Major surgical procedures require large coverage doses (such as 25 mg hydrocortisone hemisuccinate [or 0.75 mg dexamethasone] intravenously preoperatively and 100 mg [or 3 mg dexamethasone] intravenously intraoperatively), which should be tapered to replacement levels (for example, 50 mg hydrocortisone hemisuccinate intravenously every 8 hours for 24 hours, then 25 mg intravenously every 8 hours for the next 24 hours). Patients who undergo minor surgical procedures should receive moderate steroid coverage (such as 25 mg hydrocortisone preoperatively and 50 mg hydrocortisone hemisuccinate intraoperatively) and then be returned to their preoperative oral steroid preparation and dosage. Glucocorticoid coverage should be tailored to the patient's circumstances—amount of glucocorticoids received in the past, length of surgery, degree of stress, and so on—and our recommendations are meant as no more than a rough guide to safe perioperative steroid replacement.

Growth Hormone

Most of the physiologic actions of growth hormone (GH) are not produced by a direct GH target organ interaction but by mediators called GH-dependent growth factors. The most important mediator is insulin-like growth factor I (IGF-I), also known as somtatomedin C. Other, less influential growth factors include platelet-derived growth factor and insulin-like growth factor II (IGF-II), or somatomedin A.

GH deficiency causes linear growth abnormalities in children. Excessive secretion is observed in patients with pituitary adenomas (acromegaly). Acromegaly, an insidious disease, results from macroadenomas in 90% of cases and causes enlargement of the facial bones, extremities, hands, and feet, macroglossia, and hyperglycemia. Hypertension and cardiomegaly commonly develop and may lead to CHF in some patients. The diagnosis is established on the basis of persistently increased circulating GH levels and characteristic radiographic findings. Treatment, resulting in approximately 75% remission rates, involves either transsphenoidal surgery or pituitary irradiation. Since most patients undergo surgical resection, the ICU physician is confronted with potential intubation difficulties (secondary to facial bone overgrowth and macroglossia), the sequelae of

pituitary surgery (DI and secondary adrenal insufficiency), and the increased likelihood of cardiac disease.

Possible Clinical Uses for Human Growth Hormone

The therapeutic role of GH in the ICU is only now being considered. The availability of recombinant DNA–generated human GH has paved the way for research into new uses for this hormone. The protein-sparing action of GH has been demonstrated in healthy subjects receiving hypocaloric feedings, in patients with thermal injuries, during convalescence from major gastrointestinal surgery, and in malnourished postoperative patients. In the last group, daily subcutaneous injection of GH augments positive nitrogen balance after 1 to 2 days of administration. This anabolic action persists for several days after the injections are discontinued, and no long-term adverse reactions have been observed. GH therefore appears a safe and effective tool for maintaining positive nitrogen balance in critically ill patients. By limiting the quantity of hypertonic, hyperglycemic solution needed, its use may minimize the complications of parenteral nutrition. Its profound anabolic properties may prove useful in various catabolic conditions, such as thermal injury, sepsis, cancer, and other chronic disease states. Other potential clinical applications include the treatment of stress ulcers, the enhancement of immune function via the activation of cytotoxic lymphocytes, and the promotion of erythropoiesis and hemostasis. Studies have been proposed or undertaken to evaluate GH's action on wound healing and its role in the treatment of multiple–organ system failure.

Prolactin

The anterior pituitary hormone prolactin has a structure similar to that of GH. Its secretion is stimulated by central nervous system pathways, neurotransmitters (Table 16–9), hormonal agents, and physiologic stress. Its release, however, is controlled predominantly by the inhibitory effect of dopamine. Receptors for prolactin, which also bind GH, are present on lymphocytes and on cells in mammary tissue, kidney, liver, brain, prostate, testis, and ovaries. The physiologic actions of prolactin include growth, reproduction, lactation, and the development of glandular tissue. Prolactin may also play an important role in host defense by regulating the response of lymphocytes to antigenic

TABLE 16–9. Effects of Neurotransmitters on Anterior Pituitary Hormone Secretion

HORMONE	INCREASES HORMONE	DECREASES HORMONE
Adrenocorticotropic hormone	Serotonin Acetylcholine Beta adrenergic (norepinephrine)	Enkephalins
Luteinizing hormone and follicle-stimulating hormone	? Norepinephrine	Dopamine
Thyroid-stimulating hormone	Norepinephrine Serotonin	Dopamine Neurotensin
Growth hormone	Enkephalins Beta adrenergic agonist ? GABA Dopamine Serotonin Acetylcholine	Beta adrenergic antagonist Neurotensin
Prolactin	Serotonin Histamine GABA Enkephalins Vasoactive intestinal polypeptides	Dopamine Neurotensin

GABA = gamma-aminobutyric acid.

stimuli. This function is of particular interest to clinicians, since agents known to alter prolactin secretion (for example, dopamine and opiates) are used in the ICU.

Supporting the notion that prolactin helps modulate the host defense system are several animal studies identifying immunosuppression after decreases in the plasma prolactin concentration. In rats, hypophysectomy and bromocriptine therapy impair the immune response while lowering prolactin levels. The administration of prolactin or GH restores normal immune function. Furthermore, T cell dependent macrophage activation can be suppressed with bromocriptine-induced hypoprolactinemia and restored by daily intraperitoneal injections of prolactin. In mice, proliferation of T lymphocytes in response to various mitogens can also be inhibited by bromocriptine therapy. Prolactin does not alter macrophage function once activated by exposure to lymphokines, but its deficiency does appear to inhibit lymphokine secretion by lymphocytes exposed to antigen. In one study the secretion of the lymphokine gamma interferon decreased by 80% when lymphocytes exposed to antigens were first subjected to bromocriptine. The administration of prolactin restored the gamma interferon release to control levels. The clinical relevance of prolactin concentrations and immune deficiency states is being extensively investigated. Whether the experimental findings will have bearing on clinical medicine remains to be seen.

ADRENAL CORTEX

Normal Physiology

The cortex of the adrenal gland is responsible for the secretion of mineralocorticoids, glucocorticoids, and to a lesser degree sex hormones.

Aldosterone and cortisol synthesis and release are important in critical care. Understanding the biochemical pathways leading to synthesis of these hormones is necessary when discussing adrenal disease, pituitary failure, or provocative testing of adrenal function (Fig. 16–2).

Aldosterone secretion is influenced by three physiologic stimuli: the renin-angiotensin system, the serum ACTH concentration, and the serum potassium concentration. Renin is released by the juxtaglomerular apparatus of the macula densa in response to hypotension, hypovolemia, hyponatremia, certain prostaglandins, and sympathetic tone. Circulating inactive angiotensinogen is then converted by renin to angiotensin I. Angiotensin I travels through the lungs where it is transformed by angiotensin-converting enzyme (ACE) into the potent vasoactive peptide angiotensin II. Not only is angiotensin II a powerful endogenous vasopressor, it is the primary stimulus for aldosterone secretion.

Once secreted, aldosterone binds to specific receptors in the distal tubules of nephrons to promote potassium secretion and sodium reabsorption. Not surprisingly, serum sodium and potassium both alter aldosterone release. Sodium depletion leads to aldosterone synthesis and release through activation of the renin-angiotensin system, and sodium repletion inhibits this integrated response. Potassium, as might be expected, works in the opposite direction: hyperkalemia directly (not via the renin-angiotensin system) stimulates aldosterone synthesis and release, and hypokalemia inhibits it.

Glucocorticoid secretion is under the direct influence of ACTH. CRF released from the hypothalmus stimulates ACTH secretion from the pituitary gland. Via the feedback loop, glucocorticoids released from the adrenal cortex then act on the hypothalamus to inhibit further secretion of CRF. Glucocorticoids have a number of actions, apparently through binding to a specific nuclear receptor with resultant generation of messenger RNA and proteins. The clinical effects include metabolic, immune, cardiovascular, gastrointestinal, musculoskeletal, and renal system homeostasis. Glucocorticoid deficiency therefore alters nearly all organ systems (Table 16–8).

Primary Adrenal Insufficiency (Addison's Disease)

Adrenal insufficiency is simply adrenal hormonal secretion inadequate to meet physiologic requirements. Primary adrenal insufficiency, or Addison's disease, results from adrenal gland destruction or malfunction. Secondary adrenal insufficiency is a consequence of hypothalamic-pituitary disease. Primary adrenal insufficiency is idiopathic in at least 70% to 80% of cases in the United States. Of these patients, approximately 50% have antibodies against adrenal tissue (autoimmune disease). Nerup's classic article in 1974 characterized autoimmune adrenal insufficiency in a study of 106 patients with primary adrenal insufficiency. He found tuberculosis as a cause for adrenal insufficiency in only 17% of these patients, indicating an interesting epidemiologic shift from tuberculosis to autoimmune adrenalitis. Since that study further observations have been made: (1) tuberculosis is now the second leading cause of adrenal insufficiency in the United States but remains the most common cause in countries where the causative organism is endemic, and (2) autoantibodies against adrenal tissues are found in conjunction with antibodies indicating other autoimmune diseases, including antithyroid antibodies (the combination of Hashimoto's thyroiditis and Addison's disease is a fairly common occurrence and is termed Schmidt's syndrome) and antibodies against parietal cells (pernicious anemia), parathyroid gland, pancreatic B cells (diabetes), the intestinal tract (malabsorption), and the liver (chronic active hepatitis).

Other causes of Addison's disease include infiltrative processes, iatrogenesis (surgery and drugs), granulomatous diseases (coccidioidomycosis, histoplasmosis, sarcoidosis), acquired immunodeficiency syndrome (AIDS), and intrinsic functional disorders (congenital adrenal hypoplasia and hyperplasia). ICU clinicians, however, should be aware of three important causes: sepsis, hemorrhage, and trauma.

The Waterhouse-Friderichsen syndrome is adrenal hemorrhage caused when *Neisseria meningitidis* disrupts the coagulation system. Although this is the classic organism, overwhelming infection with *Staphylococcus, Haemophilus,* or *Pseudomonas* can lead to adrenal insufficiency via adrenal hemorrhage. In addition, cytomegalovirus infection and septicemia, as observed in patients with AIDS, can produce adrenal failure. Finally, metastasis from bronchogenic and breast tumors can cause primary adrenal insufficiency if at least 90% of both adrenal cortices is destroyed.

Clinical Manifestations. The prevalence of primary adrenal insufficiency in critically ill patients needs further investigation. Some authors have claimed a less than 1% incidence, whereas others report a much higher rate. Adrenal failure does occur in the ICU, is occasionally primary, and may be of prognostic importance. The ICU physician should consider adrenal insufficiency in all critically ill patients with the clinical manifestations described previously. Adrenal function should be tested in patients with refractory hypotension, electrolyte abnormalities, weakness, and gastrointestinal symptoms.

Because the hypothalamic-pituitary axis is intact in patients with Addison's disease, hypocortisolemia stimulates excessive secretion of ACTH. Since adrenocorticotropin is a potent pigmentary hormone, excessive secretion leads to hyperpigmentation of extensor surfaces and areas of trauma and scarring on the buccal mucosa, areolae, and skinfolds. This hyperpigmentation is characteristic of primary adrenal failure. Whereas secondary adrenal insufficiency produces predominantly glucocorticoid deficiency, primary disease results in both glucocorticoid and mineralocorticoid secretory loss. Loss of mineralocorticoid activity is manifest clinically as signs of salt and water depletion, orthostatic hypotension, poor skin turgor, dry mucous membranes, tachycardia, hyponatremia, hyperkalemia, and hyperchloremic metabolic acidosis.

The symptoms of adrenal insufficiency may evolve slowly but can also develop rapidly after the stress of surgery, trauma, or infection. Acute adrenal insufficiency, or addisonian crisis, may present a life-threatening emergency. Typically patients are in shock with profound volume depletion, vascular collapse, tachycardia, abdominal pain, nausea, vomiting, and diarrhea. Cerebral function deteriorates as perfusion pressure decreases, electrolyte abnormalities develop (hyponatremia), and hypoglycemia occurs. Cardiac arrhythmias ensue as a result of hyperkalemia, hypotension, and acidosis and may lead to death if these conditions, as well as the underlying adrenal insufficiency, are not corrected.

Laboratory Findings. Patients with primary adrenal insufficiency are often hyponatremic (sodium levels of 130 mEq/L or less) and hyperkalemic (potassium levels usually greater than 5 mEq/L). They may have a sodium to potassium ratio of less than 30, mild hyperchloremic metabolic acidosis (bicarbonate levels of 15 to 20 mEq/L), and mild lymphocytosis and eosinophilia. A low eosinophil count suggests primary adrenal insufficiency when found in conjunction with the other signs and symptoms of cortisol depletion.

Diagnosis. The diagnostic evaluation of adrenal insufficiency is described in a preceding section (Fig. 16–2).

Treatment. For chronic Addison's disease, glucocorticoid and mineralocorticoid replacement and treatment of the etiologic abnormality are the mainstays of therapy. Glucocorticoids are replaced to provide normal basal requirements with an additional 50% given prophylactically for mild stress and intercurrent illnesses. Since normal adults produce approximately 30 mg of cortisol and about 0.1 mg of aldosterone daily, replacement should exceed this concentration by about 50%. Glucocorticoids are given twice daily, and the synthetic mineralocorticoid fludrocortisone (Florinef) is administered once daily. Reasonable regimens for adult patients include hydrocortisone 20 to 30 mg in the morning and 10 to 15 mg in the afternoon, or prednisone 5 to 10 mg in the morning and 2.5 to 5 mg in the afternoon. Fludrocortisone is given in doses of 0.05 to 0.1 mg/d.

Acute adrenal insufficiency requires immediate therapy. Fluids containing glucose should be administered intravenously after initial blood samples are collected for blood counts and determination of electrolyte, glucose, calcium, and plasma cortisol and aldosterone concentrations. While intravenous fluids are being infused, glucocorticoids should be administered. If ACTH stimulation testing is planned, initial therapy may be dexamethasone replacement (4 mg intravenously is equivalent to 100 mg hydrocortisone). Because dexamethasone has minimal salt-retaining action (Table 16–7), hydrocortisone 50 to 100 mg intravenously every 8 hours should be administered after ACTH stimulation testing is complete. If ACTH testing is not deemed necessary, initial therapy should be hydrocortisone sodium succinate 100 to 250 mg as a bolus, followed by intravenous administration of 50 to 100 mg every 8 hours for the first 24 hours, 25 to 50 mg every 8 hours for the next 24 hours, and 25 mg every 8 hours for the third 24 hours. After that, long-term glucocorticoid replacement may begin if the patient is stable and not critically ill. Correction of fluid and electrolyte abnormalities proceeds concomitantly. If treatment is prompt, attention is given to these abnormalities, and the inciting event is treatable, the prognosis for recovery from Addisonian crisis is excellent.

Aldosterone Deficiency

Conditions that lead to isolated aldosterone deficiency are either acquired or congenital. Congenital enzyme defects may occur in the biosynthetic pathway of cortisol and aldosterone synthesis (21-hydroxylase, 11-ß-hydroxylase, and 3-β-ol-dehydrogenase) or in the specific biosynthetic pathway of aldosterone (18-hydroxylase). Both conditions are rare, but the congenital much more so. In addition, congenital insensitivity of the distal renal tubule to aldosterone, termed pseudohypoaldosteronism, rarely occurs. Hypoaldosteronism is much more likely to develop as a result of impaired renin secretion (hyporeninemic hypoaldosteronism), potassium depletion, or pharmacologic manipulation.

Hyporeninemic hypoaldosteronism accompanies aging, diabetes mellitus, and impaired renal function. It has been observed as well with multiple myeloma, interstitial nephritis, and impaired prostaglandin synthesis. In elderly and diabetic patients the probable cause is that longstanding small vessel disease and autonomic neuropathy reduce the ability of the juxtaglomerular apparatus to secrete renin in response to hemodynamic and sympathetic stimuli. In addition, a defect in the production of aldosterone (18-dehydrogenase inactivity) in response to angiotensin II infusion has been demonstrated in diabetic patients with hyporeninemic hypoaldosteronism.

ICU physicians should be aware that dopamine, when administered to sodium-depleted patients, blunts the release of aldosterone in response to angiotensin II. Also, heparin inhibits aldosterone synthesis and causes hyperkalemia in some patients. Prostaglandin inhibitors may interfere with normal renal hemodynamic regulation and thus aldosterone synthesis in patients dependent on prostanoids for adequate glomerular filtration. Furthermore, a prostaglandin feedback loop in the renin-angiotensin system alters aldosterone secretion. Although prostanoids change renal physiology in a number of ways, it is clear that prostacyclin and prostaglandin E_2 (PGE_2) stimulate renin release (and therefore angiotensin II and aldosterone) while exerting vasodilatory (prostacyclin) and diuretic (PGE_2) actions. Angiotensin II stimulates the generation of more prostaglandins, creating a fine balance of hemodynamic substances with opposing actions. It is therefore easy to create unopposed renin-angiotensin-aldosterone activity by inhibiting prostaglandin synthesis. In patients with marginal renal function who depend on prostaglandins for fluid and electrolyte homeostasis, the consequences of unopposed renin-angiotensin-aldosterone activity may be problematic.

Finally, aldosterone synthesis is impaired by ACE inhibitors, which interfere with the conversion of angiotensin I to angiotensin II.

Pharmacologic hypoaldosteronism results from suppression of renin release (beta blockers), inhibition of aldosterone synthesis (heparin, dopamine), ACE inhibition, and inhibition of renal tubular response to aldosterone's action (spironolactone). Since all of these drugs are used frequently in the ICU, the ICU physician should recognize their potential for producing hypoaldosteronism and therefore hyperkalemia.

Clinical Manifestations. Hyperkalemia is the most important clinical finding. Although mild hyperchloremic metabolic acidosis and postural hypotension occur frequently, hyponatremia may or may not be seen. Hyperkalemic distal renal tubular acidosis (RTA), or type IV RTA, develops in patients with aldosterone deficiency owing to impaired hydrogen ion excretion. The acidosis is normally mild, since these patients retain some of their renal acidifying ability.

Therefore bicarbonate replacement is often unnecessary.

In the ICU hyporeninemic hypoaldosteronism typically occurs in an elderly, diabetic patient with asymptomatic and unexplained hyperkalemia and metabolic acidosis. The diagnosis becomes more evident as the metabolic acidosis and hyperkalemia intensify after the use of a beta blocker, potassium-sparing diuretic, heparin, or dopamine.

Diagnosis. The diagnosis can be confirmed by demonstration of failure of the renin-angiotensin-aldosterone system to respond to volume depletion, confirmation of low plasma renin and aldosterone concentrations in patients known to be hypovolemic, or correction of the clinical abnormalities with mineralocorticoid replacement (fludrocortisone).

In the ICU the clinician needs only unexplained hyperkalemia to suspect hypoaldosteronism. If adrenal insufficiency is excluded, renal function is not severely impaired, drugs known to cause hyperkalemia have not been given, and exogenous potassium has not been administered, the diagnosis is likely. Inappropriately low plasma renin and angiotensin levels help to confirm the diagnosis.

Treatment. Most patients with isolated hypoaldosteronism require no specific therapy. Avoiding precipitating factors and correcting the underlying disorder are usually sufficient. Patients with diabetes or interstitial nephritis may regain appropriate renin and aldosterone secretion with control of their disease.

When long-term therapy is deemed necessary (as in persistent acidosis, hyperkalemia, and orthostasis), replacement with the mineralocorticoid fludrocortisone in doses from 0.1 to 0.3 mg/d is the preferred approach. This therapy corrects the metabolic derangements in most patients. When short-term therapy is required for hyperkalemia and acidosis, sodium bicarbonate is the initial treatment of choice. Diuresis with a thiazide diuretic can improve hyperkalemia and acidosis by promoting kaliuresis.

Hyperaldosteronism

Hyperaldosteronism may be either primary or secondary. Primary hyperaldosteronism is defined as secretion of aldosterone in excess of physiologic needs and in the absence of an identifiable stimulus. Secondary hyperaldosteronism (common in critical illness) is hypersecretion of aldosterone in response to a physiologic stimulus or pathologic condition.

Primary Hyperaldosteronism

The prevalence of primary hyperaldosteronism in the hypertensive population is between 0.1% and 2%. Primary hyperaldosteronism is caused by a unilateral adrenal adenoma in nearly 70% of cases. Adenomas are more common in women between the ages of 20 and 50 years, whereas bilateral hyperplasia is the most common form in children. The remaining 30% of cases represent bilateral adrenal hyperplasia, which is characterized by zona glomerulosa hyperplasia, hyperaldosteronism that does not coincide with the circadian secretion of ACTH, and an exaggerated response to angiotensin II infusion with markedly increased aldosterone secretion. Different mediators may account for some of the adrenal stimulation. Adrenal adenocarcinoma, a rare cause of hyperaldosteronism, usually secretes glucocorticoids or sex hormones or both in addition to aldosterone. The result is marked hypertension, hyperkalemia, and physical findings suggesting sex steroid excess. Although the pathologic diagnosis of malignancy is difficult, the finding of a very large tumor (greater than 3 cm) strongly suggests adenocarcinoma.

Clinical Manifestations.   Most patients are asymptomatic. Hypertension and hypokalemia are the cardinal features of hyperaldosteronism. Hypokalemia, caused by potassium loss in the urine via aldosterone's action on the distal tubule, leads to metabolic alkalosis. Also contributing to hydrogen ion loss in the urine is aldosterone's action in promoting hydrogen ion excretion coupled with sodium reabsorption. Symptoms, if present, are most often due to hypokalemia: weakness, cramps, polyuria, polydipsia (hypokalemia-induced nephrogenic DI), paresthesias, visual abnormalities, and arrhythmias. Tetany may occur, probably as a result of metabolic alkalosis, and Chvostek's and Trousseau's signs may be present. In addition, hypomagnesemia may contribute to the neuromuscular excitability.

Diagnosis.   Because primary hyperaldosteronism is one of the reversible causes of hypertension, the diagnosis must be considered in any patient with hypertension and spontaneous (not drug-induced) hypokalemia. The finding of normal potassium concentrations on three separate samples (drawn during normal sodium intake) excludes the diagnosis.

If persistent hypokalemia is present, measurements of plasma renin and aldosterone concentrations help to confirm the diagnosis. Before blood samples are obtained, however, adequate hydration and normokalemia must be established, since volume depletion can stimulate renin release and hypokalemia can moderately inhibit aldosterone secretion even in patients with primary aldosteronism. It is therefore necessary to discontinue diuretics, preferably for several weeks, and to ensure adequate sodium intake before the diagnosis can be made.

Measuring plasma renin activity (PRA) in the morning (after recumbency overnight) and after 3 hours in the upright position is a useful screening test. Patients with primary hyperaldosteronism demonstrate very low PRA in the morning and fail to increase PRA after assuming an upright position. In addition, PRA cannot be stimulated by furosemide-induced sodium depletion. Finding elevated or normal PRA makes primary hyperaldosteronism unlikely. An ICU patient who is well hydrated and recumbent usually exhibits low PRA, and further tests may be required to confirm the diagnosis of primary hyperaldosteronism.

Plasma aldosterone concentration or urinary aldosterone excretion should be measured in patients with low PRA. Increased urinary aldosterone excretion or plasma aldosterone concentration in a well-hydrated patient is a clue, but the diagnosis rests on the failure to suppress aldosterone (urinary or plasma) after salt loading. This test requires infusion of 2 L normal saline solution over 2 to 4 hours, which suppresses the renin-angiotensin-aldosterone system in healthy subjects, followed by plasma aldosterone determination. Finding an increased aldosterone concentration in combination with a low PRA that cannot be stimulated by the upright position or sodium depletion establishes the diagnosis of primary hyperaldosteronism.

In the ICU the diagnosis of primary hyperaldosteronism may be difficult to establish. Most ICU patients cannot tolerate fluid challenges or deprivation. The intensivist must therefore have a high index of suspicion and test for primary aldosteronism under the most reasonable conditions. Inappropriate kaliuresis, low morning PRA, and increased morning aldosterone concentration are sufficient evidence in most cases.

If primary hyperaldosteronism is confirmed, imaging of the adrenal glands with high-resolution computed tomography is the next diagnostic step. If computed tomography is nonconclusive, either magnetic resonance imaging (MRI) or adrenal scintigraphy may be helpful by demonstrating abnormal, asymmetric uptake. If the diagnosis is still obscure, selective adrenal vein sampling for aldosterone may indicate the source of excessive secretion.

Treatment. The recommended treatment for unilateral adenoma is adrenalectomy, so some patients with hyperaldosteronism enter the ICU postoperatively. Preoperatively, a reduction of blood pressure in response to spironolactone identifies patients likely to respond to surgery. Hypertension resolves in nearly 100% of patients during the 6 months after surgery, although long-term cure rates average about 70%. Before surgery, blood pressure and especially hypokalemia should be controlled for at least 1 week. This goal can be achieved with spironolactone, potassium-sparing diuretics (amiloride, triamterene), and potassium supplementation.

In patients with bilateral hyperplasia, surgical therapy, either bilateral or unilateral adrenalectomy, produces a cure rate of less than 20%. Medical therapy therefore is preferable for these patients. The mineralocorticoid antagonist spironolactone, in doses of 200 to 400 mg/d, rapidly corrects hypokalemia, although control of hypertension takes as long as 4 to 8 weeks in most patients. Other agents may be used to control blood pressure, and amiloride or triamterene may be substituted for spironolactone. In addition, dietary sodium restriction and potassium supplementation are often helpful or necessary. Nearly all patients respond to this therapy with normalization of the serum potassium level, but approximately half require additional medication for blood pressure control.

Secondary Hyperaldosteronism

An ICU physician encounters secondary hyperaldosteronism nearly every day. This condition may be appropriate (for example, when it is due to salt and volume depletion) or inappropriate (for example, when caused by renal artery stenosis or a renin-secreting tumor).

Secondary hyperaldosteronism has been clearly defined in patients with CHF, nephrotic syndrome, cirrhosis, pregnancy, and renal artery stenosis. In CHF the degree of hyperreninemia correlates with the severity of pump failure. Diminished cardiac output leads to reduced "effective" circulating blood volume (and perhaps renal perfusion pressure) and subsequent activation of the renin-angiotensin system. Angiotensin II then exerts its potent vasoconstric-

tive effects, thereby increasing afterload while it stimulates aldosterone secretion. Thus the logic behind using ACE inhibitors to treat congestive heart failure is to reduce afterload and therefore cardiac output.

In cirrhosis the importance of the renin-angiotensin-aldosterone system cannot be overlooked. Therapy with spironolactone ameliorates ascites in 80% to 90% of cirrhotic patients over a 3- to 4-week period, which suggests secondary hyperaldosteronism as a cause for volume retention in these patients. The uncertainty in these patients therefore is not whether aldosteronism is important, but why aldosterone secretion continues despite marked volume overload. Some have advocated an underfilling theory similar to the theory behind CHF-induced hyperaldosteronism. The finding of increased plasma volumes in patients with cirrhosis, however, is in direct conflict with this proposed mechanism and led to the overflow theory, which suggested a direct hepatorenal signal that leads to fluid retention when intrahepatic, or perhaps portal vein, pressure increases. Yet another theory is the peripheral arterial vasodilation theory, which suggests that diminished peripheral vascular resistance leads to overactivity of the renin-angiotensin-aldosterone system (as well as the sympathetic nervous system and ADH) via diminished renal perfusion pressure. According to this theory, hormonal secretion continues despite increased total plasma volume because the fluid and salt retention generated is insufficient to fill these enlarged vessels. In humans with cirrhosis, arteriovenous malformations have been described in the splanchnic bed, skin, and pulmonary circulation. Perhaps peripheral arterial resistance falls as a result of these malformations and fluid retention ensues. Although this situation has been demonstrated in experimental cirrhosis, additional human studies are required to confirm the vasodilation theory.

The cause of renal sodium and fluid retention in the nephrotic syndrome has been questioned as well. Patients with the nephrotic syndrome, like those with cirrhosis, tend to have normal or even increased plasma volume. There is little doubt that in some patients intravascular hypovolemia (secondary to reduced plasma oncotic pressure from hypoalbuminemia) leads to secondary hyperaldosteronism, which contributes to fluid retention. In one recent study, when nephrotic patients and control subjects were given sodium 300 mmol/d and an aldosterone antagonist (spironolactone

400 mg/d), sodium retention was reversed in the nephrotic patients but no effect was seen in the control subjects.

In renal artery stenosis the pathogenesis of secondary hyperaldosteronism is easy to understand. When stenosis occurs, perfusion pressure downstream is reduced, the vessel dilates distally, and the juxtaglomerular apparatus perceives a reduced effective circulating blood volume. Renin is therefore secreted and angiotensin II generated. Hypertension results from the vasoactive properties of angiotensin II, while salt and water retention develops from angiotensin II–induced aldosterone synthesis. The recognition of renal artery stenosis as a cause for hypertension is important because early intervention with angioplasty or surgery can reduce blood pressure and preserve renal function.

The therapy for secondary aldosteronism should be directed at the cause. CHF, cirrhosis, nephrotic syndrome, dehydration, and renal artery stenosis are all encountered in the ICU. If the underlying condition cannot be effectively reversed and aldosteronism produces unwanted clinical effects, spironolactone may be required. As in primary aldosteronism, other diuretics may be used, but circulating plasma volume should not be reduced because this is likely to stimulate further aldosterone synthesis. When volume depletion is desired (as in some postoperative patients) but hyperaldosteronism results, low-dose dopamine (0.5 to 2 μg/kg/min) may inhibit aldosterone synthesis and reverse the hypokalemia created by secondary aldosteronism.

ADRENAL MEDULLA

Normal Physiology

The primary responsibility of the adrenal medulla is epinephrine synthesis. Catecholamine release is enhanced by central nervous system stimulation through induction of tyrosine hydroxylase, the rate-limiting enzyme in catecholamine synthesis (Fig. 16–3). Dopamine acts as a neurotransmitter in the central nervous system. It is a ligand for dopaminergic receptors in the renal parenchyma and for beta and alpha receptors in the peripheral circulation. Both epinephrine and norepinephrine act as neurotransmitters, and both stimulate alpha- and beta-adrenergic receptors. Unlike epinephrine, norepinephrine is primarily synthesized, stored, and secreted by sympathetic nerve terminals.

Pheochromocytoma

Pheochromocytomas are rare tumors that secrete catecholamines (usually epinephrine), often in dangerously large quantities, producing paroxysms of arterial hypertension, tachycardia, and arrhythmia. Problems as a consequence of sudden tumor secretion may be encountered in the ICU, as a patient is being anesthetized for diagnostic radiologic procedures, during surgical resection of pheochromocytomas, or, more alarming, during anesthesia induction in a patient unsuspected of harboring a pheochromocytoma. A clear comprehension of the pathophysiology and treat-

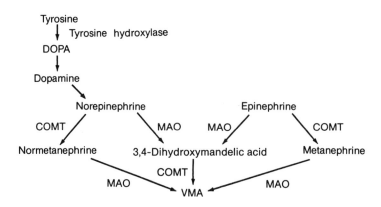

MAO = Monoamine oxidase
COMT = Catechol-o-methyl transferase
VMA = Vanillylmandelic acid

Figure 16–3.   Pathway of catecholamine release.

ment of pheochromocytomas will help the clinician avoid causing the complications of excessive catecholamine release.

Pheochromocytomas, arising from chromaffin cells of the primitive neural crest, are classified as tumors with amine precursor uptake and decarboxylation (APUD) properties. APUD tumors retain their ability to synthesize, store, and secrete various neurotransmitters (such as epinephrine, norepinephrine, dopamine, and serotonin) and peptides (such as corticotropin, endorphins, enkephalins, thyrotropin-releasing hormone, vasoactive intestinal polypeptide, calcitonin, and insulin) with physiologic activity. The majority of APUD tumors are found in the fourth through sixth decades of life. The incidence varies according to the population studied but is less than 0.1% of all hypertensive patients, for a prevalence of approximately 1 to 2:100,000 adults per year.

Pheochromocytomas most commonly occur in the adrenal glands but can also be located along the paravertebral sympathetic ganglia, usually in the abdomen. Less common locations are the neck (cervical sympathetic ganglia), thorax, and bladder wall. In adults 80% are unilateral, most commonly involving the right adrenal medulla; 10% are extraadrenal; and 10% are bilateral. In children with pheochromocytomas the frequency of bilateral tumors is 70%, with a higher prevalence of extraadrenal pheochromocytomas than in adults.

Malignancy is identified in only 10% of adult cases and an even smaller percentage of childhood cases. The differentiation between benign and malignant tumors rests on the demonstration of pheochromocytoma in sites where chromaffin cells are not usually found (lung, liver, lymph nodes, bone, muscle). There are no specific gross or microscopic pathologic features, nor are there biochemical markers that accurately define malignancy. The size and weight of the pheochromocytoma do not correlate with symptoms, and the symptoms bear no relation to malignancy.

Pheochromocytomas have been found with an increased prevalence in association with multiple endocrine neoplasia syndrome type II (MEN II). Pheochromocytomas may also be found with islet cell tumors, pituitary adenomas, carcinoid tumors, Cushing's syndrome, and aldosterone-secreting adrenal adenomas. Neurocutaneous syndromes associated with pheochromocytoma classically include von Recklinghausen's disease (neurofibromatosis) and von Hippel–Lindau disease (cerebellar hemangio-

blastoma with retinal angioma). In addition, pheochromocytomas occur more frequently in patients with ataxia-telangiectasia, tuberous sclerosis, and Sturge-Weber syndrome.

Clinical Manifestations. Most patients with pheochromocytoma are plagued by catecholamine-induced symptoms. Waves of catecholamine release produce paroxysmal symptoms in up to 50% of patients. Triggering stimuli for catecholamine release in these patients include certain movements or activity, anesthesia, drugs, surgery, and pregnancy. The most important manifestation of pheochromocytoma is hypertension, either sustained (50%) or intermittent (50%).

The majority of patients with pheochromocytoma suffer pounding severe headaches, palpitations (with or without tachycardia), and excessive, inappropriate perspiration. In fact, the triad of headache, tachycardia, and sweating in a hypertensive patient provides a 90% sensitivity and 94% specificity for the diagnosis of pheochromocytoma. Other, less common symptoms include anxiety, tumor, weakness, fatigue, postural hypotension, nausea, abdominal pain, and weight loss. Flushing is extremely rare and if present suggests a different diagnosis.

Electrocardiographic abnormalities (especially ST depression, T wave abnormalities, QT prolongation, left ventricular hypertrophy, and bundle branch block) are present in approximately 75% of patients. Supraventricular and ventricular tachyarrhythmias develop in some patients. Cardiomyopathy, either dilated or hypertrophic, is a classic finding and results not only from chronic hypertension, but also from increased catecholamine concentrations. The myofibrillar degeneration, small necrotic foci, and mononuclear cell infiltration characteristic of catecholamine-induced cardiomyopathy predispose patients to arrhythmias, pulmonary edema, and perhaps sudden death. Angina pectoris in patients with preexisting coronary disease can be accelerated during bouts of catecholamine release. Even vasospastic (Prinzmetal's) angina can be produced in patients with pheochromocytoma receiving beta blockade, apparently as a result of unopposed alpha-adrenergic receptor stimulation. Alpha-adrenergic action is also manifest as intense vasoconstriction (norepinephrine action), which leads to a contracted venous bed and eventually volume depletion. This pathophysiologic occurrence probably accounts for the occasional orthostatic hypotension and precipitous hypotension following vasodilator therapy or tumor removal. Even the adult respiratory distress syndrome (ARDS) has been associated with pheochromocytoma.

Metabolic derangements secondary to excessive circulating catecholamines are common. Frequently observed abnormalities are glucose intolerance secondary to enhanced glycogenolysis and inhibited insulin secretion (alpha-adrenergic suppression of islet cells) and lipolysis with increased concentrations of serum free fatty acids.

Important to the critical care physician is the pheochromocytoma crisis, which reflects uncontrolled, sustained catecholamine release. The resulting pressor effects lead to hypertensive encephalopathy with rapid progressive neurologic deterioration, cerebrovascular accidents, and coma. Severe arteriolar vasoconstriction produces progressive acidemia reflecting diffuse organ system hypoperfusion. If hypoperfusion continues, multiple–organ system failure develops with signs and symptoms resembling those of shock. Because of beta-adrenergic-stimulated tachycardia, beta-adrenergic changes in preload and afterload, and marked acidemia in these patients, left ventricular function and coronary artery patency play key roles in determining survival during an acute catecholamine crisis.

Diagnosis. The key to diagnosis is establishing evidence of increased catecholamine production. The critically ill patient poses a special diagnostic problem, since these patients have increased circulating catecholamine concentrations, are often receiving exogenous catecholamines, and commonly require antihypertensive and other medications that can alter the results of diagnostic studies (Table 16–10). Furthermore, the expected concentrations of urinary catecholamines and catecholamine metabolites have not been described for critically ill and postoperative patients who do not have pheochromocytoma. Nevertheless, diagnostic studies center on measurements of plasma epinephrine and norepinephrine and quantification of urinary catecholamine metabolites either overnight (when catecholamine production is at its lowest) or during a 24-hour period.

Catecholamine metabolism produces metanephrines (directly from epinephrine) and vanillylmandelic acid (VMA) (Fig. 16–3). Because VMA is produced by metabolism of both epinephrine and norepinephrine, measuring urinary excretion of VMA would logically seem to provide a highly sensitive test for pheochromocytoma. In fact, the 24-hour collection of total

TABLE 16–10. Factors That Alter Catecholamine Levels

FACTORS	EFFECTS
Stress, central nervous system disease, exertion, hypoglycemia	↑ Catecholamine concentration
Caffeine, theophylline, nicotine, vasodilators, clonidine and alcohol withdrawal, alpha and beta blockers	↑ Endogenous catecholamine excretion
Nose drops, cold formulas, bronchodilators, appetite suppressants	↑ Catecholamine concentration from exogenous administration
Alpha$_2$ agonists, calcium channel blockers, angiotensin-converting enzyme inhibitors, bromocriptine	↑ Catecholamine concentration
Aldomet, monoamine oxidase inhibitors	↓ Vanillylmandelic acid, ↓ metanephrines
Phenothiazines, tricyclic antidepressants, L-dopa	Variable changes in catecholamines and metabolites
Labetalol	Metabolite interference with all tests

↑ = increased, ↓ = decreased.

metanephrines (normal less than 1.3 mg/24 h) has proved more sensitive in clinical trials. Quantifying urinary free catecholamines (fractional catecholamine excretion) can also provide exceptional accuracy.

Most patients have increased catecholamine concentrations even during "stable" periods. Falsely increased concentrations can be found in 10% to 20% of "normal" patients, 25% of patients with essential hypertension, and patients receiving medications known to interfere with the diagnostic workup of pheochromocytoma (Table 16–10). High-pressure liquid chromatography can distinguish catecholamines from drugs that interfere with catecholamine measurement by other methods.

Because of extreme variability with changes in environmental stimuli and uncertain variability with sex, age, renal insufficiency, and other factors, single determinations of plasma catecholamines can be unreliable. Plasma catecholamine determinations therefore are usually reserved for patients with equivocal urinary catecholamine concentrations.

Once the diagnosis is made, the location of the tumor must be found. The most accurate, reliable, noninvasive technique for finding pheochromocytomas is computed tomography of the abdomen. Computed tomography detects more than 90% of tumors larger than 1 cm in diameter. MRI and monoiodobenzyl guanidine

(MIBG) scanning are also available. Arteriography (combined with computed tomography) to identify "feeding" vessels or inferior vena caval catheterization with selective venous sampling for catecholamines may aid in tumor localization.

Treatment. Treatment of a patient with pheochromocytoma begins with stabilization of the pressor actions of the endogenous catecholamines. Once the tumor is localized, surgical resection is the definitive therapy. If resection is impossible, medical inhibition of catecholamine synthesis, protection with adrenergic blockade, and radioactive tumor ablation (^{131}I-MIBG) may be attempted.

Alpha-adrenergic blockade with either phentolamine or phenoxybenzamine (beginning with 10 to 20 mg orally three or four times a day) is the initial therapy. Phenoxybenzamine has a long half-life, allowing twice-daily oral administration, and a noncompetitive mechanism of action (competitive agents can be overwhelmed by catecholamine surges). The disadvantage of these two drugs is their nonselective blockade of both postsynaptic (alpha$_1$) and presynaptic (alpha$_2$) receptors. Under normal conditions the binding of norepinephrine to the alpha$_2$ receptor leads to inhibition of further norepinephrine release (negative feedback loop). Blockade of alpha$_2$ receptors therefore leads to uninhibited catecholamine release, which occurs at the cardiac beta receptor. Tachycardia and increased contractile strength result. Prazosin, a selective alpha$_1$ blocker, allows alpha$_2$ binding and therefore feedback inhibition of norepinephrine release. Prazosin (2 to 5 mg orally twice a day) is an effective and safe agent. Alpha blockade reverses the blood volume contraction occurring in patients with pheochromocytoma. Severe hypertension during catecholamine crisis may be treated with nitroprusside, although nitroglycerin, phentolamine, prazosin, labetalol, and magnesium sulfate have also been used.

After alpha blockade is achieved, beta-adrenergic receptor blockade can be introduced to control tachycardia. Beta blockade should never be induced before alpha blockade, since it would suppress beta-mediated vasodilation while allowing alpha-mediated vasoconstriction to go unopposed, resulting in severe vasopressor activity. If a beta blocker is needed, esmolol is preferred because of its extremely short half-life. Calcium channel antagonists may prove useful.

Once pheochromocytoma has been adequately diagnosed and the patient has been protected from excessive catecholamine release, surgical excision is advisable. In the past, apparently because of decreased circulatory blood volume, patients had a precipitous drop in mean arterial pressure after resection of the tumor. The contracted venous pool resulted from prolonged alpha receptor–induced vasoconstriction. Preoperative alpha blockade with phenoxybenzamine (or other drugs) corrects the volume depletion and prevents the postoperative hypotensive events.

Drugs that increase adrenal catecholamine release (droperidol), potentiate tachycardia (atropine), cause histamine release, which increases catecholamine secretion (morphine, tubocurarine, atracurium), and sensitize the myocardium to catecholamines (halothane) should be avoided. The opioids fentanyl and alfentanil do not cause the release of histamine and therefore appear safe. Other anesthetic agents proved safe and effective (because they cause fewer cardiovascular disturbances) are etomidate, enflurane, and isoflurane. Vecuronium is the neuromuscular blocking agent of choice because it does not cause autonomic action, histamine release, or catecholamine secretion when administered to patients with pheochromocytomas.

Plasma catecholamine concentrations may abruptly increase when the tumor is manipulated during surgery. In this circumstance, and in preoperative acute catecholamine crisis, sodium nitroprusside is the agent of choice, although such agents as nitroglycerin, prazosin, labetalol, phentolamine, and magnesium sulfate have been used.

The three most important and frequently observed problems after tumor resection are increased sensitivity to opioids, hypoglycemia, and hypotension. The cause of opioid sensitivity is unknown, but severe respiratory depression has been observed with standard doses. Hypoglycemia appears to result from accelerated insulin production, which occurs because the alpha receptor inhibition of insulin release is abolished by surgery. Finally, although preoperative alpha blockade reduces the frequency of volume depletion and therefore postoperative hypotension, volume replacement exceeding measured losses is usually recommended until the vasculature regains responsiveness to catecholamines as alpha blockade wears off.

If a patient is deemed inoperable, medical treatment with alpha and beta blockade is often accompanied by alpha-methylparatyrosine inhibition of catecholamine synthesis (0.5 to 4 g/d). Radioactive MIBG has also been used with some success.

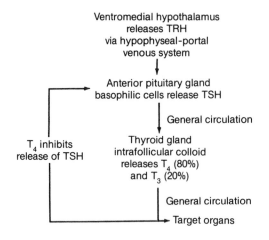

TRH = Thyrotropin-releasing hormone
TSH = Thyroid-stimulating hormone
         or thyrotropin

Figure 16—4. Negative feedback loop control of thyroid hormone.

THYROID GLAND

Normal Physiology

The thyroid gland, which normally weighs 15 to 25 g, is located in the neck overlying the trachea and below the cricoid cartilage. Its primary function is to regulate the metabolic activity of the body via the iodothyronines: 3,5,3'5'-tetraiodothyronine (thyroxine [T_4]) and 3,5,3'-triiodothyronine (T_3). These two hormones act at the cellular level to increase the speed of biochemical reactions, amount of oxygen consumption, and total energy (heat) production.

As with many other hormones, T_4 and T_3 production and release are normally regulated by a negative feedback loop (Fig. 16–4). Approximately 99% of the circulating T_4 and T_3

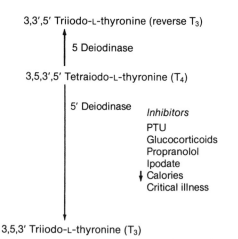

Figure 16—5. T_4 conversion to active and inactive forms.

molecules are protein bound. T_4 binds to either thyroxine-binding globulin (TBG) or thyroxine-binding prealbumin (TBPA). T_3 binds to TBG and albumin but not TBPA. This protein binding is important in determining the circulating half-life of T_3 and T_4. T_4 has a half-life of 7 days, whereas T_3 has a half-life of 24 to 30 hours.

T_3 is the more biologically active form of thyroid hormone. The majority (80%) of hormone released, however, is T_4, so it must be converted peripherally to its active form. This conversion takes place predominantly in the liver and kidneys to produce 75% of the body's supply of T_3. T_4 is converted not only to T_3, but also to a biologically inactive form called reverse T_3 (Fig. 16–5). The enzyme 5'-deiodinase, which forms T_3, is decreased in activity by starvation and critical illness.

Hyperthyroidism

Clinical Manifestations. Thyrotoxicosis occurs from increases in the secretion of iodothyronines. These hormones in turn lead to a hypermetabolic state characterized by a myriad of signs and symptoms (Table 16–11). Hyperthyroidism is four times more common in women than in men.

The most common cause of hyperthyroidism, in both the general population and the ICU, is Graves' disease (also known as diffuse toxic goiter, Parry's disease, and Basedow's disease).

Graves' disease classically involves a triad of manifestations: (1) hyperthyroidism with diffuse goiter, (2) ophthalmopathy (exophthalmos caused by an infiltrative process of the retrobulbar fat and retrobulbar edema, which can compress the optic nerve and lead to blindness), and (3) dermopathy (characterized by elevated and pruritic skin, most commonly over the tibia). It is thought to be an autoimmune disease; thyroid-stimulating antibodies are present in the majority of patients. Hyperthyroidism can occur without the presence of a goiter, especially in the elderly.

Hyperthyroidism develops in 0.2% of parturients, most commonly because of Graves' disease. This may be a difficult diagnosis to confirm, since estrogen increases the amount of TBG available, which in turn increases plasma thyroxine concentrations.

Hyperthyroidism has multiple causes (Table 16–11), including an entity called apathetic thyrotoxicosis, which occurs in the elderly. It is characterized by mental changes, atrial

TABLE 16–11. Hyperthyroidism

Signs

Goiter ⎫
Dermopathy ⎬ Classic triad of Grave's disease
Opthalmopathy ⎭
Tachycardia, tachydysrhythmias
Atrial fibrillation
Hyperkinesis
Hyperactive reflexes
Tremor
Lid lag, retraction
Thyroid bruit
Hot, moist skin
Thin, fine hair
Fatigue
Muscle weakness
Hoarseness
Impaired ability for renal concentration
Onycholysis
Congestive heart failure
Amenorrhea, oligomenorrhea
Gynecomastia
Myocardial ischemia with normal coronary arteries

Symptoms

Diaphoresis
Dyspnea
Emotional lability
Heat intolerance
Increased appetite
Nervousness
Palpitations
Weight loss
Insomnia

Causes

Graves' disease (toxic diffuse goiter, Basedow's disease, Perry's disease)
Toxic multinodular goiter
Toxic nodular goiter (Plummer's disease)
Toxic adenoma
Subacute and silent thyroiditis
Jod-Basedow disease
Pituitary tumor producing thyroid-stimulating hormone
Choriocarcinoma
Stroma ovarii
Hepatocellular carcinoma
Thyroid carcinoma
Exogenous
Pituitary resistance to thyroid hormone
Radiation-induced destruction

Treatment
Thyroid Gland

Propylthiouracil 100-400 mg q6h PO only
Methimazole 10-40 mg q6h PO or rectally
Iodide: potassium iodide 2-5 drops q8h PO, Lugol's solution 10 drops q8h PO, sodium iodide 1 g q8h IV
Lithium 300 mg q8h PO
Radioactive iodine (^{131}I) usually 70-160 μCi/g thyroid
Thyroidectomy (preserve 4-6 g of functional tissue)

Peripheral Conversion T_4 to T_3

Propylthiouracil 100-400 mg q6h PO
Glucocorticoids: dexamethasone 8-12 mg QD
Propranolol 40-60 mg q6h
Ipodate 1 g QD

Side Effects on Target Organs

Propranolol 40-60 mg q6h
Reserpine 1.0-2.5 mg QD
Guanethidine 50-150 mg QD

PO = orally.

---

fibrillation and other tachydysrhythmias, CHF, weight loss, and weakness. Thyroid adenomas, which secrete excessive amounts of thyroid hormones, cause atrophy of the normal gland by inhibiting TSH release. They are rarely malignant. Radiation-induced thyroiditis usually occurs 1 to 2 weeks after therapy for either tumor or Grave's disease. Subacute thyroiditis is usually painful and may be accompanied by a fever and flulike symptoms.

Hyperthyroidism has many atypical presentations. Atrial fibrillation may be its only sign. The likelihood of this symptom occurring in a person with hyperthyroidism increases with age and in men. Hyperthermia, caused by uncoupled oxidative phosphorylation, may also be the only sign. Angina and myocardial ischemia from coronary artery spasm with or without coronary artery disease are other possible signs of thyrotoxicosis.

Critical illness can either mask hyperthyroidism or initiate it, so the intensivist must be vigilant. The response of serum TSH to TRH administration may be reduced in semi-starvation, resembling a hypothyroid state. In addition, hyperthyroxinemia may occur without associated hyperthyroidism. Therefore the diagnosis requires not only clinical suspicion, but also correct assessment of thyroid function tests.

Diagnosis. In approximately 90% of cases of hyperthyroidism an increased serum T_4 concentration is found. Alterations in plasmaconcentrations of TBG may increase the total T_4 concentration in the absence of thyroid dysfunction. Measuring the *free* T_4 concentration differentiates hyperthyroidism from a protein binding problem. If the free T_4 level is not increased, the serum T_3 and free T_3 levels should be determined. If doubt still remains, a TRH stimulation test is indicated. A normal TSH excludes a diagnosis of hyperthyroidism, whereas an unmeasurable serum TSH concentration strongly suggests true hyperthyroidism, especially in elderly men and patients with either severe nonthyroidal disease or multinodular goiter. Patients treated with dopamine, which inhibits TSH release from the pituitary gland, may have a low but usually measurable TSH value. If the TSH is unmeasurable, hyperthyroidism or hypopituitarism is present.

Other laboratory findings associated with hyperthyroidism, although nonspecific, include abnormal results of liver function tests, mild anemia, granulocytosis, impaired glucosetolerance, and hypercalcemia (which occurs in 25% of patients).

Treatment. Treatment for hyperthyroidism is aimed at the gland itself, the peripheral conversion of T_4 to T_3, and side effects of thyroid hormone on target organs (Table 16–11). Drug therapy, aimed at attaining a euthyroid state, produces a remission in 10% to 50% of patients; therefore close observation of thyroid function is a necessity.

Two drugs, propylthiouracil (PTU) and methimazole (tapazole), are thiourea derivatives and block oxidation and iodination, as well as coupling of iodothyronines (Table 16–12) in the formation of thyroid hormone. PTU has the added advantage of blocking peripheral conversion of T_4 to T_3. These drugs are available in oral preparations, and methimazole can also be administered rectally. Side effects of PTU and methimazole include allergic reactions (usually skin rash) in 3% and 7% of patients, respectively, and agranulocytosis in 0.44% and 0.12%. PTU may also cause a vitamin K–responsive prothrombin deficiency. Intraoperative bleeding caused by thrombocytopenia and prolonged prothrombin time has been reported in surgical patients treated with PTU.

Inorganic iodides can inhibit synthesis, proteolysis, and release of thyroid hormone, with their effects lasting approximately 1 to 2 weeks. Lithium does the same but without any escape after 1 to 2 weeks. Either drug is administered 1 to 2 hours after PTU or methimazole to decrease the thyroid gland's ability to store iodide for later use. Inorganic iodide is also effective in decreasing the hypervascularity and hyperplasia associated with hyperthyroidism.

Propranolol interferes with T_4 and T_3 deiodination. Thus it and potassium iodide have been used preoperatively in patients with hyperthyroidism.

Reserpine and guanethidine are used to block peripheral effects of thyroid hormone when beta blockade is contraindicated.

Digoxin is advocated for use in patients with tachydysrhythmias until the hyperthyroidism is under control. CHF is usually refractory to digoxin treatment.

Treatment with radioactive iodine (^{123}I or ^{131}I) has the advantage of not causing the adverse sequelae associated with surgery, but it is probably contraindicated in children, adolescents, and pregnant women. The risk of subsequent hypothyroidism is greater than that after thyroidectomy, but as long as the patient receives follow-up observation, radiation-induced hypothyroidism can be easily identified and treated.

Subtotal thyroidectomy is used when radioactive iodine is contraindicated and other therapeutic modalities have failed. Acute airway obstruction may occur postoperatively because of hypoglycemia, laryngeal nerve damage, or tracheomalacia.

Thyroid Storm

Thyroid storm is rare but may occur in patients with undiagnosed or incompletely treated hyperthyroidism. The diagnosis of thyroid storm is made when thyrotoxicosis is associated with fever, tachycardia out of proportion to the fever, and central nervous system abnormalities. This problem may progress to stupor, coma, cardiovascular collapse, and death if not treated aggressively. It may mimic malignant hyperthermia and can appear intraoperatively but most often occurs abruptly within 6 to 18 hours of surgery.

An underlying cause for thyroid storm should be sought in a patient with hyperthyroidism. Infection is the most common cause unless thyroid storm occurs immediately

TABLE 16–12. Steps Leading to Production and Release of T_4 and T_3

STEP	STIMULATES	INHIBITS
Active transport of iodide	TSH	Thiocyanate, perchlorate, glucocorticoids
Oxidation and iodination of thyroglobulin (i.e., formation of MIT and DIT within the gland from iodide and tyrosine)	TSH	Propylthiouracil, methimazole, iodide
Coupling of MIT and DIT to form iodothyronines	TSH	Propylthiouracil, methimazole, iodide
Hydrolysis and release	TSH	Iodide, lithium, glucocorticoids

TSH = thyroid-stimulating hormone, MIT = monoiodotyrosine, DIT = diiodotyrosine.

postoperatively, in which case the surgery is the likely precipitant.

The treatment regimen resembles that for routine hyperthyroidism with some modifications. Adequate hydration with fluids containing glucose is necessary. Extreme fever should be treated with antipyretics, especially acetaminophen, because aspirin can increase free thyroid hormone levels. Cooling blankets may also be indicated. If oral medication can be tolerated, PTU 800 to 1200 mg followed by 200 to 300 mg every 6 hours is preferable to methimazole 80 to 100 mg followed by 30 mg every 8 hours. If not, the methimazole can be administered rectally, since neither drug is given intravenously.

Iodides should be administered 1 hour after PTU or methimazole is given (Table 16–11). Dexamethasone 2 mg every 6 hours, propranolol titrated to keep the heart rate less than 100 beats/min, and even reserpine or guanethidine may be used.

Hypothyroidism

Clinical Manifestations. Insufficient secretion of thyroid hormone, or hypothyroidism, is commonly encountered in the ICU. Hypothyroidism should not be underestimated: it can progress to coma and even death. Compounding the difficulty of its diagnosis are the nonspecific signs and symptoms (Table 16–13) and the insidious onset and progression of its clinical presentation. In a patient who has borderline thyroid function, hypothyroidism may be quickly exacerbated by a number of insults, including anesthesia, medications (sedatives, narcotics, lithium, iodides, and amiodarone), bleeding, infection, and trauma.

The common causes of hypothyroidism (Table 16–13) involve direct interference with the thyroid gland (primary hypothyroidism). The most likely causes of primary hypothyroidism are surgery and radiation therapy for hyperthyroidism. Hashimoto's thyroiditis, an autoimmune disease, leads to atrophy and scarring of the thyroid gland, which in turn leads to hypothyroidism.

Among the clinical manifestations of concern to critical care physicians are cardiovascular derangements. Cardiac output is depressed because of decreased heart rate and diminished contractility. This problem can lead to CHF, especially in patients with preexisting cardiac dysfunction. Patients do not respond well to digoxin, but if it is used, doses should be small because decreased metabolism and excretion

TABLE 16–13.   Hypothyroidism

Signs

Dry, coarse skin and hair
Alopecia
Cardiomegaly
Pericardial effusion
Hypotension
Decreased renal blood flow and glomerular filtration rate
Hypothermia
Hypoventilation
Pleural effusion
Edema of vocal cords
Enlarged tongue
Periorbital edema
Peripheral edema
Ascites
Ileus and obstruction
Dementia
Stupor
Coma
Seizures
Achlorhydria
Vitamin B_{12} deficiency
Peripheral neuropathy
Deafness

Symptoms

Dry skin
Cold intolerance
Hoarseness
Weakness
Lethargy
Weight gain
Constipation
Paresthesias
Urinary retention
Hypercholesterolemia
Hypertrigliceridemia
Sleep apnea
Hyponatremia

Causes

Primary hypothyroidism (95%)
　Autoimmune
　Postthyroidectomy
　External radiation therapy
　Radioiodine
　Medications (e.g., propylthiouracil, methimazole,
　　iodides, amiodarone, thiocyanate toxicity)
　Iodine deficiency
　Sarcoidosis
　Amyloidosis
　Tumor invasion
　Hereditary defects
Secondary hypothyroidism (<5%)
　Pituitary disorders
Tertiary hypothyroidism (<1%)
　Hypothalamic disorders
Peripheral insensitivity (<1%)

may lead to toxic effects. Pericardial effusions, in which cholesterol crystals are occasionally found, sometimes occur, but hemodynamic compromise is rare. Hypertension secondary to increased systemic vascular resistance may be encountered, and the heart may be enlarged.

Electrocardiographic changes are often nonspecific but include bradycardia, poor R wave progression, and prolonged QT interval.

Thyroid hormone replacement therapy precipitates angina pectoris in some patients. There can be diagnostic confusion, since both creatine kinase (CK) and CK-MB levels can be increased without myocardial damage in patients with hypothyroidism. Hypothyroidism has also been implicated in exacerbating atherosclerosis that may be secondary to lipid disorders.

One area of controversy is whether to treat hypothyroidism before coronary artery bypass surgery. Most experts agree that replacement therapy is indicated before elective surgical procedures on patients without cardiac dysfunction. However, since thyroid treatment may initiate angina, such therapy may be inadvisable in patients with preexisting coronary artery disease. Several investigators have found that hypothyroid patients undergoing coronary bypass surgery did well, but another group of patients has had increased perioperative complications.

An endocrine dysfunction that may exist with hypothyroidism is adrenal insufficiency. If a patient has long-standing hypothyroidism, concomitant pituitary hyperplasia may lead to ACTH deficiency. Therefore adrenocortical function should be determined if Addison's disease is suspected in a critically ill patient with documented hypothyroidism (Fig. 16–2).

A primary concern when mechanical ventilation is administered to a patient with hypothyroidism is the decreased central response to hypoxia and hypercapnia in such a patient. Compounding the respiratory difficulties may be the presence of pleural effusions or abdominal ascites, which can accompany hypothyroidism. Intubation may be difficult because of an enlarged tongue and laryngeal edema.

Another associated problem is hyponatremia caused by reduced free water excretion. Decreased bowel motility may lead to ileus or obstruction. Other abnormalities include peripheral neuropathies, deafness, hypercholesterolemia, hypertriglyceridemia, and achlorhydria, which can lead to anemia from decreased vitamin B_{12} absorption.

Amiodarone may cause hypothyroidism, probably because of its large iodine content. Long-term sodium nitroprusside infusions can also cause hypothyroidism.

Diagnosis.   Elevation of serum TSH levels is the most sensitive test for primary hypothyroidism. In secondary hypothyroidism the defect is in either the hypothalamus or the pituitary gland, and TSH levels are low. If hypothyroidism is suspected and TSH levels are equivocal, a TRH stimulation test should be performed. TRH 250 to 500 μg should be given intravenously, with serum TSH and prolactin levels measured before injection and then at 15, 30, 60, and 120 minutes after injection. Prolactin is measured to ensure that the pituitary gland responds to stimulation. These doses of TRH can cause transient increases in blood pressure. In healthy subjects the serum TSH level increases to between 5 and 25 mIU/ml during the initial 15 to 30 minutes and then returns to normal by 120 minutes. If the patient has primary hypothyroidism, the TSH level exceeds 25 mIU/ml. If TSH and prolactin concentrations are low, the deficit lies in the pituitary gland. Finally, if TSH secretion is delayed, a hypothalamic disorder is implicated. In primary hypothyroidism a serum TSH determination is usually sufficient to establish the diagnosis. A level of 5 mIU/ml or greater indicates primary hypothyroidism.

Patients with hyperthyroidism have no serum TSH response to TRH testing. This lack of response, however, is nondiagnostic, since administration of dopamine and steroids (both of which inhibit TSH release from the pituitary), catabolism, old age, and critical illness in a patient with borderline hypothyroidism may cause this pattern.

Treatment.   Thyroid hormone replacement is available as synthetic compounds of T_4 or T_3, a combination of the two, or extracts from animal thyroid. Today most patients receive synthetic compounds, most commonly T_4 (levothyroxine [Levothroid, Synthroid]), T_3 (liothyronine [Cytomel]), or a combination (liotrix [Euthroid, Thyrolar]). The therapeutic equivalents for these compounds are levothyroxine 100 μg, liothyronine 25 μg, liotrix 1 unit, and thyroid extract 1 grain.

T_4 is the more commonly used agent because this allows the body to control its own T_3 requirements. However, T_3 replacement has been advocated in critically ill patients to ensure adequate thyroid hormone levels, especially when peripheral conversion of T_4 to T_3 might be impaired.

Care must be taken in treating patients with coronary artery disease, since therapy may precipitate myocardial ischemia. Therefore replacement therapy should start slowly with daily doses of 25 μg of levothyroxine. The dose can be increased every 3 to 4 days (up to a final dose of 100 to 200 μg/d) in patients who do not exhibit electrocardiographic changes or complain of angina.

If coronary artery disease is not a concern, a starting dose of levothyroxine 100 μg/d is acceptable treatment. Dosage can be adjusted until a euthyroid state (based on serum TSH concentration) is achieved.

Myxedema Coma

The most severe form of hypothyroidism is characterized by myxedema coma. Fortunately, myxedema coma is a rare manifestation, with approximately 50% of cases occurring in hospitalized patients. Associated findings include hypothermia, hypoglycemia, respiratory acidosis, decreased level of consciousness, hypotension, and bradycardia. This is a medical emergency and carries a mortality rate of greater than 50%. Therefore the risk of treating myxedema coma is far less than the risk of missing the diagnosis. No pathognomonic tests for myxedema coma exist; the diagnosis is based on clinical findings. These include dry, scaly skin, thinning hair and eyebrows (lateral third), periorbital edema, and bradycardia. Most patients do not shiver and are hypothermic.

Treatment is thyroid hormone replacement. Before treatment, blood tests for serum TSH, reverse T_3 uptake, T_4, and cortisol levels should be performed. Supplementation should begin before the test results return. A loading dose of levothyroxine 500 μg intravenously replaces depleted thyroid stores. This therapy is followed by either 50 μg intravenously or 100 μg orally each day. Because of the risk of associated adrenal insufficiency and the high mortality rate, concomitant administration of hydrocortisone (100 to 300 mg/d) has been recommended. Clinical improvement can occur as quickly as 24 hours after the initiation of therapy.

T_3 supplementation is advocated because of its more rapid onset of action and the potential impaired peripheral conversion of T_4 to T_3, especially when treatment is supplemented by glucocorticoids. T_3 is available only in enteral form. The recommended dosage is 50 μg as a loading dose followed by 25 μg every 8 hours.

Supplementation is followed by administration of fluids and preservation of body temperature. Active rewarming should be avoided because it can precipitate vascular collapse. Many of these patients require ventilatory support because of central respiratory depression and decreased muscle strength. Infection is a common problem in patients with myxedema coma and should be treated aggressively.

Euthyroid Sick Syndrome

Of particular interest to the intensivist caring for any critically ill patient is the euthyroid sick syndrome. Within hours of major surgery or severe illness, thyroid function decreases sharply. This syndrome is manifest as a decrease in total T_4, T_3, and TSH levels, unchanged free T_4 and free T_3 levels, and increased reverse T_3 and reverse T_3 uptake. During TRH stimulation the usual response of TSH is blunted.

The question is whether the thyroid depression is a normal adaptive response or an illness necessitating treatment. Several investigators have advocated treatment, but others have failed to document improved survival with therapy.

DIABETES MELLITUS

Diabetes mellitus is present in 4% to 5% of the U.S. population. Diabetes leads to accelerated atherosclerosis, increased susceptibility to infections, peripheral and central neuropathies, ocular disease, nephropathy, and increased morbidity and mortality rates. The cardiovascular manifestations, other than artherosclerosis, include orthostatic hypotension (owing to sympathetic nerve dysfunction, which results in lack of vasoconstriction), resting tachycardia, and reduction or lack of beat-to-beat heart rate variation. Bradycardia may be refractory to atropine treatment if the vagus nerve is diseased. This is especially important when reversal agents of nondepolarizing muscle relaxants are used.

In this section we discuss the potentially lethal entities diabetic ketoacidosis (DKA) and hyperglycemic hyperosmolar nonketotic syndrome (HHNS). DKA and HHNS are severe manifestations of diabetes mellitus that usually require ICU management. Therefore they warrant special consideration here.

Diabetic Ketoacidosis

DKA is the most serious acute complication of diabetes. The mortality rate is still reported to be as high as 16%, but most intensivists find it to be less than 5%. DKA results from a relative or absolute deficiency of circulating insulin. In 50% of cases DKA is caused by medical illness, in approximately 20% to 25% by omission of insulin, and in 25% by other factors such as surgery and infection. The most common medical causes are infection, myocardial infarction, cerebrovascular accident, gastrointestinal bleeding, trauma, pancreatitis, and burns.

The pathophysiology of DKA involves not only insulin deficiency but also derangement of the counterregulatory hormones, notably glucagon. Without glucagon, glucose production may decrease by as much as 75%. Glucagon, in the absence of insulin, increases glycogenolysis, gluconeogenesis, and ketogenesis in the liver. The lack of insulin in the periphery allows the substrates for gluconeogenesis (amino acids) and ketogenesis (free fatty acids) to be delivered to the liver.

At the biochemical level, two key proteins that regulate hyperketonemia are malonyl coenzyme A (malonyl CoA) and acylcarnitine transferase. Normally (that is, when insulin/glucagon ratios are balanced), insulin increases malonyl CoA levels and decreases acylcarnitine transferase activity. This inhibits the transfer of free fatty acids into cells and prevents beta oxidation of free fatty acids to ketones. Insulin also promotes ketone utilization in the periphery.

In diabetes, when glucagon levels are high relative to insulin levels, the resultant hyperglycemia leads to an osmotic diuresis and electrolyte losses and the ketonemia causes metabolic acidosis (DKA).

Normally serum ketones are measured by the nitroprusside reaction. Unfortunately, this test measures acetoacetate and acetone but not beta hydroxybutyrate, which often is the principal ketone in DKA. Therefore initial blood ketone levels may be low. After therapy is started, beta hydroxybutyrate is oxidized to acetoacetate, thereby increasing the nitroprusside reaction, an indication of improving rather than declining status. Therefore, serial measurements of blood pH, anion gap, and serum ketones are prudent in the care of patients with DKA.

Treatment.   Therapy for DKA includes identification and treatment of the cause, as well as direct treatment of the ketosis (Table 16–14). The hallmarks of treatment are volume resuscitation and insulin administration. Volume depletion is common in DKA, with total body water deficits averaging 6 to 12 L, most of which is intracellular.

Since fluid replacement is crucial, volume is replaced with normal saline solution until either isovolemia is reached or the serum sodium level rises above 150 mEq/L, at which point hypotonic saline solution is used. Blood glucose levels are decreased by fluid resuscitation alone. When the blood glucose concentration falls to 250 mg/dl, dextrose should be added to the intravenous fluid formula. The institution of an "insulin-glucose clamp" occurs at this point when, with an insulin infusion, dextrose load is

TABLE 16–14. Treatment of Diabetic Ketoacidosis

Fluids

Give 1 L isotonic saline solution on admission followed by 1 L in 1 h, 1 L in 2 h, then 250-500 ml/h. If serum sodium level rises above 150-155 mEq/L, switch to 0.5 normal saline. When plasma glucose falls below 250 mg/dl, switch to D5W. Central hemodynamic monitoring may be required in elderly patients or those with cardiac or renal disease.

Insulin

Begin with continuous IV infusion of regular insulin 5-10 unit/h (in isotonic saline). Double infusion rate if glucose does not fall by 10% in 1 h. When plasma glucose level drops to 250 mg/dl, decrease IV infusion to regular insulin 1-3 units/h and continue until acidosis is corrected ("glucose clamp").

Potassium

Give 20 mEq/h; if oliguric, give 5-10 mEq/h; if potassium level above 6 mEq/L, stop infusion; if potassium below 4 mEq/L, increase infusion. Use continuous ECG monitoring.

Phosphorus

Give Neutra-Phos 250 mg q6h PO or potassium phosphate 0.08-0.16 mmol/kg 6 h IV. Measure serum phosphorus levels.

Bicarbonate

If arterial pH < 7.1 or bicarbonate < 5-7 mEq/L, give 1 ampule bicarbonate (44 mEq); if pH < 7.0 give 2 ampules bicarbonate (88 mEq); monitor arterial or venous pH hourly.

Magnesium

If less than 1.2 mg/dl give magnesium oxide 35 mEq q6-24h PO or magnesium sulfate or chloride 20-80 mEq/d IV. Monitor serum glucose (Chemstrip), electrolytes, arterial blood gases, anion gap, and hemodynamic and mental status.

adjusted to maintain the blood glucose at a constant level. This approach allows continued correction of ketone concentrations and pH, which usually takes twice as long as the correction of blood glucose level. Cerebral edema is a concern in treatment, and therefore precipitous drops in osmolality should be avoided. Despite conservative correction of osmolality, cerebral edema occurs in many treated patients. Symptomatic cerebral edema carries a 90% mortality.

Insulin is used to correct the primary defect in DKA. We use intravenous administration of regular insulin, starting with a bolus followed by a continuous infusion. Intramuscular or subcutaneous injections may lead to erratic absorption of insulin. Therefore we recommend the use of a continuous intravenous infusion of regular insulin until the DKA is controlled.

Insulin is unstable in alkaline solutions and thus should not be mixed with sodium bicarbonate.

Total body potassium, phosphorus, and magnesium levels are decreased in patients with DKA despite normal or increased serum values at initial examination. Potassium deficits can be as high as 5 mEq/kg. Potassium supplementation is withheld only when the serum level is 5.5 mEq/L or greater; otherwise, 10 to 20 mEq/h is normally given. If the patient is oliguric, potassium is given cautiously and potassium therapy is carefully adjusted based on serum potassium determinations. Initial hyperkalemia is attributable to intracellular shift of hydrogen ions or to direct insulin deficiency. Although not sensitive, continuous electrocardiographic monitoring is used. Electrocardiographic changes consistent with hyperkalemia are peaked T waves, decreased R waves with increased depth of the S wave, ST-T depression, and prolonged QRS and PR intervals. Complete heart block may follow these abnormalities. Progressive hyperkalemia leads to ventricular tachycardia, flutter, fibrillation, or cardiac standstill. Low serum sodium and calcium concentrations enhance these hyperkalemic effects. Conversely, hypokalemia is associated with such electrocardiographic findings as low, flat, or inverted T waves, mildly prolonged QT interval, ST-T depression, U wave, and arrhythmias, such as atrioventricular junctional rhythm or supraventricular tachycardia.

Bicarbonate treatment is slightly more complicated. A paradoxic cerebral acidemia can occur when sodium bicarbonate is administered because carbon dioxide can cross the blood-brain barrier whereas bicarbonate cannot. Other potential untoward effects of bicarbonate supplementation include augmented tissue ischemia and lactate production, impaired cardiac contractility, and rebound alkalosis after correction of hyperglycemia and ketonemia.

Another finding associated with DKA is exacerbated hyponatremia secondary to hypertriglyceridemia. Patients with DKA often have elevated serum amylase levels and may have abdominal pain implying an acute abdomen. If the suspicion of acute pancreatitis is high, the serum lipase concentration should be measured.

Despite aggressive management, complications of therapy are common and include shock, hypoglycemia, hypokalemia, hypophosphatemia, hypomagnesemia, antinatriuresis, cerebral edema, pulmonary edema, cardiac arrhythmias and infarction, and acute arterial thrombosis.

Hyperglycemic Hyperosmolar Nonketotic Syndrome

HHNS tends to occur in patients older than those with DKA, most of whom have either mild diabetes mellitus or were previously healthy. In 50% of cases a precipitating event, such as infection or dehydration, is found. The mortality rate of 40% is usually a result of concomitant disease. The pathophysiology is unknown. The hyperglycemia is greater in HHNS than in DKA, but ketonemia is less. One explanation of the lack of ketonemia is low peripheral insulin levels while the portal circulation maintains an insulin level high enough to suppress ketone formation.

Symptoms of HHNS appear after a longer time (average 12 days) than with DKA (average 3 days), leading to greater dehydration and electrolyte losses in HHNS. If the patient has neurologic symptoms, a cerebrovascular accident may be present instead. The hyperosmolar state can cause seizures, which may require treatment with phenytoin. Phenytoin may be hazardous, however, since it impairs insulin release.

Ketonuria may be associated with HHNS, but it is mild and usually secondary to starvation. An associated metabolic acidosis from lactic acid may be caused by hypoperfusion and renal insufficiency (both prerenal and renal in origin).

Treatment. The treatment of HHNS involves three steps: volume resuscitation, correction of metabolic derangements (notably hyperosmolality), and detection of the precipitating factors. The most important and first performed of these is volume repletion.

The average patient with HHNS has approximately a 25% total body water deficit. This translates into 6 to 18 L of fluid. It is customary to replace the loss with 2 to 3 L of 0.45% saline solution during the first 2 hours followed by half the body deficit during the next 12 hours (Table 16–15). Caution must be observed to avoid lowering serum osmolality too abruptly or precipitating pulmonary edema by aggressively administering fluid. Appropriate central hemodynamic monitoring is essential when caring for patients with HHNS.

Potassium repletion, as in DKA, is essential in patients with HHNS. The average requirement in the first 36 hours is 200 to 300 mEq. Serum potassium levels may decrease rapidly with fluid resuscitation, insulin therapy, correction of acidosis, and urinary losses. The standard replacement schedule for potassium

TABLE 16–15.   Treatment of Hyperglycemic Hyperosmolar Nonketotic Syndrome

Fluids

Restore intravascular volume with isotonic saline solution. Then give 2-3 L hypotonic saline (0.45%) in first 2 h followed by one half of body water deficit (0.25 × total body water in kg + urinary losses) over next 12h. Give remainder of body water deficit over next 24h. Central hemodynamic monitoring may be required in elderly or those with cardiac or renal disease.

Insulin

Begin with IV infusion of regular insulin 5-7 units/h (in hypotonic saline). When serum glucose drops to 250 mg/dl, switch fluid to D5W and decrease infusion rate of regular insulin to 1-3 units/h ("glucose clamp" technique). Maintain infusion for 24-36 h. Increase infusion rate if glucose does not fall by 10% in 1 h.

Potassium

Give 15-20 mEq/h; if oliguric, give 5-10 mEq/h; if potassium level above 6 mEq/L, stop infusion; if potassium below 4 mEq/L, increase infusion rate. Use continuous ECG monitoring.

Phosphorus

Give Neutra-Phos 250 mg q6h PO or potassium phosphate 0.08-0.16 mmol/kg/6 h IV.

Bicarbonate

If arterial pH < 7.1 or bicarbonate < 5-7 mEq/L, give 1 ampule bicarbonate (44 mEq); if pH < 7.0, give 2 ampules bicarbonate (88 mEq). Monitor arterial or venous pH hourly.

Magnesium

If less than 1.2 mg/dl give magnesium oxide 25 mEq q6-24h PO or magnesium sulfate or chloride 20-80 mEq/IV. Monitor serum glucose (Chemstrip), electrolytes, arterial blood gases, anion gap, and hemodynamic and mental status.

---

is 10 to 20 mEq/h unless initial hyperkalemia is present or the patient is oliguric. As in DKA, electrocardiographic monitoring is necessary.

Patients with HHNS are potentially more sensitive to insulin than patients with DKA. Therefore we suggest use of an intravenous regular insulin infusion starting with 5 to 7 units/h. When the serum glucose concentration reaches 250 to 300 mg/dl, the infusion is lowered to 1 to 3 units/h and the fluid is switched to 5% dextrose in water. This is continued for an additional 24 to 36 hours to correct the hyperosmolality slowly and thus prevent significant cerebral edema (Table 16–15).

The complications and causes of death are the same as noted for DKA. In one study 67% of patients who recovered, and did not use insulin before their HHNS, did not need routine insulin use.

SUGGESTED READINGS

Aaron: Cushing's disease. In Pituitary tumors: diagnosis and management. Endocrin Metab Clin North Am 1987; 705:730

Adrogue JH, Lederer ED, Suki WN, et al: Determinants of plasma potassium levels in diabetic ketoacidosis. Medicine 1986;65:163

Arieff AI: Hyponatremia associated with permanent brain damage. Adv Intern Med 1987;32:325

Arieff AI, Carroll HJ: Nonketotic hyperosmolar coma with hyperglycemia: clinical features, pathophysiology, renal function, acid-base balance, plasma-cerebrospinal fluid equilibria and the effects of therapy in 37 cases. Medicine 1972;51:73

Ayus JC, Krothapalli RK, Arieff AI: Treatment of symptomatic hyponatremia and its relation to brain damage: a prospective study. N Engl J Med 1987;317(19):1190

Braverman LE: Thyroid storm. In Krieger DT, Bordin CW (eds): Current therapy in endocrinology 1983-84. Philadelphia, 1983, BC Decker, pp 60-65

Bravo EL, Gifford RW: Current concepts: phemochromocytoma; diagnosis, localization and management. N Engl J Med 1984;311(20):1298

Chernow B, Alexander HR, Smallridge RC, et al: Hormonal response to graded surgical stress. Arch Intern Med 1987;147:1273-1278

Chin R Jr: Corticosteroids. In Chernow B (ed): The pharmacologic approach to the critically ill patient, 2nd ed., Baltimore, 1988, Williams & Wilkins, pp 559-583

Cogan E, Debieve MF, Pepersack T, Abramov M: High plasma levels of atrial natriuretic factor in SIADH. N Engl J Med 1986;314(19):1258

Eckfelt JH, Leatherman JW, Leavit MD: High prevalence of hyperamylasemia in patients with acidemia. Ann Intern Med 1986;104:362

Edes TE, Sunderrajan EV: Heparin-induced hyperkalemia. Arch Intern Med 1985;145:1070-1072

Hull CJ: Phaeochromocytoma: diagnosis, preoperative preparation and anaesthetic management. Br J Anaesth 1986;58:1453-1468

Jurney TH, Cockrell JL, Lindbert JS, et al: Spectrum of serum cortisol response to ACTH in ICU patients: correlation with degree of illness and mortality. Chest 1987;92:292

Klein I, Levey GS: Unusual manifestations of hypothyroidism following prolonged sodium nitroprusside therapy. Arch Intern Med 1984;144:123

Ladenson PW, Levin AA, Ridgway EC, et al: Complications of surgery in hypothyroid patients. Am J Med 1984;77:261

Munck A: Physiologic functions of glucocorticoids in stress and their relation to pharmacologic actions. Endocrinol Rev 1984;5:25

Murkin JM: Anesthesia and hypothyroidism: a review of thyroxine physiology, pharmacology and anesthetic implications. Anesth Analg 1982;61:371-383

Napolitano L, Chernow B: Guidelines for corticosteroid use in anesthetic and surgical stress. Intern Anesth Clin 1988;26(3):226

Schrier RW: Pathogenesis of sodium and water retention in high output and low output cardiac failure, nephrotic syndrome, cirrhosis and pregnancy. Part I. N Engl J Med 1988;319:1065

Schrier RW: Pathogenesis of sodium and water retention in high output and low output cardiac failure, nephrotic syndrome, cirrhosis and pregnancy. Part II. N Engl J Med 1988;319:1127

Schrier RW et al: Peripheral arterial vasodilation hypothesis: a proposal for the initiation of renal sodium and water retention. J Hepatol 1987;6:239-257

Senior RM, Birge SJ: The recognition and management of myxedema coma. JAMA 1971;217:61

Sheps et al: Diagnostic evaluation of pheochromocytoma. Endocrinol Metab Clin North Am 1988;17(2)

Simon HB, Daniels GH: Hormonal hyperthermia—endocrinologic causes of fever. Am J Med 1979;66:257

Teich S, Sharpe S, Chernow B: Endocrine function in the critically ill. Clin Anesthesiol 1985;3(4):1003

Tibaldi JM, Barzel US, Albin J, et al: Thyrotoxicosis in the very old. Am J Med 1986;81:619

Zaloga GP, Chernow B: Diabetic coma. In Parrillo JE (ed): Current therapy in critical care medicine, Philadelphia, 1987, BC Decker, pp 297-299

Zaloga GP, Chernow B, Smallridge RC, et al: A longitudinal evaluation of thyroid function in critically ill surgical patients. Ann Surg 1985;201:456

Zwillich CW, Pierson DJ, Hofeldt E, et al: Ventilatory control in myxedema and hypothyroidism. N Engl J Med 1975;292:662

SECTION III

SPECIFIC CRITICAL CARE TOPICS

17

OVERDOSES, INGESTIONS, AND INTOXICATIONS

NIELS LUND, MD, PhD, AND PETER J PAPADAKOS, MD

Poisoning in any form is a worldwide problem. In 1978 more than 150,000 cases were reported in the United States, and the incidence of fatal poisoning is rising steadily. Most adult poisonings tend to be deliberate, whereas childhood poisonings are usually accidental.

GENERAL CONSIDERATIONS AND ASSESSMENT

Any patient who is unconscious or delirious for unknown reasons should be considered a possible poisoning victim.

Occasionally a patient is admitted with a history of drug overdose but no symptoms. This should *absolutely not* lead to the conclusion that the patient is not at risk. Such a patient may have either ingested a low dose, or not absorbed a quantity sufficient to produce symptoms yet (Table 17–1).

Every effort should be made to obtain a history, although the histories obtained in these cases are often unclear or unreliable. In taking the history the following questions should be asked:

- To which *agent* (or agents) was the patient exposed?
- To what *amount* (dose) was the patient exposed?
- By which *route?*
- Approximately *when* did the exposure occur?

The initial clinical assessment should be performed quickly and systematically. Vital signs should be recorded at frequent intervals. The physical examination only rarely suggests a specific toxic agent (for example, hypertension from cocaine or amphetamines, hyperpyrexia from salicylates or anticholinergic drugs, increased salivation from insecticides or mushrooms). One exception is the classic cherry-red skin from carbon monoxide poisoning.

Primary attention should be directed to the support of vital functions if the patient has symptoms. Support for respiratory and cardiac function should be provided immediately. Other abnormalities that could impair ventilation or circulation (such as acid-base disorders and seizures) should be corrected.

TABLE 17–1. Toxic Agents and Characteristic Symptoms of Overdose

AGENT	SYMPTOMS AND FINDINGS
Amphetamines	Irritability, tremor, headache, diarrhea, dry mouth, tachycardia, dilated pupils, hypertension
Atropine, scopolamine	Agitation, hallucinations, dry skin and mouth, dilated pupils, blurred vision, elevated temperature
Barbiturates	Slurred speech, coma, nystagmus, ataxia, hypothermia
Narcotics	Coma, pinpoint pupils, respiratory depression
Organophosphates	Salivation, gastritis, defecation, urination, pulmonary congestion, miosis
Phenothiazines	Acute dystonia, ataxia, coma, hypothermia
Salicylates	Tachypnea, respiratory alkalosis, metabolic acidosis, pulmonary edema, elevated temperature
Tricyclic antidepressants	Dry mouth, blurred vision, urinary retention, tachycardia, arrhythmias

From Mofenson HC, Greensher J: Pediatrics 1974;54:339. Reproduced by permission of *Pediatrics*.

357

GENERAL MEASURES

General measures of support of airway ventilation, circulation, and fluid management are discussed in Chapter 2.

PHARMACOKINETICS

Effective treatment of a poisoned patient requires not only knowledge of the causative agent's mechanism of action, but also an understanding of the drug's absorption, distribution, metabolism, and elimination.

Absorption. The oral route is by far the most common route of poisoning. The level of drug found in the blood at initial examination depends primarily on the amount ingested and the rate at which it is absorbed. Stomach pH influences the rate of absorption of some drugs (for example, salicylates are more readily absorbed at a lower pH). The presence of food or the development of concretions of tablets in the stomach can inhibit absorption. The rate of stomach emptying critically affects plasma levels of drugs that are absorbed in the small intestine. Also, the drug itself may reduce gastric emptying, as occurs with alcohol, narcotics, and tricyclic antidepressants.

Distribution. Distribution is primarily determined by physicochemical characteristics, cardiac output, and tissue blood flow. The major determinants of the distribution of a drug are its lipid solubility and plasma proein binding. Lipid solubility is especially important in central nervous system deposition. Plasma protein binding is also important, since only unbound drugs can enter the tissues.

A delayed toxic effect may be seen when highly lipid-soluble drugs are first distributed to fat and subsequently redistributed into the blood. An example of this pattern is glutethimide poisoning.

Elimination. In general, drugs are biotransformed within the body. One or more transformation steps break down the active drug to inactive metabolites. Thus the drug is converted into a more easily eliminated form.

Most drugs are biotransformed in the liver and excreted through the kidneys. Therefore processes that impair heart, liver, or kidney function may depress biotransformation and elimination.

NONSPECIFIC TREATMENT

Prevention of Absorption. Most substances are absorbed within 4 hours, but some may remain in the stomach for up to 48 hours. Thus, maneuvers to prevent absorption should be considered in poisoned patients even if the ingestion occurred several hours prior to admission. These maneuvers include emesis, gastric lavage, activated charcoal, and cathartics.

Emesis. Emesis should *not* be induced in a patient who is obtunded or comatose, is having seizures, or has ingested caustic agents, hydrocarbons, convulsant agents, or small volumes (less than 10 ml/kg) of aliphatic hydrocarbons.

Ipecac syrup is the most effective emetic. Its mechanisms of action are stimulation of the medullary chemoreceptor trigger zone and gastric irritation. The dose is 10 ml in infants age 9 to 12 months, 15 ml in children 1 to 12 years, and 30 ml in patients older than 12 years. In addition, 200 to 400 ml of water should immediately follow the syrup in older children and adults. Emesis is induced within 30 minutes in 80% to 85% of patients. If vomiting has not occurred within 30 minutes, the initial dose may be repeated *except* in infants. If emesis still does not occur, gastric lavage is indicated. Apomorphine is a less desirable emetic because it may produce significant respiratory depression.

Gastric Lavage. Lavage is less effective than emesis in gastric evacuation. However, it may be useful if carried out within 4 hours of the ingestion. Lavage should be performed *only* after a cuffed endotracheal tube has been placed and the airway is protected. With the patient lying on the left side and the head lower than the rest of the body, a large (No. 32 to 36 French) fenestrated orogastric tube is inserted, preferably orally, and taped securely in place. Gastric contents are withdrawn and sent for toxicologic examination. The stomach is then lavaged with small volumes of fluid: 200 to 300 ml in adults and 100 to 150 ml in children. Tap water can be used in adults, but children *must* be given half-normal or normal saline solution to prevent water intoxication. The tube should be kept in place for administration of activated charcoal and cathartics. Emesis and lavage should *not* be used after ingestion of strong convulsants (such as strychnine) or furniture polish. Because the potential for pulmonary aspiration is high and there is a risk of lipoid pneumonia if hydrocarbon is aspirated, some physicians believe that hydrocarbon ingestion should not be treated with emesis and lavage. However, several studies indicate that emesis and lavage can be carried out safely in this situation.

Charcoal. Activated charcoal has a large surface area and adsorptive capacity. There are no contraindications for the use of activated charcoal, and it should be used early in most cases, except in poisonings caused by acids or alkali. Because of the high risk of esophageal perforations following acid or alkali ingestion, no oral treatment should be used until the integrity of the esophagus has been confirmed. The dosage is 50 to 100 g in adults and 30 to 35 g in children, mixed with 100 to 300 ml of water. Activated charcoal does not adsorb heavy metals, hydrocarbons, boric acid, mineral acids or alkalis, malathion, cyanide, alcohols, or caustic agents. Because activated charcoal readily adsorbs ipecac syrup, it should be administered only after emesis has occurred or gastric lavage has been completed.

Cathartics. The use of cathartics (sodium sulfate or phosphate, magnesium citrate or sulfate) is controversial. These substances interfere with intestinal absorption by increasing transit rate. Saline cathartics can induce hypernatremia. Cathartics are contraindicated in poisoning with caustic agents and in the presence of electrolyte imbalance. Magnesium-containing cathartics should not be used when the patient has evidence of renal failure.

ENHANCEMENT OF ELIMINATION

Renal Elimination. Elimination of drugs excreted in the urine can be enhanced by manipulating urinary pH (Table 17–2) and by increasing glomerular filtration and thus urine volume.

ALKALINIZATION. In adults an alkaline urine can be achieved by administration of sodium bicarbonate 1 to 2 mEq/kg. In children 3.5 to 5 mEq/kg should be administered over 4 hours. Urinary pH should be monitored and maintained at about 8.0.

ACIDIFICATION. Urine can be acidified by administration of ascorbic acid 500 mg to 2 g orally or intravenously or ammonium chloride 0.1 g orally or intravenously. Ammonium chloride should be administered cautiously because it may cause severe metabolic acidosis. Acid-base status should be closely monitored, and the dose regulated to prevent causing severe metabolic acidosis.

TABLE 17–2.   Drugs with Renal pH-Dependent Elimination

Weak Acids
Phenobarbitone
Salicylates
Sulfonamide derivatives
Weak Bases
Amphetamine
Ephedrine
Phencyclidine (PCP)
Pseudoephedrine
Quinine
Tocainide
Tricyclic antidepressants

From Brater DC: Drugs. 1980;19:31.

Forced Diuresis. An initial fluid load of 300 to 500 ml/h should be administered to keep urine flow at 5 to 8 ml/kg/h. Furosemide can be used to enhance diuresis. Dopamine in dopaminergic doses (0.5 to 5 μg/kg/min) may also be considered. For nephrotoxins, mannitol has been more effective in experimental models. Frequent monitoring of serum potassium, urine and blood pH, and volume status is mandatory because rapid volume expansion may result in pulmonary edema or large potassium losses in the urine.

Drugs for which forced neutral diuresis is effective are

- Aliphatic alcohol
- Meprobamate
- Lithium

Extracorporeal Removal of Toxins. If a severely intoxicated patient does not respond to supportive and specific therapy or has impairment of the normal elimination pathways, active removal of toxins may be attempted. The most effective methods are hemodialysis and hemoperfusion.

Standard hemodialysis is most useful in overdose with such drugs as

- Lithium
- Salicylate
- Alcohol
- Methanol

Hemoperfusion is superior to hemodialysis for the removal of toxins. With this method blood is percolated through either an ion-exchange resin or an activated charcoal column. Hemoperfusion is highly effective in clearing toxins that have small volumes of distribution and low clearance values. Drugs that can be removed in this way include

- Barbiturates
- Ethchlorvynol
- Glutethimide
- Meprobamate
- Methaqualone

Hemoperfusion entails the risks of hypotension, bleeding, thrombocytopenia, and leukocytopenia.

Temperature Support. Hyperthermia may complicate overdoses with certain drugs. Once severe hyperthermia (temperature greater than 40.5° C) is established, conventional cooling methods do not invariably decrease body temperature or prevent brain damage. Drugs may induce hyperthermia by increasing heat production or by decreasing heat dissipation. Heat production may be increased by either muscular hyperactivity (sympathomimetic and epileptogenic agents) or metabolic hyperactivity (salicylates). Heat dissipation may be decreased by inhibition of sweating (antichoinergics), cutaneous vasoconstriction (sympathomimetics), or interference with central temperature regulation (phenothiazines). Hyperthermia may not develop until up to 12 hours after drug intake because of delayed absorption. Treatment should be directed at the causes of heat production, primarily seizures and muscular hyperactivity. This may be accomplished with anticonvulsants, muscle relaxants, and sedatives. Sponge baths or gastric lavage with iced water may be used to reduce body temperature.

Hypothermia may be encountered in severe poisoning with barbiturates, phenothiazines, and most sedative and narcotic drugs.

SPECIFIC ANTIDOTES

Few specific antidotes for the treatment of drug overdose are available. They should obviously be used only with specific indications and *never* prophylactically. Great care should be taken when using antidotes because the duration of the antidote may be shorter than that of the primary drug. After treatment with an antidote the patient should not be released from medical care until clinicians have ascertained that the effect of the primary drug has worn off.

SPECIFIC TOXIC AGENTS

Acetaminophen. Acetaminophen is metabolized mostly through conjugation with sulfate and glucuronic acid, but also by a cytochrome P450–dependent oxidase to a potentially hepatotoxic intermediate, which is rapidly conjugated with glutathione. The nontoxic end metabolites are excreted in the urine. When large amounts of acetaminophen (more than 7.5 g) are ingested and absorbed, normal conjugation becomes saturated, resulting in increased metabolism via the cytochrome P450 pathway (Fig. 17–1). The resulting hepatotoxic effect progressively increases the half-life of acetaminophen. If severe hepatic necrosis occurs, the plasma half-life may exceed 12 hours.

Liver toxicity and death have been reported after ingestion of 6 g, but usually hepatotoxicity does not become a concern until 10 to 15 g has been ingested by an adult. Hepatotoxicity is markedly potentiated by alcohol. Diagnosis is based on the ingestion history or an elevated serum level. A serum level of 160 to 200 μg/ml at 4 hours indicates that liver necrosis may occur; if it is higher than 300 μg/ml at 4 hours, liver damage is almost certain.

Significant cardiopulmonary dysfunction is unlikely in acetaminophen poisoning. Initial treatment is directed toward prevention of further drug absorption through evacuation of the stomach and adsorption of the drug with activated charcoal. However, charcoal also adsorbs *N*-acetylcysteine, the specific antidote for acetaminophen. Forced diuresis is not effective.

Antidotes to prevent or limit liver toxicity include cysteine, methionine, and *N*-acetylcysteine. Cysteine is a glutathione precursor;

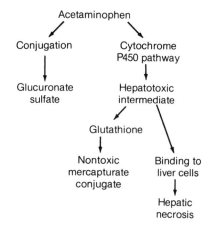

Figure 17–1. Acetaminophen metabolization.

methionine and *N*-acetylcysteine both function as glutathione substitutes. *N*-Acetylcysteine has been used with success both orally and intravenously. The substance is not available for intravenous administration in the United States. However, high concentrations may be achieved when *N*-acetylcysteine is given orally, since it is absorbed directly into the portal circulation.

The loading dose of oral *N*-acetylcysteine (Mucomyst) is 140 mg/kg, followed by 70 mg/kg every 4 hours for 4 to 18 doses. Repeat serum levels of acetaminophen and daily liver enzyme and prothrombin levels should be obtained. Rises in bilirubin, serum glutamate oxaloacetate transaminase, serum glutamate pyruvate transaminase, and prothrombin levels indicate development of liver toxicity. Blood urea nitrogen and creatinine concentrations should also be monitored because renal complications may occur.

With prompt therapy, deaths can be virtually eliminated. In most cases the findings of liver function tests gradually return to normal within several weeks.

Amyl Nitrite. Toxic effects of the following nitrites are all the same and should be treated in the same way: amyl nitrite, butyl nitrite, nitroglycerin, potassium nitrite and sodium nitrite. The patient may complain of headache and dizziness. Poisoning is manifest as cyanosis, hypoxia, respiratory failure, and coma. These patients are at high risk for vomiting and aspiration. Blood should be drawn to determine the degree of methemoglobinemia. Initial treatment is ipecac-induced emesis and gastric lavage. Oxygen should be administered to reverse the methemoglobinemia and hypoxia. If methemoglobin levels are 30% to 40% or higher, 1 mg/kg of a solution of 1% methylene blue should be given over 5 minutes intravenously. Exchange transfusions with whole blood may be necessary.

Anticholinergics. Several agents have prominent anticholinergic effects. The major anticholinergic groups are antihistamines, belladonna alkaloids, butyrophenones, phenothiazines, plant extracts, and tricyclic antidepressants. The patient has a combination of central and peripheral symptoms that result from competitive antagonism with acetylcholine at muscarinic receptors. A clinical picture of agitated psychosis in combination with signs of autonomic nervous system dysfunction (dry hot skin, supraventricular tachycardia, fever, dilated pupils, ileus, and urinary retention) strongly suggests drug intoxication.

Antihistamines and H₁-Receptor Blockers. A common feature of poisoning by antihistamines and H_1-receptor blockers is central nervous depression, which also represents the greatest threat for morbidity and death. Treatment is supportive because no specific antidote exists.

Barbiturates. Barbiturates enhance the activity of certain central inhibitory pathways. They can be divided into three groups — short acting, intermediate, and long acting — based on speed of entry to the central nervous system (CNS), onset of action and duration of action.

Specific symptoms and signs in the individual patient depend on the barbiturate involved, the amount taken, and the time since intake. Large doses of short-acting barbiturates have the greatest toxic effect and risk of death. Generally a dose 10 times or greater than the therapeutic dose will result in severe toxicity. Coma may range from mild to profound. Hypercapnic respiratory failure may be severe and result in death. Hypothermia is common. Cardiovascular collapse results from both central medullary center depression and direct myocardial and vascular effects.

The diagnosis is confirmed by high barbiturate blood levels. Coma occurs with blood levels greater than 2 mg/dl for short-acting agents, greater than 4 mg/dl for intermediate-acting compounds, and greater than 10 mg/dl for long-acting drugs.

No antidotes are available, so treatment is symptomatic and supportive. Ventilatory therapy should be guided by arterial blood gas analysis, since the patient may have close to normal blood gas concentrations even with a respiratory rate of only 2 to 4 breaths per minute. This is due to the metabolic depression exerted by barbiturates, which results in decreased carbon dioxide production. Standard ventilator settings may produce respiratory alkalosis. In addition, vigorous warming of a hypothermic patient may cause vasodilatation and hypotension or even shock. Some clinicians have suggested use of hemodialysis or hemoperfusion in severe poisoning when blood levels are 3 to 5 mg/dl (short-acting agent) or more than 10 mg/dl (long-acting agent).

Belladonna Alkaloids. Atropine and scopolamine are used individually or in combination with other agents in a wide variety of drug preparations, such as antidiarrheal agents, eye drops, sedatives, and sleeping aids. Physostigmine in a dose of 1 to 2 mg intravenously reverses CNS manifestations. This dose may have to be repeated every 1 to 2 hours. Therefore the potential risk for cholinergic toxicity should be kept in mind. Standard supportive measures should be used as needed.

Benzodiazepines. Benzodiazepines are among the most commonly prescribed drugs. Although often taken in intentional overdoses for purposes of suicide, they rarely produce serious toxicity and when taken alone almost never cause death. Overdose results in drowsiness but rarely coma.

Treatment is generally supportive. Naloxone in very large doses, theophylline 1 to 2 mg/kg intravenously, and physostigmine 1-2 mg intravenously have been recommended as antidotes to benzodiazepines. However, all of these agents have drawbacks. Flumazenil, a specific benzodiazepine receptor antagonist, has been used to treat benzodiazepine overdoses. A dose of 1 to 5 mg IV is infused until awakening occurs. Because the half-life of flumazenil (1.3 hours) is shorter than that of diazepam, repeat administration is often necessary. Since the number of benzodiazepine overdoses is increasing, some clinicians advocate giving flumazenil in the emergency department as a diagnostic and therapeutic aid. If the patient's level of consciousness increases after administration of flumazenil, at least one comnponent of the intoxication is likely to be a benzodiazepine.

Butyrophenones. Butyrophenones resemble meperidine in chemical structure and phenothiazines in clinical effects. Haloperidol and droperidol are the most commonly used compounds in this drug class. Overdose treatment is supportive.

Calcium Channel Blockers. Calcium channel blockers are increasingly used in the treatment of angina and hypertension. Overdoses of verapamil, nifedipine, and diltiazem have been reported.

Symptoms and signs of calcium channel blocker overdose include bradycardia, disturbance of arteriovenous conduction, depressed myocardial contractility, decreased cardiac output, and hypotension. Drugs used for treating calcium channel blocker toxicity include atropine, calcium, dopamine, epinephrine, isoproterenol, and norepinephrine. In patients who cannot tolerate beta-adrenergic stimulation, atropine and calcium are the preferred agents. In a study of dogs, treatment of calcium channel blocker overdose with 4-aminopyridine gave good results.

Caustic Agents. Poisoning with caustic agents usually occurs when infants and children ingest them by mistake. The most common sources are drain and toilet bowl cleaners and dishwasher detergents. These are available in both solid and liquid forms. Liquids are more dangerous because they are easily consumed.

Pain occurs immediately on ingestion of caustic agents. Burned areas, such as lips, tongue, and upper airway, become edematous. Edema may result in airway obstruction. The pulse may become rapid and weak from translocation of intravascular fluid into the damaged tissue, respirations are shallow, and shock is common. Late effects include infection, as well as perforation of the esophagus or stomach (after at least a week). Perforation in the mediastinum, with immediate sharp pain, occurs soon after ingestion. Even if the course initially seems benign, esophageal strictures may develop weeks later.

Emesis or lavage is *contraindicated.* The poison should be *immediately diluted* by drinking water. Neutralizing solutions of alkali or acids should *not* be given because they may generate heat-producing reactions. Milk should not be given because it may confuse interpretation of findings at esophagoscopy. Endoscopy is indicated whenever caustic agents are ingested to determine whether the esophagus is intact. Severe esophageal burns are not always accompanied by mouth burns. Contaminated clothing should be removed and the skin washed. If esophageal lesions are found, corticosteroid therapy is started: prednisone 60 mg/d in four divided doses for 4 days and thereafter in gradually decreasing doses over 2 to 3 weeks. If evidence of perforation or fever is present, a broadspectrum antibiotic should be given. Intravenous therapy is instituted until oral fluids can be tolerated.

Chloral Derivates. Chloral hydrate, chloral betaine, and triclofos sodium all produce the same active metabolite: trichloroethanol. Chloral hydrate is rapidly absorbed from the gastrointestinal tract, especially when taken as a liquid and when taken in combination with ethyl alcohol. Chloral hydrate is metabolized so fast that it is almost undetectable in plasma. However, its metabolite, trichloroethanol, has a half-life of up to 14 hours. Lethal doses reported vary from 4 to 30 g. An ingestion of more than 5 g should be considered dangerous.

Symptoms are similar to those of barbiturate intoxication. However, chloral hydrate may cause epigastric distress, nausea, vomiting, hemorrhagic gastritis, and esophageal strictures. Supraventricular and ventricular arrhythmias, jaundice, and renal damage have also been described.

Treatment is the same as for barbiturates (see preceding discussion).

Cocaine. Cocaine is a powerful sympathomimetic that inhibits epinephrine and norepinephrine reuptake at presynaptic receptor sites and results in end-organ hypersensitivity. It increases dopamine activity in the CNS by increased release of dopamine and blockade of reuptake. It also probably increases serotonin activity in the CNS through an effect similar to that of dopamine. Cocaine is different from amphetamines in that it has local anesthetic effects, its duration is shorter, and cardiac arrhythmias and convulsions are more likely with acute toxicity. It is metabolized in the liver and in plasma by cholinesterase and excreted in the urine. Urine excretion is not dependent on either urine pH or volume.

Intoxication follows a biphasic pattern: rapid progression from mild to intense CNS stimulation followed by an abrupt CNS depression. CNS effects are dose related. Initial symptoms are euphoria, reduced feeling of fatigue, restlessness, confusion, and delirium. Higher doses lead to headache, nausea, vomiting, twitching of small muscles (fingers and face), tremors, hyperreflexia, and generalized seizures. Hyperpyrexia is also common and probably results from hypermetabolism and vasoconstriction. When blood levels become very high, stimulation can suddenly change to depression with cardiorespiratory failure, hyporeflexia, and coma.

Treatment is supportive. If the intoxicated patient survives for more than 3 hours after the overdose, the prognosis is usually good. Protection of the airway and maintenance of adequate ventilation are the highest priorities. Seizures usually respond well to intravenously administered diazepam. Hypertension, tachycardia, and arrhythmias normally respond to propranolol 1 to 8 mg intravenously as needed. Severe hypertension may require treatment with nitroprusside. Hyperpyrexia should be treated with cooling blankets and antipyretics.

A large oral intake of cocaine (which is unusual) is treated with gastric lavage and activated charcoal (see preceding discussion). Flushing nasal mucosa to remove unabsorbed cocaine is absolutely contraindicated, since this maneuver may increase absorption.

Codeine. Codeine makes up approximately 0.5% of raw opium. It is widely used as both an analgesic and an antitussive. The analgesic effect of 120 mg of codeine given intramuscularly is equal to that of 10 mg of morphine. In contrast to morphine, codeine is rapidly absorbed when given orally. It is metabolized in the liver and excreted in the urine.

Symptoms and signs are similar to those of other narcotics and include pinpoint pupils, drowsiness, spasticity, shallow respirations, and respiratory failure. The lethal dose of codeine is approximately 800 mg in a person who has not developed tolerance to the drug.

Treatment for codeine overdose is the same as for morphine (see later discussion of morphine). However, when codeine is ingested orally, emesis or gastric lavage or both should be used, followed by administration of activated charcoal.

Ethchlorvynol. Ethchlorvynol is a CNS depressant similar to the barbiturates. Clinical symptoms of overdose are also similar to those seen in barbiturate overdose. However, in contrast to barbiturates and glutethimide, the duration of coma can be prolonged.

No specific antidote is available. Supportive treatment is the same as for barbiturates.

Ethyl Alcohol. Ethanol is one of the most abused drugs in the world. The use of alcohol is a contributing factor in 50% of home and automobile accidents in the United States. Ethanol is metabolized to acetaldehyde in the liver. This is the rate-limiting step, and it is critically dependent on alcohol dehydrogenase. The enzyme becomes saturated at blood levels between 13 and 30 mg/dl. Thus a 75 kg human can metabolize 7 to 10 g of alcohol per hour. Judgment becomes impaired at a blood level of 20 to 30 mg/dl, and at approximately 150 mg/dl most people are grossly intoxicated. Death is common when the level exceeds 400 to 500 mg/dl. Ethanol intoxication also produces a variety of metabolic derangements, including abnormal glucose metabolism, electrolyte abnormalities, acid-base disturbances, changes in serum osmolality, and abnormalities in temperature regulation.

The diagnosis is based on blood alcohol level. An odor of alcohol does not necessarily imply ethanol intoxication, nor does it indicate that the coma is ethanol induced.

Treatment is support for the patient and prevention of complications while ethanol is being metabolized. Aspiration, dehydration, shock, and respiratory failure should be prevented. In cases of life-threatening intoxication (greater than 400 mg/dl), some clinicians suggest using hemodialysis to remove the agent rapidly.

Glutethimide. Glutethimide is a CNS depressant with rapid absorption from the gastrointestinal tract. It is metabolized in the liver to several active metabolites. Some of the metabolites have half-lives of more than 24 hours, and they also undergo enterohepatic recirculation. A dose of 5 g produces toxic effects, and 10 to 20 g is potentially lethal.

Clinical signs and symptoms are the same as for barbiturate overdose. There is no antidote for glutethimide, so treatment is supportive and directed at symptoms.

Hallucinogens.   See the discussions of LSD, marijuana, and phencyclidine.

Heroin.   See the discussion of morphine.

Lithium.   Lithium salts have been used for the past 40 years, primarily to treat manic-depressive disorders. The therapeutic dose of lithium often overlaps the toxic dose. The goal is to keep the blood level of lithium at 0.4 to 1.2 mEq/L. Blood levels higher than 1.4 mEq/L produce toxic symptoms. The most common toxic effects are nausea and diarrhea. A fine resting hand tremor indicates impending intoxication.

CNS signs of intoxication include weakness, slurred speech, ataxia, increasing tremor, and drowsiness. Renal complications include nephrogenic diabetes insipidus and interstitial nephritis, either of which may lead to electrolyte imbalance.

Treatment is supportive and directed at symptoms. Normal urine output must be restored with fluid therapy and may require osmotic diuretics and intravenous sodium bicarbonate. Serum electrolyte levels should be carefully monitored and corrected. In severe intoxication hemodialysis is the treatment of choice.

LSD.   The mechanism of action of LSD is an agonistic effect at presynaptic serotonin receptors in the midbrain, which releases postsynaptic cells from tonic inhibition. Perception, perspective, proprioception, sense of time, vision, and body image are altered. Mood swings can be dramatic, ranging from anxiety, depression, and dread to elation. Motor system effects include hyperreflexia, increased motor tone, tremor, and ataxia. Autonomic nervous system effects include mydriasis, hypertension, tachycardia, nausea, palpitations, hyperpyrexia, sweating, hyperglycemia, and urinary frequency. Since acute intoxication is manifest as alterations in cognitive function and judgment, patients are usually brought to hospitals because of an accident, a panic reaction, or attempted suicide.

The manifestations of LSD intoxication usually resolve spontaneously within 12 hours. Treatment is therefore primarily supportive. If the patient is extremely agitated, a benzodiazepine can be administered in standard dose.

Marijuana.   Marijuana is the third most commonly abused drug (after alcohol and cigarettes) among high school seniors in the United States. The drug is distributed mainly to lipid-rich tissues, most notably the brain. Excretion is via the urine and occurs over a period of days.

Signs and symptoms include euphoria, relaxation, altered balance and coordination, increased reaction time, altered time perception, impaired short-term memory, increased appetite, dry mouth, mild tachycardia, hypertension, and conjunctival redness. Panic and paranoia are the most common major adverse reactions. Patients usually respond to reassurance, although the use of a tranquilizer may occasionally be necessary. Acute medical emergencies and deaths have not been reported.

Meperidine.   In contrast to morphine, meperidine has a high degree of oral bioavailability. Duration of action is 2 to 4 hours, somewhat shorter than that of morphine. Meperidine is widely distributed throughout the body and metabolized primarily in the liver. In the absence of pain an intramuscular dose of 0.5 to 1 mg/kg significantly decreases ventilatory response to an increased carbon dioxide tension in 20 to 60 minutes. Intravenous administration of 1.5 mg/kg can produce significant respiratory depression within 5 minutes. Cardiovascular effects include decreased peripheral arterial and venous resistance and increased pulmonary vascular resistance. CNS symptoms include hyperirritability with twitching, spasticity, and tachypnea. Treatment is the same as for morphine overdose.

Meprobamate.   Meprobamate is a CNS depressant similar to the barbiturates. Signs of acute overdose include coma, respiratory depression, and hypotension. Development of adult respiratory distress syndrome has been described. The lethal dose is approximately 40 g. Treatment is similar to that described for barbiturates.

Methadone.   Methadone is a synthetic agent used both as an analgesic and in treatment of narcotic addiction. Unfortunately, it has also become one of the more common agents for acute narcotic overdose. At a dosage of 40 to 80 mg/day methadone produces effects similar to those of morphine (miosis, constipation, nausea, vomiting, and urinary retention). It also produces significant respiratory depression at therapeutic doses. In contrast to morphine, methadone is very effective when given orally. Although highly bound to plasma protein, it is still extensively distributed to the tissues.

Clinical signs and symptoms of overdose are similar to those of morphine (see the succeeding discussion). As little as 40 to 50 mg may produce coma and respiratory depression in an adult in whom tolerance has not developed. Pulmonary edema is a common finding. Treatment is identical to that for morphine overdose.

Methaqualone. Although methaqualone depresses the CNS in a way similar to barbiturates, it can also produce CNS stimulation. This is expressed as delirium, hyperreflexia, hypertonicity, myoclonus, and seizures. A dose of 2.5 g produces coma, and 8 g is generally considered a lethal dose. Signs of CNS overactivity may help differentiate methaqualone overdose from other hypnotic-sedative overdoses. Treatment is the same as for barbiturates with one exception: seizures should be treated not with barbiturates but with phenytoin or possibly a benzodiazepine.

Morphine. Morphine, the prototypic narcotic, is an opium alkaloid. Its mechanism and locus of action have not been completely elucidated. Morphine is not very effective when given orally because of biotransformation during gastrointestinal absorption. It is converted to inactive metabolites (by *N*-demethylation and especially glucuronidation) in the liver and other tissues. The resulting water-soluble products are excreted in the urine. The dose-related adverse effects of morphine include CNS depression, decreased respiratory responsiveness to carbon dioxide, decreased cough reflex, nausea, and vomiting. Morphine also produces miosis and stimulates release of antidiuretic hormone from the hypothalamus. The hypotensive effect of morphine and related opiates is intensified by concomitant administration of phenothiazine tranquilizers. Neonates, especially premature babies, have not developed the metabolic pathways to eliminate morphine and other opiates and are unusually sensitive to them.

Treatment of morphine overdose, as with all narcotic overdoses, includes support of respiration and the use of naloxone. The common starting dose of naloxone is 0.4 mg intravenously every few minutes as needed.

Oxycodone. Oxycodone, an effective oral narcotic, is a semisynthetic derivative of morphine. Treatment of oxycodone intoxication is as in morphine overdose.

Naloxone. Naloxone has an almost pure narcotic antagonist effect, without significant agonist action. It is virtually free of the undesirable effects of the other narcotic antagonists. Its onset of action is extremely rapid when it is given intravenously. However, if narcotic reversal is too dramatic, hypertension, arrhythmias, and pulmonary edema may develop. The duration of antagonism by naloxone (15 to 20 minutes) is usually not as long as the duration of the narcotic responsible for the overdose. Therefore clinical vigilance and repeated doses of naloxone may be necessary.

Pentazocine. Pentazocine is an analgesic drug with potency similar to morphine. The *N*-allyl derivative of phenazocine, pentazocine has weak opiate antagonist but strong opioid agonist properties and is widely used in treatment. Overdose may produce symptoms similar to those of morphine and meperidine overdose. Pentazocine causes respiratory depression, sedation, dizziness, and nausea and should be used with caution in patients with raised intracranial pressure and respiratory or liver disease. Hallucinations or psychotonic effects ("active thoughts," dreaming, feeling of impending doom, depersonalization) have been reported with overdose. Pentazocine may also cause dysphoria rather than euphoria. It is capable of inducing withdrawal in narcotic abusers. Pentazocine overdose is reversible by naloxone but not by other narcotic antagonists.

Phenacetin. Phenacetin is found in many over-the-counter pain preparations. Although one of its metabolic byproducts is acetaminophen, its concentration in the liver is generally insufficient to produce hepatic necrosis and failure. The most prominent manifestation of phenacetin overdose is methemoglobinemia. Hemolysis may also occur. Massive overdoses of phenacetin are associated with cyanosis, respiratory depression, and cardiac arrest. Evidence of renal dysfunction (oliguria, anuria, brown urine) and liver dysfunction (jaundice, elevated liver enzyme concentrations) may also be found. Emergency treatment should include measures to remove the drug from the body, such as emesis, gastric lavage, and activated charcoal.

If methemoglobin levels are greater than 30% to 40%, methylene blue in a dose of 1 mg/kg should be given intravenously over a 10-minute period. If the levels remain elevated, the dose should be repeated in 1 hour.

Phencyclidine. Phencyclidine (PCP) is a synthetic amphetamine. It is a readily available street drug made in home laboratories. PCP induces a state of CNS excitation and central autonomic hyperactivity manifest as mood changes (usually euphoria but sometimes depression), anxiety, sensory distortions, visual hallucinations, delusions, depersonalization, dilation of the pupils, hypertension, and increased body temperature.

Reassurance that the bizarre thoughts, visions, and sounds are due to a drug and not to a "nervous breakdown" usually suffices to calm the patient. Short-acting barbiturates or minor tranquilizers, such as chlordiazepoxide or diazepam, may help reduce the anxiety.

Phenothiazines. The antipsychotic phenothiazines have three clinically important subgroups: aliphatics (chlorpromazine), piperazines (fluphenazine, trifluoperazine, perphenazine), and piperidines (thioridazine). The pharmacologic and toxicologic properties of the phenothiazines are qualitatively similar, but the relative potency and toxicity depend on the chemical substitution. Adverse effects include drowsiness, sedation, hypotension, reduction of convulsive seizure threshold, ocular and skin pigmentation, hepatotoxicity, blood dyscrasias, and extrapyramidal symptoms, including akathisia, dystonia, tremors, and rigidity. Phenothiazines may produce abnormalities in myocardial repolarization and induce arrhythmias. Treatment of severe reactions with diphenhydramine 50 mg intravenously or benztropine 2 mg intravenously is usually effective.

Propoxyphene. Propoxyphene is a narcotic that is related to morphine but more closely to methadone. It is clinically useful alone as an analgesic but is commonly combined with aspirin or acetaminophen. The drug's toxicity resembles that of other narcotic analgesics. It may cause sedation, nausea, and dizziness. CNS depression can be profound, but the drug does not cause significant respiratory depression. Treatment of overdose is similar to that of morphine overdose.

Salicylate. The most common cause of accidental poisoning continues to be the ingestion of aspirin (acetylsalicylic acid). The most toxic salicylate is oil of wintergreen (methylsalicylate). This compound is found in many products, such as liniments and solutions used in hot vaporizers.

Ingestion of 10 to 30 g of aspirin has been reported fatal in adults. The early symptoms of salicylism are related to CNS stimulation: vomiting, tinnitus, hyperpnea, hyperactivity, hyperthermia, and seizures. As the poisoning worsens, CNS depression, respiratory failure, and cardiovascular collapse develop. Salicylate-induced hyperpnea decreases carbon dioxide tension and plasma carbonic acid levels. The resultant alkalosis stimulates renal excretion of large quantities of base in the form of bicarbonate. Sodium, potassium, and large amounts of organic acids are lost in the urine along with bicarbonate. Blood pH tends to normalize in adults, but acidosis develops in young children and neonates. This appears to be due to the toxic effects of salicylate and loss of buffer-base.

Treatment of overdose should include early evacuation of the stomach. Oral administration of sodium bicarbonate is contraindicated because it increases salicylate absorption. If severe acidosis is present after urinary output has been established, sodium bicarbonate can be given intravenously. Potassium restoration is therefore essential for successful alkalinization of the urine. Vitamin K, 25 mg in a single intramuscular or intravenous dose, is given for bleeding caused by hypoprothrombinemia. Hemodialysis should be considered if the patient's condition appears to be deteriorating despite aggressive medical support.

Thioxanthenes. The thioxanthenes resemble the phenothiazines in chemical structure, absorption, metabolism, excretion, and chemical effects. Fever, fatigue, and drowsiness are the most common adverse effects. Treatment of overdose is supportive.

Tricyclic Antidepressants. Acute poisoning with tricyclic antidepressants (TCAs) can produce a complex, life-threatening clinical situation. The therapeutic/toxic ratio for these agents is low. A dose of 2000 mg of imipramine has been reported to be lethal. TCAs are metabolized primarily in the liver and excreted via the kidneys. Drug half-lives range from 10 to 20 hours for imipramine to 80 hours for protriptyline. The clinical presentation may include CNS toxic effects, such as hallucinations, choreoathetosis, myoclonus, seizures, or dystonia that progresses to coma and respiratory depression. Anticholinergic effects, such as dilated pupils, dry mucosae, and urinary retention, may be evident. However, the major management problems involve the heart. TCAs may induce direct myocardial depression or intractable ventricular arrhythmias. Early cardiac effects include supraventricular tachycardia and prolongation of the QRS complex. Cardiac toxicity may progress to hypotension and cardiac arrhythmias (atrial fibrillation, complete atrioventricular block, ventricular ectopy, and ventricular tachycardia).

Treatment of ventricular ectopy is complicated by the heart's underlying hyperactivity and by the fact that patients remain at risk for days. Type I antiarrhythmic agents, such as procainamide, quinidine, and disopyramide, are contraindicated because their effects are similar to those of the tricyclic antidepressants. Phenytoin and propranolol have been recommended. Atrioventricular conduction problems should be treated with standard methods, including insertion of a pacemaker for high-level blocks. Because TCAs interfere with normal function of the adrenergic synapse, response to adrenergic agonists may be severely impaired. Standard methods to remove the drug from the gastrointestinal tract should be pursued because the anticholinergic side effects slow gastrointestinal motility and delay absorption. Hemodialysis and hemoperfusion appear useless.

The treatment of neurologic effects is controversial. The anticholinesterase inhibitor physostigmine usually reverses the anticholinergic effects of TCAs.

ENVIRONMENTAL TOXINS

Ethylene Glycol. Ethylene glycol, a major constituent of antifreeze, is another alcohol that produces toxic effects similar to those of methanol. Treatment is similar.

Methyl Alcohol. Methyl alcohol, like other alcohols, produces significant CNS depression. It is rapidly absorbed via the gastrointestinal tract and skin and is metabolized to formaldehyde. Toxic effects include nausea, vomiting, metabolic acidosis, retinal damage with blindness, cerebral edema, and cardiovascular collapse. The two main treatment approaches are the administration of ethanol, which favorably competes with methanol for the enzyme alcohol dehydrogenase, and the removal of methanol and its metabolites via hemodialysis.

Organophosphates. Organophosphorous insecticides are widely used in modern agriculture. They are among the most poisonous materials commonly used for pest control. Their toxic actions to humans are similar and also similar to the effects of the chemical warfare agents known as nerve gases. The most common, parathion, is a yellow to dark brown liquid of low vapor pressure that is insoluble in water. Parathion is available commercially as the active ingredient of various dusts, wettable powders, emulsifiable concentrates, and aerosols. Parathion and its relatives inhibit the enzyme cholinesterase in all parts of the body by phosphorylating the active site. Severe respiratory distress eventually appears in major intoxications. Mucus secretion, bronchospasm, and pulmonary edema are common.

Three major principles of treatment are artificial ventilation when indicated, administration of atropine in large doses to control the cardiovascular and visceral actions of the poison, and injection of pralidoxime chloride (2-PAM) or a related systemic anticholinesterase antidote.

Petroleum Distillates. A group of straight or branched chain aliphatic hydrocarbons is produced by the fractional distillation of petroleum. Major toxic effects of these agents include chemical pneumonitis and CNS dysfunction manifest as lethargy and stupor. Rare effects are coma and cardiovascular, hepatic, renal, and bone marrow toxicity.

The major therapeutic decision in the management of an acute poisoning is whether to remove the material from the stomach. In general, emesis or lavage should be used only for large-volume intake or for a mixed ingestion including aromatic hydrocarbons or insecticides. Corticosteroids and prophylactic antibiotics are of no benefit and should not be administered.

Plants. Plants and fungi are responsible for the most common intoxications treated in poison control centers. Between 5% and 10% of emergency room evaluations for poisonings are related to this class.

The initial treatment of the patient is the same as for any serious poisoning or ingestion: stabilization of the airway and the respiratory and cardiovascular systems. Because the list of plants and fungi is long, specific treatments should be guided by the poison control center recommendation. (A list of current emergency telephone numbers can be found in the *Physicians' Desk Reference* immediately after the table of contents.)

SUGGESTED READINGS

Comstock EG, Boisaubin EV: Guide to management of drug overdose. In Physicians' desk reference. Oradell, NJ, 1990, Medical Economics Co, p. 2473

Freas GC: Poisoning. In Chernow B (ed): The pharmacologic approach to the critically ill patient, ed. 2. Baltimore, 1988, Williams & Wilkins, p. 743

Goodman LS, Gilman A (eds): The pharmacological basis of therapeutics. New York, 1985, Macmillan

18

CRITICAL CARE MANAGEMENT OF TRAUMATIZED PATIENTS

COLIN F. MACKENZIE, MD

ASSESSMENT OF TRAUMATIC INJURY

Assessment of injury is essential for allocation of therapeutic resources, prediction of outcome, and comparison of trauma care delivery. Since trauma mortality and morbidity are functions of both injury severity and quality of medical care, survival rates and quality of care among facilities, emergency medical services, and states or countries can be compared only if the statistical analysis controls for patient injury severity. The development of scoring systems in trauma care has enabled clinicians, epidemiologists, and health service researchers to obtain objective evidence for allocation and evaluation of trauma care services.

Several indexes of injury currently in use compare the extent of and outcome from injury. These include the Glasgow Coma Scale, Injury Severity Score, Anatomic Index, Trauma Score, and the revised Acute Physiology and Chronic Health Evaluation Index (APACHE II). These indexes permit numeric descriptions of the overall severity of injury in patients who have multiple injuries and physiologic derangements. The Glasgow Coma Scale (GCS) is incorporated into many of the other indexes and is a simple index useful for assessing head-injured patients (see Chapter 5). The Trauma Score, based on systolic blood pressure, respiratory rate, respiratory effort, capillary refill, and GCS, has been shown to be a good predictor of survival from blunt trauma. The Trauma Score is useful to identify anomalous outcomes in the management of patients with multiple sites of trauma. The Injury Severity Score (ISS) excludes patients dead on arrival and has been

used successfully to compare outcome from trauma in different states and countries. Patients with ISS in excess of 20 should receive specialized trauma critical care. Twelve variables make up the APACHE II scoring system. The score and the acute risk of death rise on the basis of initial physiologic abnormality, chronic health problems, and advanced age. APACHE II is not specifically designed for trauma patients but is used to assess severity of disease. The indexes used for assessment of injuries and their limitations are summarized in Table 18–1.

RESPIRATORY MANAGEMENT

Problems with Traditional Respiratory Care in Trauma Patients

Many trauma patients are unable to tolerate the traditional approaches to prevention of hypoxemia and lung collapse. Unconsciousness, loss of laryngeal reflexes, facial injury, and lack of cooperation make incentive spirometry, intermittent positive-pressure breathing (IPPB), and face mask continuous positive airway pressure (CPAP) or positive end-expiratory pressure (PEEP) ineffective. Critical illness following trauma frequently requires tracheal intubation and mechanical ventilation. The alternatives for managing common respiratory complications after trauma are described in the following paragraphs.

Mobilization

Several therapeutic maneuvers may be used to minimize respiratory dysfunction in the trauma patient with bone fractures. The sim-

TABLE 18–1. Indexes Used for Assessment of Injury and Prediction of Outcome or Severity of Disease

INDEX	COMMENT
Glasgow Coma Scale (GCS)	Brainstem reflexes not analyzed; no left/right differentiation in motor response; facial trauma and tracheal intubation restrict assessment of eye opening and verbal response
Injury Severity Scale	Excludes patients dead on arrival; ranking of severity based on subjective impressions; correlates well with outcome only in patient groups with low mortality; combination of moderately severe injuries may result in a higher score than a fatal head injury
Anatomic Index	Most useful when assessing patients with blunt trauma and head injury such as may occur in road traffic accidents; index correlates with outcome when mortality rate is in excess of 20%
Trauma Score	Includes GCS so has same limitations; may be useful as a mechanism for assessment of patient triage and to identify anomalous outcomes in treatment of patients with multiple trauma sites
APACHE	Not specifically designed for trauma patients; score is changed by therapeutic intervention during initial resuscitation; determination of score begins only when patient reaches an ICU; requires a mixed patient population; not good at predicting individual patient outcome

plest is mobilization. Early fracture reduction is essential to facilitate mobilization postoperatively. Traction devices should allow side-to-side turning and postural drainage while maintaining bone alignment. Such devices include internal and exoskeletal fixation, Neufeld's and Buck's traction, and spinal rods. Coordination of respiratory care among critical care specialist, orthopedist, neurosurgeon, and general surgeon is mandatory. The critical care specialist must synthesize these specialists' individual ideal wishes and with the help of physical therapists must attempt to minimize restrictions on mobilization.

Chest Physiotherapy

Chest physiotherapy is used prophylactically and therapeutically to clear secretions and reverse atelectasis in trauma patients. Chest physiotherapy includes postural drainage, which positions the affected lung lobe or segment uppermost. While the patient is in one of the 11 specific postural drainage positions, manual external chest percussion and vibration are carried out. The tracheobronchial tree is suctioned to remove any loosened secretions, and coughing is encouraged. Indications for therapy include deterioration of clinical and radiologic findings concerning the chest, hypoxemia, acute atelectasis, early pneumonia, and lung contusion.

Chest physiotherapy is useful for prophylaxis in patients who have chronic sputum-producing lung disease and are immobilized because of trauma. Obese patients and those with depressed levels of consciousness also benefit from prophylactic maneuvers to expand the lung and clear secretions after trauma. Patients with smoke inhalation and aspiration of gastric contents require chest physiotherapy. The acutely quadriplegic patient has a shorter recovery and is less likely to require tracheostomy if prophylactic chest physiotherapy is employed.

Chest physiotherapy is beneficial even for patients with sternal, rib, and clavicular fractures (Fig. 18–1). Chest physiotherapy improves ventilation/perfusion relationships with lung contusion. Compared to outcome reports from other centers use of chest physiotherapy reduces the mortality rate when used in combination with mechanical ventilation and PEEP.

Chest physiotherapy is useful in reversing acute atelectasis. It is also beneficial in the early stages of pneumonia-like conditions in patients with trauma. The advantages of chest physiotherapy over bronchoscopy are that detrimental cardiopulmonary changes occur less frequently and no physician participation is required. Bronchoscopy is usually less efficacious and more hazardous than chest physiotherapy when the patient has low lung compliance, poor gas exchange, and air bronchograms visible on chest roentgenogram.

Flail Chest

Flail chest is a descriptive term for the paradoxic movement of a thorax segment that occurs with respiration. The flail segment moves in with inspiration as subatmospheric pressure is generated in the pleura and moves out with exhalation and positive pleural pressure. Because positive-pressure mechanical ventilation prevents generation of subatmospheric pressures greater than -5 cm H_2O, paradoxic movement of the flail segment is reduced during positive-pressure respiration. The so-called internal pneumatic stabilization provided by positive pressure stabilizes the flail segment. Additional PEEP may be required to reduce hypoxemia.

A

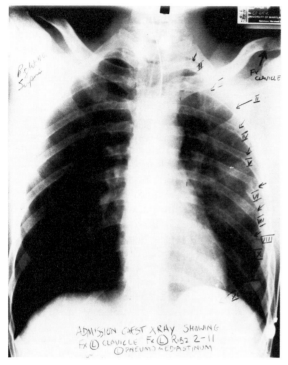

B

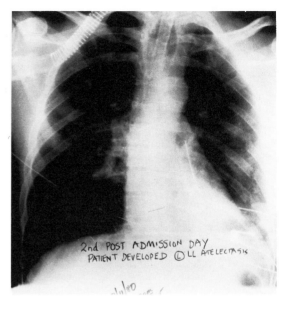

C

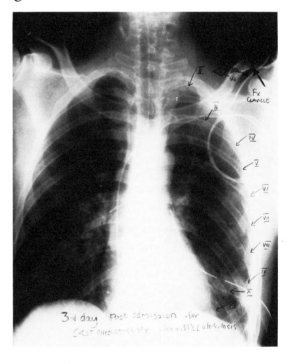

Figure 18–1. **A,** Admission portable chest roentgenogram taken in the anteroposterior supine position shows fractures of left clavicle and ribs 2 to 11. A pneumomediastinum, most visible around the aortic knob, is present in the left lung. A left lung contusion is apparent underlying fractured ribs 5 to 7. **B,** A left lower lobe segmental atelectasis developed the day after admission, and the patient became hypoxemic despite controlled mechanical ventilation and routine turning and suctioning. A chest tube was placed in the left lung but the pneumomediastinum persisted. A pulmonary artery catheter was placed to exclude cardiac causes for deteriorating pulmonary function (see Fig. 18–1, *C*). **C,** Chest physiotherapy, including postural drainage, percussion, coughing, and tracheal suctioning, was carried out despite the clavicular fracture, multiple rib fractures, pneumomediastinum, and deteriorating pulmonary function. This chest roentgenogram was taken within 12 hours of a single treatment with chest physiotherapy and shows clearance of the left lower lobe atelectasis and radiologic improvement in the left lung contusion. Respiratory function improved, and the patient was extubated 5 days after admission.

Flail chest reduces functional residual capacity (FRC), resulting in alveolar collapse. Vital capacity (VC) is reduced, and efforts to increase minute ventilation are inefficient, increasing work of breathing and oxygen consumption. The determinant of need for tracheal intubation and mechanical ventilation is the degree of underlying lung injury that accompanies the flail chest.

Patients with little underlying lung injury may be satisfactorily managed without mechanical ventilation if adequate analgesia is provided with epidural local anesthetics and narcotics. Oxygen administration and breathing exercises with supportive coughing may be all that are required to maintain a clear chest. Intercostal nerve blocks are not a satisfactory way to provide analgesia because they are too short lived and potentially complicated by iatrogenic pneumothorax (see Chapter 28).

The major goal in the management of flail chest is prevention of secretion retention and infection. A question is whether physical maneuvers to clear secretions should be performed on a patient with a flail chest. Fractured ribs are displaced during inspiration, exhalation, and turning, both with mechanical ventilation and during spontaneous ventilation. The rib displacement that occurs during coughing, defecation, sitting up, and lying down may be considerably more than can be achieved with chest physiotherapy maneuvers such as chest percussion. No one would dispute that the jagged edge of a fractured rib is hazardous, but the additional hazard associated with percussion is overrated. When correctly performed by a trained therapist, chest percussion is not forceful because the air trapped in the cupped hand cushions the hand's impact. Novice therapists and nontherapists may perform percussion incorrectly, which should be especially avoided in the patient with flail chest. Chest percussion may be most beneficial in the management of flail chest, since it is frequently the lung underlying the rib fractures that requires the therapy (Fig. 18–1). Chest vibration is a more forceful maneuver in which the chest wall is manually compressed. Vibration should not be performed over rib fractures.

Application of positive pressure is the mainstay of ventilatory management. Some authorities advocate CPAP administered through a face mask. The duration of positive pressure application is determined by the amount of thoracic injury, the patient's pulmonary status before the injury, and the presence of trauma to other systems. Face mask CPAP is frequently not well tolerated. Intermittent mandatory ventilation (IMV) is also sometimes inappropriate for a large-segment flail, since paradoxic movement occurs during generation of subatmospheric pressures with spontaneous respiration. Controlled mechanical ventilation with PEEP is still the "gold standard" against which other therapies for flail chest are compared.

Lung Contusion

Hemorrhage and interstitial and pulmonary edema occur in lung contusion. The cause may be rapid deceleration associated with falls or high-speed automobile accidents. Blast injury or high-velocity missiles can also cause lung contusion. The mechanism in most cases is rapid deceleration that causes sudden compression and expansion or an implosion effect in lung parenchyma.

In the early stages of lung contusion no radiologic evidence of lung damage may be apparent, particularly when the patient has been rapidly evacuated by helicopter from the accident scene. The patient may not have fractured ribs or any external signs of injury. Contusion is one of the common results of blunt chest trauma. The diagnosis of lung contusion is based on five criteria: (1) history of blunt chest trauma, (2) appearance of radiologic infiltrates that have a nonsegmental distribution and are commonly seen 6 or more hours after injury (Fig. 18–2),

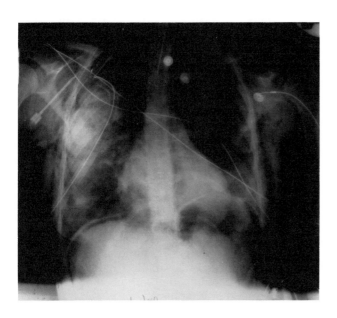

Figure 18–2. Admission film of a 28-year-old woman transported by helicopter directly from a road traffic accident. A contusion is present in the right lung. A right mainstem bronchus rupture and diffuse subcutaneous mediastinal pericardial and subdiaphragmatic air also appear in this erect portable chest roentgenogram.

(3) bloody tracheal secretions on suctioning of the tracheobronchial tree, (4) crackles on auscultation of the chest, and (5) progressive hypoxemia.

Radiologic evidence often underestimates the extent of lung contusion. Rib fractures and external signs of injury correlate poorly with lung injury found at autopsy. Hypoxemia results from intraalveolar hemorrhage, atelectasis, and parenchymal edema. Chest physiotherapy is efficacious in managing the atelectasis and retention of bloody secretions that occur with lung contusion. The patient should be examined carefully for transbronchial aspiration of blood after chest physiotherapy. If this occurs, the opposite "good" lung segment should be treated with postural drainage, chest percussion and vibration, and removal of loosened bloody secretions by suction. Transbronchial aspiration is most likely to occur when coagulopathy accompanies blunt trauma and may confuse the radiologic diagnosis of lung contusion by showing a segmental distribution. Lung laceration and traumatic cysts may accompany severe lung contusion. If the blood within the contused lung is not removed, it acts as a culture medium, leading to infection as a common sequela.

Fluid management of the patient with a lung contusion remains controversial. Some advocate diuretics, fluid restriction, and use of plasma, blood, and albumin to maintain colloid pressure. I have found that restriction is ineffective and increases the incidence of other organ failure. In most level I trauma centers fluid therapy is monitored by a fluid challenge technique guided by measurement of pulmonary wedge pressure and cardiac output. The fluid challenge is described later in the section on assessment of cardiac reserve. Cardiac output and tissue oxygen delivery are adjusted with the fluid challenge while respiratory dysfunction is minimized with careful monitoring of wedge pressure. The mortality rate from lung contusion at my institution was reduced to 10% of 132 consecutive patients with lung contusion when these fluid management techniques were used with positive-pressure ventilation and chest physiotherapy. This compares favorably with the 20% to 50% mortality rates reported by other medical centers.

Airway Disruption

Several mechanisms for airway disruption have been proposed. Compression of the thoracic cage may cause widening of the transverse dimensions, producing lateral traction on the airway. If the glottis is closed at the moment of impact, airway compression between the sternum and vertebral column causes airway rupture. Another theory suggests that rapid deceleration of the lung causes torsion and shearing, which are greatest at the carina. A combination of these mechanisms may well occur. Bronchoscopy is the most reliable means of establishing the site, nature, and extent of airway disruption and should be performed when the diagnosis is suspected.

After penetrating trauma, airway injury is usually obvious. Blunt trauma involving rapid deceleration should raise the suspicion of airway rupture. A vertical partial tear in the membranous portion or complete transection of the mainstem bronchus may occur (see Fig. 18–2). The history and physical and radiologic examinations reveal dyspnea, pneumothorax, pneumomediastinum, and subcutaneous emphysema. A collapsed lung cannot be reexpanded despite tube thoracostomy and pleural drainage. Rupture of a mainstem bronchus occurs in 80% of patients with airway disruption; rupture of the trachea occurs in 15%. Fractures of the first, second, or third rib are present in 53% of patients with bronchial rupture. More than 80% of traumatic airway ruptures occur within 2.5 cm of the carina.

Thoracotomy is indicated to repair the rupture unless the patient is too unstable or the bronchial tear involves less than one third of the bronchial circumference and the air leak can be controlled by tube thoracostomy. In one study half of cases of airway rupture were undiagnosed until 1 month after injury. This state of affairs should clearly be avoided by early diagnosis with fiberoptic bronchoscopy. With delayed diagnosis bronchial stenosis and infected bronchopleural fistula make management difficult. Double-lumen tracheal tubes, endobronchial intubation, high-frequency ventilation, and endobronchial insufflation are used as means to maintain ventilation, occlude the tear, or reduce airway pressure and airway leakage.

Pneumothorax

Pneumothorax may occur secondary to trauma. At my level I trauma center it was the most frequently missed diagnosis in the field management of patients who died after motor vehicle accidents. Details of pathophysiology, diagnosis, and therapy for pneumothorax are presented in Chapter 3.

Hemothorax

Traumatic pneumothoraces are usually associated with some degree of hemothorax. Clinical findings indicating pleural fluid include diminished chest movement, tracheal deviation from the fluid if this is voluminous, and absence of palpable breath sounds. Stony dullness to percussion may clear when the patient is turned if the pleural fluid is not loculated (so-called shifting dullness). Breath sounds are absent over fluid, but bronchial breathing is heard above the fluid. A thoracotomy is required if the hemothorax is greater than 1000 ml or loss of at least 150 ml/h continues for 4 or more hours.

Ruptured Diaphragm

The mechanism for ruptured diaphragm is thought to be abdominal trauma accentuated by tensing of the abdominal musculature. Victims aware of an impending crash carry out the Valsalva maneuver. Other authorities have suggested that diaphragm ruptures occur more frequently in thoracic trauma. In 44 patients treated for diaphragm rupture over 5 years at a level I trauma center, 75% of ruptures were on the left side, eight were on the right side, and two were through the central tendon. The liver seems to protect the right hemidiaphragm. All but one of these diaphragm ruptures were caused by motor vehicle accidents.

Clinical signs and symptoms include tachypnea, cyanosis, tracheal shift, diminution in breath sounds, and bowel sounds on auscultation of the chest. In practice, these classic signs are rarely seen. More frequently, nonspecific findings such as associated chest and abdominal injuries and hypotension lead to a suspicion of diaphragm rupture. Chest roentgenograms are helpful, although in the previously mentioned series it established the diagnosis in only 32% (14 of 44 patients). Other means of diagnosis were by egress of peritoneal lavage fluid through a chest tube and as an incidental finding at surgery. Diagnostic peritoneal lavage was positive in only 50% of patients. In about 7% of patients the diagnosis of ruptured diaphragm is initially missed. If the diagnosis is in doubt, it can be confirmed by contrast studies or computed tomographic (CT) scans. Only 43% of patients (19 of 44) had herniation of viscera into the left side of the chest. Treatment is surgical repair to prevent visceral herniation, incarceration, and strangulation. Other complications include wound infection, diaphragmatic abscess, and pneumonia.

Bronchopleural Fistula, Empyema, and Lung Abscess

Bronchopleural fistula, empyema, and lung abscess are considered together because they are often concurrent events after trauma. A lung contusion gives rise to a traumatic cyst, which becomes infected and develops into a lung abscess. The lung abscess may rupture into the pleura, causing an empyema. The empyema drains through an empyema tube, and a bronchopleural fistula may occur. A scenario can also be envisioned in which a traumatic rupture of the airway is the primary traumatic insult. This becomes infected, resulting in lung abscess and empyema. Chest physiotherapy is highly successful in draining a lung abscess that communicates with the tracheobronchial tree.

Empyema may occur as a complication of pneumococcal pneumonia. Lung abscess may also be caused by infection with capsular type 3 pneumococcal pneumonia. *Staphylococcus aureus, Klebsiella pneumoniae, Pseudomonas aeroginosa,* and *Haemophilus influenzae* are the major organisms causing empyema and lung abscess following trauma.

CARDIAC MANAGEMENT

Cardiac trauma is a frequently suspected but seldom proved result of blunt trauma. Cardiac dysfunction is, however, a major management problem.

Assessment of Cardiac Reserve

The fluid challenge is an objective method of determining reserve cardiac function. In association with other clinical signs the fluid challenge can be used to determine the need for fluid infusion, fluid restriction, or inotropic support. In its simplest form only a central venous pressure monitor is required. In its most sophisticated form the fluid challenge uses cardiac output and blood gas measurements before and after challenge guided by pulmonary artery and wedge pressure readings. Starling function curves of the left and right sides of the heart may be constructed. The four outcome possibilities following fluid infusion of crystalloid or colloid are shown in Figure 18–3. Fluids are given with a 50 ml syringe at a rate of 50 ml/min in 250 ml increments. Fluid infusion continues until wedge or central venous pressure rises at least 2 mm Hg above the prechallenge pressure and remains elevated for 5 minutes after fluid infusion ceases.

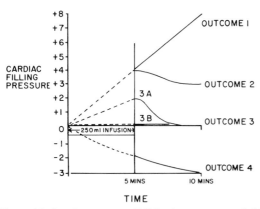

Figure 18–3. Outcome possibilities in response to fluid challenge. (From Mackenzie CF et al: J Neurosurg 1985;62:843-849.)

In outcome 1, wedge pressure rises and, 5 minutes after infusion ceases, cardiac filling pressure remains elevated without any increase in cardiac output. This response indicates that the heart has limited reserve function and is unable to increase contractility to respond to the increased cardiac filling pressures. Further infusion is expected to result in acute pulmonary edema. The therapeutic indication this response dictates is to restrict further fluid infusion and reduce myocardial depressant agents, such as morphine. If the trend continues, the use of inotropic agents, such as intravenous dopamine, to increase myocardial contractility should be considered.

In outcome 2, wedge pressure rises 3 to 4 mm Hg or more but then falls within 5 minutes to a level 2 mm Hg above the baseline. This response indicates that myocardial contractility is adequate for the increase in cardiac preload. The suggested treatment is to infuse fluids and maintain cardiac filling pressures within this range for optimum cardiac function and tissue oxygen supply.

In outcome 3, wedge pressure is unchanged (3B in Fig. 18–3) or rises immediately but then falls to the baseline (3A) following fluid challenge. This response indicates that the patient has considerable reserve cardiac function and that a greater circulating volume could be tolerated. The indication for therapy, if the patient is oliguric or has evidence of poor tissue perfusion (acidosis or low mixed venous oxygen tension), is not to give inotropic agents, but rather to infuse fluid until the ventricular function curve demonstrated in outcome 2 is obtained.

In outcome 4, wedge pressure is initially unchanged with fluid infusion, but systemic arterial pressure rises with increasing increments of fluid and the pulse rate falls. After an infusion of 500 ml or more, WP falls to a level 2 to 3 mm Hg below the baseline and cardiac output is increased. Although this response is uncommon (less than 5% of patients), it suggests that improved myocardial perfusion and cardiac function occur as a result of either systemic vasodilation caused by rapid fluid infusion or slowing of the heart rate. The Frank-Starling function curve shifts to the left, and cardiac output increases with decreased filling pressures. Further therapeutic intervention is usually not required because the increased cardiac output improves oxygen delivery and tissue perfusion.

The fluid challenge technique is useful in a variety of traumatic injuries (Fig. 18–3 and Table 18–2). If pulmonary edema occurs during fluid challenge, fluid infusion should be stopped. The patient is placed sitting up if possible, and oxygenation is monitored. If

TABLE 18–2. Physiologic Changes Before and After Resuscitation from Shock in Eight Patients

VARIABLE	BEFORE RESUSCITATION	AFTER RESUSCITATION	p VALUE
$\dot{V}_{DS}/\dot{V}_{T}$	46.0 ± 9.40	40.0 ± 13.70	< .05
$\dot{Q}_{S}/\dot{Q}_{T}$ (%)	18.1 ± 4.25	15.1 ± 3.80	< .05
Part (mm Hg)	77.0 ± 18.20	106.0 ± 22.30	NS
CI (L/min/m²)	3.9 ± 1.97	5.2 ± 2.27	< .05
$Paco_2$ (mm Hg)	36.1 ± 7.53	36.1 ± 7.75	NS
Cao_2 - $C\bar{v}o_2$ (ml/dl)	4.9 ± 2.20	4.5 ± 2.10	NS
Cao_2 × Qt (ml O₂/min)	1076.0 ± 32.80	1526.0 ± 39.10	< .05
$\dot{V}o_2$ (ml O₂/min)	325.0 ± 18.00	421.0 ± 20.50	< .05

From Mackenzie CF, Shin B: Crit Care Med 1980; 8:271.

An average volume of 700 ml (range 250 to 1400 ml) of plasma protein solution was given over 20 minutes until shock was reversed and wedge pressure remained elevated 2 mm Hg above baseline.

$\dot{V}_{D}/\dot{V}_{T}$ = dead space, $\dot{Q}_{S}/\dot{Q}_{T}$ = intrapulmonary shunt, Part = mean arterial pressure, CI = cardiac index, Cao_2 × $\dot{Q}_{T}$ = O₂ delivery, $\dot{V}o_2$ = oxygen consumption, NS = not significant.

necessary oxygenation is improved by increasing the inspired oxygen fraction. If the patient has a tracheal tube, positive pressure is applied to restore the Starling forces across the alveolar capillary membrane and reverse transudation of fluid into the alveolus. If before fluid challenge the patient is known to have limited reserve cardiac function (flat Starling function curve), leg raising and pneumatic trouser inflation are reversible means of increasing cardiac filling pressures in combination with fluid challenge. Should cardiac failure or pulmonary edema result, the increased cardiac filling pressures are readily reversible by deflation of the trousers or lowering of the legs. In mechanically ventilated patients, endpoints for fluid challenge include failure of cardiac output to rise, elevation of mixed venous oxygen saturation above 75%, and wedge pressure of 25 mm Hg or evidence of pulmonary edema, such as a sudden fall in lung/thorax compliance.

Shock

Hypovolemic shock is depletion of intravascular volume with failure of physiologic compensatory mechanisms and inadequate blood flow to organs. Tissue and cellular oxygen delivery and consumption are impaired. Traumatic shock includes the physiologic deficits found in hypovolemia. In addition, hemorrhage causes anemia, restricting oxygen carriage. Tissue injury contributes to shock by causing microemboli and release of vasoactive substances, including kinins, prostanoids, leukotrienes, and endorphins. The cell membrane requires adenosine triphosphate (ATP) to function and maintain homeostasis across the cell. Production of ATP requires oxygen and glucose transport to the cell, and this mechanism fails during shock. Intracellular lactate levels rise and pH falls. Free radicals accumulate after ischemic cell injury and may damage the cell membrane, enzyme systems, and mitochondria. Shock is a continuum of pathophysiologic changes that become progressively severe unless the causative factor is treated and resuscitation is undertaken. Hypovolemic patients have rapid, shallow breathing and may have normal or low blood pressure. Tachycardia and peripheral vasoconstriction are present. Cardiac filling pressures are maintained by constriction of the venous capacitance vessels, but cardiac output is low. The patient is oliguric and has pale, clammy skin. If mixed venous saturation is monitored, it is lower than normal because of low cardiac output. Capillary refill time is prolonged. In young adults blood pressure is not a good indicator of shock because sympathoadrenal responses cause vasoconstriction and maintain normal blood pressures. In severe shock decompensation occurs. Patients usually do not suddenly "crash"; rather it is the clinician who fails to recognize the compensated state of shock.

Diagnosis of shock is usually based on clinical findings. Additional factors accompany shock depending on the cause. In hypovolemic shock, clinical signs include narrow pulse pressure, low cardiac output, oliguria, pale clammy skin, and increased peripheral resistance. In septic shock many of the signs result from release of vasoactive peptides or lysosomal enzymes from damaged, ischemic, or infected tissue. Vasodilation and increased capillary permeability and vascular capacity occur in septic shock. Metabolic acidosis, fall in platelet count, and coagulopathy may also accompany shock.

Therapy and investigation of the cause of shock should occur simultaneously. The goals of therapy are to restore circulating volume, optimize cardiac filling pressure, and increase oxygen delivery to the ischemic tissues. Oxygenation should be supplied via face mask or if indicated by tracheal intubation and administration of 100% oxygen. At least two large-bore (14-gauge or larger) intravenous tubes should be inserted for rapid infusion. Multiple intravenous sites above and below the diaphragm on the right and left sides of the body ensure circulating volume replacement.

Many centers use single infusion sites and large-bore intravenous tubing (5 mm inner diameter compared with the standard 3.2 mm inner diameter) in conjunction with short French 8- to 10-gauge catheters. Infusion rates of 1200 to 1400 ml/min can be obtained. In hemorrhagic and traumatic shock blood should be transfused to maintain hematocrit values of about 30%. Coagulation should be monitored, and if necessary fresh-frozen plasma and platelets administered. The endpoint of rapid volume infusion is reversal of the clinical signs of shock.

Monitoring should include blood pressure, venous pressure, urinary output, creatinine clearance, hematocrit, hemoglobin level, arterial and mixed venous blood gas concentrations, coagulation profile, and electrolyte levels. If shock remains despite rapid volume infusion and evidence of diminished cardiac reserve is found, dopamine or dobutamine 2 to 15 µg/kg/min is administered to improve ventricular function. If the patient's condition does not stabilize rapidly, a pulmonary artery catheter should be inserted. In septic shock the source of the sepsis must be found and treated with appropriate antibiotics and drainage when indicated. In hemorrhagic shock the bleeding should be controlled by external pressure and surgical intervention.

One group of researchers examined $\dot{V}/\dot{Q}$ relationships after experimental hemorrhage using the Wagner-West multiple insert gas technique. Their data show that a homogeneous shift of $\dot{V}/\dot{Q}$ occurs in hemorrhagic shock to a higher mean $\dot{V}/\dot{Q}$ in all lung regions. The dead space is increased in shock and decreases with resuscitation. With successful reversal of shock, cardiac output increases and pulmonary blood flow delivers more carbon dioxide to the alveolus so that end-tidal carbon dioxide and mixed expired carbon dioxide increase. After resuscitation, end-tidal carbon dioxide more nearly equals arterial carbon dioxide. Intrapulmonary shunt decreases with shock but increases with resuscitation.

When the fluid challenge technique described previously was used on eight patients in a trauma critical care unit, cardiorespiratory function was measured before and after resuscitation from shock. Shock was defined in these patients as a systolic blood pressure less than 100 mm Hg and mixed venous oxygen partial pressure ($P\bar{v}_{O_2}$) less than 35 mm Hg. An average of 700 ml (range 250 to 1400 ml) colloid (Plasmanate) was given in 20 minutes. The findings are summarized in Table 18–2. Mean blood pressure rose, and shunt fell significantly from 18.1% to 15.1%. Cardiac index (CI) rose from 3.9 to 5.2 L/min/m^2. Arterial carbon dioxide tension (Pa_{CO_2}) and arteriovenous oxygen content difference ($Ca_{O_2} - C\bar{v}_{O_2}$) were unchanged despite the significant changes in cardiac output, intrapulmonary shunt ($\dot{Q}s/\dot{Q}T$), and dead space (V_{DS}/V_T). The probable explanation for the lack of change in Pa_{CO_2} and $Ca_{O_2} - C\bar{v}_{O_2}$ that resuscitation restored perfusion to previously ischemic tissues so that increased oxygen consumption and carbon dioxide production resulted.

Why there should be differences between the animal and human model is not clear. One explanation may be that the humans did not have hemorrhagic shock. Cardiac output was high, and therefore the heterogenous distribution of $\dot{V}/\dot{Q}$ may merely have resulted from loss of autoregulatory pulmonary vasoconstrictor reflexes. In the animals with hemorrhagic shock the change in $\dot{V}/\dot{Q}$ was homogeneous.

Drugs Used in Shock and Following Trauma

NALOXONE

Naloxone is a specific and highly selective antagonist of the μ opiate receptor. Beta-endorphin levels are increased following trauma and contribute to the pathophysiology of shock. Naloxone reverses hypotension, and this action is stereospecific. Only the L form of naloxone is active, suggesting that specific, probably central receptors are involved. In dogs, naloxone increases mean arterial blood pressure and improves left ventricular contractility, stroke volume, and cardiac output with no effect on heart rate or pulmonary wedge pressure. Acidosis, with elevated lactate levels and low body temperature, limits the pressor response to naloxone. A bolus of 0.3 mg/kg is followed by a continuous infusion to produce vasoactive effects. Several anecdotal reports have described benefit from naloxone in hemorrhagic shock, but no study has shown benefits in humans.

STEROIDS

In experimental hemorrhagic shock methylprednisolone 30 mg/kg 1 hour before and up to roughly ½ hour after blood loss, in association with adequate volume replacement, significantly improves survival. However, when steroids are given later, hemodynamic or metabolic effects are not consistently reproducible. Glucocorticoids may therefore be of benefit if given in the field within ½ hour of injury, but their usefulness by the time the patient reaches a hospital is more controversial. Recent studies showed no benefit of corticosteroids in improving outcome from severe sepsis or septic shock. However, other authors found that steroid treatment resulted in an overall mortality rate of 10.5% (9 of 86 patients) compared with 38.4% (33 of 86) in a control group receiving saline solution. In my institution steroids are not routinely used in therapy for shock.

OTHER PHARMACOLOGY AGENTS

Other, more recent therapies for shock include antibody therapy and treatment with fibrinolytic enzymes. Antilipopolysaccharide reduces mortality and morbidity rates in gram-negative bacterial infections. In conjunction with conventional therapy it may reduce the current 50% mortality rate in humans. Therapeutic fibrinolysis can be achieved by administration of urokinase and streptokinase. In human studies 47% of patients receiving streptokinase therapy survived refractory shock from trauma and infection and adult respiratory distress syndrome (ARDS). Since survival in shock patients with ARDS is reported to be only 4% to 21%, streptokinase therapy may be beneficial.

Myocardial Ischemia

During shock, neural, humoral, metabolic, and peripheral vascular changes progressively disrupt myocardial contraction. Cardiac dysfunction has been verified experimentally and clinically. Laboratory studies of the mechanisms of shock have documented impaired coronary perfusion and myocardial ischemia. Recent reports suggest that endogenous opiates and free radical–generating systems may be involved. Other hypotheses include reduction in myocardial perfusion pressure, production of circulatory depressant factors, and altered myocardial responsiveness to sympathetic stimulation. Subcellular mechanisms suggest that the excitation-contraction coupling processes of the heart are affected. Potential mechanisms include impaired myocardial substrate utilization, hypoglycemia, disseminated intravascular coagulation, and altered prostaglandin-thromboxane systems. Many complex, multifunctional relationships are involved. To date, no single mechanism is postulated to cause myocardial depression.

Myocardial Contusion

Blunt chest trauma is the usual cause of myocardial contusion. The injury should be suspected in any patient with high-speed injuries to the anterior chest, particularly if sternal fracture occurs. Often ventricular dysrhythmias, ischemic electrocardiographic changes, and chest pain (in a conscious patient) occur. The contused area is analogous to an ischemic, hypokinetic or akinetic area of myocardium in myocardial infarction. The heart may therefore be subject to pump failure and require inotropic support and antiarrhythmic drugs such as lidocaine.

Diagnosis of myocardial contusion should be made, since its presence affects anesthetic and critical care management. Diagnostic techniques include electrocardiography, which shows nonspecific ST and T wave changes, sinus bradycardia, premature beats, and heart block. No diagnostic test specific for cardiac contusion has a high degree of accuracy. Myocardial injury

is likely if the MB component of creatine phosphokinase (CPK) is 5% or more of the total CPK concentration and lactic dehydrogenase (LDH) and LDH_2 levels are elevated. Radionuclide scanning is not helpful in diagnosing myocardial contusion. Two-dimensional echocardiography and radionuclide angiography, the diagnostic tools of choice, show depression in the ejection fraction or evidence of dyskinesia. Transmural infarction from blunt cardiac injury is a rare entity. Serial electrocardiograms should be obtained for 3 to 4 days and serial measurements of CPK and LDH isoenzymes performed if myocardial contusion is suspected.

The therapy for myocardial contusion is directed at its complications. Observation, electrocardiographic monitoring, and appropriate therapy for dysrhythmias may be required. If cardiac failure develops, management is with pulmonary artery catheterization and inotropic support. A pacemaker may be used to control heart block, and an intraaortic balloon pump is employed to support extreme cardiac dysfunction. Myocardial oxygenation should be optimized by intravascular volume support, maintaining a hemoglobin level of 12 to 15 g/dl. Pulmonary support should be optimal.

If surgery and anesthesia are required, a pulmonary artery catheter should be inserted. Elective surgery should be postponed until cardiac evaluation is complete. Pulmonary artery catheters are also inserted in patients with myocardial contusion when they are receiving mechanical ventilation, have multiple injuries, and have evidence of cardiac or renal insufficiency.

The diagnosis of myocardial contusion is often suspected but rarely proved. Seventeen patients (10%) had myocardial contusion found at autopsy among 173 consecutive deaths following helicopter transport to the hospital after road accidents. An electrocardiogram should be obtained in survivors 3 to 4 weeks after myocardial contusion to rule out infarction. Long-term follow-up with radionuclide angiography is indicated to detect ventricular aneurysms and infarction.

Cardiac Tamponade

Penetrating trauma is the most common cause of cardiac tamponade, although it may occur in association with blunt chest trauma and rupture of the thoracic aorta. Tamponade occurs when the pericardium contains sufficient volume to prevent the ventricles from filling adequately during diastole. Stroke volume and cardiac output fall, and hypotension occurs. The heart sounds are distant, and neck veins are distended. Pericardiocentesis relieves the tamponade but is only a temporary measure. Intravenous fluid should be given to maintain high cardiac filling pressure.

Cardiac tamponade is diagnosed by pulmonary artery catheterization, electrocardiography, echocardiography and chest roentgenogram, which shows cardiomegaly. Pulmonary artery catheterization shows low cardiac output and stroke volume, equalization of pulmonary artery and ventricular diastolic pressures, and a right ventricular diastolic/systolic pressure ratio > 1:3. Central venous and wedge pressures are elevated. An electrocardiogram shows decreased voltage and may show electrical alternans. An echocardiogram shows pericardial fluid.

Hemorrhagic tamponade requires a thoracotomy. Subacute tamponade (effusion) is managed initially with pericardiocentesis. The effusion is drained by pericardial window if needle aspiration fails to relieve the tamponade. The chronic presence of blood, inflammation, or infection in the pericardium results in constrictive pericarditis. Definitive management of constrictive pericarditis is removal of the pericardium.

Fat Embolus

Pulmonary embolization may follow trauma because of fat, thrombus, or air. Thromboembolism and air embolus are described elsewhere in the text. Fat embolus is specifically related to bony injury from surgery or trauma. The fat emboli syndrome consists of tachypnea, mental changes, cough, fever, and hemorrhagic petechiae on the upper chest, axilla, and subconjunctiva. Fat embolization may result from globules entering through open venous channels either from the marrow at a fracture site or by release of chylomicrons from fat stores in response to circulating catechol levels. The fat globules are filtered in the pulmonary capillaries where serum lipase hydrolyzes them. A characteristic pulmonary infiltrate is seen on chest roentgenogram. The hydrolysis products can damage the endothelium directly or indirectly by triggering the kinin cascade. The cause of the syndrome is uncertain. Some authors suggest that corticosteroids are beneficial in resolving pulmonary injury secondary to fat emboli. Steroids' mechanism is postulated to be the usual one of promoting proliferation and maturation of type II pneumocytes. Early operative fixation of long bone fractures is important in reducing the incidence of fat embolization syndrome.

In my experience in a level I trauma center only two patients showed fat embolization out of 5427 admissions over 5 years. Bony injuries underwent early fixation. Patient mobilization and turning were aggressively encouraged and carried out. Circulating volume and cardiac function were optimized by fluid challenge. These factors may help prevent fat embolism. If fat embolism occurs, management is supportive and includes mechanical ventilation and PEEP to reduce the accompanying respiratory dysfunction.

VASCULAR INJURIES

Aorta and Great Vessel Injuries

The patient with a ruptured thoracic aorta has usually received a high-speed injury. However, the patient may show no evidence of external chest trauma. Other extrathoracic injuries frequently accompany rupture of the aorta. In one study 65% of patients with ruptured aorta required early exploratory laparotomy. A true erect chest roentgenogram is the simplest means of excluding the diagnosis of aortic injury. If an ill-defined aortic knob or widened superior mediastinum is found, aortography should be performed. Surgical repair is indicated if the diagnosis is confirmed. Penetrating injury to the aorta and great vessels usually results in hemothorax and death before the patient reaches the hospital.

Extremity Vascular Injuries

A palpable distal pulse does not exclude proximal arterial injury. When a pulse deficit does occur in conjunction with ischemic changes, an arterial injury is almost always found. Blunt trauma and a popliteal artery pulse deficit are likely to be associated with arterial injury because of the lack of collateral vessels for the popliteal artery. Pulses can be properly evaluated only after shock is corrected and dislocation and fractures are reduced. The diagnosis of vascular spasm is one of exclusion. Exploratory surgery is the only way to diagnose spasm accurately.

Injuries Associated with Vascular Compromise

About 7.5% of first rib fractures are associated with vascular injuries. Indications for angiography include brachial plexus palsy and associated rib fractures or shoulder trauma. Isolated first rib fractures without neurovascular clinical findings do not require angiography. Penetrating vascular injuries can usually be managed with end-to-end anastomoses or lateral sutures. Blunt arterial injuries are less amenable to simple surgical techniques and frequently require resection and grafting.

HEAD INJURIES

Head injury is the most frequent cause of mortality following trauma. The GCS is widely used as a simple and reproducible means of assessing level of consciousness. Survival of head-injured patients with blunt trauma is directly correlated with GCS score (Table 18–3). Many neurotrauma centers use GCS as the basis of initial clinical management. Critical care management of head injury is discussed in Chapter 5 and is directed at reducing brain swelling and controlling intracranial pressure. The management aim of neurotrauma critical care is to provide the best environment for dysfunctional neurons to recover. This is achieved by adequate cerebral perfusion (at least 18 ml/100 g tissue/min), optimum oxygenation, and suitable nutrition. About one fourth of head-injured patients do well with conventional management, and another one fourth die despite aggressive critical care. In the remaining half the outcome is determined by critical care interventions.

Epidural Hematoma

The incidence of epidural hematoma is 5% to 15% in fatal head injuries. Provided therapy is rapid, epidural hematoma is a surgically correctable lesion with return to normal or near normal neurologic function. The classic clinical presentation of loss of consciousness followed by a lucid interval occurs in only one third of cases. Only 30% to 50% of patients with epidural hematoma have pupillary abnormalities. Epidural hematomas occur in 90% of patients with skull fractures. Lack of abnormalities on a CT scan does not rule out the development of delayed epidural hematoma or the need for serial neurologic examinations. CT scanning must be repeated in patients with significant neurologic deterioration. The management of epidural hematoma is rapid surgical removal.

Subdural Hematoma

Subdural hematoma (SDH) is common in severe head injury, occurring in 26% to 63% of such patients. Simple SDH is caused by shearing forces that tear bridging vessels, resulting in a subdural collection of blood. Simple SDH represents 45% of all acute SDHs and has a 21% mortality rate. Complicated SDH includes contusion or laceration of the underlying brain. Complicated SDHs make up 41% of all SDHs and have a mortality rate greater than 50%. The presence of multiple or bilateral SDHs or multiple cerebral lacerations increases the

TABLE 18–3. Survival of Head-Injured Patients with Blunt Trauma by Glasgow Coma Score (Excluding Cardiac Arrests)

GLASGOW COMA SCORE	BLUNT TRAUMA		TOTAL TRAUMA	
	NO.	MORTALITY (%)	NO.	MORTALITY (%)
3	30	80	60	80
4	16	31	28	46
5	15	40	22	46
6	18	22	27	26
7	18	6	23	4
8	17	6	24	13
9	12	0	21	0
10-14	266	5	369	7
15 ± transient loss of consciousness	668	2	1,015	2
TOTAL	1060		1589	

From Siegel JH, Dunham CM: Trauma, the disease of the 20th century. In Siegel JH (ed): Trauma: emergency surgery and critical care. New York, Churchill Livingstone, pp 1-32.

mortality rate from 50% to 90%. Decerebrate posturing and SDH are associated with a 78% mortality rate. The management of SDH depends on the clinical presentation, volume of hematoma, and swelling of the underlying cortex. Frequently after surgical removal of clot, management is directed at reduction of cerebral swelling secondary to cortical contusion.

Skull Fracture

The importance of skull fracture lies in its recognition, association with epidural hematoma, and communications with sinuses and cerebrospinal fluid. Linear fractures are important if they cross major vessels, such as the middle cerebral artery. Compound fractures of the skull or base have distinct presentations, treatments, and complications. Depressed skull fractures require therapy when the depression is greater than the thickness of the skull. Compound skull fractures may communicate with air through a scalp laceration, or a fracture in the base of the skull may communicate with the sinus cavities. Compound depressed skull fractures are a neurosurgical emergency. Infection may occur if the dura is lacerated. Removal of devitalized tissues is necessary to prevent bacterial contamination.

Cerebrospinal Fluid Leak

A persistent cerebrospinal fluid leak may develop after base of skull fractures. The dura overlying the base of the skull is easily torn. The subarachnoid space is then in direct contact with paranasal sinuses or the middle ear, resulting in rhinorrhea or otorrhea. The continual risk of meningitis necessitates monitoring of temperature, white blood cell count, and mental status. Prophylactic antibiotics are not used, since they do not prevent meningitis and their use could result in development of resistant organisms if infection does occur.

Cerebrospinal fluid leaks are managed by positioning the patient with head up whenever possible, monitoring the volume of leak, and searching for signs of infection. The majority of leaks stop without therapy within a week. If the leak persists, daily lumbar taps are used to remove 30 to 60 ml spinal fluid. After 3 days if the leak persists, continuous spinal drainage is used. If these maneuvers fail, the leak should be found and closed surgically.

Prognosis Following Head Injury

The GCS provides an estimate of severity of head injury survival, and neurologic outcome and determines initial clinical management. The major criticisms of the GCS are that it does not analyze brainstem reflexes or differentiate between left and right sides in motor response and that facial trauma or tracheal intubation make eye opening or verbal responses difficult to assess. Using the combination of GCS and CT scan as the basis for a specific diagnosis (such as SAH, SDH, and contusion) improves outcome determination compared with GCS data alone.

Multimodal evoked potentials (MMEPs) including somatosensory (SEPs), visual (VEPs), and brainstem auditory (BAEPs), are now used to characterize brain injury following trauma. MMEPs are thought to be the best indicators of prognosis, accurately predicting 1-year outcome in 80% of patients. Old age, intracranial pressure greater than 20 mm Hg, GCS less than 8, and fixed and asymmetric pupils are associated with poor prognosis. In descending order of accuracy as sole predictors of outcome are MMEPs, age, intracranial pressure, GCS, and pupils.

SPINAL CORD INJURY

Critical care management of patients with spinal cord injury depends on the completeness and level of neurologic deficit, how recently the injury occurred, and the extent of other trauma sustained at the time of cord injury. Only if neurologic deficit accompanies the injury does management of respiratory and cardiac function differ from normal. Spinal shock occurs when motor and sensory function is lost below the level of the cervical or high thoracic spinal cord lesion. The patient has flaccid paralysis, absence of deep tendon, abdominal, and Babinski reflexes, and retention of urine and feces. Spinal shock is accompanied by cardiovascular dysfunction resulting in hypotension and occasionally hypertension and bradycardia. Spinal shock may last 3 days to 6 weeks.

Respiratory Function

The effects of spinal cord transection on respiratory function can be predicted from Figure 18–4, which displays the spinal segmental innervation of the inspiratory and expiratory muscles of respiration. The important muscles of expiration have thoracic segmental innervation;

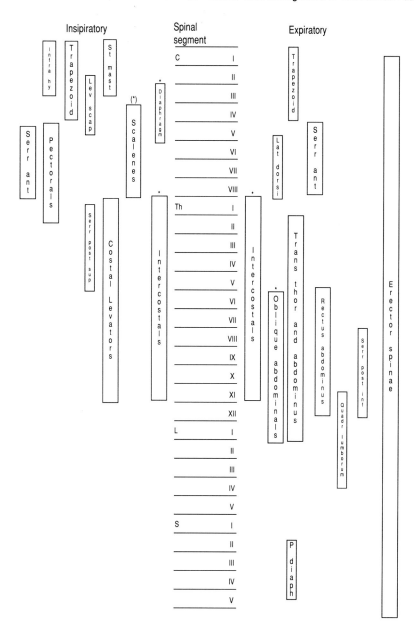

Figure 18–4.   Spinal segmental innervation of the inspiratory muscles *(left)* and expiratory muscles *(right)*. (From Fugl-Meyer, AR: Scand J Rehab Med 1971;3:141-150.)

therefore, in cervical spinal cord transection, loss of expiratory function is expected and can be measured. The diaphragm is the principal muscle of inspiration, and its movement accounts for more than two thirds of the air that enters the lungs during quiet breathing. The diaphragm is partially denervated with a C5 cord transection, and respiratory function is grossly impaired with a C4 level lesion. For spinal cord injury above C4, mechanical ventilatory support is usually mandatory in the acute phase. A complete neurologic deficit in the cervical cord paralyzes the intercostales, levatores costarum, and serratus posterior superior muscles, which elevate and abduct the ribs, enlarge the thorax, and facilitate the action of the other inspiratory muscles.

VC may be as low as 100 ml after cervical spinal cord injury but is usually between 350 and 1500 ml. The average VC of 30 patients with complete motor quadriplegia (levels C3 to C7) reported in the literature was 1300 ml. Cervical spinal cord transection may reduce expiratory flow and expiratory reserve volume to 40% of normal levels. Expiratory flow rates of 10 L/s or 600 L/min are required to produce an effective cough. Following spinal cord injury at C5, expiratory flow may be as little as 2 L/s. This loss of expiratory power results in an increase in residual volume of 140% to 200% predicted normal levels. The ineffective cough, inadequate expansion, and incomplete emptying of the lungs result in secretion retention and inadequate gas exchange. Respiratory function tests may be used to predict the need for tracheal intubation and mechanical ventilation.

Indications for Tracheal Intubation and Mechanical Ventilation

Tracheal intubation and mechanical ventilation may be necessary because cervical spine neurologic deficits result in inadequate alveolar ventilation, causing carbon dioxide retention. In addition, because respiratory function is subnormal and the patient cannot cough effectively, secretions are incompletely cleared from the lungs and the potential for respiratory complications increases greatly. Oxygenation may therefore be compromised. The need for tracheal intubation and mechanical ventilation is assessed by simple respiratory function tests. The guidelines in Table 18–4 may be used as indications for intubation in the acute phase of quadriplegia.

Arterial oxygen should be greater than 60 mm Hg when the patient is breathing room air, and oxygen should be given to maintain PaO_2 at about 100 mm Hg. A chest roentgenogram should show no signs of atelectasis or infiltrate. Intrapulmonary shunt may be assessed by determining the PaO_2/FIO_2 ratio. If this value is less than 250 (equivalent to about 15% shunt) and $PaCO_2$ rises above 45 mm Hg, tracheal intubation should be performed and mechanical ventilation instituted. Atelectasis appearing on chest roentgenogram within 12 hours of cord transection usually means that the patient

requires mechanical ventilation. Poor respiratory function as outlined in Table 18–4 usually means that the patient will require mechanical ventilation within 12 to 24 hours. If a trend toward pulmonary dysfunction is apparent, intubation should be performed before respiratory distress occurs. In the critical care unit, if the patient has no evidence of hypotension or acute respiratory distress, tracheal intubation is carried out with the assistance of topical anesthesia and fiberoptic laryngoscopy. If the patient has acute respiratory distress, a resuscitator bag provides ventilation and oxygenation.

In quadriplegia or paresis, the simple pulmonary function tests outlined in Table 18–5 are an appropriate monitor of progression for the patient who requires mechanical ventilation. I have used controlled mechanical ventilation with a time-cycled, volume-preset ventilator initially for all acute high cervical spine injuries, since this mode of ventilation optimally inflates the lung at all times. IMV or assisted ventilation frequently provides inadequate lung expansion because of the spontaneous breaths between the mandatory or assisted cycles. Inadequate lung expansion, in the early states of quadriplegia when intensive care and invasive lines are required, may give rise to undesirable respiratory complications, such as atelectasis, pneumonitis, and pneumonia. In the later stage of recovery IMV is useful in respiratory muscle training.

Serial pulmonary function testing indicates when weaning from mechanical ventilation is indicated. VC and maximum inspiratory and expiratory pressures are indicators of the ability to maintain spontaneous ventilation. With more sophisticated equipment or measurement of flow, the efficacy of the patient's cough can be determined by measuring expiratory flow. Intrapulmonary shunt can be determined approximately by PaO_2/FIO_2 or the alveolar-arterial oxygen difference and, together with measure-

TABLE 18–4. Indications for Intubation and Mechanical Ventilation in Acute Quadriplegia

INTUBATION CRITERIA	VALUE INDICATING NEED FOR INTUBATION
Maximum expiratory force	$< +20$ cm H_2O
Maximum inspiratory force	< -20 cm H_2O
Vital capacity	< 15 ml/kg or < 1000 ml
PaO_2/FIO_2	< 250
Chest roentgenogram	Atelectasis or infiltrate

TABLE 18–5. Weaning Criteria for Removal from Mechanical Ventilation and Interval Measurements of Respiratory Function in Quadriplegic Patients

WEANING CRITERIA/ MEASUREMENT	ACCEPTABLE VALUE FOR REMOVAL
Maximum inspiratory force	> -20 cm H_2O
Maximum expiratory force	$> +20$ cm H_2O
Vital capacity	> 1000 ml or > 15 ml/kg
Expiratory flow	> 10 L/s (level dependent)
PaO_2/FIO_2	> 250
VD/VT	> 0.55
Lung/thorax compliance	> 30 ml/cm H_2O

ment of dead space (V_{DS}/V_T), may be used to assess the adequacy of gas exchange. Lung/thorax compliance can be easily calculated at the bedside and indicates the pressure changes the patient must generate for each breath. Some values used in weaning adult quadriplegic patients from mechanical ventilation are shown in Table 18-5.

A quadriplegic patient must be adequately prepared, both physically and mentally, for removal from mechanical ventilation. The physical requirements include adequate nutrition and metabolic status. Supplementary hyperalimentation may be necessary, and the patient should be in electrolyte balance. Infection, which may be masked because of the lack of temperature control in quadriplegic patients, should be treated. Fluid management must ensure that the patient is neither volume underloaded nor volume overloaded in relation to cardiac and renal function. Mechanical impairments to breathing such as gastric distention, too tight a halo vest, or inappropriate positioning should be avoided during spontaneous breathing. The patient should be prepared psychologically by reassurance that help is at hand if breathing difficulty occurs and by an explanation of what to expect during the weaning process.

IMV rates in patients with C4-6 level lesions can be gradually reduced to decrease dependence and provide respiratory muscle training. Cuirass ventilators, negative-pressure jackets, or rocking beds enable some patients with cervical cord injuries to remain out of the hospital by providing support when respiration is impaired during sleep. An increasing number of ventilator-dependent quadriplegic patients can be cared for at home with family support.

Chest Physiotherapy

Both spontaneously breathing and mechanically ventilated quadriplegic patients need prophylactic physiotherapy to prevent atelectasis and pneumonia. Chest physiotherapy includes postural drainage, chest wall percussion and vibration, tracheal suctioning, and breathing exercises. Specific active and passive range of motion exercises are also carried out. Because quadriplegic patients have decreased VC, total lung capacity, expiratory reserve volume, and forced expiratory volume, pulmonary complications are common. In addition, paralysis of the trunk and extremity muscles makes patients unable to turn themselves and cough. Diaphragm function is limited by abdominal and

intercostal muscle paralysis. During the first 3 months following acute quadriplegia, death is most frequently due to pulmonary complications; chest physiotherapy greatly reduces the incidence of such complications.

In the acute phase after injury, chest physiotherapy is made easier by a bed that can be positioned head up, head down, prone, or supine. The Stryker Frame permits such positioning. Other users advocate the Rotorest bed, but the Rotorest allows access to only four of the 11 postural drainage positions, complicates nursing procedures, and causes decubitus ulcers and tissue breakdown from continuous rotation. In contrast, the Stryker Frame allows seven of the 11 postural drainage positions, assessment of skin integrity over the whole body, and protection of bony prominences. The hydraulic Stryker Frame can be operated by one person.

Cough and Glossopharyngeal Breathing

Cough in quadriplegic patients can be improved by glossopharyngeal breathing (GPB), or "frog breathing." The muscles of the mouth, pharynx, and larynx are used as a respiratory pump to inflate the lungs in a similar manner to the respiratory movements of frogs and other amphibians. In quadriplegic patients VC increases from 11% to 50% of predicted normal with use of an average of 20 glossopharyngeal breaths of 80 ml each. GPB results in increased lung volume and better cough and mucous clearance than with unaided breathing.

Patients may take from a day to several months to master GPB taught by a physical therapist. Once the technique is mastered, several weeks are needed before the patient has enough strength and endurance to cough effectively. With GPB, quadriplegic patients can speak loudly and longer, cough, be free of mechanical ventilatory support, and increase their physical and social activity. In summary, GPB is a breathing substitute that requires none of the ordinary muscles of respiration and no mechanical equipment. GPB improves VC, lung/thorax compliance, expiratory flow, cough, and speech.

Cardiac Function

Sympathetic denervation that accompanies high spinal cord injuries changes cardiac function and therefore fluid management and cardiac assessment. Cord transection results in loss of the thoracolumbar outflow and sympathetic nervous system control over the heart and peripheral circulation. Therefore monitoring of cardiac function is important in the acute phase of spinal shock. During spinal shock the patient requires close monitoring to prevent cardiac decompensation. When circulating volume is depleted, the quadriplegic patient is unable to maintain cardiac filling pressures by sympathetically induced constriction of the venous capacitance vessels. Arteriolar constriction cannot maintain blood pressure. The normally innervated heart responds to overtransfusion with tachycardia and sympathetically induced increased contractility. A quadriplegic patient's heart is less able to deal with such an increase in venous return, and acute pulmonary edema may develop. This is a widely reported and common cause of death during the early course of quadriplegia. In one study of 44 patients with cervical spine injury, 30 died within 11 days of the onset of quadriplegia and 20 had severe pulmonary edema. Interruption of sympathetic innervation or respiratory failure was thought to be the mechanism, although neurogenic and humoral influences on the pulmonary capillary were not excluded. In another study overreplacement of intravascular volume led to the sudden development of pulmonary edema in four of nine quadriplegic patients.

The pulmonary artery catheter is important in monitoring the patient during the acute phase of quadriplegia. In my institution all patients with complete cervical cord injuries and unstable incomplete lesions have pulmonary artery catheterization during the critical 48 to 72 hours after injury. Once cardiac function is assessed and optimized, central venous pressure monitoring suffices. If the patient requires surgery while still in spinal shock, a pulmonary artery catheter is inserted for perioperative management. The pulmonary artery catheter may be used to assess reserve cardiac function and the need for vasoactive drugs and to optimize cardiac output and tissue perfusion by means of the fluid challenge technique described earlier. Data from 22 patients with acute quadriplegia are shown in Figure 18–5 and demonstrate that about 30% of individuals in spinal shock have left ventricular dysfunction. Recovery of neurologic function is thought to benefit from improved tissue oxygen delivery occurring after optimization of cardiac function.

Medical, nursing, and paramedical personnel working with quadriplegic patients must be aware that rapid changes in body position may have both cardiac and respiratory effects. During spinal shock, head elevation causes a sudden decrease in cardiac filling pressure, a fall in

cardiac output, and possibly cardiac arrest. Ace bandages around the lower extremities, abdominal binders, G suits, or military antishock trousers (MAST) may be used to minimize orthostatic hypotension. Sudden change into the head-down position, because of loss of sympathetic cardiovascular innervation, may precipitate acute myocardial failure with pulmonary edema. In spinal shock and until vasomotor tone returns, body position changes must be performed gradually and with careful monitoring of arterial and venous pressures.

Inotropic Support

Hypotension may directly impair spinal cord perfusion. Therefore treatment of low blood pressure on admission is extremely important and may determine neurologic recovery. However, after the first 24 hours an episode of hypotension to a mean arterial pressure of 60 mm Hg is unlikely to change neurologic outcome when urine output is adequate, mixed venous saturation is normal, and no evidence of lactic acidosis is present. Quadriplegic patients show considerable fluctuation in blood pressure following spinal cord injury. Intervention with inotropic agents should occur only after fluid challenge and then should follow specific guidelines. If reduced creatinine clearance (less than 50 ml/min), decreased mixed venous oxygen saturation (less than 70%), lactic acidosis, or deterioration in the level of neurologic function is resistant to fluid administration, inotropic support may be beneficial.

Isoprotenerol, a beta agonist, has positive inotropic and chronotropic actions that may make it the agent of choice in a quadriplegic patient with bradycardia. Atropine 0.02 mg/kg has a rapid onset and a duration of action of only 10 to 15 minutes, making its use appropriate when cardiac function is changing rapidly. Intravenous atropine is indicated in quadriplegic patients who are bradycardic, acutely hypotensive, and in cardiac failure with pulmonary edema. Atropine reverses hypotension and elevates cardiac output and tissue oxygen delivery. In a bradycardic quadriplegic patient, atropine may reverse cardiac failure and allow time for more definitive treatment by infusions of centrally acting inotropic agents. Atropine should be used with caution in patients with myocardial ischemia or valvular lesions because tachycardia may precipitate cardiac failure or severely compromise myocardial perfusion.

Dopamine has less chronotropic effect than isoproterenol. This may be advantageous, since

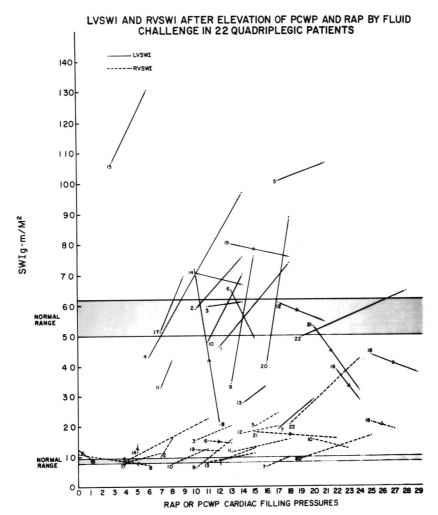

Figure 18–5. Left ventricular stroke work index (LVSWI) and right ventricular stroke work index (RVSWI) (g-m/m²) before and after elevation of wedge pressure (PCWP) and right atrial pressure (RAP) in 22 quadriplegic patients. LVSWI is plotted against PCWP, and RVSWI is plotted against RAP. Individual patient curves are represented by case number. RVSWI is shown as a dashed line, LVSWI as a continuous line. Arrows on the lines represent direction with fluid challenge. An average volume of 520 ml (range 250 to 1500 ml) of plasma protein solution was given over 12 minutes. (From Mackenzie CF et al: J Neurosurg 1985;62:843-849.)

in certain groups of patients, such as those with myocardial ischemia or mitral stenosis, tachycardia may severely reduce myocardial perfusion or result in cardiac failure. Dopamine has advantages over other inotropic agents at low doses (5 µg/kg/min) because it is thought to improve renal perfusion selectively. Dobutamine, a similar agent, may be useful when dysrhythmias are a problem.

Despite the lack of physiologic indications, some authors continue to advocate use of alpha-adrenergic agonists in spinal cord injury. I believe that their use should be avoided completely and that, in hypotensive quadriplegic patients, circulating volume should be optimized by fluid challenge. If hypotension, olig-

uria, and evidence of poor tissue perfusion remain following fluid administration and elevation of cardiac filling pressure to 18 mm Hg, inotropic agents, not vasoconstrictors, are indicated.

Autonomic Hyperreflexia

Autonomic hyperreflexia is characterized by acute generalized sympathetic activity in response to an endogenous or exogenous stimulus below the level of a T7 or higher spinal cord transection. In traumatic paraplegia during World War I, cutaneous, proprioceptive, and visceral stimuli were found to trigger this reflex response. Precipitants of autonomic hyperreflexia include cold and hot cutaneous stimuli, urinary catheterization, bladder irrigation, urinary retention, enemas, gastric distention, and acute pyelitis. In addition, rectal examination or manual disimpaction, muscle stretching, positioning, or surgical procedures performed without adequate anesthesia may precipitate autonomic hyperreflexia.

Symptoms of autonomic hyperreflexia include severe headache, sweating, nasal obstruction, desire to vomit, blurring of vision, and complaints of feeling flushed. The signs are hypertension, bradycardia, dysrhythmias, sweating, and gooseflesh. Sweating rarely extends below T10 and is most marked at the level of the lesion. Sweating below the level of transection is more likely to be part of the general sympathetic response. Cutaneous vasodilation occurs above and vasoconstriction below the spinal cord injury. Additional signs include changes in skin and rectal temperature, convulsions or loss of consciousness, cessation of respiration, visual field defects, and signs of cerebrovascular accident.

The original explanation of autonomic hyperreflexia was proposed by Kurnick, who described the neural pathways of bladder stimulation. The afferent limb of the reflex is the pelvic nerves, posterior columns, and spinothalamic tract. The efferents are the autonomic fibers to blood vessels and viscera. The splanchnic outflow of T5-11 is probably the most important. Somatic efferent nerves may also be involved. Vasoconstriction and visceral contraction appear below the level of spinal cord injury, and muscle spasms may occur. The massive vasoconstriction below the level of the lesion is associated with a rise in plasma norepinephrine and dopamine beta hydroxylase levels. Normally, hypertension that follows peripheral vasoconstriction stimulates the carotid and aortic arch baroreceptors, resulting in vasodilation, bradycardia, and blood pressure reduction. In quadriplegic patients, because the higher centers no longer inhibit the spinal reflex, vasodilation does not occur and the hypertension is not relieved. The blood pressure increase stimulates the afferents from the aortic and carotid baroreceptors, which pass in the ninth and tenth cranial nerves to the vasomotor center. Efferents from the vasomotor center pass in the tenth cranial nerve, causing bradycardia. Cardiac dysrhythmias may result from this vagal hyperactivity. Adrenal medulla secretion seems to be unchanged. Plasma norepinephrine, but not epinephrine, levels increase. Dopamine beta hydroxylase concentration is also elevated, suggesting that sympathetic overactivity is the cause of the cardiovascular changes.

In the ICU or chronic care facility, autonomic hyperreflexia may occur in association with a nonsurgical stimulus. Use of general anesthesia to prevent autonomic hyperreflexia is inappropriate. Pharmacologic means of prevention and control include the use of ganglionic blockers, alpha-adrenergic antagonists, and drugs acting directly on the vessel wall, such as sodium nitroprusside. Dysrhythmias resulting from autonomic hyperreflexia may be controlled with beta blockers. Stimuli known to provoke the response should be avoided, and sedation may be helpful to control the patient's anxiety.

Medical Management

Steroids

The efficacy of glucocorticosteroids in the treatment of spinal cord trauma remains controversial. The use of steroids in both experimental and clinical head injury has yielded conflicting results. At least 12 animal studies of spinal cord injury have been reported; 10 indicate that steroids are beneficial in enhancing recovery when the cord lesion is partial. When the lesion is severe and complete, recovery does not occur with glucocorticosteroids.

Steroid-treated patients with complete lesions do not have enhanced recovery. In patients who have complete motor paralysis with some sensory sparing, steroids have no benefit. In a group of patients with severe partial cord injury, however, those receiving steroids (methylprednisolone or dexamethasone) had recovery indices at 1 year of 83%, whereas patients who did not receive the medication had a recovery rate of 68%, similar to the experimental models.

Consequently, in many neurotrauma units, all cord-injured patients begin receiving steroids on admission. If the deficit remains complete on the motor examination after 3 days, the steroids are stopped, since the risk of gastrointestinal bleeding or infection is considerable. If the patient has any motor function distal to the injury site, the steroid medication is continued for 7 to 10 days and then tapered over the next 7 to 10 days.

Naloxone

Improvement in spinal cord blood flow may reduce or even reverse the ischemic changes resulting from spinal shock and may improve neurologic recovery. Following spinal cord injury, spinal cord blood flow is compromised and hypotension accompanies spinal shock. Endogenous opiates have been implicated as mediators of hypotension, hypothermia, and hypoventilation following spinal cord injury in rats. A 10 mg/kg intravenous bolus of naloxone provided the best neurologic recovery in experimental spinal cord injury in animals and when used in human studies. It has not been proved that naloxone influences long-term outcome, but it may speed the attainment of best neurologic recovery and therefore improve rehabilitation.

Thyrotropin-Releasing Hormone

Thyrotropin-releasing hormone (TRH) is reported to enhance recovery in cats with partial cord injury. TRH is an ergotropic substance that promotes central nervous system activation. Six cats were given TRH hourly for 5 doses after a contusion injury. The recovery in animals with partial lesions who received the drug was nearly 100%. Control animals had only 80% recovery. If the recovery had been followed longer, the difference between the treated and nontreated groups might have been small.

TRH elevates systemic blood pressure in animals; an increase in perfusion pressure to areas of focal ischemia may enhance recovery. TRH has not been tested against other drugs that act directly on the heart and have little action in the central nervous system. No substantial evidence for benefit in humans exists.

PERIPHERAL NERVE INJURIES

Management of peripheral nerve injuries requires early diagnosis, complete evaluation, and appropriate investigations and decisions to perform surgery.

Brachial Plexus Injury

The brachial plexus originates from the roots of C5-T1. C5 gives rise to deltoid function, C6 to biceps, C7 to triceps, C8 to deep flexors of the forearm, and T1 to the intrinsic muscles of the hand and fingers. Injury to the brachial plexus results in failure of abduction and loss of elbow extension and flexion. Injuries to the forearm, wrist, and hand most commonly involve the median and ulnar nerves.

Peripheral Nerve Repair

Repair of a peripheral nerve injury is delayed whenever soft tissues and bones are extensively injured. Primary nerve repair, especially of digital nerves, is considered in clean lacerations. If exploration reveals nerve stumps that are contused or irregular, repair is delayed 4 to 6 weeks. When an upper extremity fracture is associated with a peripheral nerve injury, exploration is not indicated, since 75% of the nerves recover spontaneously. In gunshot wounds the nerve disruption is often greater than anticipated and repair is delayed. If the brachial plexus is explored for an associated vascular injury, the extent of injury to the plexus can be assessed.

If nerve endings are not found at the initial exploration or the patient is not explored, electromyelography (EMG) is performed at 3 weeks to determine the status of neural function. Nerve exploration is indicated for neurolysis or repair within 4 weeks if the nerve was found to be transected and was not repaired at the time of admission. Exploration also should be carried out if EMG and clinical examination 8 to 12 weeks after injury reveal poor or absent nerve conduction because of entrapment, resection, or failure of the initial repair.

INTRAABDOMINAL INJURY

The most common intraabdominal injury is spleen trauma, followed by liver trauma (Table 18–6). Splenorrhaphy rather than splenectomy is the surgical procedure of choice because of increased susceptibility to pneumococcal infection after splenectomy. A high mortality rate is associated with severe blunt trauma to the liver, especially with major stellate fractures or avulsions of the hepatic vein or tears in the hepatic vena cava. Late deaths from hepatic injury are caused by sepsis, hepatic failure with coagulopathy, renal failure, respiratory failure, and multiple organ failure. An important finding among patients who die after intraabdominal trauma is that more than 80% have severe associated extraabdominal trauma.

Pancreatic injury may not be recognized initially, especially in an unconscious patient. Epigastric pain, tenderness, or guarding together with ileus and cardiovascular instability may suggest pancreatic injury. The serum amylase level is elevated and continues rising. Peritoneal lavage and CT scans may reveal no abnormalities.

TABLE 18-6. Incidence of Abdominal Organ Injury from Blunt Trauma in 870 Patients Requiring Operative Intervention (1978-1982)

ORGAN INJURED	NUMBER OF PATIENTS	% OF TOTAL WITH INJURY
Spleen	367	42.2
Liver	310	35.6
Retroperitoneal hematoma	127*	14.6
Serosa and mesentery of bowel	113†	13.0
Diaphragm	44	5.1
Bowel wall rupture	41	4.7
Small bowel	30	3.4
Colon	11	1.3
Bladder	28‡	3.2
Kidney	23	2.6
Mesenteric vascular (SMA or SMV)	17	2.0
Vena cava or iliac vein	9	1.0
Ovarian cyst rupture	9	1.0
Stomach	2	<0.1
Pancreas	2§	<0.1
Duodenum	1‖	<0.1
Aorta	1	<0.1

*Not associated with major retroperitoneal organ injury.
†Injuries requiring repair or bowel resection.
‡All but one associated with pelvic fracture.
§Eight additional injuries in association with splenectomy.
‖Six paraduodenal hematomas.
SMA = superior mesenteric artery or vein (SMV).
Data from Cox EF: Blunt abdominal trauma: a 5-year analysis of 870 patients requiring celiotomy. Ann Surg 1984;199:467.

Management of pancreatic injury includes operative intervention, resection of devitalized tissue, adequate external drainage, and control of hemorrhage. The most common complications are fistula, pseudocyst, delayed hemorrhage, abscess formation, and pancreatitis.

Small bowel injuries result in abdominal pain and peritonitis. Gastric decompression is performed and antibiotics are given before and after surgery. Colon injury is associated with relatively higher mortality and morbidity rates because of the high bacterial content of the large bowel. Preoperative and postoperative antibiotic coverage is given for anaerobic and aerobic organisms. Injury to the kidney, ureters, and bladder is not detected by peritoneal lavage because these organs are located extraperitoneally. Urinalysis, cystography, intravenous pyelography, and CT scanning are the diagnostic tools for examination of the urinary tract.

Renal lacerations, expanding renal hematomas, and renal pedicle or pelvis injuries require surgical exploration. Minor renal contusions, lacerations without contrast dye extravasation, and intrarenal lacerations without evidence of disruption of the renal capsule generally are managed conservatively with observation for signs of hypertension, blood loss, and infection.

Surgical exploration may be required for patients with transcortical lacerations that cause minor dye extravasation, for subscapular hematomas, or if hypertension develops after renal injury. After discharge all patients with renal trauma should receive follow-up monitoring for development of infection, hypertension, fistulas, urinomas, or ureteral obstruction.

Traumatic ureteral injuries are uncommon. Diagnosis is based on intravenous pyelography. Primary repair may be possible, or stents can be placed and brought out through a nephrostomy or cystostomy. Bladder injury is suspected in patients with hematuria and an associated pelvic fracture. A cystogram confirms the diagnosis. Bladder contusions are managed with urinary catheter decompression and irrigation to remove clots. Bladder ruptures require surgical repair.

Complications

Infection giving rise to abscess formation is the major complication of intraabdominal trauma. Wound dehiscence may occur in obese, malnourished, or elderly patients. Diabetes and the use of corticosteroids are associated with an increased infection rate. Clinical manifestations include fever, elevated white blood cell count, pain, abdominal or rectal mass, purulent drainage from wounds, and bacteremia with gut flora. Diagnostic findings include the presence of free air, displaced abdominal viscera, and an ileus pattern on abdominal roentgenogram. CT scanning may help establish the diagnosis. Preoperative antibiotics and volume resuscitation are required before surgical drainage. Wound healing is assisted by adequate nutrition.

MUSCULOSKELETAL INJURY

Assessment of orthopedic injuries includes examination of vascularity, soft tissue, neurologic status, and bone and joint trauma. The management goals are early stabilization of fractures, debridement of devitalized tissue, provision of nutrition, and infection control.

In the postoperative period the optimum orthopedic management permits side-to-side turning and mobilization. Bone stabilization reduces the need for pain medication and minimizes release of marrow products into the circulation. Pulmonary function is greatly improved by internal fixation or use of external traction devices. Femoral, tibial, radial, ulnar, and humeral injuries can be managed with external or internal fixation. Pelvic fractures with retroperitoneal hematoma and major displacement are usually managed with external fixation. Both internal and external fracture stabilization allow postural drainage positioning and chest physiotherapy. Neufeld's traction is a compromise that minimizes the respiratory complications of prolonged immobilization. However, it is not ideal because it does not rigidly immobilize the fracture site.

Compartment Syndromes

Compartment syndromes may occur in the forearm and leg. Excessive pressure within the dense fascial compartments compresses capillaries and produces ischemia of muscles and nerves. The syndromes may develop because of revascularization after ischemia, bleeding, or venous occlusion. Examination shows a tense limb, tenderness, motor weakness, hypesthesia, and a diminished pulse. Compartmental manometry is diagnostic. Treatment is fasciotomy.

HYPOTHERMIA

Hypothermia is associated with massive transfusion, exposure, and spinal cord injury. Hypothermia impairs citrate and lactate metabolism, shifts the oxyhemoglobin dissociation curve to the left, delays drug metabolism, increases blood viscosity, and impairs red blood cell deformability. In the critical care unit, central rewarming by heated humidification of inspired gases is the therapy of choice. Intravenous fluids should be warmed and acid-base status monitored if profound hypothermia has occurred. Cardiac dysrhythmias, coagulopathies, hepatic and renal failure, pancreatitis, and diabetes-like syndromes may result from hypothermia. Many patients respond to rewarming with marked vasodilation and relative hypovolemia. Monitoring of cardiac reserve by central venous catheterization is advisable.

MASSIVE BLOOD TRANSFUSION

Massive transfusion is usually defined as the infusion of 10 or more units of blood within 24 hours. The indication for blood transfusion is restoration or maintenance of oxygen-carrying capacity. Complications associated with massive transfusion include coagulopathy, citrate intox-ication, and hypothermia. Hypokalemia, hyperkalemia, acidosis, and alkalosis are reported as complications of massive transfusion. In my experience hypokalemia and alkalosis are more likely to occur. Packed red blood cells are potassium deficient after storage, and gluconeogenesis stimulates insulin release. The result of these factors is that potassium moves into the cells, reducing serum levels. Alkalosis occurs because shock impairs the kidneys' ability to excrete bicarbonates. Citrate (a bicarbonate precursor) and mechanical hyperventilation increase the pH and amount of potassium entering the cell. Hypocalcemia may occur with very rapid infusion at rates greater than 1 ml/kg/min for long periods and can be corrected by intravenous calcium chloride. Calcium deficiency prevents clotting and decreases cardiac contractility. The use of micropore filters remains controversial. Microaggregates of platelets, white blood cells, and fibrin have been implicated in causing posttransfusion pulmonary dysfunction. In my experience micropore filters are a logistic hazard because they prevent rapid blood infusion, so I routinely use 170 μm macropore filters without obvious detrimental effects on lung function.

If massive hemorrhage or shock is present despite rapid infusion of 1500 to 2000 ml of plasma protein fraction (PPF) and no cross-matched or type-specific blood is available, type O Rh-positive packed red blood cells are given. Blood is given if the hematocrit value is less than 30% and systolic blood pressure is less than 100 mm Hg after PPF infusion. Group O is the universal donor, containing neither plasma antibodies nor cell antigen of a major ABO group. In a 22-month period at my institution 343 patients received 1945 units of type O Rh-positive blood without hemolytic or major transfusion reactions even though 170 patients were of blood groups other than O. However, of the 47 Rh-negative patients, 36 developed anti-Rho (D) antibody. Type-specific or cross-matched blood is used as soon as it is available. Use of non-cross-matched type O Rh-positive blood may be lifesaving.

Autotransfusion can provide an immediately available source of blood and reduce the demands placed on the blood bank. The risk of infection is avoided, viable platelets and labile factors are retained, and metabolic alterations of stored blood are avoided. Blood may be collected from the thorax or abdomen. Bacteremia following autotransfusion is reduced by restriction of the technique to patients whose wounds are free from fecal contamination.

Several commercially available cell saver devices can be used for autotransfusion.

Blood may be warmed with a heating coil, by means of a countercurrent system such as the Level One rapid transfusion system (Level One Technologies), and by use of heating blankets and warmed inspired gases. Heat lamps and elevation of ambient temperature also reduce the adverse effects of hypothermia.

Coagulopathy

Coagulopathy is diagnosed by monitoring of platelet count, prothrombin time (PT), partial thromboplastin time (PTT), and fibrinogen after at least every 10 units of blood. Disseminated intravascular coagulation may occur. Hepatic ischemia, shock, and hypothermia impair coagulation. Acidosis reduces platelet aggregation, and sepsis produces thrombocytopenia.

Therapy for coagulopathy involves controlling sources of hemorrhage by using digital external pressure, inflatable splints, or a MAST suit as appropriate. Little scientific evidence supports prophylactic component therapy with fresh-frozen plasma (FFP) and platelets. If the source of bleeding is controlled and a specific coagulopathy is diagnosed on the basis of the coagulation profile, component therapy is used. If coagulopathy develops during massive transfusions and the platelet count is less than 100,000, platelet infusions are helpful. FFP is not helpful in most cases unless the PT and PTT are greater than 1½ times control values. The risk of hepatitis after FFP should be weighed against the benefits to coagulation. About 90% of current FFP use is inappropriate. Thrombocytopenia in association with sepsis is reversed by finding and directing therapy to the site of infection.

MYOGLOBINURIA

Myoglobinuria results from ischemia with muscle contusion. Persistent myoglobinuria suggests a continuing focus of muscle necrosis. Necrotic tissue should be sought and removed. Renal function deteriorates unless urinary output is maintained with fluid infusion and diuretic therapy with mannitol. Bicarbonate infusion may help prevent precipitation of myoglobin in the renal tubules. If rhabdomyolysis occurs, 5% dextrose 1000 ml with bicarbonate 100 mg and mannitol 25 g may help prevent renal failure.

SUGGESTED READINGS

Assessment of Traumatic Injury

Baker SP, O'Neill B: The injury severity score: an update. J Trauma 1976;16:882-885

Champion HR, Sacco WJ, Hunt TR: Trauma Severity Scoring to predict mortality. World J Surg 1983;7:4-11

Champion HR, Sacco WJ, Lepper RC: An anatomic index of injury severity. J Trauma 1980;20:197-202

Knaus WA, Draper EA, Wagner DP, et al: Apache II — a severity of disease classification system. Crit Care Med 1985;13:818-829

Mackenzie CF: Advances in trauma emergency care. In Anaesthesia review 4. Edinburgh, 1986, Churchill Livingstone, pp 135-145

Mackenzie CF: Anesthesia for traumatized patients. ASA refresher course lecture No. 252, 1988, pp 1-6

Teasdale G, Jennett B: Assessment of coma and impaired consciousness: a practical scale. Lancet 1974;2:81-84

Respiratory Management

Mackenzie CF: Clinical indications and usage of chest physiotherapy: anatomy, physiology, physical examination and radiology of the airways and chest. In Mackenzie CF (ed): Chest physiotherapy in the intensive care unit, 2nd ed. Baltimore, 1989, Williams & Wilkins, pp 53-92

Mackenzie CF: Physiological changes following chest physiotherapy. In Mackenzie CF (ed): Chest physiotherapy in the intensive care unit, 2nd ed. Baltimore, 1989, Williams & Wilkins, pp 215-250

Thoracic and Abdominal Injury

Cox EF, Siegel JH: Blunt trauma to the abdomen. In Siegel JH (ed): Trauma emergency surgery and critical care. New York, 1987, Churchill Livingstone, pp 883-910

Hedley-Whyte J, Burgess GE, Feeley TW, Miller MG: High-speed blunt injuries. In Applied physiology of respiratory care. Boston, 1976, Little, Brown & Co, pp 183-198

Kirsh MM: Acute thoracic injuries. In Siegel JH (ed): Trauma: emergency surgery and critical care. New York, 1987, Churchill Livingstone, pp 863-882

Mackenzie CF, Shin B, Fisher R, Cowley RA: Two year mortality in 760 patients transported by helicopter from the road accident scene. Am Surg 1979;45:101-107

Shin B: Lung contusion. In Cowley RA, Conn A, Dunham CM (eds): Trauma care, vol 1. Philadelphia, 1987, JB Lippincott Co, pp 126-150

Shin B, Mackenzie CF, Chodoff P: Is IMV superior to controlled ventilation in the management of flail chest? Crit Care Med 1979;7:138

Shin B, McAslan TC, Hankins JR, et al: Management of lung contusion. Am Surg 1979;45:168-175

Shock

Bone RC, Fisher CJ, Clemmens TP: A controlled clinical trial of high dose methylprednisolone in the treatment of severe sepsis and septic shock. N Engl J Med 1987;317:653-658

Bowen JC, Rees M: Endogenous opiates in shock. In Hardaway RM (ed): Shock, the reversible stage of dying. Littleton, Mass, 1987, PSG Publishing Co, pp 505-511

Dunham CM, Cowley RA: Shock trauma/critical care handbook. II. Shock. Rockville, Md, 1986, Aspen Publishers, pp 81-91

Gaffin SL: Antibody therapy for shock. In Hardaway RM (ed): Shock, the reversible stage of dying. Littleton, Mass, 1987, PSG Publishing Co, pp 511-516

Hardaway RM, Williams CM: Influence of steroids on hemorrhagic and traumatic shock. J Trauma 1987; 27:667-670

Parker JL, Jones CE: The heart in shock. In Hardaway RM (ed): Shock, the reversible stage of dying. Littleton, Mass, PSG Publishing Co, 1987, pp 348-366

Robinson NB, Chi EY, Robertson HT: Ventilation perfusion relationships after hemorrhage and resuscitation: an inert gas analysis. J Appl Physiol 1983; 54:1131-1140

Veterans Administration Systemic Sepsis Cooperative Study Group: Effect of high dose glucocorticoid therapy on mortality in patients with clinical signs of systemic sepsis. N Engl J Med 1987;317:659-665

Ruptured Aorta

Ayella RJ, Hankins JR, Turney SZ, Cowley RA: Ruptured thoracic aorta due to blunt trauma. J Trauma 1977; 17:199

Dunham CM, Cowley RA: Thoracic injuries. In Shock trauma/critical care handbook. Rockville, Md, 1986, Aspen Publishers Inc, pp 145-200

Vascular Injury

Sodestrom CA: The diagnosis of extremity vascular injuries caused by blunt trauma. In Cowley RA, Conn A, Dunham CM (eds): Trauma care. Philadelphia, 1987, JB Lippincott Co.

Head Injury

Geisler F, Salcman M: The head injury patient. In Siegel JH (ed): Trauma: emergency surgery and critical care. New York, 1987, Churchill Livingstone, pp 919-946

Matjasko J, Pitts L: Controversies in severe head injury management. In Matjasko J, Katz J (eds): Controversies in neuro anesthesia and neurosurgery. Orlando, Fla, 1986, Grune & Stratton, Inc, pp 181-232

Spinal Cord Injury

Head M, Riddoch G: The autonomic bladder, excessive sweating and some other reflex conditions in gross injuries of the spinal cord. Brain 1917;40:188-263

Kurnick NB: Autonomic hyperreflexia and its control in patients with spinal cord lesions. Ann Intern Med 1956;44:678-686

Mackenzie CF, Shin B, Krishnaprasad D, et al: Assessment of cardiac and respiratory function during surgery on patients with acute quadriplegia. J Neurosurg 1985; 62:843-849

Mackenzie CF, Ducker TB: Cervical spinal cord injury. In Matjasko J, Katz J (eds): Controversies in neuroanesthesia and neurosurgery. Orlando, Fla, 1986, Grune & Stratton, Inc, pp 77-134

McMichan JC, Michel L, Westbrook PR: Pulmonary dysfunction following traumatic quadriplegia: recognition, prevention and treatment. JAMA 1980;243:528-531

Meyer GA, Berman IR, Doty DB, et al: Hemodynamic responses to acute quadriplegia with or without chest trauma. J Neurosurg 1971;34:168-177

Woolman L: The disturbance of circulation in traumatic paraplegia in acute and late stages: a pathological study. Paraplegia 1965;2:213-216

Fluid Management

Mackenzie CF, Shin B, Krishnaprasad D, et al: Assessment of cardiac and respiratory function during surgery on patients with acute quadriplegia. J Neurosurg 1985; 62:843-849

Patterson A: Massive transfusion. Int Anesthesiol Clin 1987;25:61-74

Peters RM: Fluid resuscitation and oxygen exchange in hypovolemia. In Siegel JH (ed): Trauma: emergency surgery and critical care. New York, 1987, Churchill Livingstone, pp 157-180

Shin B, Mackenzie CF, McAslan TC, et al: Postoperative renal failure in trauma patients. Anesthesiology 1979; 51:218-221

Shin B, Mackenzie CF, Helrich M: Creatinine clearance for early detection of posttraumatic renal dysfunction. Anesthesiology 1986;64:605-609

19

BURNS

WILLIAM R. FURMAN, MD

Victims of major burns suffer a unique form of trauma in which the organ system primarily affected is the integument. Intensive care is often required to treat the respiratory, hemodynamic, and multisystem complications of burn injury and the many surgical procedures required. This chapter discusses the critical care of burn patients with an emphasis on aspects that are unique among critically ill patients.

GENERAL CONSIDERATIONS

The general approach to burn treatment begins with a delineation of the location and severity of the primary and all associated injuries. Burn injuries are described according to their depth and extent. The depth of destruction of the skin and underlying structures is classified as first, second, or third degree to indicate a superficial, partial-thickness, or full-thickness burn, respectively (Table 19–1). If structures beneath the skin, such as muscle or fascia, are burned, the term "fourth degree" is sometimes used. In terms of management and prognosis, it is more useful to distinguish first- and superficial second-degree burns from those that are deeper (deep second, third, and fourth degree) and to observe whether inhalational injury is present. Deep second-, third-, and

fourth-degree burns either do not heal spontaneously or do so with such poor cosmetic and functional results that surgical debridement and grafting are required in their management.

The extent of injury is the percentage of the body surface area (BSA) that has received second- or third-degree burns; first-degree burns are ignored in this determination. Detailed charts such as the one in Figure 19–1 are used to delineate the burned areas and determine their extent. A rough estimate can be made by applying the "rule of nines," in which 9% is assigned to each of 11 body parts (head and neck, each arm, upper anterior trunk, lower anterior trunk, upper posterior trunk, lower posterior trunk, each thigh, and each leg and foot). The term "major burn" applies to deep second- and third-degree burns involving greater than 15% to 20% of the BSA and to those associated with an inhalational injury.

The prognosis for survival after a burn is roughly inversely proportional to the total extent of deep second- and third-degree burns. The mortality rate is greatest in infants and in the elderly, and inhalational injury increases the risk of death from major burns by 30% to 40%. Other injuries, such as fractures and blunt abdominal trauma, incurred with the burn may worsen the prognosis.

The prognosis and treatment of burns is generally not differentiated according to type of

TABLE 19–1. Burn Characteristics by Wound Depth

	DEPTH (DEGREE)		
	FIRST	**SECOND**	**THIRD**
Surface	Warm	Wet, bullae	Dry
Color	Red	Pink, mottled	White, charred
Sensation	Sensitive	Very sensitive	Anesthetic
Examples of causes	Sunburn	Flash burns, scald (spilled)	Flame, scald (immersion), electrical

THE FRANCIS SCOTT KEY MEDICAL CENTER
a Johns Hopkins Health System member institution

BALTIMORE REGIONAL BURN CENTER

ADMISSION BURN EVALUATION SHEET

Date of Admission: _____   Weight: _____

AREA	PERCENT OF BURN					SEVERITY OF BURN		TOTAL PERCENT
	0-1 Year	1-4 Years	5-9 Years	10-15 Years	ADULT	2°	3°	
Head	19	17	13	10	7			
Neck	2	2	2	2	2			
Ant. Trunk	13	17	13	13	13			
Post. Trunk	13	13	13	13	13			
R. Buttock	2½	2½	2½	2½	2½			
L. Buttock	2½	2½	2½	2½	2½			
Genitalia	1	1	1	1	1			
R.U. Arm	4	4	4	4	4			
L.U. Arm	4	4	4	4	4			
R.L. Arm	3	3	3	3	3			
L.L. Arm	3	3	3	3	3			
R. Hand	2½	2½	2½	2½	2½			
L. Hand	2½	2½	2½	2½	2½			
R. Thigh	5½	6½	8½	8½	9½			
L. Thigh	5½	6½	8½	8½	9½			
R. Leg	5	5	5½	6	7			
L. Leg	5	5	5½	6	7			
R. Foot	3½	3½	3½	3½	3½			
L. Foot	3½	3½	3½	3½	3½			
				Total				

Code: Blue areas indicate 2°
Red areas indicate 3°

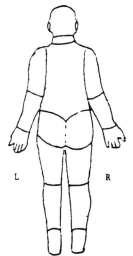

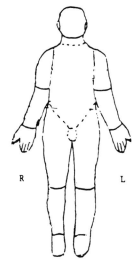

L   R   R   L

Figure 19–1.   Baltimore Regional Burn Center Admission Burn Evaluation Sheet.

injury (thermal, chemical, electrical, or radiationinduced), except that the mortality rate from high-voltage (greater than 1000 volt) electrical injuries tends to be increased relative to the percentage of the BSA affected. This is because the electrical current passes through, and seriously injures, muscles, fascia, and viscera, while the superficial structures dissipate the energy and effects of thermal, chemical, and radiation exposures. Electrical current produces heat energy proportional to the current squared in deep structures. This energy is especially detrimental if the voltage is high enough to produce a large current flow.

The care of burn patients has three phases: immediate resuscitative, debridement and grafting, and reconstructive. Critical care management is required during the first two phases. The first phase extends from the time of hospital admission to the initiation of surgical debridement and burn wound grafting. This period usually spans 2 to 4 days. The second phase continues from that point until all the burn and surgical wounds have healed.

RESUSCITATIVE PHASE

The primary concerns at the moment of hospital admission of a burn patient are assessment of the airway and treatment of respiratory compromise. After airway management, priorities include cardiopulmonary resuscitation, monitoring and vascular access, fluid resuscitation, and initial care of the burned areas.

Airway Management

Respiratory dysfunction is common in critically ill patients, and burn victims are no different in this regard. Overwhelming pulmonary infection, pulmonary edema, or adult respiratory distress syndrome (ARDS) may develop anytime during recovery from burns and may necessitate endotracheal intubation. Four causes of respiratory dysfunction are most commonly encountered in the resuscitative phase of burn care: carbon monoxide poisoning, upper airway edema, subglottic thermal and chemical burns, and chest wall restriction.

Carbon monoxide (CO) is a colorless, odorless gas that causes asphyxia at relatively low concentration because it binds to hemoglobin 200 times more readily than oxygen. CO is emitted during combustion and is a major concern to victims trapped in closed space fires (buildings, automobiles). CO may cause cerebral hypoxia, unconsciousness, and ultimately death, depending on the degree of exposure.

CO poisoning in burn patients requires immediate recognition and treatment to prevent hypoxic tissue death (neural tissue is especially sensitive). It is diagnosed and quantitated by measurement of the arterial blood carboxyhemoglobin level, which is expressed as percent saturation of hemoglobin (Saco). Saco of more than 15% is usually toxic, and over 50% is almost always lethal. CO poisoning should be suspected in all victims of thermal injury, especially those in fires in confined spaces. Hypoxic patients may complain of headache, shortness of breath, nausea, or angina pectoris and may be tachypneic, irritable, or delirious, but they are not cyanotic. In such cases arterial blood gases and Saco should be measured to distinguish between hypoxemia (low Pao$_2$) and CO poisoning. CO poisoning cannot be diagnosed by standard (two-wavelength) pulse oximetry, but newer three-wavelength devices are being developed for this purpose.

Removal of CO begins as soon as exposure to the gas is terminated. If the patient breathes room air (21% oxygen), the half-time of elimination is about 4 hours, but if 100% oxygen is administered, it can be decreased to 40 minutes. Intubation is indicated whenever the level of consciousness is depressed. In addition, when high oxygen concentrations are required, an endotracheal tube is more reliable than a mask. If pharmacologic intervention is needed to facilitate intubation, burn patients require no special consideration early in the course. The hypersensitivity to succinylcholine they develop (see later discussion) is not evident in the first 8 to 12 hours, and a standard rapid-sequence intubation protocol may be used.

Upper airway edema develops within 24 hours of exposure to heated inspired gas mixtures. All supraglottic tissues may be affected, and swelling, if untreated, may be so severe that complete inspiratory obstruction results. This potentially lethal problem should be anticipated if the victim was burned in a closed space fire (the same situation in which CO poisoning is suspected) or if hoarseness, facial or intraoral burns, an injected tongue, or sooty oral and nasal secretions are observed.

Significant upper airway edema may rapidly lead to laryngeal structures so deformed as to be unrecognizable. The conservative approach is intubation whenever upper airway swelling is a risk, but this results in unnecessary discomfort for a number of patients whose airway never would have become obstructed. An alternative is to select patients who are at risk but lack facial and intraoral burns, perform nasopharyngoscopy at frequent (2-hour) intervals, and intubate at the first sign of erythema or swelling of glottic and supraglottic structures. Such a departure from the most conservative approach can be made only if the airway can be examined repeatedly during the first 24 hours. Pulmonary flow-volume loops may also be performed and repeated at intervals as a means of diagnosing inspiratory obstruction, but they are no substitute for direct examination.

Like asphyxia, upper airway edema occurs before any abnormal responses to neuromuscular blocking agents can develop. Accordingly, depolarizing muscle relaxants can be used to facilitate intubation if the potential for obstruction is recognized and treated at an early stage. A rapid-sequence intubation is often the best choice in such a situation.

Once advanced swelling has occurred, the intubation technique must preserve spontaneous respiratory efforts until the airway has been secured. Both awake oral intubation (direct laryngoscopy) and awake nasal intubation (over a fiberoptic bronchoscope) are acceptable techniques. However, with either method, airway manipulation can worsen obstruction. Therefore, if complete obstruction occurs before intubation is accomplished, emergency cricothyroidotomy may be necessary. Alternatively, inhalational induction of anesthesia with halothane and 100% oxygen can be carried out, and direct laryngoscopy can be performed under general anesthesia.

Upper airway swelling usually subsides in 3 to 4 days, after which extubation can be considered. Unintended extubation before that time is potentially lethal because of the difficulty of reintubation. The endotracheal tube should be securely fixed in place, and sedatives, nondepolarizing muscle relaxants, and limb restraints should be used as needed.

Tracheobronchial (subglottic) thermal burns do not occur unless live steam or burning gases are inhaled. Otherwise, the heat in the inspired gas mixture is dissipated in the upper airway (where thermal injury does take place). Chemical inhalational injury is common, however, especially with fires in buildings containing plastic and synthetic materials. When burned these substances emit toxic fumes, such as hydrogen chloride, a combustion product of polyvinyl chloride, which has both pulmonary and myocardial toxic effects in the first 48 hours.

The sequence of events in inhalational pulmonary injury generally begins with a decrease in pulmonary defenses because of impaired mucociliary clearance and reduced alveolar surfactant activity. Caustic products of combustion also stimulate release of chemotactic substances, such as histamine, kallikreins, and serotonin, producing mucosal tissue injury and edema. After a few hours, airway obstruction from bronchospasm, mucosal edema, and sloughed epithelium (pseudomembranous tracheobronchitis) causes regional atelectasis and intrapulmonary shunting. Hyaline membrane formation, followed by interstitial and alveolar pulmonary edema, occurs with worsening gas exchange.

Fluid and protein shifts in the early postburn period may also lead to pulmonary edema, especially in patients with severe inhalational exposure or with antecedent pulmonary or cardiac disease. Early intubation and mechanical ventilation with positive end-expiratory pressure (PEEP) are often required. Corticosteroids and prophylactic antibiotics have not proved beneficial. Antibiotics should be used only to treat documented infections. Bronchoscopy is seldom helpful in the treatment of lobar atelectasis because it does nothing to eliminate the pulmonary tissue injury that causes airway obstruction.

Circumferential chest wall burns can produce chest wall edema, leading to a restrictive ventilatory defect, usually in the first 24 hours. Inflating the lungs may be nearly impossible, even at very high inspiratory pressures, until escharotomy (surgical excision of the chest wall and subcutaneous tissues) is performed. This condition is usually diagnosed after intubation has been performed and mechanical ventilation has begun because of respiratory failure. The principal signs are a lack of inspiratory movement of the chest wall and a continually rising level of peak inspiratory pressure. During escharotomy the thoracic compliance improves almost instantly, and ventilatory pressure typically declines before the procedure is complete. This procedure is typically performed under neuroleptanalgesia or ketamine anesthesia with a nondepolarizing muscle relaxant.

Succinylcholine

When intubation is performed during the first 8 to 12 hours after burn injury, succinylcholine may be used. Later, exaggerated potassium release from muscle occurs when patients with 20% or greater burns are given succinylcholine, making them susceptible to hyperkalemic arrhythmias and death. The mechanism is an increase in acetylcholine receptors on the muscle membrane, which probably does not begin before the second day and is greatest between 5 and 60 days after burn injury. Although succinylcholine may be safely used in the first 2 days, the usual recommendation is to abjure its use after 8 to 12 hours and not to use it again until all the burn wounds have been covered with healed graft.

A nondepolarizing muscle relaxant (NDMR) is used for facilitating intubation when succinylcholine is contraindicated. However, burn patients require higher doses of NDMRs than other patients do to achieve the same result. Resistance to NDMRs is greatest between 5 and 60 days after the burn and increases with burn size. In burn patients potency of these drugs may be reduced by as much as 80% (five times the usual dose must be given to achieve the desired effect). The succinylcholine-produced increase in acetylcholine receptors that causes hyperkalemia also may be the cause of the observed resistance to NDMRs. If a rapid-sequence intubation is selected to reduce the risk of aspiration of gastric contents, very large doses of muscle relaxants are required to achieve early and complete relaxation. Pancuronium or vecuronium, as much as 0.8 mg/kg, is used for this purpose in some medical centers, and the relatively minor inconvenience of prolonged relaxation is considered acceptable.

Fluid Resuscitation

All burn victims need large volumes of sodium-containing fluid because of tissue edema, which results from an increase in capillary permeability in the burned area. Several formulas are used to estimate the fluid requirement during the first 24 hours. Most physicians prescribe intravenous crystalloid 2 to 4 ml/kg body weight for every 1% of BSA burned, with care individualized after the first day. Victims at the extremes of age, those with larger burns (greater than 30% BSA), and those with high-voltage electrical burns often require fluids in great excess of the calculated needs.

The most commonly used resuscitation formula is the Parkland formula, which prescribes lactated Ringer's solution during the first 24 hours: 4 ml/kg body weight for each 1% burn. One half of this is given during the first 8 hours after the burn, and the remainder is given over the next 16 hours. However, the formula is only a guide to therapy, and care must be individualized based on the patient's clinical response. Colloid is generally not given in the first 24 hours after the burn.

Hypoproteinemia, resulting in edema of all tissues, often occurs in the first 24 to 48 hours. The Parkland formula, like most fluid replacement formulas, includes colloid 0.5 ml/kg body weight for each 1% BSA burned given during the second 24 hours, but whether this measure improves survival remains controversial.

After the first 24 to 48 hours the adrenal response to stress usually causes increased potassium excretion (up to 300 mEq/d) and severe sodium retention. Large amounts of free water

and potassium may be required, and sodium administration should be guided by electrolyte monitoring.

Burn victims require secure venous access for administration of the large amounts of fluid used for initial resuscitation, nutritional support, and intraoperative management during debridement and grafting procedures. This need is often best met in patients with large burns by inserting a multilumen catheter into a large vein (femoral, subclavian, or internal jugular) at the time of admission.

The adequacy of the initial fluid resuscitation must be continually assessed by observation of the patient's weight, vital signs, urine output, skin turgor, and mental status. If hypotension or oliguria occurs, myocardial depression (caused by mediators released in patients with large burns) should be considered and monitoring of central venous and pulmonary artery pressure may be required. Nonburned areas are preferred for insertion of all lines to reduce the risk of bacterial contamination.

Initial Burn Care

Topical care of burn wounds begins after resuscitation has been initiated. If possible, the patient should be immersed in water ("tubbed") to assist in removing the remaining dead skin and cleansing the wounds. Hypotensive patients and intubated patients may be too unstable to transfer to the tub room and may need to be cleansed in bed.

Washing is especially important for the treatment of burns caused by chemicals or radioactive substances if these are still on the skin at admission. One common injury requiring skin cleansing is a burn caused by tar used in road and roofing work. The tar is both hot (thermal burn) and caustic (chemical burn). It adheres to the skin and hairs and must be scraped away, often with a razor, as quickly as possible. If the patient cannot tolerate the discomfort involved in this procedure, intravenous narcotics, sedatives, or ketamine may be required.

After the burn wound is cleansed, burn dressings are applied. Topical antimicrobial agents are used to control burn wound sepsis, even though they do not completely eradicate the bacteria. The choice of agent varies among burn centers, but those most often used are mafenide (a methylated sulfonamide) and silver sulfadiazine (principally a vehicle for delivering silver into the burn wound).

Mafenide offers excellent control of burn wound flora but has several disadvantages. It is readily absorbed into the bloodstream and produces significant carbonic anhydrase inhibition, which leads to metabolic acidosis. The metabolic breakdown products of mafenide present an osmotic load, producing an osmotic diuresis, and an acid load, which worsens the metabolic acidosis. Hyperventilation is required to buffer this acid load. In the presence of superimposed respiratory disease or inhalation injury, this may lead to respiratory failure. Mafenide also produces pain at the application site and causes an allergic skin rash in up to 7% of patients.

Silver sulfadiazine is less effective in bacterial control than mafenide but does not produce pain on application. Propylene glycol is absorbed into the bloodstream from the silver sulfadiazine vehicle. The presence of propylene glycol in the serum and urine is not harmful, but it complicates efforts to monitor fluid resuscitation by measuring serum osmolality and urine specific gravity. A minor side effect of silver sulfadiazine is leukopenia, which lasts 2 to 4 days but appears to have no clinical significance.

Fasciotomies are required when a compartment syndrome develops in an extremity. This complication is frequently associated with electrical burns and results from the massive necrosis of tissue. If the patient's condition is too unstable for safe transport to the operating room, the procedure can be performed in the ICU in much the same manner as a chest wall escharotomy (see the preceding discussion).

DEBRIDEMENT PHASE

After the initial resuscitation, patients with deep second- or third-degree burns undergo a series of debridement and grafting operations until their wounds are completely covered. Like most critically ill patients, burn victims are at risk for renal failure, gastrointestinal bleeding, altered metabolism, malnutrition, infection, and altered immunity. Unlike most critically ill patients, however, they undergo a series of operative procedures. This section covers some manifestations of organ system failure that are peculiar to burn patients and discusses preoperative preparation and postoperative intensive care management.

Renal Failure

Renal failure occurs in up to 30% of burn patients. In addition to the usual causes in critically ill patients, such as prerenal azotemia

and nephrotoxic antibiotics, burn patients are susceptible to chemical nephritis from inhaled products of combustion, such as sodium bichromate, and to a form of polyuric renal failure characterized by a low fractional excretion of sodium. The latter form usually begins 2 to 3 weeks after the burn and may be severe enough to require dialysis.

Acute tubular necrosis may be associated with myoglobinuria if significant muscle injury has taken place. Myoglobinemia and myoglobinuria often occur after high-voltage electrical and lightning injuries and can also be found in victims of thermal burns. Although the mechanism of toxicity has not been defined, the current treatment is diuresis with mannitol and furosemide and alkalinization of the urine until the pigmenturia has cleared.

Gastrointestinal Bleeding

Like other ICU patients, burn patients are at high risk for ulceration of the lining of the stomach and duodenum. The association of peptic ulceration with burns has been given the eponym Curling's ulcer. Histamine blockers (H_2 blockers) may be used to decrease acid production in the gastrointestinal tract. However, the clearance of these agents (cimetidine and ranitidine) is accelerated in burn victims, necessitating a reduction in the dose interval from every 8 hours to every 6 hours in many patients. A good way to monitor the efficacy of this therapy is to measure the gastric pH during treatment.

Hypermetabolism

Burn patients are hypermetabolic and have an increased nutritional requirement. Early aggressive alimentation by the enteral route if possible, and intravenously if needed, controls catabolism and supports immune function. Positive nitrogen balance should be established as early as possible after the burn, especially in patients with burns greater than 20% of the BSA.

Perioperative Management

Surgery and perioperative care should be performed in warm environments, and heat loss minimized in every way possible. Radiant lamps, warmed intravenous fluids and inspiratory gases, and meticulous attention to covering the patient are required in the care of these patients. Thermoregulation is abnormal after major burns, and burn patients need environmental temperatures higher than those preferred by the ICU staff. A temperature in excess of 25° C is desirable, despite the inconvenience of working in a hot room; some institutions routinely maintain their ICUs and operating rooms at 33° C.

For safe anesthetization of a burn patient, provision must be made for monitoring, intravenous access, and ventilatory support during the entire time spent outside the ICU. This includes the periods of transfer to and from the operating room, as well as that of the operative procedure. Decisions about how to monitor the electrocardiogram and blood pressure or whether additional intravenous catheters, arterial lines, or a pulmonary artery catheter is needed should be made before surgery, and action should be taken in the ICU rather than the operating room, where time is at a premium and staff are relatively scarce.

Ideally, the patient should go to the operating room with a functioning arterial catheter or a limb designated for blood pressure monitoring by cuff and with enough intravenous lines of adequate caliber to continue the fluid resuscitation and to administer medications and blood as required during surgery. Secure central access is often needed for administration of blood products because the degree of loss during debridement and grafting can be extensive and even life threatening. An estimate may be obtained by predicting that 3% of the blood volume will be lost for every 1% of the BSA excised. For example, the excision and grafting of 16% of the BSA may require replacement of about one half of the patient's blood volume over as little as 1 hour. The venous access must therefore permit transfusion of at least this much blood, and some patients' needs will exceed this estimate. In a large patient the requirement may be as great as 1 unit of packed red blood cells every 5 minutes.

A laboratory examination is indicated near the time of surgery, with particular attention to electrolyte levels, hematocrit, platelet count, indicators of renal function, and arterial blood gas concentrations. Because current surgical practice advocates aggressive early debridement as a means of controlling burn wound sepsis, laboratory abnormalities do not usually lead to postponement of surgery. Rather, they provide information that indicates the need for modifying the management plan to correct electrolyte abnormalities or for transfusing blood or platelets before surgery.

If renal function is found to be declining, volume status should be reassessed, and choices and dosage of pharmacologic agents may need to be changed. If oxygenation or ventilation is deteriorating, cardiac function is reassessed and ventilatory management is adjusted in an effort to stabilize the patient before surgery. The goal is not to delay surgery, but rather to make adjustments that will permit a safe operation, even in the face of changing pathophysiologic conditions.

Legitimate reasons to delay surgery usually involve life-threatening developments, such as arrhythmias, hypotension, or respiratory failure so severe as to preclude safe transport to the operating room.

Postoperative Management

The postoperative care of the burn patient includes management of hemodynamic support, pain control, and ventilation. After debridement and grafting surgery, many burn patients are tachycardic, hypotensive, or both, for several reasons. First, they tend to suffer considerable pain in their donor and graft sites, and as they regain consciousness, they hurt. Second, because thermoregulation is abnormal after major burns, they often shiver, increasing their heart rate and cardiac output. Third, blood loss during burn surgery is difficult to estimate accurately. Despite the best efforts of the operative team, blood and crystalloid repletion can be inadequate. Fourth, debridement of colonized or infected burn wounds may release humoral factors that cause hypotension by reducing systemic vascular resistance.

Pain is constant, and the only effective treatment is narcotic analgesics. Burn patients are not believed to be resistant to narcotics, but they do require large amounts to treat their discomfort. Health care providers remain reluctant to provide adequate pain relief, usually because they are under the misapprehension that narcotic addiction will result from overly liberal use of these drugs. To date no evidence has been presented to support this notion, and several retrospective studies have concluded that providing pain relief to burn-injured patients does not cause persons nonaddicted before injury to become addicts. The only way to determine whether analgesia is sufficient is via the patient's verbal report: patients with chronic pain may lack the physiologic (pupillary dilation, sweating, tachycardia, tachypnea) and objective (grimacing, crying) behavioral signs ordinarily associated with acute pain. After surgery narcotics should be administered as needed until the patient reports relief.

Burn injury leads to an increase in metabolic rate, the magnitude of which increases as burn size increases. In addition, the injury itself increases heat loss because of skin disruption. After surgery and transport from the operating room, body temperature often falls, leading to shivering and an oxygen requirement increased as much as fivefold. This in turn increases cardiac rate and output in direct proportion to the increase in oxygen consumption.

An assessment of the patient's volume status is always necessary after burn surgery. The vital signs, filling pressures (if available), urine output, hematocrit, and blood values must be measured as they would for any critically ill surgical patient. Because of the potential for massive blood loss and large fluid shifts, the hematocrit value often changes during the immediate postoperative period, necessitating consideration of further transfusion. This does not necessarily mean that the intraoperative blood component therapy was inadequate, but rather may reflect the time required for equilibration after surgery. Ongoing blood loss also occurs, especially if the patient has a coagulopathy.

Burn wound sepsis is an important cause of perioperative hypotension and is one of the chief causes of death in burn patients. Debridement of infected areas can lead to hypotension during or after surgery. As for other critically ill patients, vasopressors and inotropic agents may be used to treat septic shock, but no outcome studies have ever shown that raising the blood pressure in this manner improves outcome.

Like other ICU patients, burn patients are weaned from mechanical ventilatory support when their general condition is improving and the condition that required respiratory intervention has resolved. The decision to wean and extubate should not be based simply on recovery from anesthesia, but rather should be made in the context of the patient's overall care plan. When the patient has a large burn or an associated inhalational injury, extubation between successive operative procedures may be neither prudent nor feasible. In such cases continued sedation or even early tracheostomy may be a better plan. A tracheostomy is better tolerated than an oral or nasal endotracheal tube, and the risk of adverse outcome from displacement is far less.

SUGGESTED READINGS

Furman WR: Major burns. In Rogers MC, (ed): Current practice in anesthesiology. Philadelphia, 1988, BC Decker Inc, pp 310-313

Furman WR, Stiff JL: Burn anesthesia. In Stene JK, Grande CM (eds): Trauma anesthesia. Baltimore, 1991, Williams & Wilkins, pp 286-300

Haponik EF, Munster AM (eds): Respiratory injury: Smoke inhalation and burns. New York, 1990, McGraw-Hill Book Co

Martyn JAJ: Clinical pharmacology and drug therapy in the burned patient. Anesthesiology 1987;65:67-75

Martyn JAJ (ed): Acute management of the burn patient. Philadelphia, 1990, WB Saunders Co

20

TEMPERATURE DISTURBANCES

DANIEL I. SESSLER, MD

Homeothermic species require a nearly constant internal body temperature. When internal temperature deviates significantly from normal, metabolic function deteriorates. Under normal conditions the human thermoregulatory system maintains central body temperature within 0.5° C of "normal," which is approximately 37° C. Hypothermia results from cold exposure alone or combined with drugs or illnesses that impair thermoregulation. During anesthesia and surgery, hypothermia is commonly caused by anesthetic-induced inhibition of thermoregulation and exposure to a cold operating room environment. Shivering-like tremor characterizes recovery from general anesthesia. Fever is a physiologic response to infection but may also result from noninfectious stimulation of the immune system or from drug toxicity. Hyperthermia can also occur in extreme environmental heat. Whether "appropriate" or not, hyperthermia significantly increases metabolic demand and may require treatment. The prevention and management of such temperature-related complications are improved by an understanding of normal and drug-influenced thermoregulation.

NORMAL THERMOREGULATION

Thermoregulation is similar to many other physiologic control systems in that the brain uses negative feedback to minimize perturbations from normal values. Temperature is centrally regulated, principally by the hypothalamus, but is based on signals derived from nearly every type of tissue, including other parts of the brain, the spinal cord, deep central tissues, and the skin surface. Thermoregulatory information is processed in three phases: afferent thermal sensing, central regulation, and efferent response.

Afferent Thermal Sensing

Temperature information is obtained from thermally sensitive cells throughout the body. Cold signals travel to the hypothalamus and other central structures primarily via A-delta nerve fibers, whereas information about warmth travels by unmyelinated C fibers. Receptors for warmth increase their firing rates when temperature increases, and cold receptors do so when temperature decreases. Most ascending thermal information traverses the spinothalamic tracts in the anterior spinal cord, but no single spinal tract is critical for conveying thermal information.

Central Thermoregulation

The hypothalamus regulates temperature by comparing integrated thermal inputs from the skin surface, neuroaxis, and deep tissues with threshold temperatures for heat and cold (Fig. 20–1). When the integrated input from all sources exceeds one of the thresholds, responses are initiated to maintain adequate body temperature. The slope of response intensity versus the difference between thermal input and the threshold temperature is referred to as the gain of that response. The difference between the lowest warm and highest cold thresholds indicates the thermal sensitivity of the system. The interthreshold range (temperature range over which no regulatory responses occur) typically is 0.5° C. Thus, although the brain presumably detects temperature changes within this range, changes do not trigger

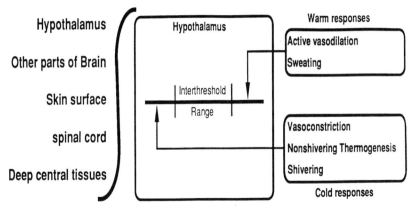

Figure 20–1. Thermoregulatory control mechanisms. Mean body temperature is the integrated thermal input from a variety of tissues, including the brain, skin surface, spinal cord, and deep central structures. Mean body temperature below the threshold for response to cold provokes vasoconstriction, nonshivering thermogenesis, and shivering. Mean body temperature exceeding the hyperthermic threshold produces active vasodilation and sweating. No thermoregulatory responses are initiated when mean body temperature is between these thresholds (interthreshold range). (From Sessler DI: Temperature monitoring. In Miller RD [ed]: Anesthesia, ed. 3. New York, Churchill Livingstone, 1990, pp 1227–1242.)

regulatory responses until they reach one of the thresholds. These relationships are illustrated in Figure 20–2.

How the body determines absolute threshold temperatures is unknown, but the thresholds vary daily in both sexes (circadian rhythm) and monthly in women by 0.5° C. Exercise, food intake, infection, hypothyroidism, hyperthyroidism, anesthetic and other drugs (including alcohol, sedatives, and nicotine), and adaptation to cold and warmth alter threshold temperatures. Central regulation is intact from infancy but may be impaired in elderly or extremely ill patients.

Efferent Responses

The hypothalamus responds to temperatures exceeding the appropriate threshold via effector mechanisms that increase metabolic heat production or alter environmental heat loss. Each thermoregulatory effector has its own threshold and gain, so an orderly progression of responses and response intensities occurs in proportion to

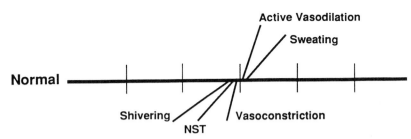

Figure 20–2. Thresholds and gains for thermoregulatory responses in awake humans. The vertical lines represent different effector responses, and the dark horizontal line shows central body temperature. The intersection of each line with the temperature scale is the threshold, and the slope indicates the gain of that response. Thermoregulatory sensitivity is shown as the distance between the first cold response (vasoconstriction) and the first warm response (active vasodilation); temperatures within this range do not elicit thermoregulatory compensation. Actual thresholds in nonanesthetized individuals are closer (0.2° C) than illustrated, and the gains are higher. The slope of the line representing shivering is relatively small because of the broad range of shivering intensity, which increases in proportion to hypothermia. Nonshivering thermogenesis *(NST)* is not triggered until vasoconstriction is nearly complete. The slope of the line representing vasoconstriction is steep because the response is an "all-or-nothing" phenomenon. Because each thermoregulatory effector has its own threshold and gain, there is an orderly progression of responses, and response intensities in proportion to need. (From Sessler DI: Temperature monitoring. In Miller RD [ed]: Anesthesia, ed. 3. New York, Churchill Livingstone, 1990, pp 1227–1242.)

need. The major effector mechanisms in humans are behavioral regulation, cutaneous vasoconstriction, nonshivering thermogenesis, shivering, active vasodilation, and sweating. Energy-efficient effectors, such as vasoconstriction, generally are maximized before metabolically costly responses, such as shivering, are initiated.

The combined efficacy of thermoregulatory responses determines the environmental temperature range the body can tolerate without changing central temperature. When specific effector mechanisms are inhibited (for example, when shivering is prevented after administration of muscle relaxants), the tolerable environmental range is decreased but temperature remains normal unless other effectors cannot compensate for the imposed stress. Behavioral regulation (as by dressing appropriately, modifying environmental temperature, and voluntary movement) is the most important effector mechanism.

Cutaneous vasoconstriction decreases heat loss via convection and radiation from the skin surface. Total skin blood flow is divided into nutritional (capillary) and thermoregulatory (arteriovenous shunt) components. The arteriovenous shunts are anatomically and functionally distinct from the capillaries supplying nutritional blood to the skin. Consequently, vasoconstriction does not compromise the needs of peripheral tissues. Shunt flow is mediated primarily by norepinephrine (released by presynaptic adrenergic nerve terminals), which binds alpha$_2$ receptors that are sensitized by local cooling and inhibited by local temperatures of 35° C or greater. Circulating norepinephrine binds alpha$_1$-adrenergic receptors, which are not sensitive to local temperature.

Nonshivering thermogenesis increases metabolic heat production without producing mechanical work. Skeletal muscle and brown fat tissue are the major sources of nonshivering heat. The metabolic rate in both tissues is controlled primarily by the circulating norepinephrine concentration. Since thermoregulatory shivering is not fully effective at birth, nonshivering thermogenesis is the infant's primary response to hypothermia. It increases heat production approximately 100% in infants but only 25% to 40% in adults.

Shivering increases metabolic heat production by approximately 200% in adults. Shivering is energy inefficient and produces surprisingly little heat. The body uses it only as a last defense against hypothermia (that is, its activation

threshold is below that for vasoconstriction and nonshivering thermogenesis).

PERIOPERATIVE HYPOTHERMIA

Mild hypothermia (central temperatures between 33° and 36° C) is common intraoperatively because anesthetics depress metabolic heat production and central thermoregulation and because patients lose heat to a cold operating room environment. Anesthetics produce immediate vasodilation that allows cool peripheral blood to mix with warm central blood, causing central temperatures to decrease by 1° C. Central body temperature then decreases linearly for 2 to 3 hours (as heat is lost to the environment) until thermal steady state is achieved. By definition, thermal steady state occurs when metabolic heat production equals heat loss to the environment. In a passive thermal steady state, heat production and loss are balanced without thermoregulatory intervention. An active steady state occurs when patients become sufficiently hypothermic to trigger thermoregulatory responses, decrease heat loss to the environment, and increase metabolic heat production.

General anesthesia decreases the threshold temperatures triggering responses to hypothermia by 2.5° C and probably increases the threshold temperatures initiating responses to hyperthermia by a comparable amount (Fig. 20–3). Widening the interthreshold range (decreasing the sensitivity of the thermoregulatory system) produces a broad temperature range over which active thermoregulatory responses are absent intraoperatively. Within this range patients are poikilothermic and body temperature changes are determined passively by the difference between metabolic heat production and heat loss to the environment.

The only thermoregulatory responses available to an anesthetized, paralyzed, hypothermic patient are vasoconstriction and nonshivering thermogenesis. Patients who become sufficiently hypothermic during surgery (for example, central body temperatures of 34.5° C) undergo a profound peripheral cutaneous vasoconstriction and increase their systemic oxygen consumption by 20%. The temperature at which vasoconstriction and nonshivering thermogenesis occur is the thermoregulatory threshold for the anesthetic agent in the dose or concentration administered.

The thermoregulatory threshold in healthy

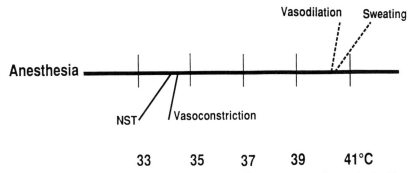

Figure 20–3. Thresholds and gains for common thermoregulatory responses in anesthetized humans. For explanation see Figure 20–2. Shivering is not shown because it is inhibited by muscle relaxants and local effects of inhaled anesthetics. The thresholds for vasoconstriction and nonshivering thermogenesis are lowered to approximately 34.5° C (depending on anesthetic type and dose). The effects of anesthetics on active vasodilation and sweating are unknown, but the thresholds are probably several degrees above normal. (From Sessler DI: Temperature monitoring. In Miller RD [ed]: Anesthesia, ed. 3. New York, Churchill Livingstone, 1990, pp 1227–1242.)

adult patients given halothane-oxygen or nitrous oxide–fentanyl anesthesia for elective donor nephrectomy is 34.5° C. During isoflurane anesthesia for the same procedure this threshold decreases 3° C for each percent of end-tidal concentration and is inversely proportional to the inhaled concentration (Fig. 20–4). The vasoconstriction threshold in infants anesthetized with halothane differs little from that in adults but is associated with a greater increase in oxygen consumption (consistent with the increased role of nonshivering thermogenesis in nonanesthetized infants). The effect of narcotics, such as fentanyl, on thermoregulation is unresolved because these drugs affect animals differently from humans.

Central thermoregulation remains intact during regional anesthesia, providing some protection from hypothermia. However, hypothermia may occur because of anesthetic depression of regional thermal afferent input and efferent responses, such as vasoconstriction and shivering,

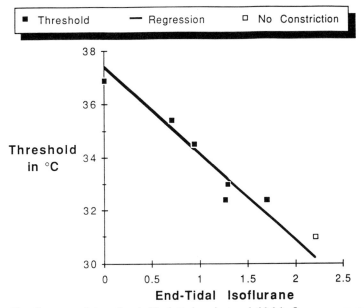

Figure 20–4. The thermoregulatory threshold plotted against end-tidal isoflurane concentration. In this illustration the thermoregulatory threshold is the central temperature at which the skin surface temperature gradient (forearm-fingertip) equalled 4° C. The dark line is the least-squares regression calculated with data only from subjects in whom vasoconstriction occurred: Threshold = $37 - 3 \cdot$ [isoflurane]; $r = -0.96$. (From Støen R, Sessler DI: Anesthesiology 1990; 72:822-827.)

or because of excessive heat loss to the operating room environment.

Hypothermia also may be deliberately induced to confer protection during operations, usually cardiac procedures, that increase risk of tissue ischemia or hypoxia. During such surgeries an inadequate tissue oxygen supply may force cells to use anaerobic metabolism, which is both inefficient and unlikely to provide adequate energy. Since hypothermia reduces the metabolic rate in all cells, it generally provides greater protection against ischemia and hypoxia than drugs, such as barbiturates, that selectively reduce metabolic rate only in neurons. The lower metabolic rate decreases cell energy needs and toxic waste production by anaerobic metabolism. Since patients deliberately made hypothermic usually are nearly fully rewarmed following surgery, their thermal management is generally similar to that of patients with mild perioperative hypothermia.

The physiologic changes induced by hypothermia are completely reversible. Patients who are still hypothermic postoperatively usually rewarm within several hours, even without specific intervention. Since there is little evidence that mild hypothermia is dangerous, this rate of recovery is usually acceptable. Additional warming may be necessary if thermoregulatory responses to cold (vasoconstriction and shivering) cause excessive hemodynamic or metabolic stress or if thermoregulatory effectors are sufficiently inhibited by disease or administration of drugs, such as muscle relaxants or vasodilators, to prevent natural rewarming.

Central body temperature increases only when metabolic heat production exceeds heat loss to the environment. Normally about 85% of metabolic heat is lost through the skin by convection, conduction, and radiation. These losses are determined by the difference between skin surface temperature and ambient temperature (conduction increases linearly, but radiation is a higher-order function). Thus increasing temperature surrounding the skin best preserves metabolic heat. Because burns are likely at temperatures greater than 40° C, actually transferring heat through the skin is dangerous. Instead, temperature surrounding the skin should be increased to 35° to 40° C. Moderate temperature increases over a large amount of skin are more effective than large temperature increases in small areas.

One of the best methods of warming the skin surface is the Bair Hugger (Augustine Medical, Eden Prairie, Minn.), which circulates warm air through channels in a blanket. The resulting shell of warm air around the patient transfers some exogenous heat and prevents loss of metabolic heat. Although radiant warmers permit better access to the patient than an encircling blanket, they are less efficient because they do not prevent convective heat loss, which may account for half the total heat loss. Placing a circulating water blanket under the patient is only minimally effective because the bed mattress already provides good insulation; these blankets are more effective when placed *over* the patient.

The thermoregulatory role of hands and feet is to dissipate excess metabolic heat. Blood flow through peripheral arteriovenous shunts in patients whose thermoregulatory shunts are open is 10 times greater than metabolic needs, resulting in considerable heat loss. Consequently, in patients whose thermoregulatory vasoconstriction is inhibited by residual anesthetic drugs or vasodilators, covering the hands and feet speeds rewarming.

TEMPERATURE MEASUREMENT SITES

Thermoregulatory responses are determined from the integrated temperature of many tissues, but most of the input comes from deep abdominal and thoracic tissues, the spinal cord, and the brain. Thus no single temperature can be considered a "gold standard." In practice, temperatures are usually divided into central and skin surface monitoring sites. Because temperatures in the central tissues are similar, an estimate of thermal input from all of these tissues can be obtained by measuring a single temperature adjacent to the tympanic membrane or in the esophagus, pulmonary artery, or rectum.

The type of thermometer (mercury-in-glass, thermistor, or thermocouple) is unimportant so long as it has an adequate functional range and is properly used. Digital electronic thermometers usually are the most practical because they can be left in place to provide continuous measurements.

POSTOPERATIVE TREMOR

Shivering-like tremor occurs in 40% of patients during recovery from anesthesia. The major risks to patients include a 200% increase in metabolic demand and exacerbated postoperative pain. Electromyographic (EMG) analysis of tremor patterns in patients recovering from isoflurane anesthesia reveals two patterns: a clonic (5 to 7 Hz) activity similar to that produced by pathologic clonus and plantar flexion–induced clonus, and a more common, tonic activity that resembles normal shivering (Fig. 20–5). Because clonic activity is not a component of normal thermoregulatory shivering, these data suggest the existence of at least two types of postoperative tremor, one of which is not simply normal shivering.

Both clonic and tonic postoperative tremors occur most often at intermediate residual anesthetic concentrations (for example, 0.1% to 0.3% end-tidal isoflurane). All of this tremor is preceded by peripheral vasoconstriction (as is normal shivering). Hypothermia is required to trigger both types of tremor. Although the clonic tremor is not normal thermoregulatory shivering, it may represent a primitive spinal thermoregulation that is normally suppressed by the hypothalamus.

Patients who become sufficiently hypothermic to trigger intraoperative thermoregulatory responses are likely to continue doing so postoperatively. However, efferent responses including shivering may be altered by high concentrations of residual anesthetic (producing abnormal EMG patterns). When postoperative hypothermic patients have very low residual anesthetic concentrations, they initiate appropriate responses to cold, including vasoconstriction and normal shivering.

Treatment of postoperative tremor remains empirical because the cause is still unclear.

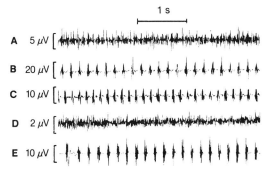

Figure 20–5. Typical electromyographic (EMG) signals from the soleus muscle during, *A,* normal cold-induced shivering; *B,* pathologic clonus in a patient with spinal cord transection; *C,* postanesthetic spontaneous EMG clonus; *D,* postanesthetic tonic EMG activity; and *E,* postanesthetic clonus induced by plantar flexion. The traces shown in *C, D,* and *E* are from the same patient. Tonic EMG activity (75% of the signal) superficially resembles normal shivering. Pathologic clonus (25% of the signal), spontaneous EMG clonus, and flexion-induced clonus have a similar, rhythmic, 5 to 7 Hz, "on-off" bursting pattern that is not a component of normal shivering. (From Sessler DI, Israel D, Pozos RS, et al: Anesthesiology 1988;68:843-850.)

Maintaining strict intraoperative normothermia does prevent postoperative tremor. In contrast, skin surface warming prevents and rapidly treats tremor following general anesthesia, even in hypothermic patients. Intravenously administered narcotics are not generally effective in treating postoperative tremor, but meperidine (10 to 20 mg) is an exception. Meperidine's effect on tremor may not be mediated by μ opiate receptors.

ACCIDENTAL HYPOTHERMIA

First reported more than 400 years ago, hypothermia has probably been known far longer. Accidental hypothermia is arbitrarily defined as a central temperature of 35° C or less unrelated to medical intervention. It occurs when the thermoregulatory system fails to compensate for decreased environmental temperature. When environmental stress is extreme, hypothermia occurs despite normal thermoregulation. Even competent thermoregulatory effectors cannot long compensate for high wind velocity, cold water immersion, or extremely low temperatures. Hypothermia may also occur in mild environments when thermoregulation is impaired by drugs, illness, or old age.

The exposure of young, healthy adults to the normal range of cold conditions rarely results in hypothermia because the thermoregulatory system can compensate for a wide range of ambient temperatures. Infants, however, are at particular risk because their low mass and high skin surface area increases heat loss to the environment. The elderly are also susceptible because their decreased muscle mass and decreased energy reserves decrease the adequacy of shivering and vasoconstriction. Thin people are more likely to become hypothermic than those in whom fat provides better thermal insulation. Large burns and major trauma also predispose to hypothermia by increasing heat loss to the environment.

Most often, accidental hypothermia results from exposure to moderate environmental stress combined with ineffective thermoregulation. Medical conditions that directly inhibit central thermoregulation include infections, malnutrition, and hypoglycemia. Hypothalamic strokes and tumors also may destroy thermoregulatory function, resulting in a "poikilothermia syndrome"; these patients (who otherwise function normally) are susceptible to severe hypothermia or hyperthermia even in moderate environments.

Cardiorespiratory illnesses are predisposing factors to hypothermia because they impair thermoregulatory effectors, particularly shivering in response to cold stimuli. Hypothyroidism may lead to hypothermia because metabolic heat production is lower than normal. The physiologic responses to hypothermia are also impaired in malnourished, exhausted, acidotic, hypoglycemic, and paraplegic individuals.

Although nearly lethal plasma concentrations of ethanol cause direct vasodilation, moderate plasma ethanol concentrations cause vasodilation by depressing central thermoregulation. Ketamine and the benzodiazepines also inhibit central thermoregulation. Barbiturates, phenothiazines, and narcotics decrease body temperature in a cold environment. This mechanism of action is unclear and probably results from a combination of peripheral effects (such as direct vasodilation) and central thermoregulatory impairment. Drugs that inhibit central thermoregulation usually do so by increasing the interthreshold distance, resulting in a range over which individuals are poikilothermic. Hypothermia (rather than hyperthermia) more commonly results because cold stress is more common than excessive warmth. Cocaine and amphetamines are exceptions in that they frequently produce centrally mediated hyperthermia.

Since behavioral regulation is normally the most important response to suboptimal environmental temperatures in humans, inhibition of this response increases the risk for accidental hypothermia. Behavior-altering drugs, such as psychotropics, and dementia impair the behavioral response to thermal stimuli, predisposing the person to hypothermia.

Clinical Signs and Symptoms. The physiologic changes induced by hypothermia are virtually without exception reversible, and function returns to normal when euthermia is reestablished. Mild hypothermia (33° to 35° C) is most notable for regulatory responses (in victims with intact thermoregulation). Peripheral vasoconstriction decreases cutaneous blood flow 10-fold, significantly reducing heat lost to the environment. Nonshivering thermogenesis increases metabolic rate 25% to 40% in adults and 100% in infants, but this augmentation is small compared with the 200% increase produced by shivering. Minute ventilation increases in proportion to the metabolic rate, but victims do not become hypercarbic or hypoxemic. Cold exposure produces an osmotic diuresis that is not reversed by antidiuretic hormone. Cerebral function is well maintained during mild hypothermia, but confusion develops at body temperatures near 33° C.

Hypothermia (in the absence of shivering and nonshivering thermogenesis) decreases metabolic rate by 8% per degree centigrade. The clinical findings in moderate and severe hypothermia usually reflect this decrease. Thus most physiologic functions are diminished during hypothermia. Whole body oxygen demand decreases, and oxygen consumption in tissues with higher than normal metabolic rates is especially reduced. Cerebral blood flow decreases but in proportion to the brain's metabolic needs. Consciousness is lost at 28° C. Primitive reflexes such as gag, pupillary constriction, and monosynaptic spinal reflexes remain intact until 25° C. Nerve conduction decreases with falling temperature but peripheral muscle tone increases, resulting in rigidity and myoclonus at temperatures near 26° C.

Moderate hypothermia decreases heart rate and increases contractility; stroke volume is well maintained. At temperatures less than 28° C, sinoatrial pacing becomes erratic and ventricular irritability increases. Fibrillation usually occurs between 25° and 30° C, and electrical defibrillation is usually ineffective at these temperatures. Coronary artery blood flow decreases but, as in the brain, in proportion to need and without causing tissue ischemia. In severe hypothermia a combined respiratory and metabolic acidosis develops, suggesting peripheral ischemia, which is surprising because peripheral oxygen transport appears adequate.

Respiratory strength is diminished at central temperatures less than 33° C, but the ventilatory carbon dioxide response is minimally affected. Hepatic blood flow and function also decrease, significantly inhibiting metabolism of most drugs. Bowel peristalsis decreases at temperatures below 34° C, and paralytic ileus develops at central temperatures below 28° C. Blood viscosity and hematocrit values gradually increase, and coagulation is progressively impaired at temperatures less than 33° C. Hyperthermia produces hyperglycemia. However, hypoglycemia (from alcohol injection or diabetes) frequently predisposes to development of accidental hypothermia.

Diagnosis. Since temperature inaccuracies of 1° C or less are unlikely to influence diagnosis or therapy, the choice of monitoring site does not warrant excessive concern. Mercury-in-glass thermometers usually do not read sufficiently low temperatures to permit diagnosis of accidental hypothermia. However, most electronic thermometers (thermistor or thermocouple) function over a wide temperature range and have various probes suitable for different monitoring locations. Digital electronic thermometers also are more convenient than mercury models because they can be used continuously to evaluate the rewarming of hypothermia victims.

Tympanic, nasopharyngeal, esophageal, bladder, and rectal temperatures have been used to monitor hypothermia. Rectal temperatures (at a 10 cm depth) are convenient but may misrepresent central temperature if hypothermia develops rapidly because they are slower to reflect this temperature change. The result may be an initial temperature reading above actual and an underestimated rate of recovery. Consequently, rectal temperatures are sometimes considered intermediate rather than central. Tympanic thermometers must be inserted carefully (to obtain accurate values and avoid perforating the eardrum) but correlate extremely well with pulmonary artery and brain temperature. Distal esophageal temperatures also correlate well with other central temperature measurements. Bladder temperature is similar to rectal temperature (and is therefore intermediate) when urine flow is low but equals pulmonary artery (and thus central) temperature when flow is high. Because bladder temperature is strongly influenced by urine flow, it is rarely clinically useful. Oral and axillary temperatures are not useful in hypothermia victims.

More difficult than the diagnosis of hypothermia per se is identification of treatable predisposing factors and associated illness, especially frost-bite. Because hypothermia produces analgesia, even severe injuries may not provoke complaints. Careful physical examination and a history including degree and duration of exposure, the victim's age, and known predisposing illnesses facilitate the diagnosis of injury and the search for coexisting conditions. State of consciousness has both diagnostic and prognostic value. Fully conscious victims of hypothermia typically survive, even with minimal therapy (unless killed by an underlying, predisposing disease). Since hypothermia itself does not produce unconsciousness until central temperature decreases to 28° C, stupor or unresponsiveness in victims with higher temperatures indicates an underlying problem, such as hypoglycemia, intoxication, or stroke.

Severe hypothermia is associated with profound bradycardia (10 beats/min) and shallow respiration (two breaths/min). Cardiopulmonary resuscitation is probably unnecessary in hypothermic patients with spontaneous respiration and intact circulation, even when bradycardia is extreme.

Treatment and Prognosis. Patients with moderate or severe hypothermia should be treated in an ICU and monitored for arrhythmias, electrolyte disturbances, increased intracranial pressure, vascular volume, urine production, and underlying disease. Because infections are common in survivors of accidental hypothermia, antibiotics are probably warranted. Although thermoregulatory shivering speeds rewarming, it should be inhibited (by administration of 10 to 20 mg meperidine) because its metabolic demand offsets that advantage.

Initial central temperatures often underestimate hypothermia because rapid cooling combined with vasoconstriction exaggerates the difference between central and peripheral temperatures in hypothermia victims. Following transport to a warm environment, redistribution of central heat to the cold periphery can further decrease central temperature several degrees. This "after-drop" normally occurs in the first 15 minutes following rescue and may be aggravated by aggressive peripheral warming that causes locally mediated vasodilation. More serious is the hemodynamic instability caused by rapid vasodilation. Hypotension may be exacerbated by the release of lactic acid and other products of ischemia. Acidosis may contribute to cardiac irritability.

Hypothermia victims may be rewarmed by passive, active surface, or active central methods. When most metabolic heat loss to the environment is prevented by passive insulation of the skin surface, central body temperature increases 1° C per hour. This rewarming rate is usually sufficient for mild hypothermia, and the method is free of risks. Active skin surface warming via immersion in water at 42° to 43° C increases central temperature 5° C per hour. The disadvantages of this method include limited access to the subject and the need to move and dry the person before attempting defibrillation, both of which make cardiopulmonary resuscitation difficult. This technique poses the greatest risk of acidosis and hypotension caused by locally mediated peripheral vasodilation.

Hypothermia severe enough to require active rewarming (that is, less than 30° C) may warrant a central warming technique that does not produce rapid peripheral vasodilation. Although extracorporeal circulation has been used, peritoneal lavage is nearly as effective, considerably safer, and more readily available. One or two peritoneal catheters, flushed with normal saline solution at 40° C at a rate of 10 L/h, increases central temperature 5° C per hour. Other central warming methods, such as inhalation of warm gases, warmed intravenous fluids, diathermy, mediastinal lavage, and warm water enemas, and passive peripheral methods, such as hot water bottles, are ineffectual or pose risks that exceed their possible benefits.

HYPERTHERMIA

Hyperthermia occurs when the hypothalamus regulates at a higher temperature than normal (fever) and during periods of extreme environmental heat (heat stroke) or excessive metabolic heat production (for example, malignant hyperthermia; see next section).

Heat Stroke

Central temperature normally increases 1° to 2° C during exercise. This increase is regulated and occurs even in cool environments. Heat stroke results when a warm and humid environment, combined with exercise and inadequate fluid intake, overcomes the ability of centrally mediated effectors to lose heat. Hyperthermia (central temperatures of 40° C or more) and intravascular volume depletion result. In mild cases tachycardia is combined with orthostatic vital signs; severe heat stroke is indicated by frank shock.

Treatment is supportive and consists of moving the victim to a cool environment and rehydration. In hypotensive patients rehydration should be intravenous; typically several liters is required. Electrolyte disturbances may accompany severe heat stroke. Active cooling is not necessary; intact central regulation rapidly decreases temperature when physical exertion stops and the victim is placed in a cool environment.

Fever

In the 1940s, fever was shown to be mediated by soluble "endogenous pyrogens" released during immune stimulation. The factors have since been identified as interleukin-1, tumor necrosis factor, interferon-alpha, and macrophage inflammatory protein-1. This mechanism differs from "normal" thermoregulation, which is not dependent on circulating factors, and explains why drugs such as aspirin decrease fever but do not influence normal body temperature.

Endogenous pyrogens produce a coordinated increase in the thermoregulatory threshold temperatures, causing the body to defend an abnormally high central temperature. The usual thermoregulatory effectors (vasoconstriction, nonshivering thermogenesis, and shivering) are used to increase metabolic heat production and decrease heat loss to the environment. Maintaining a high temperature is a greater metabolic stress than that resulting from the passive increase in metabolic rate of 7% per degree centigrade caused by simply being at a higher temperature.

Fever develops in infected mammals, birds, reptiles, and fish (reptiles and fish use behavioral regulation to control body temperature). It is unlikely that such a metabolically expensive response would have been retained in so many species for so long without providing significant benefit. (Obviously, fever may be maladaptive in individual cases.) Phylogeny suggests that fever developed hundreds of millions of years ago to assist immune function. Studies in the 1960s and 1970s demonstrated a greater mortality rate when fever was prevented in infected lizards (by denying them access to a warm environment or by administration of aspirin). Aspirin administration also increases the mortality rate in infected mammals. The protective effects of fever result from increased immune and cytotoxic function, not a direct effect on bacterial or viral pathogens. Specifically, fever increases neutrophil and macrophage motility and activity, activates T lymphocytes, causes secretion of antibacterial chemicals, and decreases serum iron (which is required for bacterial growth).

Mild hyperthermia appears to facilitate immune function. Therefore treatment of fever is best reserved for cases in which it causes excessive metabolic demand, produces patient discomfort, or approaches dangerous levels (central temperature more than 40° C). When treatment of fever is appropriate, it is guided by the knowledge that fever results from central regulation and that most of the metabolic stress is caused by the body's effort to maintain a high temperature. Thus, although vigorous cooling lowers body temperature, it has a high metabolic cost and causes patient discomfort. A better approach is to treat the underlying immune stimulation or inhibit central mediation of fever.

Most fever is due to infection; in critically ill patients aggressive treatment of infection is usually warranted in any case. Antibiotics and, when necessary, surgery should be aggressively instituted in patients with severe fever. The second line of therapy is administration of antipyretic medications, including aspirin and nonsteroidal antiinflammatory drugs. Non-infection-related fever (such as that secondary to tumor, rheumatoid disease, allergic reactions, or tissue necrosis) is also best approached by treating the underlying cause and, when necessary, inhibiting central fever mediation. In some of these diseases, steroids and diphenhydramine (Benadryl) are helpful.

MALIGNANT HYPERTHERMIA

Malignant hyperthermia is an acute hypermetabolic syndrome triggered by succinylcholine and the potent inhalation anesthetics. The perioperative onset of malignant hyperthermia may be fulminant and its course rapid. Symptoms include skeletal muscle rigidity, hypercarbia, and fever, which can progress within 30 minutes to a premorbid state in which the arterial pH is as low as 6.6 and the temperature 108° C. The in vitro caffeine-halothane contracture test for susceptible muscle remains the only proven way to diagnose malignant hyperthermia. Intravenous administration of dantrolene sodium inhibits triggering of the syndrome and provides effective treatment.

Triggering Drugs. The only well-documented triggering agents for malignant hyperthermia in humans are succinylcholine and the potent inhalation anesthetics. Caffeine, hypercarbia, hypercalcemia, digoxin administration, exercise, and stress are not causes. In the porcine model that best represents human malignant hyperthermia, the syndrome is triggered by alpha-, but not beta-, adrenergic agonists. Although none of the vasopressors has been shown to trigger this syndrome in susceptible humans, isoproterenol may be the safest drug for treating susceptible patients who require arterial blood pressure support.

A clinically similar syndrome, neuroleptic malignant syndrome, is expressed as hypermetabolic fever triggered by the use of psychotropic drugs, such as phenothiazines, tricyclic antidepressants, and monoamine oxidase inhibitors. Positive caffeine contracture muscle biopsies in some patients with neuroleptic malignant syndrome suggest a pathophysiology similar to that of malignant hyperthermia. Successful treatment of the neurolept syndrome with dantrolene also suggests some clinical kinship.

Signs and Symptoms. The symptoms and signs of malignant hyperthermia result from skeletal muscle hypermetabolism and injury.

Malignant hyperthermia usually occurs during the first 2 hours of anesthesia but has also appeared after prolonged anesthesia and during recovery. Occasionally it occurs many hours after surgery.

The first symptoms of malignant hyperthermia crises are sinus tachycardia, hypertension, and tachypnea, followed by the emergence of cyanotic areas and patches of bright red flushing on the patient's skin. Generalized, rigor mortis-like skeletal muscle rigidity occurs in approximately 30% of crises, usually associated with a more fulminant course. Central thermoregulation remains intact during malignant hyperthermia. Hyperthermia occurs because continuous muscle contracture generates more heat than the body can dissipate to the environment. Although fever is a relatively late finding, temperature can increase at a rate of 1° C every 5 minutes, rising above 46° C. In other cases fever is minimal.

Treatment and Prognosis. Current recommendations for treating acute malignant hyperthermia include discontinuation of triggering drugs, lung hyperventilation with 100% oxygen, and immediate intravenous administration of dantrolene 2.5 mg/kg. If all symptoms (rigidity, acidosis, and tachycardia) do not disappear within 30 minutes of the initial dantrolene dose, an additional 2.5 mg/kg should be administered every 30 minutes (to a maximum of 10 mg/kg) until symptoms resolve.

Arterial blood gas and serum electrolyte levels should be measured frequently to aid management. Urine should be checked for myoglobinuria at least once. If the clinical and laboratory findings return to normal with dantrolene therapy, cooling measures are not needed. Intravenous administration of dantrolene should be continued at 2.5 mg/kg every 6 hours for approximately 24 hours following a severe crisis. Mild or aborted episodes of malignant hyperthermia require less dantrolene.

DANTROLENE. The elimination half-life of dantrolene during anesthesia is approximately 9 hours. The drug is metabolized in the liver primarily to 5-hydroxydantrolene, which is pharmacologically similar to the parent compound, and has a half-life of approximately 15 hours. Hepatoxicity can occur with prolonged oral use but has never been reported during the treatment of hyperthermic crises.

Dantrolene increases the contraction activation threshold voltage in susceptible and normal muscle, prevents the depolarization of susceptible muscle by halothane, and decreases intracellular calcium concentration. These effects are partially reversed by calcium, although they do not resemble the changes apparent with calcium channel blockers. Nevertheless, the toxicities of diltiazem-dantrolene and verapamil-dantrolene appear to be synergistic, causing hyperkalemia and cardiac arrest. In contrast, the combination of nifedipine and dantrolene appears to be safe.

Sedation and Analgesia in Susceptible Patients. Elective surgery is not contraindicated in patients known to be susceptible to malignant hyperthermia. Both regional and general anesthetics can be administered safely, although unnecessary stress should be avoided with either technique. Any type of conduction anesthesia with any type of local anesthetic is acceptable, including lidocaine and other amide local anesthetics. Susceptible patients can safely be given narcotics, nitrous oxide, benzodiazepines, ketamine, and etomidate. Barbiturates inhibit triggering of malignant hyperthermia, as do the nondepolarizing muscle relaxants.

Diagnostic Tests. The in vitro caffeine-halothane contraction test developed by Kalow and Britt in 1970 is the only widely accepted test for malignant hyperthermia. The diagnosis is established by evaluating a fresh, intact muscle segment for contraction in response to halothane and caffeine, which have little effect on normal muscle. The test is difficult to perform and interpret. Consequently, it is not a routine procedure and is available at only approximately 20 medical centers in the United States and Canada.

Average creatine phosphokinase activity is 152 IU in susceptible patients, 93 IU in first-degree relatives, and only 43 IU in normal subjects. However, in any particular patient neither the creatine phosphokinase activity nor the combination of this activity and family history is sufficient to confirm or exclude the diagnosis of malignant hyperthermia. Recently observed differences between normal and susceptible tissues may provide a basis for minimally invasive tests.

Counseling. Patients who have had a typical hyperthermic crisis and their family members must be considered susceptible until a biopsy proves otherwise. These patients should be told about malignant hyperthermia, must inform their anesthesiologists that they may be susceptible, and should wear a medical alert bracelet. They may also be referred to the Malignant Hyperthermia Association of the United States* to receive additional information and a monthly

* P.O. Box 191, Westport, CT 06881-0191 (203) 655-3007.

bulletin. The association maintains a 24-hour physician referral service to assist with crisis and elective management, including referral for muscle biopsy.

Most anesthesiologists respond to even slight fever, tachycardia, and hypercapnia by changing to a nontriggering anesthetic technique; many also administer dantrolene. Increased awareness and early treatment have decreased the number of severe crises and substantially reduced the mortality rate. They have also introduced a diagnostic dilemma: although these patients may be susceptible, they are more likely to have experienced only a febrile reaction from excessive heating, tissue trauma, pyrogen release, drug administration, or blood incompatibility.

Patients whose symptoms are more indicative of malignant hyperthermia should be told that they may be susceptible but that muscle biopsy is necessary to ascertain the diagnosis. A biopsy is not mandatory because malignant hyperthermia has few if any manifestations except during anesthesia. The decision to perform a biopsy should be made jointly by the anesthesiologist and the patient and must take into account the expense and inconvenience of the in vitro contracture test and the probability that minimally invasive tests will soon be available. Since nontriggering anesthetics are safe, susceptible patients can still undergo elective surgery and lead otherwise normal lives.

Pathophysiology. The biochemical changes of malignant hyperthermia are limited to skeletal muscle and hematologic tissues. Triggering of susceptible muscle takes place during excitation-contraction coupling. Although the mean sarcoplasmic reticulum membrane potential in susceptible muscle is normal, contraction occurs at -86 mV, whereas normal muscle must be depolarized to -54 mV to initiate a contraction. This is significant because the potent inhaled anesthetics depolarize susceptible, but not normal, muscle by 5 to 15 mV, which is sufficient to cause a contraction. Succinylcholine depolarizes both normal and susceptible muscle but triggers only susceptible muscle. A two-site excitation-contraction coupling mechanism has been proposed with succinylcholine, halothane, and dantrolene acting at the first site and caffeine acting at the second site (Fig. 20-6).

Once susceptible muscle has been triggered, contraction begins and is maintained by a complex series of biochemical changes. The primary defect may be an increase in phospholipase-A_2 activity, which in turn increases

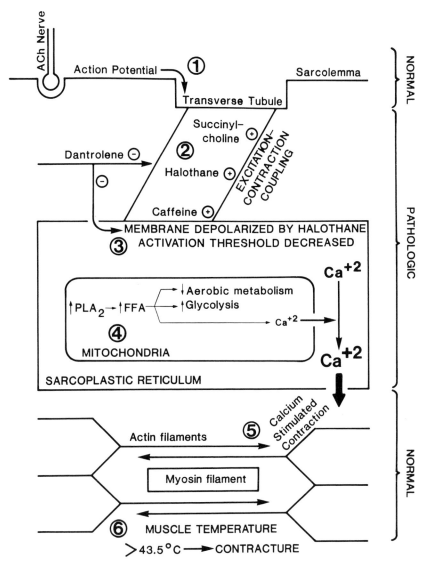

Figure 20–6. *1,* An action potential from the neuromuscular junction is propagated into a transverse tubule. *2,* The signal is transferred to sarcoplasmic reticulum by excitation-contraction coupling. The process is enhanced by succinylcholine, halothane, and caffeine but inhibited by dantrolene. *3,* The threshold of sarcoplasmic reticulum activation is lowered sufficiently in susceptible patients that small depolarization caused by halothane stimulates calcium release. Both effects are alleviated by dantrolene. *4,* Elevated phospholipase-A_2 *(PLA$_2$)* activity increases concentration of free fatty acid *(FFA)*. This results in decreased aerobic metabolism, compensatory increase in glycolysis, and release of mitochondrial calcium. *5,* The increased myoplasmic calcium concentration binds troponin. Actin and myosin then interact, causing contraction. *6,* At a muscle temperature greater than 43.5° C, calcium is no longer required for actin-myosin interaction and contraction becomes an irreversible contracture. (From Sessler DI: J Pediatr 1987;109:9-14.)

mitochondrial free fatty acid release. In the presence of free fatty acid, calcium release from the sarcoplasmic reticulum is increased and reuptake is inhibited. Calcium released by the sarcoplasmic reticulum allows actin and myosin fibers to interact. In late stages, when the muscle temperature rises above 43.5° C, actin-myosin binding is no longer calcium dependent and the muscle contraction becomes irreversible.

CONCLUSION

Temperature is among the most jealously guarded physiologic parameters in mammals. Normally body temperature is maintained by a complex but effective system. Temperature deviating significantly from normal may result from appropriate changes in thermoregulation, such as fever in response to infection; ineffective thermoregulation, as during anesthesia; extreme environmental exposure, such as accidental hypothermia; or excessive metabolic heat production, such as malignant hyperthermia. By understanding the pathophysiology of these diseases, clinicians can optimally diagnose and treat temperature disturbances.

ACKNOWLEDGEMENT: I gratefully acknowledge the editorial assistance of Winifred von Ehrenburg.

SUGGESTED READINGS

Davatelis G, Wokpe SD, Sherry B, et al: Macrophage inflammatory protein-1: a prostaglandin-independent endogenous pyrogen. Science 1989;243:1066-1068

Guze BH, Baxter LR Jr: Current concepts: neuroleptic malignant syndrome. N Engl J Med 1985;313:163

Kluger MJ: Is fever beneficial? Yale J Biol Med 1986; 59:89-95

Lonning PE, Skulberg A, Abyholm F: Accidental hypothermia: review of the literature. Acta Anaesthesiol Scand 1986;30:601-613

Paton BC: Accidental hypothermia. Pharmacol Ther 1983;22:331-377

Satinoff E: Neural organization and evolution of thermal regulation in mammals. Science 1978;201:16-22

Sessler DI: Malignant hyperthermia. J Pediatr 1986; 109:9

Sessler DI, Israel D, Pozos RS, et al: Spontaneous postanesthetic tremor does not resemble thermoregulatory shivering. Anesthesiology 1988;68:843-850

Sessler DI, Olofsson CI, Rubinstein EH: The thermoregulatory threshold in humans during nitrous oxide–fentanyl anesthesia. Anesthesiology 1988;69:357–364.

21

PSYCHOLOGIC STRESS IN THE INTENSIVE CARE UNIT

ROBERT A. VESELIS, MD, and GRAZIANO C. CARLON, MD

To patients and families, and even to physicians with little critical care experience, the ICU environment is alien, complex, cold, and frightening. Furthermore, its physical components and its staff are perceived through the confusion of critical illness and the threat of imminent death. Reality is distorted by emotions, and interactions among individuals reflect the stress created by fear, anger, and denial. All physicians should consider the psychologic dimension of medicine, but it probably is never more significant than in critical care medicine. In the ICU the equally fearsome components acute illness and chronic illness coexist; with each new day the patients and their families anxiously hope for signs of improvement and become discouraged and demoralized by the absence of visible progress. Those emotionally involved with the patient incessantly reinterpret such generic words as "stationary" or "unchanged," often distorting them beyond recognition and making them the basis for unreasonable hopes or unwarranted despair.

Lucid personal accounts by health professionals who have been patients in ICUs emphasize the feelings of despair, alienation, and abandonment that affect even the best informed and most balanced persons when they are powerless, at the mercy of machines and individuals with whom they cannot communicate. In this artificial environment the human psyche is subjected to unusual and noxious stimuli, globally defined as stressors; individuals respond to these pressures by developing symptoms of stress, with which they must then deal.

SOURCES OF STRESS FOR THE PATIENT

In the ICU, as everywhere else in the health system, the patient should be the focus of attention. The ethical justification for medicine, from its major discoveries to its most trivial day-to-day application, is to provide patients with the care they need and want.

Traditionally physicians have been custodians of their patients' freedom of choice. When medicine had little to offer from a scientific standpoint, physicians attached a great deal of importance to their personal relationships with patients; the physician counseled, advised, and consoled but was never an impersonal administrator of therapeutic regimens the patient did not understand and therefore could not knowingly accept. In the last century, and especially the last few decades, the tumultuous progress of medical science has placed physicians in a position to treat and even eradicate most of the diseases that have afflicted humankind since its origin. Inebriated by these admirable successes, physicians may become oblivious of their primary obligation and perceive that their goal is the cure of the disease, rather than the physical and emotional well-being of the patient.

The dangers of this distorted priority are nowhere more real than in ICUs, where technology reigns and patients are often incapable of communicating their anxieties, feelings, and desires. Critical care health providers may see the patient as an appendage of the illness, the means to use the scientific marvels at their

413

disposal, rather than the end of their efforts. This subversion of all humanistic thinking, from Kant to modern-day philosophers, has been aptly described by H.A.F. Dudley: "too often physical triumph is the pinnacle of our aspirations; psychological destruction the nadir of our success."

The major causes of stress, as perceived by the patient, have been determined by interviewing former ICU patients. The most highly ranked stressors are related to the nature of the ICU environment; they include immobilization, isolation, lack of information and communication, noise, sensory overload with subsequent sensory deprivation, lack of sleep, and depersonalization. Dependence on technology for life support is not inherently a major stressor, even though ventilator-dependent patients may be seriously harmed by their communication difficulties.

Noise is one of the most significant and intractable problems for ICU patients. Noise levels can be as high as 90 dB, comparable to a Boeing 707 jet plane at takeoff; they usually average 55 to 60 dB, as loud as a busy cafeteria, and are present day and night. Furthermore, the sounds are usually meaningless to patients and are monotonous and continuous, characteristics that increase patients' psychologic discomfort. Even though many of the devices used in the ICU generate significant noise, the largest contribution comes from the activity of the hospital staff.

Although noise is a stressor in its own right, in the ICU it is often a component of a far broader source of serious discomfort, sensory overload. This condition is created by the presence of multiple stimuli, which bombard the sensory organs at a rate that prevents the central nervous system from processing and organizing them. Thus the information that reaches the patient is chaotic and results in sensory overload, a condition experienced as a state of crowding and confusion that affects judgment and ability to communicate. The absence of recognizable sensory input ultimately results in sensory deprivation; in the midst of bright lights and continuous noise the patient becomes virtually isolated from the environment, with potentially severe psychologic consequences.

In addition to sensory deprivation, limited communication can contribute to the patient's social isolation. Interpersonal exchanges are short and unsatisfactory; the average time of contact between ICU patients and events taking place in their environment, including verbal or nonverbal exchanges with the hospital staff, is

less than 2 minutes. Even for healthy individuals, that period is insufficient to understand and respond to complex stimuli. Furthermore, patients are often immobilized by paralyzing agents, heavy sedation, physical restraints, or loss of neuromuscular strength or coordination. Physical dependence increases the patient's perception of social isolation and creates severe stress.

Sleep deprivation is also a common complaint of ICU patients who are not comatose or heavily sedated; even when they finally fall asleep, their electroencephalographic patterns are very different from those associated with the classic sleep stages. Inadequate or insufficient sleep is a recognized source of stress that leads to inability to concentrate, irritability, confusion, depression, and even hallucinations. The resulting disorientation may be erroneously attributed to organic reasons.

Physicians and other health professionals, projecting their own concerns, rate the onset of a life-threatening disease as a major source of stress for ICU patients. Interestingly, however, patients attach less significance to the global concept of illness and are far more disturbed by the small but constant irritations of ICU care, such as pain, thirst, tracheal suctioning, and uncomfortable positions. These problems particularly affect ventilator-dependent patients; they are subjected to a greater number of unpleasant interventions than most other hospital patients and are less capable of communicating their discomfort to the staff. Thus they experience significant frustration, anger, and anxiety, which may precipitate true psychotic behavior, including suicidal attempts.

The concept that ICU care, the most advanced modality of life support available to patients, could cause a severe, self-destructive mental disorder may be difficult to accept. However, this problem has been well documented and, not surprisingly, is especially serious in the many patients admitted to the ICU for attempted suicide. ICUs provide attentive therapy for physical problems, but the realities of staffing and bed turnover preclude prolonged stays and close attention to deeply rooted psychiatric problems. The patient is usually discharged before psychologic care can begin and remains at the same or even greater risk of committing suicide. A special medical and ethical problem occurs when a patient with no psychiatric history develops suicidal tendencies during or after a stay in the ICU. The patient's psychosis may manifest itself through the adamant refusal of minor treatments, which are nevertheless lifesaving; complex questions of patient competence that have not been directly addressed can then be raised.

Many patients remain conscious during part or all of their ICU stay. Cares and concerns of ordinary life are not always obliterated by drugs, extreme illness, or the introspection caused by the imminence of death. Economic considerations, in particular, may represent a serious psychologic burden to patients. ICU bills may be staggering, insurance may be inadequate or unavailable, income may be diminished or lost entirely. The patient may fear, sometimes reasonably, that the price for survival is financial ruination. This source of stress may be equally intense for the patient's family, especially when the patient is the major or sole breadwinner. Destitution may follow the patient's death, since often the highest ICU costs are generated by the patients who do not survive. The family may direct anger at the patient for lack of any other target; guilt and desperation soon develop, and these stressful emotions may severely strain family unity.

Economic problems are not the only source of tension for a family whose member has been admitted to the ICU. Conflicts that had been successfully dealt with before may reappear with unexpected force. Coping mechanisms fail, and negative feelings toward the patient may become apparent, significantly adding to everyone's stress. Fortunately, this problem does not occur frequently, and most families remain cohesive and supportive through serious adversity. When it does happen, however, it is difficult to resolve, since the involvement of people outside the family adds unpredictable dimensions to their quarrels.

PATIENTS' RESPONSE TO STRESS

In addition to the physical responses to stress, such as vasoconstriction, potentiated ototoxic effects of some drugs, and stimulation of the pituitary-adrenal axis, severe psychologic disturbances may occur. The clinical significance of mental stress should never be underestimated. In one study 7% of the patients admitted to a surgical ICU required psychiatric consultation. As compared with other patients without overt psychiatric problems, this group remained in the ICU longer, required more frequent support with mechanical ventilation, and had a higher incidence of cardiac arrest and a higher mortality rate. Although cause and effect could not be unequivocally established in that study,

provocative questions about the role of psychosomatic illness in the ICU were raised.

Aberrant responses observed in ICU patients that cannot be attributed to organic or pharmacologic causes are sometimes defined as "ICU psychosis." The cause of this disease entity, which still lacks complete definition, includes the stressful conditions mentioned before, such as sensory overload and sleep deprivation. The symptoms include impairment of the cognitive process, global clouding of consciousness, a diminution of the ability to think, perceive, and remember, and depression, sometimes so severe as to mimic a catatonic state. These symptoms were first described in patients who had had open heart surgery; at that time the proposed cause was microembolization from cardiac bypass. It soon became apparent, however, that the explanation was inadequate, since many factors could contribute to the syndrome and sometimes organic causes could be eliminated.

In support of the theory of a primary mental illness, symptoms similar to those described in ICU psychosis have been demonstrated in prisoners kept under strict isolation and in shipwrecked sailors. Those individuals, subjected to conditions of sensory deprivation presumably comparable to those in a busy ICU, reported severe impairment of their ability to think and reason, disorientation, gross disturbances in sensation, and vivid perceptual experiences including hallucinations and delusions. In ICU patients unpredictable stimuli appear to cause the most severe discomfort, perhaps because protective mechanisms cannot be activated. The presence of underlying organic deficits certainly aggravates ICU psychosis. Brain-damaged patients are more vulnerable to sensory overload and sensory deprivation, and conditions that alter subjective perceptions, such as administration of sedative medications or metabolic abnormalities, may also increase the incidence of psychosis. These theories find support in the observation that both older patients and "overalert" patients, who allow excessive sensory input, are more prone to ICU psychosis.

Some researchers have suggested that ICU psychosis is an attempt to create a barrier to an uncontrollable environment, which is overloading the patient's ability to process information. Others have placed greater emphasis on the severe sleep disturbances that occur in almost all ICU patients. In normal volunteers, sleep deprivation does not necessarily cause psychosis, but rather a lack of attention during monotonous tasks. However, in the ICU, with its many other sources of stress, sleep deprivation may well be an important cause of psychosis. A vicious circle of sensory overload, sensory deprivation, sleep deprivation, agitation, and psychosis can easily develop. In critically ill patients, sleep deprivation may have serious physiologic consequences because it can affect the central control of ventilation.

TREATMENT OF PSYCHOLOGIC DISTURBANCES

Psychologic problems of ICU patients are usually recognized when they include physical symptoms (agitation, confusion, hallucinations). Unfortunately, the ICU staff is not trained to identify, much less treat, psychiatric manifestations when they appear as a minor personality disorder or excessive introversion. Usually the staff recognizes the problem only when it begins to affect the patient's physical well-being. At that point the easiest and often the only method of treatment is pharmacologic. Secondary safety interventions often are also necessary, including forcible immobilization to prevent patients from injuring themselves or the staff. Although usually unavoidable, these measures are distasteful and may contribute to the patient's social isolation and depersonalization, ultimately sustaining the cycle of ICU psychosis.

Pharmacologic Treatment

The general goals of pharmacologic treatment should always include relief of physical discomfort, especially pain. The agents selected should also be useful in acute psychosis and when necessary should induce deep sedation and amnesia. Haloperidol is commonly used because it effectively controls even the most agitated patient, although conditions of acute psychosis may require the administration of large amounts over short periods. In most cases therapy begins with intravenous or intramuscular doses as low as 1 mg. The dosage can then be increased to 2 to 5 mg every 8 hours, depending on response, although patients with severe agitation may require as much as 50 mg over 1 to 2 hours to achieve adequate control. Haloperidol has relatively minor side effects during short-term administration, although malignant neuroleptic syndrome has been reported even after a few doses. In elderly patients haloperidol and other neuroleptics may cause extrapyramidal symptoms. Therefore these drugs are absolutely contraindicated in patients with Parkinson's disease. In rare cases haloperidol precipitates cardiac arrhythmias, which could be dangerous in critically ill patients. There is no firm evidence that haloperidol or any other neuroleptic agent antagonizes the effects of dopamine on renal receptors; but in patients receiving low doses of dopamine for enhancement of renal perfusion, absence of response could theoretically be attributed to the concomitant administration of haloperidol. When depression is a major problem, especially in conscious, alert patients who will require prolonged ICU stay, tricyclic antidepressants can be used. Some of the drugs in this category also have a soporific effect and help to normalize sleeping patterns.

Most commonly the goals of therapy are to sedate a patient who is not necessarily psychotic and possibly to induce amnesia for the traumatic experiences of critical illness. In the ICU continuous sedation is often desirable and at times indispensable. The goals of this intervention include prevention of injuries and facilitation of support modalities, such as mechanical ventilation. Sedation has become increasingly important as paralyzing agents have fallen into disfavor. Although effective sedation can undoubtedly be maintained with discrete administration of many different agents, continuous intravenous administration is useful in a busy ICU because it significantly reduces the frequency of medical or nursing interventions to assess the sedation level or administer additional doses. Furthermore, drugs properly administered by continuous infusion maintain stable blood levels and therefore produce consistent and predictable clinical effects.

Thiopental was one of the first substances used for continuous infusion in critically ill patients. Although this drug had well-recognized adverse effects, it was commonly used in operating rooms and therefore was familiar to physicians. Also, thiopental induces deep sleep and amnesia in virtually all patients at doses of 25 to 250 mg/h. This universal efficacy eludes all other drugs used in the ICU, although their far greater safety has greatly reduced the role of thiopental as a sedative for critically ill patients.

Benzodiazepines are the agents most frequently used to sedate ICU patients. A complete review of their pharmacology is beyond the scope of this chapter, but we emphasize that the drugs in this group are not interchangeable. Sedation in the ICU has many, sometimes conflicting goals: the ideal agent should have rapid onset, predictable duration of action, and rapid elimination even in the presence of hepatic and renal dysfunction; it should have a specific antagonist so that rapid reversal is possible; it should provide all desired effects without the need for supplemental substances; it should not induce cardiovascular instability or respiratory depression; it should have a high therapeutic index; it should be stable in solution; and it should not interact with other substances during simultaneous infusion.

The perfect agent does not yet exist, although midazolam, a drug whose use is increasing, has many of the required qualities. Midazolam has no active metabolites and lower tissue accumulation than with most benzodiazepines; therefore its pharmacodynamics are more predictable. It is water soluble and is relatively inert when infused through the same venous access site with many of the drugs used in critically ill patients. In healthy volunteers the half-life of midazolam is short (1½ to 3½ hours), but it can be extended to as long as 22 hours in patients with decreased blood flow to the liver. In rare cases it causes respiratory depression; deaths from apnea have been reported in patients receiving the drug for endoscopic procedures. Thus patients who are breathing spontaneously should be closely supervised after intravenous administration of midazolam. Hypotension may also follow midazolam administration; the drug can potentiate the negative inotropic effects of some narcotics and, like any other sedative administered to critically ill patients, may reverse the peripheral vasoconstriction induced by agitation. Vigilance and immediate interventions to correct rapid shifts in intravascular volume distribution must accompany the administration of midazolam, or any other hypnotic or narcotic drug, in critically ill patients. Despite these disadvantages, midazolam is useful and safe in the management of agitated ICU patients. It can be administered by continuous infusion at a rate of 1 to 20 mg/h, or in intermittent doses of 2.5 to 5 mg every 2 to 3 hours. Tolerance may develop rapidly and necessitates higher doses. Our patients have been able to open their eyes and follow simple commands while receiving midazolam doses as high as 500 mg/d.

Narcotics are the other class of drugs extensively used in critically ill patients. The oldest narcotic, morphine, remains one of the most commonly used. However, its already considerable cumulative effects may be magnified in critically ill patients, especially in the presence of decreased splanchnic flow or renal function. Of the newer narcotics, sufentanil has an important role in the management of critically ill patients. This drug has hypnotic and analgesic properties and therefore has many of the required characteristics of the ideal ICU sedative. Its onset of action is rapid, its pharmacokinetics predictable, and its cumulative effect less pronounced than that of morphine or fentanyl. It does, however, induce severe respiratory depression, especially at the higher doses required for administration as a single agent, and therefore should be used only in patients receiving mechanical ventilation. Muscular rigidity, affecting primarily the chest wall muscles, has also been described. Since sufentanil may depress the cardiovascular system when administered with midazolam, that combination, although extremely effective in maintaining sedation and analgesia, should be used prudently. Usually an intravenous infusion of sufentanil 20 to 100 µg/h induces sedation.

Many other substances also maintain sedation in critically ill patients: diazepam, meperidine, alfentanil, methadone, etomidate, and propofol, to mention just a few. While the drug selection is left to the physician, some considerations can be universally applied. The response to sedative drugs varies greatly among patients and in a single patient at different stages of the illness; accordingly, dosage should be adjusted to produce the desired effect rather than on the basis of theoretical considerations. Organ dysfunction may prolong the duration of action, especially when the kidneys or liver is affected. Thus recovery time may be unexpectedly long, and neurologic damage may not be definitely assessed until the levels of the sedative agents are demonstrably too low to affect the function of the central nervous system. Many agents have summative or even potentiating effects that are not restricted to their sedative action but may also affect other organ systems, especially cardiovascular and respiratory functions. Finally, the goal of therapy should be clearly defined before a drug is selected. For instance, when pain control rather than hypnosis is the desired effect, techniques that do not affect the level of consciousness should be considered, such as patient-controlled analgesia or epidural administration of narcotics.

Other Treatment

During the acute phase of illness, drugs are the easiest or even the only method of therapy available for psychologically disturbed patients, since psychotherapy cannot be provided without communication, which is often difficult with ICU patients. Frequently, when patients can express themselves effectively, they are also ready for discharge from the ICU. However, many patients are fully conscious and aware of their surroundings but must remain in the ICU, sometimes for a prolonged period, because of the nature of their illness. Every effort should be made to minimize the psychologic discomfort associated with their condition. Social contacts with the conscious patient must be maintained at all costs; this is one of the most effective, and too often neglected, methods of providing psychologic balance. Patients should feel that they are still members of the community where they live, no matter how restricted their field of activity. The staff should talk to the patients and attempt to elicit responses, either verbally or through other means. Newspapers, radio, and television provide needed windows on the outside world and should be made readily available. Families should be allowed prolonged visiting periods unless their presence clearly disturbs the patient. Indeed, relatives and friends should never be perceived as annoyances who disturb the orderly flow of activities in the ICU, but as major contributors to the patient's well-being.

The ICU staff must develop special communication skills when dealing with patients, especially those who are conscious and alert although severely ill. They must present information in a manner easy to understand, usually discussing one concept at a time, to avoid worsening sensory overload. Also, they must be patient in eliciting answers from a patient who cannot talk. The staff must understand the frustration of any alert individual who can only mouth words to express relatively complex concepts, since intubation or other conditions prevent the emission of understandable sounds. Lip reading is not a skill taught in medical or nursing school, and all critical care practitioners know the limitations of this form of communication. Written communication may be equally impractical. Even excluding patients who have language barriers, are poorly literate, or are too young to write, the fine muscular coordination needed to write legibly can be seriously impaired in a critically ill patient. Furthermore, patients are often lying in positions poorly suited for comfortable writing, they may have uncorrected vision problems, since glasses are usually banished from ICUs, and they may be unwilling or unable to invest the time and energy required for a written conversation. Frustration, anger, and anxiety can build quickly and interfere with the relationship between patients and staff members, or even families, unless those who are not diseased accept that the burden of establishing and maintaining communication falls almost exclusively on them.

SOURCES OF STRESS FOR THE STAFF

Thus far we have discussed the responsibility of the ICU staff and the strenuous efforts required to provide adequate physical and psychologic care to patients with life-threatening illnesses and extraordinary support needs. Care providers in the ICU may have serious difficulties coping with the stress of treating such a demanding patient population. Ignoring the staff's problems, or expecting that they will be resolved through discipline and sense of duty exclusively, is absurd. The best evidence of the inanity of such wishful thinking is the intractable shortage of ICU nursing staff and the high turnover rate, which reaches 70% to 80% a year in some ICUs. The results are increased costs, lower standards of care, and reduced availability of ICU beds, clearly a poor combination to address the problems of extreme illness.

Many, diverse components contribute to the stress experienced by the ICU staff. They must continually make critical decisions, with little margin of error. Crisis conditions may persist for prolonged periods or recur repeatedly with short remissions. Similar conditions are experienced by soldiers on the battlefield, when hostilities continue unremittingly week after week and precipitate a psychologic battle fatigue marked by depression, feelings of inevitable defeat, anger, and finally desertion of duty. Legal and ethical uncertainties often trouble professionals already stressed by the absence of definitive scientific solutions to many clinical problems. Friction arises among ICU care providers and even more often between them and members of other services. Perhaps the most significant source of stress is the constant presence of death, often accentuated by prolonged, senseless intensive care support of terminally ill patients. To understand the frustration and anger experienced by the ICU staff, the reader might picture the reaction of surgeons who were continually required against their best judgment to perform complex surgical procedures on patients who would inevitably die on the operating table. The very concept is unthinkable, yet it represents a daily experience for most ICU practitioners. The reactions include feelings of worthlessness, loss of control, depression, and withdrawal from the problems of the patient, resembling the symptoms of battle fatigue.

Ultimately the patients suffer because their isolation and attendant disorientation increase.

Staff members may also identify with dying patients, who may remind them of relatives, friends, or even themselves. They may form close emotional ties with a patient, which makes it hard to provide objective care and to accept death when it occurs. Inevitably, staff members are also confronted with their own mortality, especially when patients close to them in age or other identifiable circumstances die. Those deaths may be magnified in significance, creating a perception of hopelessness even when objective data do not support it.

Although death is always present in hospitals, the vast majority of physicians encounter it infrequently and can avoid extended involvement with patients during their final days and hours. For most medical and even surgical specialties, in-hospital mortality rates are measured in minute fractions of a percent; in the ICU, mortality rates are commonly 20% to 30% and may reach 60% to 70% in some groups of patients. Many health professionals cannot derive enough comfort from the often astounding successes of critical care medicine to compensate for the inevitable, frequent failures.

To add to the anguish of ICU physicians and nurses, the allocation of critical care resources is often capricious and therefore so is the decision of who will survive and who will die. As previously mentioned, an inordinate amount of useless effort must be invested in clearly hopeless cases; a possible although not inevitable consequence is that care is not available, or is inadequate, for patients who would greatly benefit. The notorious case of Susan von Stetina, who unnecessarily suffered irreversible brain damage after a disconnection of her mechanical ventilator went unrecognized for many minutes, is a sobering reminder of the consequences of attempting to provide care beyond the ICU's resources. Critical care practitioners are placed in double jeopardy. On one side, hospital administrators insist on cost curtailment and ration resources by postponing acquisition of supplies and equipment or enforcing staff shortages, without openly stating that their goal is reduction of services. On the other side, government agencies, the legal system, and the media thunder and threaten if care is withheld. The result is a trial by ordeal in which the health professional can only lose.

While physicians must operate in a nonsupportive, if not outright hostile, environment, patients are being accorded increasing autonomy. Ethically this attitude is irreproachable. Its primary goal is to prevent misguided health care providers from forcing extraordinary therapies on patients who clearly refuse them. Like many statements of principle that choose to ignore the realities of human nature, however, the guidelines for autonomy do not address the issue of patients who abuse the limited resources of medical care. In reality, many more ICU patients request continued care, even though their prognosis is poor, than demand cessation of support.

Since openly restricting care against the patient's wishes is not considered acceptable and rationing is not officially sanctioned (indeed, its existence is usually denied), subterfuge becomes a tempting alternative. Critical care physicians may try to use their superior understanding of the limits and potentials of pharmacologic and mechanical remedies to restrict care, even though the most aggressive support measures appear to continue. From an ethical viewpoint this conduct can only be condemned. The concept that the end, fairly allocating scarce resources, justifies the means, deceiving patients and colleagues, is unacceptable. The only route to a just distribution of care is to emphasize the scientific aspects of decision making. On that basis, physicians can argue that they are not obligated to respect the patient's wishes, or to offer the patient choices, when medical treatment is futile. This position has deep historical and philosophical roots; even Hippocrates, in his oath, enjoined physicians from attempting to treat hopeless conditions, lest they be considered charlatans. Interestingly, however, when critical care practitioners can formulate rules to decide when to limit care, they often base the decision on physiologic functional outcome, a subjective concept with which the patient may not agree, rather than on survival and recovery of mental function, objective conditions with which it is far more difficult to argue.

The deep feelings aroused by these conflicting positions suggest that firm guidelines for decision making in critical care will not be soon forthcoming. Philosophic and ethical writings on these subjects will continue to fill countless volumes, but if they follow the pattern established thus far, they will have no practical significance because they will only identify the problems without suggesting practical solutions.

Conscious and subconscious expectations by families and patients may place additional stress on nurses and physicians. We all harbor idealized images of health professionals. Even though we may rationally accept that they are simply human beings, with weaknesses, flaws, and prejudices like those of any other person, we greet any deviation from the idealized role with disillusionment, disappointment, and loss of confidence. Health care providers should approach this perception problem with the frank admission that the science of medicine and the knowledge of its providers have well-defined limits. However, the temptation is to try to live up to the magnified expectations of patients and families, to enjoy their awe and admiration. Critical care practitioners, who can cover themselves with the protective cloak of complex technology, may be most likely to succumb to this attitude, which is inevitably self-defeating. Even though physicians may at times be able to project the image of powerful individuals who can master forces and devices unavailable to common mortals, the price of this narcissistic satisfaction is unacceptable. Failures and mistakes inevitably occur and become apparent even to those who cannot understand the technology of critical care medicine, precipitating a crisis of confidence. Furthermore, physicians who aspire to a superhuman condition relinquish the right to display such emotions as grief, discomfort, anguish, or uncertainty; this repression of basic psychologic needs inevitably leads to severe frustration, and considerable stress.

Relationships with other health professionals in the ICU may add to the stress of care providers. Nurses are rightfully resentful when their contribution to patient care is offhandedly dismissed as less important than that of physicians. ICU physicians and nurses clearly differ in their perceptions of the significance of this problem. When questioned, nurses commonly indicate discomfort with the decision-making process in the ICU and suggest that consultations among health professionals regarding patient care are inadequate. Physicians, on the other hand, believe that there is nearly complete harmony in the ICU, reflecting the bias generated by their greater control of treatment plans. The consequence of a professionally dissatisfied nursing staff is a high turnover, which ultimately limits physicians' ability to implement the therapeutic plans so independently formulated.

Relationships with health professionals outside the ICU may also be a significant source of stress for critical care practitioners. Disagreement on therapeutic interventions or prognostic evaluation is common. Nonetheless, physicians with no training in critical care may have the authority to order treatments that conflict with the most current principles of management. In other instances, unrealistic expectations of recovery, based on the behavior of the primary disease rather than on the degree of vital organ failure, may inspire rescue fantasies in the physician-of-record. This physician may perceive a skeptical critical care staff as hostile; the inevitable negative outcome only reinforces the perception that the patient did not receive all the support possible. The family may pressure the primary physician to "do everything," even though nothing may be available beyond comfort and compassion, which should never be denied. The conflict created by demands that cannot be met may result in unpredictable behavior and therefore additional conflicts.

Even though the art of healing is one of the oldest human endeavors, the science of medicine spans only a few decades. Many people can remember a time when hospitals were places where hapless individuals, who did not have a home where they could pass away with dignity, went to die. As a matter of fact, many more patients die in hospitals today than in the past, but virtually every one of them is admitted with the expectation that their illness will be identified, understood, and treated. As success becomes common, those who are excluded may perceive that they have been unfairly singled out because their physician was incompetent or negligent. Thus the pressures experienced by patients, families, and health professionals have no historical precedent.

New needs result in innovative solutions; to accommodate the heightened anxieties of patients and families, many hospitals have added professional patient representatives to their staffs. These individuals translate medicine into comprehensible terms and guide patients through the often bewildering maze of procedures and regulations of a modern hospital. Even though many other health professionals claim to be patient advocates, they may have conflicts of interest that cause the patient to distrust them. Physicians and nurses who actively treat the illness, for instance, may be suspected of pursuing their own goals rather than the patient's wishes. Paternalism is disappearing in the relationship between care givers and care receivers; although this is possibly desirable, a new type of interaction must be developed to replace it. In all aspects of life, individuals who have a significant personal involvement with a problem cannot be objective about it; the intervention of a third, unbiased party can frequently prevent conflicts or resolve them before they escalate beyond control, to the detriment of all parties.

The patient representative is of course most useful when serious stress is most likely, and when the gap between medical information and patients' ability to comprehend it is greatest. Thus ICUs are prime areas for patient representatives, who can act as a bridge between sophisticated technology and complex pharmacology on one side and the human needs of anguished patients and families on the other.

To conclude on an optimistic note, we should note that, despite the numerous conditions that generate psychologic stress in critical care health professionals, many develop coping mechanisms and continue in practice for many years without becoming cynical and callous. Technologic advances increasingly require that critical care medicine be practiced as an independent specialty by professionals who have no other responsibilities. Efforts should be made to improve working conditions in the ICU and also to identify the individuals who have the character and mental attitude that can most effectively deal with the conflicts, disappointments, and defeats that are as much a part of critical care as dazzling technologic and pharmacologic accomplishments.

SUGGESTED READINGS

Abram MB: President's Commission for the Study of Ethical Problems in Medicine and Biomedical and Behavioral Research: deciding to forego life-sustaining treatment. Washington, DC, 1983,. US Government Printing Office.

Bentley S, Murphy F: Perceived noise in surgical wards and in intensive care areas: an objective analysis. Br Med J 1977;2:1053

Bloom G: Some thoughts on the value of saving lives. Theoret Med 1984;5:241-51

Brett AS, McCullough LB: When patients request specific interventions: defining the limits of the physician's obligation. N Engl J Med 1986;315:1347-51

Critical Care Committee of the Massachusetts General Hospital: Optimum care for hopelessly ill patients. N Engl J Med 1976;295:362-367

Danis M, Gerrity MS, Southerland LI, Patrick DL: A comparison of patient, family, and physician assessments of the value of medical intensive care. Crit Care Med 1988;16:594-600

Dudley A: Affective disturbances in patients in intensive care. In Walker WF, Taylor DE (eds): Intensive care. Edinburgh, 1975, Churchill Livingstone

Eisendrath SJ, Link N, Matthay M: Intensive care unit: how stressful for physicians? Crit Care Med 1986;14:95-98

Falk SA, Woods NF: Hospital noise — levels and potential health hazards. N Engl J Med 1973;289:774-81

Glass DC, Singer JE: Urban stress: experiments on noise and social stressors. New York, 1972, Academic Press, Inc

Knaus WA: Rationing, justice and the American physician. JAMA 1986;255:1176-1181

Kornfeld D: Psychiatric complications of open-heart surgery. N Engl J Med 1965;273:287-292

Miller JG: Information overload and psychopathology. Am J Psychiatry 1959;116:695-704

Parker MM, Schubert W, Shelhamer JH, Parrillo JE: Perceptions of a critically ill patient experiencing therapeutic paralysis in an ICU. Crit Care Med 1984;12:69-71

Redding JS, Hargest TS, Minsky SH: How noisy is intensive care? Crit Care Med 1977;5:275-276

Riggio RE, Singer RD, Hartman K, Sneider R: Psychological issues in the care of critically-ill respirator patients: differential perceptions of patients, relatives, and staff. Psychol Rep 1982;51:363-369

Sands S, Ratey JJ: The concept of noise. Psychiatry 1986;49:290-297

Smith C: In need of intensive care — a personal perspective. Intensive Care Nurs 1987;2:116-122

Walton DN: Death and dying in medicine: what questions are still worth asking? Theoret Med 1984;5:121-139

Youngner S, Jackson DL, Allen M: Staff attitudes towards the care of the critically ill in the medical intensive care unit. Crit Care Med 1979;7:35-40

MULTIPLE ORGAN SYSTEM FAILURE

PHILIP D. LUMB, MB, BS

Critical care medicine has been criticized for not having improved the morbidity and mortality rates of a number of illnesses. Recently the high cost of maintaining patients in intensive care facilities has been publicized, and increasing restrictions have been placed on health care reimbursement in the face of rising costs of medical care. If the ICU census is investigated, the proportion of older patients with a larger number of preexisting chronic medical condition is greater than previously when age often excluded patients from admission to the ICU. Also, early posttrauma resuscitation based on military management protocols and rapid access to organized medical care have increased the number of critically ill patients arriving in the hospital and surviving for the first several hours after injury and admission. Unfortunately, prolonging initial survival alone only escalates hospital costs and increases the frustration surrounding critical illness for patients' families and medical personnel. This chapter explores some of the current thoughts surrounding the pathophysiology of critical illness and discusses present concepts and future research into appropriate patient management.

Multiple organ system failure (MOSF) is identified as a disease of critical care medicine because progressive organ failure following catastrophic illness or severe trauma can be recognized only in the setting of rapid access to sophisticated resuscitative and supportive medical care. This syndrome was first recognized in the 1960s and was associated with the development of organized protocols for early resuscitation and establishment of trauma centers. Like adult respiratory distress syndrome (ARDS) earlier, it has become the *bête noire* of critical

care medicine. Unfortunately, the diagnosis does not specify a unifying pathologic process, and in some instances the nomenclature is used without adequate justification because definitions are imprecise. Obviously this diminishes the chances of appropriate clinical investigation. Hypotheses regarding primary metabolic-nutritional, mediator, septic, and hormonal mechanisms of MOSF abound, but as far as therapy for this syndrome is concerned, few fundamental changes have occurred. New generations of antibiotics are available with greater efficacy and lower failure rates in vitro, more detailed resuscitation protocols are used with recent alterations in the use of vasoconstrictor and inotropic agents, and new, highly sophisticated mechanisms for supporting pulmonary, renal, and cardiac function have been developed, but none of these has altered the overall mortality rate. These results have stimulated discussion and research into different directions, as well as the realization that a new approach to therapy is needed, since improved results are likely to elude current practice.

Financial stimuli for improvements in care abound. Patients with hypermetabolism and multiple organ failure stay in the critical care unit an average of 21 days at an approximate cost of $85,000. Patients discharged from the ICU have a prolonged rehabilitation, frequently as long as 10 to 12 months. Rehabilitation primarily involves the reestablishment of muscle mass and neuromuscular function. Its estimated cost is in the range of $300,000.

A common criticism is that a large proportion of medical resources is expended in the last few months of some patients' lives and that recognition of these cases could save a large sum of money. At present the predictors for survival are inadequate to allow prospective restriction of care in most instances.

DEFINITIONS

Discussion of the features of MOSF requires an understanding of the most common presentations of the syndrome and acceptance of definitions common to all aspects of the disease. Respiratory insufficiency and associated mechanical ventilatory requirement are considered a common denominator of MOSF. Cerra (1988) defines acute lung injury as an "alteration of alveolar structures associated with a clinically significant impairment of the gas-exchange apparatus following exposure of the lung to any noxious environmental or endogenous agent." Furthermore, he divides acute lung injury into three classes: "(1) ARDS [in which] patients have an appropriate antecedent history, severe hypoxemia despite high concentrations of supplemental oxygen (Pao_2/Fio_2 less than 200 mm Hg), diffuse infiltrates on chest x-ray films, no precipitating pulmonary infection, and no other explanation for acute respiratory distress. [Most investigators would also require demonstration of reduced pulmonary compliance and a wedge pressure less than 18 mm Hg.] (2) Acute lung injury [in which] patients fail to meet the strict inclusion criteria for ARDs, yet manifest a similar clinical picture and x-ray findings and have no other explanation for respiratory distress, and (3) severe acute lung injury as defined, but resulting from diffuse pulmonary infection."

Classification and identification of the incidence and severity of MOSF are hampered by the lack of uniform diagnostic criteria for inclusion of the other organ systems, even though their function may be compromised. During the development of a data collection and management system in the surgical ICU, one of the most difficult tasks has been standardizing the system dictionary to permit entry of specific diagnoses into the data base for prospective therapeutic trials and accurate retrospective analysis. Definitions of renal, liver, cardiac, gastrointestinal, hematologic, and central nervous system failures are inadequate and confusing.

Liver failure is generally defined on the basis of hyperbilirubinemia (bilirubin level at least twice the upper limit of normal). Enzyme changes are usually not included in the definition because they do not reflect function. Kidney failure is usually defined as an acute elevation of serum creatinine concentration above baseline values by 50% to 150% and to an absolute level greater than the upper limit of normal. Cases are subclassified as nonoliguric (24-hour output greater than 400 ml) or oliguric (less than 400 ml). Creatinine clearance is a more appropriate basis for diagnosis, but the baseline value is often not available. Gut failure is present when enteral feeding is not tolerated. This may be manifest as failure of gastric emptying, progressive gastrointestinal tract distention, or diarrhea. Sepsis syndrome is usually defined as hyperthermia, leukocytosis, hypermetabolism, and a hyperdynamic cardiovascular response. The last is characterized by high cardiac output and low systemic vascular resistance. Coagulation system failure is generally defined as the presence of thrombocytopenia, or prolongation of prothrombin time (PT) and activated partial thromboplastin time (aPTT), hypofibrinogenemia, elevated concentrations of fibrin degradation products (FDP), or prolongation of bleeding time. Disseminated intravascular coagulation (DIC) is the best-defined symptom of coagulation failure. Its hallmarks are hypofibrinogenemia, elevated FDP, and morphologic evidence of red blood cell damage. This is accompanied by prolongation of PT and aPTT and clinical evidence of bleeding from sites of trivial trauma. Central nervous system failure is manifest as agitation, delirium, obtundation, coma or seizures without known drug cause, or ischemic or mass lesion. Cardiac failure exists when right or left ventricular filling pressures exceed values that maximize stroke volume or stroke work and when systemic perfusion is inadequate to meet metabolic needs. Vascular failure is sometimes defined as the inability to sustain adequate organ perfusion pressures and blood flow despite total systemic oxygen delivery adequate to meet metabolic needs without excessive oxygen extraction.

The reader should recognize the imprecision, lack of agreement, and often lack of objectivity in the preceding definitions. When two or more of these system failures coexist, multiple organ system failure (MOSF) is diagnosed.

Many authors have tried to describe the syndrome of MOSF. Review articles tend to agree that in the absence of a specific cause, preventive treatment is crucial. The deficits must be corrected, the failing systems must be supported, and the still functioning systems must be maintained. However, as DeCamp and Demling (1988) noted, "the syndrome currently affects a wide variety of critically ill or injured patients. The mortality rate is well in excess of 60%. . . . The term *sepsis syndrome* also is used to reflect the fact that infection, although frequently present, is not essential for initiating or perpetuating progressive organ failure. A systemic inflammatory response modulated by a cascade of soluble protein and lipid mediators seems to be the final common pathway linking the sepsis syndrome with MOSF." The prime issue facing critical care practitioners remains the support of individual organ systems, despite a lack of physiologic knowledge, and the prevention of sequential organ system failure by provision of homeostatic environment in which the components of cellular reconstruction are provided in appropriate quantities.

POTENTIAL MEDIATORS

A major difficulty in discussing the recent advances in the management of the sepsis syndrome and its relationship to MOSF is the proliferation of data on a variety of mediators. Although these mediators are recognized as having potentially great significance in the future management of critical illness, at present they have only theoretical potential. The significance of the stress response to critical illness is highlighted by a recent review article that details the following mediators of the stress response: endogenous opioid peptides, tumor necrosis factor, interleukin-1, eicosanoids, cortisol, and the actions of the sympathetic nervous system.

Endogenous Opioid Peptides

The discovery of multiple opiate peptides and receptors during the last few years has improved understanding of the biologic actions of this class of compounds. These include "the modulation of behavior, antinociception, ventilatory drive, vasomotor tone, heart rate, temperature, metabolism, and immunity" (Cheung and Chernow, 1989). Studies using specific opiate analogs and antagonists have been performed to elucidate these effects. Opioid receptors are found in the brain, spinal cord, and some peripheral sites. The main storage sites for these compounds are the brain, hypothalamus, pituitary gland, and adrenal medulla. The interest in opiate peptides increased after reports that naloxone could reverse the hypotension associated with endotoxic shock. However, despite multiple subsequent studies that confirm the original beneficial findings in a variety of shock states, including hypotension associated with neurogenic shock, the response is transient and no

increases in long-term survival have been reported. The quantities of naloxone required are significant, and patients who receive this therapy may become agitated and difficult to manage because of reversal of the antinociceptive effects of the endogenous opiates. However, when exogenously administered narcotics may contribute to hemodynamic instability, the use of a low-dose, continuous naloxone infusion titrated to hemodynamic response may be beneficial. The actions of naloxone are thought to be due to its interaction with endogenous catecholamine and opioids, although the positive cardiac effects may be due to prevention of the release of myocardial depressant factor. Future research may lead to the development of a specific agonist capable of reversing the vascular depressive effects without affecting the antinociceptive effects of the endogenous opioids. One such compound being studied is thyrotropin-releasing hormone. At present, however, no effective therapeutic options are based on this work.

Inflammatory Mediators

Complement

A number of mediators have been implicated in the inflammatory response following trauma. Bacteria, endotoxin, and injured tissue itself can stimulate an inflammatory reaction. The systemic response to these mediators results in end organ injury and hastens the resulting syndrome of MOSF. Activation of the complement cascade is an integral part of the inflammatory response to infection and tissue injury. Subsequent neutrophil attraction, margination onto endothelium, and activation with release of oxygen radicals and protease result in local tissue damage.

Coagulation Cascade

Local and systemic activation of the clotting cascade results in microvascular coagulation that produces further cell damage and tissue injury. Platelet-activating factor released from leukocytes, macrophages, endothelium, and platelets has received a great deal of research attention. Interesting work using isolated rabbit lung perfusion techniques is attempting to elucidate the actions of platelet-activating factor, which is known to cause aggregation of both platelets and neutrophils and stimulation of the arachidonic acid cascade.

Eicosanoid System

Arachidonic acid metabolism is involved in the initial response to tissue and cellular injury, which leads ultimately to the hyperdynamic septic state. However, research on modulating the response has failed to reduce morbidity and mortality rates.

Tumor Necrosis Factor

Recently attention has been focused on lymphocyte- and macrophage-derived peptide hormones known as lymphokines and monokines, respectively. Tumor necrosis factor (TNF, cachectin) is a polypeptide product of activated macrophage. Elevated levels of this compound are associated with higher mortality rates in critically ill patients with sepsis. Also, TNF seems to be responsible for some of the toxic manifestations observed in septic shock. Infusion of TNF in experimental animals reproduces the hemodynamic and metabolic state observed in more conventional septic preparations, such as the cecal perforation model.

Interleukin

Interleukin-1 (IL-1) is a well-studied monokine that is released with infection or inflammation and promotes fever, neutrophilia, and hepatic acute-phase protein production. The early release of IL-1 may be beneficial in sepsis because it stimulates local tissue protective actions. However, evidence also suggests that a circulating IL-1-like substance alters metabolism by enhancing muscle proteolysis and increasing peripheral amino acid oxidation in patients with sepsis and organ failure. This information, like much research data, is beguiling, but the current applicability is small.

Cellular Immunity

An additional area of interest is the changes in cellular immunity in patients with sepsis and multiple organ failure and the implications of these observations for future treatment. A group of Japanese investigators studied changes in total lymphocyte count, lymphocyte cell surface markers (OKT3, OKT4, OKT8, and B1), serum complement factors C3 and C4, immunoglobulins IgG, IgA, and IgM, ceruloplasmin, and transferrin in nine postoperative patients with sepsis and multiple organ failure. Five patients in the group survived. A comparison of the immune responses of the survivors

and nonsurvivors revealed striking differences, with serial levels of C3, C4, ceruloplasmin, and transferrin increased in survivors but not in nonsurvivors. The authors concluded that these changes in cellular immunity may represent another manifestation of multiple organ system failure.

CONCLUSION

A pessimist might consider critical care medicine a failure because of the inability of currently available therapeutic measures to decrease deaths from sepsis and trauma. However, the recognition of multiple system organ failure has led to many improvements in resuscitative and supportive techniques over the past 20 to 30 years. As knowledge about the interactions of the various mediators increases and therapeutic maneuvers to modify their synthesis and distribution are developed, critical care may rely less on acute resuscitation and more on stabilizing the circulation after protective agents have been administered. Studies of calcium channel blockers in the treatment of head injury raised this possibility, although subsequent research has failed to confirm early optimism and enthusiasm. Possibly future practitioners will recognize modern antibiotic therapy as a temporizing measure rather than a curative one and will consider its use one of the greatest impediments to progress in patient care in the latter half of the twentieth century. These clinicians may be able to intervene in tissue injury by primary measures designed to modify the end organ effects of mediators rather than relying on passive organ support and normal physiologic, reparative activities to increase survival.

Greater research sophistication is providing new insight into changes at the cell molecular level that may determine the success of resuscitation. For example, research using differential complementary DNA (cDNA) screening has found that increased synthesis of mRNA coding for fibrinogen is consistent with the increased levels of circulating fibrinogen noted in shock. According to Deutschman et al. (1989), "screening for differential gene expression has also identified changes in the synthesis of mRNA's whose products were either previously unidentified or unrecognized as relevant to shock/resuscitation states. The technique of screening for differential gene expression may be used to investigate alterations in most tissues and changes induced by many common therapeutic interventions or disease states. As such, the technique may have wide applicability in studying the response to anesthesia, surgery and critical illness."

The preceding highlights a problem in critical care research: it has been conducted with available clinical monitors and therefore is restricted in scope. Only recently have investigators begun to seek control of the available technology and direction of its future development. For example, it is possible that the great attention paid to hemodynamic detail is based more on the ability to monitor arterial pressure and cardiac output than on a specific requirement for this information. If other monitoring devices and techniques, such as noninvasive cardiac output devices, pulse oximetry, the Niroscope, and differential gene mapping, had been available earlier, current thought would probably be oriented in a different direction. The management of multiple organ failure must be regarded as a future therapeutic challenge rather than a failure.

Critical care practitioners have been frustrated with the reality of progressive organ failure in patients whose therapy appears to be succeeding until suddenly the increased requirements for supportive therapy become evident. Although the expectation remains high that current research efforts will provide new insight into the problem and new therapeutic agents, present management strategies remain remarkably similar to those of the past. New technologic sophistication is not the answer to improving patient survival, although close attention to the details of all aspects of critical care practice may help.

SUGGESTED READINGS

Abraham E, Shoemaker WC, Bland RD, et al: Sequential cardiorespiratory patterns in septic shock. Crit Care Med 1983;11:799-804

Borzotta AP, Polk HC: Multiple system organ failure. Surg Clin North Am 1983;63:315-336

Bromley HR, Frei LW, Nelson LD, Shoemaker WC, panelists, and Reines HD, moderator: Expert exchange: how much perfusion is enough? In Cerra FB (ed): Perspectives in critical care. St Louis, 1988, Quality Medical Publishing, pp 31-44

Cerra FB: Multiple organ failure syndrome. In Cerra FB, (ed): Perspectives in Critical Care. St Louis, 1988, Quality Medical Publishing, pp 1-30

Chernow B, Roth BL: Pharmacologic support of the cardiovasculature in septic shock. In Sibbald WJ and Sprung CL (eds): Perspectives on sepsis and septic shock. Fullerton, Calif, 1986, The Society of Critical Care Medicine, p 183

Cheung AT, Chernow B: The stress response to critical illness. In Chernow B, Todres ID (eds): Problems in anesthesia. Philadelphia, 1989, JB Lippincott Co, pp 165-179

Clowes G, George B, Villar C: Muscle proteolysis induced by a circulating peptide in patients with sepsis or trauma. N Engl J Med 1983;308:545-552

Cox SC, Norwood SH, Duncan CA: Acute respiratory failure: mortality associated with underlying disease. Crit Care Med 1985; 13:1005-1008

Curtis MT, Lefer AM: Protective actions of naloxone in hemorrhagic shock. Am J Physiol 1980; 239:H416

Debets JMH, Kampmeijer R, van der Linden MPMH, et al: Plasma tumor necrosis factor and mortality in critically ill septic patients. Crit Care Med 1989;17:489-494

Decamp MM, Demling RH: Posttraumatic multisystem organ failure. JAMA 1988;260:530-534

Deutschman CS, Cabin DE, Delgado EM, et al: Differential complementary DNA (cDNA) screening identifies induction of fibrinogen gene expression following shock/resuscitation. Anesthesiology 1989;71:A168

Dinarello C, Mier J: Lymphokines: current concepts. N Engl J Med 1987;316:379-386

Filkins JP: Monokines and the metabolic pathophysiology of septic shock. Fed Proc 1985;44:300-304

Fry DE: Multiple system organ failure. Surg Clin North Am 1988;68:107-122

Henao F, Aldrete JS: Multiple systems organ failure: is it a specific entity? South Med J 1985;78:329-334

Holaday JW, Faden AI: Naloxone reversal of endotoxin hypotension suggests role of endorphins in shock. Nature 1978;275:450-456

Nishijima MK, Takezawa J, Hosotsubo KK, et al: Serial changes in cellular immunity of septic patients with multiple organ-system failure. Crit Care Med 1986; 14:87-91

Reines HD, Halushka PV, Cook JA, et al: Lack of effect of glucocorticoids upon plasma thromboxane in patients in a state of shock. Surg Gynecol Obstet 1985;160:320-322

Repine JE, Tate RM: Oxygen radicals and lung edema. Physiologist 1983;26:78-82

Shoemaker WC, Appel PL, Kram HB: The role of oxygen transport patterns in the pathophysiology, prediction of outcome, and therapy of shock. In Bryan-Brown CW, Ayres SW (eds): New horizons: oxygen transport and utilization. Anaheim, Calif, 1987, The Society of Critical Care Medicine, pp 65-92

Shoemaker WC, Appel PL, Waxman K, et al: Clinical trial of survivors' cardiorespiratory patterns as therapeutic goals in critically ill postoperative patients. Crit Care Med 1982;10:398-404

Wilkinson JD, Pollack MM, Glass NL, et al: Mortality associated with multiple organ system failure and sepsis in pediatric intensive care unit. J Pediatr 1987;3:324-328

Zaloga GP, Chernow B, Zajtchuk R, et al: Diagnostic doses of protilerin (TRH) elevate BP by non-catecholamine mechanisms. Arch Intern Med 1984;144:1149

23

CARDIOPULMONARY RESUSCITATION

CHARLES W. OTTO, MD

Resuscitation from cardiac arrest in the hospital depends on the rapid response of a well-trained team that usually includes nurses, respiratory care technicians, and pharmacists, as well as physicians. The critical care physician is often expected to be a primary member of the hospital cardiopulmonary resuscitation (CPR) team. The team must act in coordination and communicate readily. Promoting teamwork by providing a common framework of knowledge and approach to the cardiac arrest victim is the goal of advanced cardiac life support (ACLS) courses sponsored by the American Heart Association. The critical care physician must be thoroughly familiar with ACLS protocols to function within the team. Team leadership also requires up-to-date and in-depth knowledge of physiology, pharmacology, and alternative techniques of CPR. The purpose of this chapter is not to reiterate the protocols taught in ACLS courses but to provide some of the scientific background on which these protocols are based. The chapter focuses on cardiac arrest. Other circumstances requiring cardiovascular support, such as shock and dysrhythmias not associated with cardiac arrest, are covered in other chapters.

Approximately 40% of patients with in-hospital cardiac arrest are resuscitated, and of these, 25% survive to discharge. The best initial resuscitation rates are found in the ICU, whereas the best survival rates are in patients whose arrest occurs in the emergency department. The in-hospital success is similar to resuscitation and survival rates from out-of-hospital arrest in cities with rapid response emergency medical systems. In out-of-hospital arrest the factors most important to good outcome are a short arrest time before CPR, rapid defibrillation, and good coronary perfusion during CPR. A better outcome might be expected in

the hospital because of rapid response and application of ACLS by an expert team. However, the illnesses of hospitalized patients reduce their likelihood of survival. An arrest victim in the hospital is also more likely to be elderly, a factor that may reduce survival. Furthermore, the cause of arrest in hospitalized patients is less frequently ventricular fibrillation secondary to myocardial ischemia, the most common cause of out-of-hospital arrest and the cause associated with the best outcome. In resuscitation attempts, attention to the details of CPR is important. However, it should always be remembered that CPR is directed at the symptoms of arrest, not the cause. So much attention should not be paid to the mechanics of CPR that search for a treatable cause of the arrest is forgotten.

DO NOT RESUSCITATE ORDERS

Standards of medical and nursing practice dictate that CPR be performed on any patient suffering cardiac arrest without specific orders to the contrary. Since nearly every patient admitted to a critical care unit has a potentially life-threatening illness, the response, should cardiac arrest occur, must be considered. Do not resuscitate (DNR) orders may be appropriate for patients with terminal diseases and a limited life expectancy, regardless of the intercurrent illness necessitating intensive care, and for patients whose immediate illness requiring ICU admission is associated with an extremely high mortality rate. If possible the physician should discuss DNR orders with the patient and follow the patient's wishes. If the patient cannot participate directly in such decisions, family members should be consulted in an attempt to determine the patient's wishes. The physician must make clear to all involved that DNR orders are not orders to withhold treatment. Forgoing or withdrawing life-sustaining therapy is a separate decision from withholding resuscitation attempts once death has occurred. A related issue when DNR orders are written is the response to unexpected cardiac arrest associated with an iatrogenic complication, such as tension pneumothorax. If CPR will be instituted in such circumstances (DNR orders notwithstanding), the physician should inform the patient and family of this.

PHYSIOLOGY OF VENTILATION DURING CARDIOPULMONARY RESUSCITATION

In the absence of an endotracheal tube, the distribution of gas to the lungs and stomach during mouth-to-mouth or bag-valve-mask ventilation is determined by the relative impedance to flow into each compartment (that is, the opening pressure of the esophagus and the lung/thorax compliance). Although data on airway pressures during cardiac arrest are sparse, esophageal opening pressure is believed to resemble that found in anesthetized individuals (approximately 20 cm H_2O) and lung/thorax compliance may be reduced. Insufflation of air into the stomach leads to gastric distention, impeding ventilation and increasing the danger of regurgitation and gastric rupture. Keeping inspiratory airway pressures low deters gastric insufflation. A major cause of increased airway pressures and gastric insufflation is partial airway obstruction by the tongue and pharyngeal tissues. Management of the obstructed airway is covered in previous chapters. However, it should be pointed out that many individuals have a difficult time using a bag-valve-mask apparatus. Tidal volumes are often greater with mouth-to-mouth and mouth-to-mask ventilation than with a resuscitation bag. Better ventilation is obtained with two individuals, one maintaining the airway and mask and another using both hands to squeeze the bag. Ensuring adequate ventilation is imperative when a resuscitation bag is being used.

Even with an open airway, a relatively long inspiratory time is necessary to give significant tidal volumes at low inspiratory pressures. Since recommended tidal volumes are 0.8 to 1.2 L/breath, 1½ to 2 seconds may be necessary. The most recent standards published by the American Heart Association recommend that 1

TABLE 23–1.   Order of Priorities During Cardiopulmonary Resuscitation*

1. Diagnose fibrillation and defibrillate
2. Open airway
3. Begin ventilation
4. Perform chest compressions
5. Administer oxygen
6. Provide intravenous access
7. Administer epinephrine
8. Assess adequacy of circulation
9. Intubate

*Assuming all equipment and expertise are available. If not, move to next priority until they become available.

to 1½ seconds be allowed for ventilation by pausing after every five chest compressions during two-rescuer CPR. Pressure applied to the anterior arch of the cricoid cartilage (Sellick maneuver) can prevent air from entering the stomach at airway pressures up to 100 cm H_2O. This is a useful adjunct for preventing gastric insufflation during CPR in the hospital where other people are available to perform the maneuver.

Endotracheal intubation is the best way to ensure adequate ventilation without gastric distention. It should be performed whenever a resuscitation attempt lasts longer than a few minutes and an individual trained in intubation techniques is available. However, intubation should not be performed until adequate ventilation (preferably with supplemental oxygen) by other means and circulation by chest compressions have been established. Defibrillation (where appropriate) should not be postponed for intubation (Table 23–1). Once an endotracheal tube is in place, ventilation can proceed without concern for gastric distention or synchronizing ventilation with chest compressions. Performing ventilation and chest compression simultaneously probably does not improve outcome and may be harmful. However, blood flow slows rapidly when chest compressions are stopped and resumes slowly. Consequently, following endotracheal intubation, no pause should be made for ventilations and ventilation should be approximately 12 breaths/min without regard for the compression cycle.

PHYSIOLOGY OF CIRCULATION DURING CLOSED CHEST COMPRESSION

Two theories of the mechanism of blood flow during closed chest compression have been proposed. They are not mutually exclusive, and which predominates in humans continues to be investigated.

Cardiac Pump Mechanism

The original description of closed chest cardiac massage in 1960 suggested that the heart was compressed between the sternum and spine, resulting in increased intraventricular pressure, closing of the atrioventricular valves, and ejection of blood into the lungs and aorta. During the relaxation phase, negative intrathoracic pressure caused by expansion of the thoracic cage facilitates blood return and aortic pressure results in aortic valve closure and coronary perfusion. Support for this theory comes from echocardiography studies in animals showing reduction in ventricular size and mitral valve closure with chest compression during the early stages of CPR. In addition, CPR techniques that incorporate sternal compressions, compared with techniques that raise intrathoracic pressure without sternal compressions, result in better tissue blood flow and survival in animals.

Thoracic Pump Mechanism

A few early investigators questioned the cardiac pump mechanism, and many physicians have questioned the ability of rescuers to depress the sternum adequately in very large individuals. In 1976 a report was published of a patient undergoing cardiac catheterization who simultaneously developed ventricular fibrillation and an episode of cough-hiccups. With every cough-hiccup a significant arterial pressure was noted. The patient never lost consciousness even though CPR was not performed. This description of "cough CPR" led to further studies and to the concept of the thoracic pump mechanism. According to this theory, all intrathoracic structures are compressed equally by the increase in intrathoracic pressure resulting from sternal compression. Backward flow through the venous system is prevented by valves in the subclavian and internal jugular veins and by dynamic compression of the veins at the thoracic outlet. Thicker, less compressible vessel walls prevent collapse on the arterial side. The heart acts as a passive conduit with the atrioventricular valves remaining open during chest compression.

Numerous studies and observations support the thoracic pump mechanism. Angiography has shown that during a cough blood can flow through the left heart into the aorta without cardiac compression. Maneuvers that raise intrathoracic pressure (simultaneous ventilation and chest compression or abdominal binding) increase arterial pressure and carotid blood flow more than standard CPR. Artificial circulation adequate to maintain viability can be accomplished with simultaneous ventilation and inflation of vests surrounding the chest and abdomen in experimental animals.

Fluctuations in intrathoracic pressure clearly play a significant role in blood flow during CPR. The cardiac pump mechanism probably also contributes under some circumstances. Which mechanism predominates varies from victim to victim and even during the resuscitation of the same victim.

Distribution of Blood Flow

Cardiac output is severely depressed during CPR, ranging from 10% to 33% of prearrest values in experimental animals. Total blood flow also tends to decrease with time during closed chest compression, although changes in technique and the use of epinephrine may help sustain cardiac output. Nearly all of the cardiac output is directed to organs above the diaphragm. Brain blood flow may be 90% of normal and myocardial blood flow 20% to 50% of normal, while lower extremity and abdominal visceral flow is reduced to less than 5% of normal. All flows tend to decrease with time, but the relative distribution of flow does not change. Epinephrine improves flow to the brain and heart while flow to organs below the diaphram is unchanged or further reduced.

PHYSIOLOGY OF GAS TRANSPORT DURING CARDIOPULMONARY RESUSCITATION

The circumstances of no flow during cardiac arrest and low flow during CPR severely perturb the normal physiology of gas transport (Table 23–2). This discussion assumes that cardiac arrest occurs in a patient being mechanically ventilated through an endotracheal tube and that ventilation is maintained constant. With the onset of ventricular fibrillation and cessation of blood flow, oxygen (O_2) uptake from the inspired gas stops and carbon dioxide (CO_2) excretion in the exhaled gas rapidly approaches zero as the functional residual

TABLE 23–2. Changes in Gas Transport During Cardiopulmonary Resuscitation*

CO_2 excretion[†]	Reduced
Arterial Blood	
CO_2 content	Reduced
CO_2 tension	Reduced
O_2 content	Normal or slightly reduced for FIO_2
O_2 tension	Normal or slightly reduced for FIO_2
Mixed Venous Blood	
CO_2 content	Unchanged or increased
CO_2 tension	Increased
O_2 content	Reduced
O_2 tension	Reduced

*Assuming adequate ventilation is provided through an endotracheal tube.
†As measured by carbon dioxide elimination from the lungs.
CO_2 = carbon dioxide, O_2 = oxygen, FIO_2 = fraction of inspired oxygen.

capacity is washed out by continued ventilation.* Since end-tidal CO_2 is a reflection of the CO_2 in alveolar gas, it also rapidly approaches zero. At the tissue level, continued metabolism depletes meager tissue O_2 stores, resulting in a tissue O_2 deficit and CO_2 excess. Tissue pH is reduced because of buffering of the excess CO_2. Because there is no blood flow, these changes in O_2 and CO_2 at the tissue level and in the lung are not reflected in arterial or venous blood. Blood gases measured during cardiac arrest without CPR are unchanged from prearrest values.

If normal circulation is restored by rapid defibrillation, cellular metabolism returns to normal but the tissue O_2 deficit and CO_2 accumulation remain. More oxygen moves into the tissues from the blood than usual, and more CO_2 diffuses into venous blood. Mixed venous blood (sampled in the right ventricle or pulmonary artery) has a lower O_2 content and higher CO_2 content than normal, resulting in increased O_2 uptake and CO_2 excretion even though tissue O_2 consumption and CO_2 production may be normal. With constant ventilation the increase in

* Under conditions of steady-state metabolism, hemodynamics, and ventilation, O_2 uptake from inspired gas and CO_2 excretion in exhaled gas are equal to total body O_2 consumption and CO_2 production, respectively. In the non–steady state conditions of cardiac arrest and CPR, a similar relationship may not exist. Hence the terms "O_2 uptake" and "CO_2 excretion" more accurately reflect what is being measured than the more common terms "O_2 consumption" and "CO_2 production."

CO_2 being returned to the lungs causes a temporary rise in alveolar, end-tidal, and arterial CO_2. Within a short time the O_2 deficit is satisfied, the excess CO_2 is removed, and respiratory physiologic variables return to normal.

During the low flow state of CPR, CO_2 excretion (expressed as milliliters of CO_2 per minute in exhaled gas) is decreased from prearrest levels approximately to the same extent as cardiac output is reduced. Although decreased cellular metabolism may be partially responsible, the reduced CO_2 excretion probably is due primarily to shunting of blood flow away from the lower half of the body. The exhaled CO_2 reflects only the metabolism of the part of the body that is being perfused. In the nonperfused areas, CO_2 accumulates during CPR. When normal circulation is restored, the accumulated CO_2 is "washed out" and a temporary increase in CO_2 excretion is seen.

Although CO_2 excretion is reduced during CPR, the mixed venous partial pressure of CO_2 ($P\bar{v}CO_2$) is usually increased. Two factors account for this elevation. Buffering of acids reduces serum bicarbonate. Consequently, the same blood CO_2 content (milliliters CO_2 per deciliter blood) results in a higher $P\bar{v}CO_2$. In addition, mixed venous CO_2 content is frequently, but not invariably, elevated. When flow to a tissue is reduced, not all the CO_2 produced is removed, and CO_2 accumulates, raising the tissue partial pressure of CO_2. This allows more CO_2 to be carried in each aliquot of blood, and mixed venous CO_2 content increases. If flow remains constant, a new equilibrium is established in which all CO_2 produced in the tissue is removed but at a higher venous CO_2 content and partial pressure.

During CPR the arterial CO_2 content and partial pressure ($PaCO_2$) are usually reduced. This reduction accounts for most of the increased arterial/venous CO_2 difference observed during CPR. Even though venous blood may have an increased CO_2 level, the marked reduction in cardiac output with maintained ventilation results in efficient CO_2 removal. An additional result of decreased pulmonary blood flow is that many nondependent alveoli are not perfused and therefore have no CO_2 in the alveolar gas. End-tidal CO_2 level (a measure of mixed alveolar CO_2) is low and correlates poorly with arterial CO_2. However, end-tidal CO_2 level does correlate well with cardiac output during CPR. As flow increases, more alveoli become perfused, alveolar dead space is diminished, and end-tidal CO_2 measurements rise.

INFLUENCE OF TIME

For many years it has been taught that irreversible brain damage occurs if blood flow is not restored within 4 minutes. Recent studies in animals suggest that good neurologic outcome may be possible after cardiac arrest up to 15 minutes if good circulation is promptly restored. In practice, survival from cardiac arrest still depends on rapid resuscitation. Outcome is improved when bystanders begin CPR. The best rates of survival from ventricular fibrillation occur when basic CPR is begun within 4 minutes and defibrillation is applied within 8 minutes. Witnessed arrests have a better outcome than unwitnessed arrests. The importance of early defibrillation has been recognized only in recent years. Defibrillation should take precedence over all other resuscitative efforts if the diagnosis of ventricular fibrillation can be made and defibrillation equipment is available (Table 23–1).

Standard CPR is effective only for a limited period. Despite the occasional success of prolonged resuscitation efforts, standard CPR sustains most patients for only 15 to 30 minutes. If resuscitation has not occurred in that time, the results are dismal. Therefore in recent years considerable effort has been spent in attempting to find new techniques that provide better blood flow during CPR and thus better survival.

ALTERNATIVE TECHNIQUES OF CIRCULATORY SUPPORT

A number of alternatives to standard external chest compression have been investigated in recent years. However, none has proved superior to the standard technique, and all must still be considered experimental. According to the thoracic pump theory, maneuvers that increase intrathoracic pressure during chest compression should improve blood flow and pressure. Consequently, several techniques using different methods to raise intrathoracic pressure have been studied, including abdominal binding, military antishock trousers, simultaneous ventilation and compression, interposed abdominal compression, and pneumatic vest CPR. Early results with a number of these techniques indicated improved aortic pressures and common carotid blood flows. However, subsequent studies failed to demonstrate consistently improved resuscitation success or survival. The increase in aortic pressures seen with these techniques was expected to improve myocardial perfusion. Unfortunately, raised intrathoracic pressure causes an increase in right atrial and intraventricular pressure that is comparable to or greater than the increase in aortic pressure. The result is no improvement or actual diminution in coronary perfusion pressure and myocardial blood flow. The increased intrathoracic pressure caused by these techniques is associated with a rise in intracranial pressure so that the improvement in cerebral blood flow has been small or none despite increased common carotid artery flow.

An alternative technique, commonly called high-impulse CPR, is based more on the cardiac pump mechanism. In this experimental model, relatively short compressions with moderately high force result in cardiac output that is directly related to the rate of compressions. The optimal cardiac output and coronary blood flow are obtained with 120 compressions per minute. Only recently has this technique received much attention. To date, comparisons with the standard technique have not shown a clear improvement in resuscitation and survival.

In contrast to the closed chest techniques, two invasive maneuvers have maintained cardiac and cerebral viability during long periods of cardiac arrest in animals. Open chest cardiac massage and cardiopulmonary bypass through the femoral artery and vein using a membrane oxygenator can provide better hemodynamics and myocardial and cerebral perfusion than closed chest techniques. Prompt restoration of blood flow and perfusion pressure with cardiopulmonary bypass can provide resuscitation with minimal neurologic deficit after 20 minutes of fibrillatory cardiac arrest. However, to be effective, these techniques must be instituted early, probably within 15 to 20 minutes. If open chest massage is begun after 30 minutes of ineffective closed chest massage, survival is no better even though hemodynamics are improved. The need to institute these invasive maneuvers early in an arrest obviously limits the application. When arrests occur in the hospital or ICU, the expertise necessary to apply these techniques may be available. However, practitioners are appropriately reluctant to apply such invasive maneuvers until it is clear that closed chest techniques are ineffective. Unfortunately, at that point invasive methods may be too late to be successful. Before invasive procedures can play a greater role in modern CPR, a way must be developed to predict, early in the resuscitation, which patients will respond to closed chest compressions.

ASSESSING THE ADEQUACY OF CIRCULATION DURING CARDIOPULMONARY RESUSCITATION

Palpation of a pulse in major blood vessels is the traditional method of assessing the efficacy of closed chest compressions. However, the palpable pulse primarily reflects systolic blood pressure, and mean blood pressure correlates better with cardiac output. Moreover, successful resuscitation correlates with myocardial blood flow, aortic diastolic pressure, and coronary perfusion pressure in experimental animals. During standard CPR in dogs an arterial diastolic pressure of 40 mm Hg is usually associated with successful resuscitation. Studies of alternative CPR techniques with increased intrathoracic pressure have revealed that a more accurate measure is the coronary perfusion pressure, defined as the difference between arterial and right atrial diastolic pressures. In dogs the critical coronary perfusion pressure for resuscitation is approximately 25 mm Hg. In the ICU many patients suffering cardiac arrest have intraarterial and venous pressure monitors already in place. They provide a useful means for judging the adequacy of chest compressions. Although the critical aortic diastolic and coronary perfusion pressures for humans are not known with certainty, the animal numbers can be used as a guide. If the aortic diastolic pressure is less than 40 mm Hg or the aortic diastolic minus the right atrial diastolic pressure is less than 25 mm Hg, efforts should be made to improve chest compressions and additional epinephrine should be administered to raise the pressure. Pressures above these levels do not ensure success. Damage to the myocardium from the underlying disease may preclude survival no matter how effective the CPR efforts. However, pressures below these levels are associated with poor results even in patients who might be saved.

Although invasive pressure monitoring may be ideal, exhaled end-tidal CO_2 is an excellent noninvasive guide to the effectiveness of standard CPR. Its use is based on the observation that myocardial blood flow and successful resuscitation are highly correlated with cardiac output during CPR. As discussed in the section on gas transport, CO_2 excretion during CPR with an endotracheal tube in place is flow dependent rather than ventilation dependent. Since alveolar dead space is large during low flow conditions, end-tidal CO_2 is low. If cardiac output increases, more alveoli are perfused and end-tidal CO_2 rises. Within a wide range of cardiac outputs during CPR, end-tidal CO_2 correlates with cardiac output, coronary perfusion pressure, initial resuscitation, and survival. A recent retrospective study demonstrated that no patient with an end-tidal CO_2 less than 10 mm Hg could be successfully resuscitated. In the absence of invasive pressure monitoring, end-tidal CO_2 monitoring can be used to judge the effectiveness of chest compressions. Attempts should be made to maximize end-tidal CO_2 by alterations in technique or drug therapy. Of course, since sodium bicarbonate liberates CO_2, which is excreted through the lungs, the end-tidal CO_2 values are temporarily useless after bicarbonate administration. However, end-tidal CO_2 values stabilize within 5 minutes of bicarbonate administration.

DEFIBRILLATION

The longer ventricular fibrillation continues, the more difficult defibrillation is and the less likely successful resuscitation becomes. The fibrillating heart has a high oxygen consumption, which increases myocardial ischemia and decreases the time to irreversible cell damage. Thus conversion of ventricular fibrillation to a rhythm capable of restoring spontaneous circulation should be the first priority of any resuscitation attempt (Table 23–1). The only effective treatment of this rhythm is electrical defibrillation, and the sooner it is applied, the higher the rate of successful resuscitation. The amplitude (coarseness) of the fibrillatory waves on an electrocardiogram may reflect the severity and duration of the myocardial insult and thus have prognostic significance. As the myocardium becomes more ischemic, fibrillation becomes less vigorous, the electrocardiographic pattern becomes finer, and defibrillation becomes more difficult. Manipulation of the pattern with drugs, such as epinephrine, does not affect success of defibrillation. Consequently, defibrillation should not be postponed for any other therapy but should be carried out as soon as fibrillation is diagnosed and the equipment is available. The precordial thump, although rarely successful, can be tried while a defibrillator is awaited. It should not be used for a conscious patient with ventricular tachycardia unless a defibrillator is immediately available, since it is as likely to induce fibrillation as normal rhythm. Blind defibrillation should be tried in adults if no monitoring is available. This should rarely be necessary, since modern defibrillators have built-in monitoring capability with the paddles used as electrodes.

Defibrillation is accomplished by current passing through a critical mass of myocardium, causing simultaneous depolarization of the myofibrils. The output of a defibrillator is indicated in energy units (joules or watt-seconds). The relationship between energy and current is given by the following equations:

$$\text{Energy (joules)} = \text{Power (watts)} \times \text{Duration (seconds)} \quad \text{(Eq. 1)}$$

$$\text{Power (watts)} = \text{Potential (volts)} \times \text{Current (amperes)} \quad \text{(Eq. 2)}$$

$$\text{Current (amperes)} = \frac{\text{Potential (volts)}}{\text{Resistance (ohms)}} \quad \text{(Eq. 3)}$$

Rearranging and substituting produces this relationship of energy, current, and impedance (resistance):

$$\text{Current (amperes)} = \sqrt{\frac{\text{Energy (joules)}}{\text{Resistance (ohms)} \times \text{Duration (seconds)}}} \quad \text{(Eq. 4)}$$

The actual energy delivered by a defibrillator varies inversely with the impedance between the paddle electrodes. The energy setting on most modern defibrillators indicates the energy that will be delivered when discharged into a 50 ohm load. Even at a constant delivered energy, Equation 4 demonstrates that as impedance between the electrodes increases, the delivered current decreases. Therefore optimum success of defibrillation is obtained by keeping transthoracic impedance as low as possible.

Transthoracic impedance during defibrillation varies from 15 to 150 ohms among patients. Important factors in reducing transthoracic impedance are shown in Table 23–3. Resistance decreases with increasing paddle size, although concern has been expressed that large paddles spread the current over too great an area to be successful. The greatest impedance is between the metal electrodes and skin. Saline-soaked gauze pads and electrocardiographic electrode creams reduce impedance. Paste specifically formulated for defibrillation provides the least resistance. Firm pressure of at least 11 kg improves impedance, partly by improving electrode-skin contact and partly by expelling air

TABLE 23–3. Factors Reducing Transthoracic Impedance During Defibrillation

Large paddle electrode size (≥ 8 cm diameter)
Defibrillation paste
Firm pressure on electrodes (≥ 11 kg)
Defibrillation during exhalation
Successive shocks

from the lungs. Since air is a poor conductor, defibrillation should always be performed during the expiratory phase of ventilation. Transthoracic impedance decreases with successive shocks, although the clinical importance of this factor has been questioned. This may partially explain why additional shocks of the same energy may succeed when previous shocks did not.

The incidence and severity of myocardial damage from defibrillation in humans are not known. In animals, high-energy shocks, especially if repeated at close intervals, result in dysrhythmias, electrocardiographic changes, and myocardial necrosis. Consequently, it would seem prudent to keep energy levels as low as possible during defibrillation. However, if energy is too low, the delivered current may be insufficient for defibrillation, especially when transthoracic impedance is high. A general relationship exists between body size and effective defibrillation energy. Children need less energy than adults, approximately 0.5 to 2.0 J/kg. However, over the size range of adults, body size does not seem to be a clinically important variable. Current evidence suggests that most adults can be defibrillated with energy levels of 200 joules or less, which is insufficient to cause myocardial injury. However, if two or three shocks at this energy level are unsuccessful, subsequent attempts should be made at 300 to 360 joules.

DRUGS IN TREATMENT OF CARDIAC ARREST

Catecholamines and Vasopressors

Vasopressors are the only drugs universally accepted as useful in resuscitation from cardiac arrest. Epinephrine has been the primary vasopressor used. Its efficacy lies entirely in its alpha-adrenergic properties. Peripheral arteriolar vasoconstriction increases aortic diastolic pressure, causing an increase in coronary perfusion pressure and coronary blood flow. It is tempting to invoke the cardiac-stimulating, beta-adrenergic properties in explaining epinephrine's success. However, animal studies have demonstrated that all drugs with strong alpha agonism (epinephrine, norepinephrine, phenylephrine, methoxamine, dopamine) are equally successful, whereas pure beta agonists (isoproterenol, dobutamine) are unsuccessful. Alpha-adrenergic blockade precludes resuscitation with epinephrine, whereas beta blockade has no effect. Although beta activity of epinephrine increases the amplitude of fibrillatory waves, epinephrine has no effect on the success of, or energy necessary for, defibrillation. Survival and neurologic outcome studies have not shown a difference between epinephrine and pure alpha drugs in CPR.

The beta-adrenergic effects of epinephrine are potentially deleterious during cardiac arrest. Epinephrine increases oxygen consumption and decreases the endocardial/epicardial blood flow ratio in the fibrillating heart. Myocardial lactate production does not change following epinephrine administration during CPR, suggesting that the improved blood flow and oxygen delivery are matched by an increased oxygen demand. The pure alpha-adrenergic agents do not increase myocardial oxygen consumption. Epinephrine has been shown to increase cerebral blood flow during CPR in several studies. Studies of the efficacy of pure alpha agents in improving cerebral blood flow have shown conflicting results.

The effectiveness of epinephrine during CPR is probably related to a reduction in myocardial ischemia because of improved blood flow caused by the raised coronary perfusion pressure during closed chest compressions. Although other alpha-adrenergic drugs may provide the same effect without the theoretical adverse beta-adrenergic effects, no other drug has been shown in animal or clinical studies to be superior to epinephrine. The standard dose of epinephrine is 1 mg intravenously every 5 to 10 minutes during arrest. However, the range of individual response is wide and this dose may be too low. If pressure or end-tidal CO_2 monitoring suggests that cardiac output and perfusion pressures are too low during CPR, additional doses of epinephrine should be given.

A number of drugs, including epinephrine (diluted to 1 mg/10 ml), may be given via the endotracheal tube. Some studies have shown a good pharmacologic effect when circulation is intact. However, during CPR the absorption is erratic and the effect unpredictable. For all drugs used in CPR the preferred route is intravenous. Central administration is best, although upper extremity peripheral administration also gives good results. Onset of action with peripheral injection may be speeded if the drug is followed by a bolus of fluid to help force it to the central circulation.

Sodium Bicarbonate

Sodium bicarbonate has been the second most used drug during CPR. Its liberal use began with early reports that sodium bicarbonate improved resuscitation success in animals, that acidosis lowered the fibrillation threshold, and that respiratory acidosis impaired physiologic response to catecholamines. More recently, concern has been expressed that sodium bicarbonate could be harmful during CPR. As discussed in the section on physiology of gas transport during CPR, tissue acidosis during CPR is caused primarily by low blood flow and accumulation of CO_2 in the tissues. Metabolic acidosis, as indicated by blood lactate levels, develops slowly during CPR in both experimental animals and humans. Intravenously administered sodium bicarbonate combines with hydrogen ion, liberating CO_2. The arterial CO_2 tension ($Paco_2$) is temporarily elevated until the excess CO_2 is eliminated through the lungs. CO_2 readily diffuses across cell membranes, whereas bicarbonate diffuses much more slowly. Thus sodium bicarbonate administration could result in a paradoxic worsening of intracellular acidosis. Direct evidence of this occurring during CPR is lacking. However, depressed cardiac muscle function is known to result from intracellular acidosis and to occur more rapidly with elevations in $Paco_2$ tension than with metabolic acidosis. One study also found that bicarbonate administration during CPR in dogs resulted in cerebrospinal fluid (CSF) acidosis because CSF Pco_2 increased while CSF bicarbonate levels remained unchanged. However, two recent studies found no change in CSF pH after bicarbonate administration. Studies in recent years have not found that sodium bicarbonate improves resuscitation or survival.

In contrast to the lack of conclusive evidence that bicarbonate improves outcome or that it increases intracellular acidosis, other adverse effects of aggressive bicarbonate administration are well documented. Hypernatremia, hyperosmolarity, and metabolic alkalosis are common during and after CPR when bicarbonate is used, and these abnormalities are associated with a low resuscitation rate and poor survival. Therefore current knowledge suggests that sodium bicarbonate should be used judiciously, if at all, during CPR. It is probably unnecessary in resuscitations lasting less than 15 minutes. It may be useful if a known preexisting severe metabolic acidosis is present. In prolonged resuscitations, if blood gases indicate a severe metabolic acidosis by a low calculated bicarbonate or marked base deficit, bicarbonate administration may be tried. If it is used, increases in $Paco_2$, and thus tissue CO_2, may be reduced by giving the bicarbonate slowly rather than by rapid intravenous bolus. When sodium bicarbonate is administered, drug interactions must be avoided, especially the precipitation of $CaCO_3$ that occurs when calcium chloride is administered in an intravenous line with bicarbonate.

Atropine

Atropine sulfate, a muscarinic blocker, enhances sinus node automaticity and atrioventricular conduction by its vagolytic effects. It is frequently used during cardiac arrest associated with an electrocardiographic pattern of asystole or slow idioventricular rhythm. However, the predominant cause of asystole and electromechanical dissociation (EMD) is severe myocardial ischemia. Heightened parasympathetic tone probably contributes little to these rhythms during cardiac arrest in adults. Studies in humans and animals provide little evidence that atropine actually improves outcome. The most important means of treating these rhythms is to improve myocardial oxygenation by improving coronary perfusion. Therefore the first priority should be chest compressions and epinephrine to improve coronary perfusion pressure. When EMD is present, especially with a supraventricular rhythm or narrow QRS complexes, mechanical causes of poor cardiac filling (cardiac tamponade, tension pneumothorax, and severe hypovolemia) should be sought. Since asystole and EMD have a dismal prognosis and atropine has minimal adverse effects, it can be tried as a second-line drug in refractory arrest with these rhythms. The most important side effects of atropine occur only if resuscitation is successful. After the usual 1 to 2 mg intravenous dose, mydriasis may occur, confounding neurologic examination. Occasionally a rapid sinus tachycardia is present following resuscitation when atropine is given. A dose of 2 mg is fully vagolytic in most adults.

Isoproterenol

In contrast to atropine, isoproterenol is contraindicated during cardiac arrest. Isoproterenol has been used in cardiac arrest when the electrocardiogram shows a slow rhythm, especially idioventricular rhythm. The primary cause of such a rhythm is myocardial ischemia. As a pure beta-adrenergic agonist, isoproterenol increases myocardial oxygen consumption while reducing aortic diastolic pressure and coronary blood flow. Therefore it is counterproductive to myocardial resuscitation. The only possible use of isoproterenol is after successful resuscitation to temporarily speed up a slow perfusing rhythm while awaiting placement of a pacemaker. The widespread availability of temporary transvenous pacemakers and increasing availability of external pacemakers make even this use of the drug rarely necessary. If isoproterenol is used for this indication, great care must be taken that the drug does not increase myocardial ischemia, leading to recurrent arrest.

Calcium Salts and Calcium Channel Blockers

Because calcium increases myocardial contractility and enhances ventricular automaticity under normal physiologic circumstances, it has been used for years as a treatment for asystole and EMD. An early report of success in four children following open heart surgery was bolstered by animal studies demonstrating moderate success with calcium chloride in asphyxial arrest. However, the children were probably hypocalcemic, and the animal studies showed that alpha- and mixed-adrenergic agonists were more effective than calcium. More recently, dangerously high calcium levels (up to 18.2 mg/dl) have been reported during CPR in humans. Studies of dogs with asystole or EMD following defibrillation found that administering calcium did not result in resuscitation or improve electromechanical coupling during pacing. Retrospective studies and prospective clinical trials of calcium and placebo in out-of-hospital arrest with asystole and EMD have shown no improvement in resuscitation or survival. Consequently, the current evidence suggests that calcium is useful in cardiac arrest only if the arrest is precipitated, or contributed to, by severe hyperkalemia, severe hypocalcemia, or calcium channel blocker overdose. If calcium is used, the chloride salt in a dose of 2 to 4 mg/kg is preferred because it produces higher and more consistent levels of ionized calcium than other salts.

At the opposite extreme from calcium administration during CPR is the suggestion that calcium is harmful and that calcium channel blockers should be given. With anoxia or ischemia, cellular phosphate energy stores are rapidly depleted, allowing a large shift of calcium into cells. The high intracellular calcium concentration may result in vasoconstriction following resuscitation, impeding reperfusion of the heart and brain. High intracellular calcium concentrations activate enzyme systems, which can cause further cellular damage, especially in the presence of oxygen during reperfusion. Despite these theoretical considerations, no studies have been conducted on the effects of calcium channel blockers on myocardial damage or function when used during or after cardiac arrest. Experimental studies have focused primarily on the brain. In animals treatment with lidoflazine, flunarizine, verapamil, or magnesium sulfate increases cerebral blood flow after resuscitation. Neurologic function in dogs is improved by lidoflazine following ventricular fibrillation but not following asphyxia-induced cardiac arrest. Nimodopine improves neurologic function in an experimental model of global brain ischemia and in patients with subarachnoid hemorrhage. A recently completed multicenter trial did not demonstrate a beneficial effect of lidoflazine on neurologic outcome in comatose survivors of cardiac arrest. Overall, there is no convincing evidence that calcium channel blockers improve outcome from cardiac arrest. The vasodilation and negative inotropism and dromotropism caused by these drugs make their safe use in cardiac arrest questionable.

Lidocaine and Bretylium

Lidocaine and bretylium tosylate are used during cardiac arrest to aid defibrillation when ventricular fibrillation is refractory to electrical countershock therapy or when fibrillation recurs following successful conversion. However, no antiarryhthmic agent has proved superior to electrical defibrillation or more effective than placebo in the treatment of ventricular fibrillation. Lidocaine is primarily an antiectopic with few hemodynamic effects. It tends to reverse the reduction in ventricular fibrillation threshold caused by ischemia or infarction, but it may also increase the defibrillation threshold. Bretylium has been called a primary antifibrillatory drug because it reduces the chances for reentry between ischemic and normal areas of myocardium. In contrast to lidocaine, bretylium has significant hemodynamic effects. When given intravenously, it releases norepinephrine from adrenergic nerve endings, causing tachycardia, hypertension, and increased contractility when the circulation is intact. Blockade of both uptake and release of norepinephrine at the nerve terminal begins after about 20 minutes and peaks 45 to 60 minutes following administration. This blockade can lead to profound hypotension. Bretylium also reverses the reduction in fibrillation threshold caused by ischemia, but in contrast to lidocaine, it reduces or does not change the defibrillation threshold.

Despite some apparent electrophysiologic advantages and anecdotal reports of chemical defibrillation with bretylium, controlled randomized trials comparing lidocaine and bretylium have failed to demonstrate a difference in resuscitation or survival from out-of-hospital ventricular fibrillation. Because of the demonstrated adverse consequences of hypotension caused by bretylium, it is not recommended as first-line treatment during CPR. Its use should be reserved for fibrillation refractory to defibrillation and lidocaine or for recurrent fibrillation uncontrolled by lidocaine.

POSTRESUSCITATION CARE

The major factors contributing to the high in-hospital mortality rate after successful resuscitation are progression of the primary disease and cerebral damage resulting from the arrest. It may be in this postresuscitation period that critical care physicians have the greatest impact on outcome. Active management in this period appears to mitigate postischemic brain damage and improve neurologic outcome. Although a significant proportion of patients have severe neurologic deficits following resuscitation, aggressive support of brain function does not seem to increase the numbers of patients surviving in vegetative states. Most severely damaged patients die of multisystem failure within 2 weeks.

When flow is restored following a significant period of global brain ischemia, three stages of cerebral reperfusion occur in the ensuing 12 hours. Immediately after resuscitation there are multifocal areas where no reflow occurs. Within an hour a global hyperemia appears, followed quickly by prolonged global hypoperfusion. Intracranial pressure elevation is uncommon following resuscitation from cardiac arrest, although severe ischemic injury can lead to edema during the ensuing days.

Postresuscitation support is focused on providing stable oxygenation and hemodynamics to minimize any further cerebral insult (Table 23–4). Any patient who is comatose or semiconscious after resuscitation should be maintained with mechanical ventilation for several hours to ensure adequate oxygenation and ventilation. Restlessness, coughing, or seizures should be aggressively treated with appropriate medications, including neuromuscular blockers if necessary. Pao_2 should be maintained above 100 mm Hg, and moderate hypocapnia (Pco_2 25 to 35 mm Hg) may be useful. Hemodynamic management is directed to maintaining or

TABLE 23–4. Postresuscitation Support for Optimal Neurologic Outcome

Oxygenation

Maintain arterial oxygen tension >100 mm Hg with supplemental oxygen and/or positive end-expiratory pressure

Ventilation

Ensure $Paco_2$ ≤40 mm Hg during spontaneous ventilation

Mechanical ventilation for patients who are comatose or semiconscious for at least 2-6 h—maintain $Paco_2$ 25-35 mm Hg

Hemodynamics

Ensure normal plasma volume—moderate volume expansion may be used

Brief (5 min) hypertension to MAP 120-140 mm Hg immediately after resuscitation desirable

Maintain MAP 90-110 mm Hg with volume expansion, inotropes, or vasopressors as needed

Avoid hypotension

Avoid severe, prolonged or repeated hypertension

Control of Restlessness, Straining, and Seizures

Narcotics for awake patient in pain

Benzodiazepines, barbiturates, or other sedatives

Nueromuscular blockers, if necessary, during mechanical ventilation

Phenytoin, barbiturates, or diazepam for seizures

Metabolic

Moderate hemodilution to hematocrit 30%-35%

Serum osmolality 280-300 mOsm unless treating elevated ICP

Glucose 100-300 mg/dl

Normal electrolytes and acid-base status

Maintain normothermia

Intracranial Pressure

Elevate head of bed 20-45 degrees

If ICP monitoring is used, maintain ICP <15 mm Hg and coronary perfusion pressure >50 mm Hg

---

$Paco_2$ = arterial carbon dioxide tension, MAP = mean arterial pressure, ICP = intracranial pressure.

improving cerebral blood flow. Blood volume should be kept normal or expanded with non-blood solutions. Moderate hemodilution to a hematocrit value of 30% to 35% may be useful. Five minutes of moderate hypertension (mean arterial pressure 120 to 140 mm Hg) may help overcome the initial cerebral no-reflow phenomenon. Hypertension frequently occurs without additional therapy because of the effects of epinephrine given during CPR. Thereafter, blood pressure should be carefully controlled in the normotensive to slightly hypertensive range (90 to 110 mm Hg mean arterial pressure) by means of volume loading, inotropes, or vasopressors as needed. Because cerebral autoregulation of blood flow is severely attenuated,

hypotension dramatically reduces cerebral perfusion. Severe prolonged or recurrent hypertension should also be avoided because it worsens the neurologic outcome. Intracranial pressure monitoring, in the absence of specific indications, has not improved outcome. If intracranial pressure is measured, cerebral perfusion pressure should be maintained greater than 50 mm Hg. Unless the presence of intracranial hypertension is known or strongly suspected, serum osmolality should be maintained in the normal range (280 to 300 mOsm). Hyperglycemia during cerebral ischemia increases neurologic damage. Although the effect of high serum glucose concentration in the postresuscitation period on outcome is unknown, glucose levels should be kept between 100 and 300 mg/dl.

General supportive care to produce optimal cerebral oxygenation and perfusion improves outcome, but specific pharmacologic therapy directed at brain preservation has not had further benefit. Initial animal trials of barbiturates were encouraging, but a large multicenter clinical trial of thiopental given after cardiac arrest found no improvement in neurologic status. Barbiturates are used in the postresuscitation period only as an adjunct for controlling intracranial hypertension or seizures. The recent enthusiasm for calcium channel blockers seems to parallel the experience with thiopental. Neurologic improvements found in animal studies are not being reproduced in clinical trials. Currently no evidence shows that any specific pharmacologic agent improves neurologic outcome following cardiac arrest.

PROGNOSIS

The ultimate prognosis of a comatose survivor of CPR is important for caregivers and family alike. In a retrospective study of out-of-hospital arrest victims, the likelihood of awakening could be correlated with findings at admission. If pupillary light response and spontaneous eye movements were absent and the motor response to pain was absent or extensor posturing, the patient had only a 5% chance of ever awakening. The better these signs on admission, the greater the chance of awakening. A companion study found that the chance of ever awakening fell rapidly in the days following arrest. If the patient was not awake by 4 days after arrest, the chance of ever awakening was less than 20%. All those awakening had marked neurologic deficits. Most patients who recover completely show rapid improvement in the first 48 hours. The severity of the neurologic injury is correlated with the level of creatine kinase BB found in the CSF. Peak values are reached 48 to 72 hours after arrest, and levels of 25 IU or more are associated with severe neurologic damage.

SUGGESTED READINGS

Abramson NS, Safar P, Detre KM, et al: Randomized clinical study of cardiopulmonary-cerebral resuscitation: thiopental loading in comatose cardiac arrest survivors. N Engl J Med 1986;314:397

American Heart Association: Textbook of advanced cardiac life support. Dallas, 1987, The Association

American Heart Association: Standards and guidelines for cardiopulmonary resuscitation (CPR) and emergency cardiac care (ECC). JAMA 1986;255:2905

Berenyi KG, Wolk M, Killip T: Cerebrospinal fluid acidosis complicating therapy of experimental cardiopulmonary resuscitation. Circulation 1975;52:319

Bishop RL, Weisfeldt ML: Sodium bicarbonate administration during cardiac arrest: effect on arterial pH, pCO2, and osmolality. JAMA 1976;235:506

Coon GA, Clinton JE, Ruiz E: Use of atropine for bradysystolic cardiac arrest. Ann Emerg Med 1981;10:462

Criley JM, Blaufuss AH, Kissel GL: Cough-induced cardiac compression: self-administered form of cardiopulmonary resuscitation. JAMA 1976;236:1246

Edgren E, Terent H, Hedstrand U, Ronquist G: Cerebral spinal fluid markers in relation to outcome in patients with global cerebral ischemia. Crit Care Med 1983;11:4

Eisenberg MS, Bergner L, Hallstrom A: Cardiac resuscitation in the community: importance of rapid provision and implications for program planning. JAMA 1979;241:1905

Ewy GA: Alternative approaches to external chest compression. Circulation 1986;74(suppl IV):IV-98

Ewy GA: Electrical therapy for cardiovascular emergencies. Circulation 1986;74(suppl IV):IV-111

Haynes RE, Chinn TL, Copass MK, Cobb LA: Comparison of bretylium tosylate and lidocaine in management of out of hospital ventricular fibrillation: a randomized clinical trial. Am J Cardiol 1981;48:353

Kay JH, Blalock A: The use of calcium chloride in the treatment of cardiac arrest in patients. Surg Gynecol Obstet 1951;93:97

Kouwenhoven WB, Jude JR, Knickerbocker GG: Closed-chest cardiac massage. JAMA 1960;173:1064

Longstreth WT, Diehr P, Inui TS: Prediction of awakening after out-of-hospital cardiac arrest. N Engl J Med 1983;308:1378

Longstreth WT, Inui TS, Cobb LA, Copass MK: Neurologic recovery after out-of-hospital cardiac arrest. Ann Intern Med 1983;98:588

Mattar JA, Weil MH, Shubin H, Stein L: Cardiac arrest in the critically ill. II. Hyperosmolal states following cardiac arrest. Am J Med 1974;56:162

Melker RJ: Recommendation for ventilation during cardiopulmonary resuscitation: time for change? Crit Care Med 1985;13:882

Michael JR, Guerci AD, Koehler RC, et al: Mechanisms by which epinephrine augments cerebral and myocardial perfusion during cardiopulmonary resuscitation in dogs. Circulation 1984;69:822

Mullie A, Lust P, Penninck J, et al: Monitoring of cerebrospinal fluid enzyme levels in post-ischemic en-

cephalopathy after cardiac arrest. Crit Care Med 1981;9:399

Olson DW, Thompson BM, Darin JC, Milbrath MH: A randomized comparison study of bretylium tosylate and lidocaine in resuscitation of patients out-of-hospital ventricular fibrillation in a paramedic system. Ann Emerg Med 1984;13:807

Otto CW: Cardiovascular pharmacology II: the use of catecholamines, pressor agents, digitalis, and corticosteroids in CPR and emergency cardiac care. Circulation 1986;74(suppl IV):IV-80

Otto CW, Yakaitis RW, Ewy GA: Effects of epinephrine on defibrillation in ischemic ventricular fibrillation. Am J Emerg Med 1985;3:285

Otto CW, Yakaitis RW: The role of epinephrine in CPR: a reappraisal. Ann Emerg Med 1984;13:840

Redding JS, Pearson JW: Evaluation of drugs for cardiac resuscitation. Anesthesiology 1963;24:203

Rudikoff MJ, Maughan WL, Effrom M, et al: Mechanisms of blood flow during cardiopulmonary resuscitation. Circulation 1980;61:345

Sanders AB, Atlas M, Ewy GA, et al: Expired PCO2 as an index of coronary perfusion pressure. Am J Emerg Med 1985;3:147

Sanders AB, Ewy GA, Bragg S, et al: Expired PCO2 as a prognostic indicator of successful resuscitation from cardiac arrest. Ann Emerg Med 1985;14:948

Sanders AB, Otto CW, Kern KB, et al: Acid-base balance in canine model of cardiac arrest. Ann Emerg Med 1988;17:667

Sessler DI, Mills P, Gregory GA, et al: Bicarbonate administration does not cause a paradoxical brain intercellular acidosis during recovery from hypoxic lactic acidosis. Anesthesiology 1986;65:A442

Stueven HA, Thompson BM, Aprahamian C, et al: Lack of effectiveness of calcium chloride in refractory asystole. Ann Emerg Med 1985;14:630

Stueven HA, Thompson BM, Aprahamian C, et al: The effectiveness of calcium chloride in refractory electromechanical dissociation. Ann Emerg Med 1985;14:626

Stueven HA, Tonsfeldt DJ, Thompson BM, et al: Atropine in asystole: human studies. Ann Emerg Med 1984;13:815

Taffet GE, Teasdale TA, Luchi RJ: In-hospital cardiopulmonary resuscitation. JAMA 1988;260:2069

Weaver WD: Calcium-channel blockers and advanced cardiac life support. Circulation 1986;74(suppl IV):IV-94

Weaver WD, Cobb LA, Dennis D, et al: Amplitude of ventricular fibrillation waveform and outcome after cardiac arrest. Ann Intern Med 1985;102:53

Weaver WD, Hill D, Fahrenbruch CE, et al: Use of the automatic external defibrillator in the management of out-of-hospital cardiac arrest. N Engl J Med 1988;319:661

Weil MH, Grundler W, Yamaguchi M, et al: Arterial blood gases fail to reflect acid-base status during cardiopulmonary resuscitation: a preliminary report. Crit Care Med 1985;13:884

Weil MH, Rackow EC, Trevino R, et al: Difference in acid-base state between venous and arterial blood during cardiopulmonary resuscitation. N Engl J Med 1986;315:153

Weisfeldt JL, Bishop RL, Greene HL: Effects of pH and pCO2 on performance of ischemic myocardium. In Roy PE, Rona G (eds): Recent advances in studies on cardiac structure and metabolism, vol. 10. Baltimore, 1975, University Park Press, p 355

Yakaitis RW, Ewy GA, Otto CW, et al: Influence of time and therapy on ventricular defibrillation in dogs. Crit Care Med 1980;8:157

24

POSTOPERATIVE INTENSIVE CARE OF TRANSPLANTATION PATIENTS

AKE GRENVIK, MD, KEITH L. STEIN, MD, AND DAVID J. KRAMER, MD

HISTORICAL BACKGROUND

The first successful solid organ transplantation took place in 1954 at the Peter Bent Brigham Hospital in Boston, where a kidney was removed from a donor and reimplanted into his identical twin. Ten years later, Hardy et al. and Starzl et al. reported the first successful human lung and liver transplantations, respectively. In 1966 Lillehei and associates performed the first pancreas transplantation. In 1967 the first human heart transplantation was completed by Barnard in Capetown, using the technique developed in animals by Shumway et al. at Stanford University. The Stanford group also designed a more complex method for combined heart and lung transplantation in animals and in 1981 accomplished one of the first successful human heart and lung transplantations, although this type of transplantation had already been performed in a child by Cooley in 1968.

BRAIN DEATH

Although a living donor was used for the first kidney transplantation, the lung, liver, and pancreas were all procured from just deceased donors immediately after cardiac function stopped. Obviously this could not be the donor's condition for the spectacular heart transplantation, in which a vital organ was removed from a heart-beating cadaver. This donor was certified dead based on cessation of brain function as characterized by Mollaret and Goulon in 1959 in their description of "le coma dépassé."

Organ donors for transplantation may be in any of three categories: living individuals, brain-dead cadavers, or non-heart-beating cadavers. The ethically and physiologically preferred donor condition is brain death. In 1968 a Harvard committee identified the brain-dead state as an irreversible coma with unreceptivity and unresponsivity, cessation of spontaneous breathing, absence of all central nervous system reflexes, and an isoelectric electroencephalogram. In 1981 the President's Commission for the Study of Ethical Problems in Medicine and Biomedical and Behavioral Research published detailed guidelines for the definition of brain death, which are currently accepted as the "gold standard" in the United States. These guidelines state that "an individual with irreversible cessation of all functions of the entire brain, including the brain stem, is dead." Cessation is recognized as the absence of cerebral and brainstem functions. Irreversibility is acknowledged when the cause of coma is established and is sufficient to account for the loss of brain functions, the recovery of any brain function is not possible, and the absence of brain function persists for an appropriate observation period or trial of therapy.

BRAIN-DEAD ORGAN DONOR MANAGEMENT

The greatest limitation to transplantation surgery is organ shortage. The donor pool necessary to meet current transplantation needs is estimated to be 10,000 to 15,000 per year in the United States alone. Depending on the age criteria used, an estimated 12,500 to 27,000 potential organ donors die each year in this country. Only 15% to 20% of these deaths result in organ donation.

Essentially all brain-dead organ donors are in ICUs at the time of death certification. Inadequate donor management in the ICU before organ procurement contributes to the shortage of organs for transplantation. Early donor recognition, rapid and accurate declaration of brain death, and optimal physiologic maintenance of these potential donors are all important to prevent waste of scarce resources and improve outcome of transplantation surgery.

LOGISTIC PROBLEMS

Although the frequency of double- and multiple-organ transplants is increasing, the vast majority of recipients have end-stage single-organ failure. Typically these recipients do not need emergency transplantation. However, because of the limited longevity of procured organs and the need to minimize ischemic injury to the transplanted organ, the procedure becomes an emergency when a donor organ is available. Current preservation techniques permit the following time limits for hypothermic ischemia: kidney 48 to 72 hours, liver 24 hours, pancreas 24 hours, heart 6 hours, and lung 4 hours.

The postmortem surgical recovery of organs for transplantation is described in detail elsewhere. The principles are the same regardless of the organs being recovered. However, for multiple-organ procurement that includes the heart, the donor midline incision starts at the suprasternal notch and ends at the symphysis. The major vessels are identified, and cannulas are placed in the abdominal aorta, inferior vena cava, and portal vein. Circulation is arrested by infusion of hypothermic cardioplegic solution into the aortic root. Cold crystalloid solution, most commonly Euro-Collins or University of Wisconsin solution, is then flushed through the abdominal organs. The heart is usually removed first, followed rapidly by the other organs. Several procurement teams from different transplantation centers may be involved in multiple-organ procurement. These teams communicate frequently with their base hospitals for optimal timing of the recipient operation.

In managing the recipient's postoperative treatment, the ICU physician needs information about the donor's condition in the ICU at a usually distant hospital before organ procurement and in the operating room during this procedure. This information includes the donor's hemodynamic stability, especially if circulatory shock or cardiac arrest with resuscitation occurred; duration and quantity of medication, such as vasoactive drugs; and metabolic stability, such as control of diabetes insipidus and renal function before organ procurement. Other necessary data include the length of cold ischemia time during transportation and before implantation in the recipient and the anesthesiologic and surgical techniques used in transplantation.

KIDNEY TRANSPLANTATION

Since kidney transplantation began in 1954, more than 100,000 kidneys have been transplanted in the United States alone. Of the almost 10,000 kidneys transplanted each year, 20% are from living related donors and 80% are from brain-dead organ donors. At the end of the 1980s, graft survival reached almost 90% with living related donors and 70% for cadaver kidneys. Patient 1-year survival, however, is much higher and reaches 95% to 100% in prominent transplantation centers.

The number of kidney transplant procedures in the United States is expected to double to nearly 20,000 per year during the 1990s, since end-stage renal disease develops in approximately 22,000 Americans each year and the quality of survival and cost compete favorably with long-term dialysis. Renal transplant patients with no complications do not need postoperative intensive care. However, a variety of both early and delayed complications occur commonly after kidney transplantation and may necessitate ICU admission.

The standard surgical technique is a heterotopic retroperitoneal implantation in the left or right lower quadrant of the abdomen (Fig. 24–1). The usual renal vascular connections are performed through end-to-side anastomosis with the external iliac artery and vein. The ureter is similarly anastomosed end to side with the urinary bladder, a so-called ureteroneocystostomy. Normally no stents or drains are used. Postoperative surgical complications usually involve one of the two blood vessels or the ureter.

Arterial complications include thrombosis and disruption of the anastomosis. These complications most often are technical, but arterial thrombosis may also be seen in acute rejection. Arterial thrombosis causes pain, tenderness, hematuria, and oliguria. Such symptoms necessitate reexploration, which occasionally saves the transplanted kidney. Most often, however,

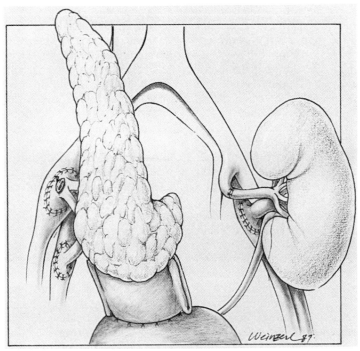

Figure 24–1. Implantation of a kidney in the left lower quadrant, with anastomoses of the renal artery and vein to the iliac vessels and the ureter to the bladder. The pancreatic implantation in the right lower quadrant similarly illustrates anastomoses for the pancreatic arterial supply and venous drainage, as well as a short portion of the duodenum anastomosed to the bladder, side to side. (From Groth CG [ed]: Pancreatic transplantation. Philadelphia, 1988, WB Saunders Co.)

allograft nephrectomy is necessary. Symptoms of a ruptured arterial anastomosis include sudden severe pain, local swelling, cessation of urine production, and hypovolemic shock. This complication also necessitates emergency reexploration with allograft nephrectomy and repair of the iliac artery.

Venous thrombosis is less common than arterial but also most frequently the result of technical difficulties. The patient has severe pain, swelling, oliguria, and gross hematuria. This complication necessitates allograft nephrectomy.

The ureter receives its blood supply from the renal artery. Utmost caution should be exercised during the renal procurement to minimize damage to this blood supply. Impaired perfusion results in ureteral ischemia and necrosis, the latter causing urinary leakage, usually at the ureteroneocystostomy site. Swelling of the ipsilateral leg and genitalia and persistent drainage of serous fluid from the wound are indications of possible urinary leak. Operative repair with internal stenting of the ureter may be necessary.

Fluid accumulation around the kidney may be diagnosed by ultrasonography and may represent a hematoma, abscess formation, urinoma from ureteral leakage, or a lymphocele caused by transection of lymphatic vessels in the area. All of these conditions necessitate surgical drainage to preserve kidney function.

HEART TRANSPLANTATION

Thirty years have passed since Lower and Shumway reported on their experimental cardiac transplantations in dogs. In that time heart transplantation has become a routine procedure performed in more than 170 medical centers in the United States. In 1988 approximately 1600 hearts were transplanted in the United States and 2400 worldwide. The results are excellent, with more than 80% 1-year survival in the most prominent transplantation centers.

End-stage cardiac disease resulting in New York Heart Association class IV symptoms, including an ejection fraction of less than 20%, is an indication for heart transplantation. These patients are in the final stages of cardiomyopathy, most often caused by idiopathic, ischemic, or valvular heart disease and less commonly the result of viral myocarditis, amyloidosis, or sarcoidosis. Transplant recipients are increasingly older; patients up to 65 years of age are accepted at many centers. These patients are so sick that candidates on the waiting list for this procedure at Stanford University, who did not receive a heart in time, had a 1-year mortality rate of 95%.

During procurement the donor heart is arrested with cardioplegic solution and preserved with Euro-Collins solution. After removal the heart is placed in cold crystalloid solution at 4° C and transported in an insulated sterile container to the transplantation center. Implantation of the donor heart into the recipient, following removal of the native heart, starts with a left atrial anastomosis. Anastomoses of the right atrium, the pulmonary artery, and finally the ascending aorta are then performed. Portions of both atria of the native heart are left in the recipient to simplify the two atrial anastomoses and minimize direct manipulation of the four pulmonary veins and the two venae cavae. The coronary arteries of donor heart are also retained to avoid delicate anastomoses of these vessels. Only the four anastomoses described are necessary to complete a heart transplantation (Fig. 24–2).

Whereas orthotopic heart transplantation involves removal of the native heart, heterotopic transplantation permits its retention by side-to-side or piggyback connection of the donor heart to the native heart. In this technique, developed in Capetown, the transplanted donor heart assists the failing native heart. The rotated donor heart is placed in the right lower chest and connected to the native heart through anastomoses similar but not identical to those for orthotopic heart transplantation. These anastomoses are left atrium to left atrium, right atrium to right atrium, aorta to aorta end to side, and pulmonary artery end to side. The last usually necessitates an interpositioned graft to bridge the distance between the two pulmonary arteries (Fig. 24–3).

The potential immediate postoperative complications are similar to those with conventional cardiac surgery, including bleeding from any anastomosis or cannulation site, cardiac tamponade, and unilateral or bilateral phrenic nerve paralysis. Pulmonary and systemic emboli are rare in conventional cardiac surgery during the immediate postoperative period but occur with orthotopic heart transplantation, probably from formation of mural thrombi in the donor atria. Mural thrombus formation in the left atrium and ventricle of the native heart in orthotopic heart transplantation has a different cause but is a more common complication. In patients receiving a heterotopic heart, atelectasis forms in the right lower lobe because the donor heart is competing for space in this area of the chest.

Donor hearts are scarce in relation to the large number of patients needing transplantation. Patients deteriorating rapidly while awaiting a heart transplant are treated with an intraaortic balloon pump or occasionally with a single or bilateral ventricular assist device or total artificial heart. These devices are not totally implantable, since they require connection to an extracorporeal power source. This has increased the infection rate after cardiac transplantation when a ventricular assist device or total artificial heart is used as a bridge to transplantation. Bleeding has also been more common after these complicated and multiple procedures.

A problem after all heart transplantations is interpretation of the electrocardiogram (ECG). Patients receiving orthotopic heart transplants may have two P waves, one emanating from remaining portions of the native right atrium and the other from the donor heart. With heterotopic heart transplantation

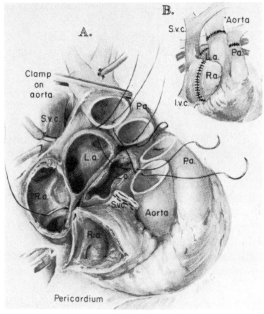

Figure 24–2. The four anastomoses required for heart transplantation, showing posterior remnants of the recipient left and right atrium anastomosed directly to the left and right atrium, respectively, of the donor heart. This is followed by end-to-end anastomosis of the aorta and pulmonary artery between donor heart and recipient. The completed anastomoses are shown in the right upper corner insert. (From Shoemaker WC et al [eds]: Textbook of critical care, ed 2, Philadelphia, 1989, WB Saunders Co.)

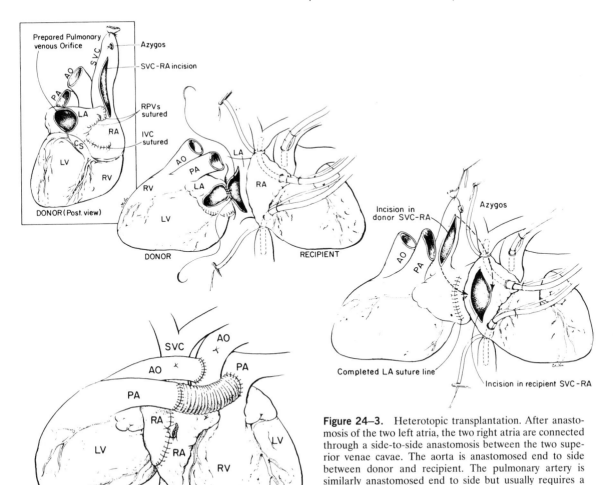

Figure 24–3. Heterotopic transplantation. After anastomosis of the two left atria, the two right atria are connected through a side-to-side anastomosis between the two superior venae cavae. The aorta is anastomosed end to side between donor and recipient. The pulmonary artery is similarly anastomosed end to side but usually requires a short graft to bridge the distance between donor and recipient. (From Shoemaker WC et al. [eds]: Textbook of critical care, ed 2, Philadelphia, 1989, WB Saunders Co.)

the postoperative ECG with its chaotic appearance may be particularly difficult to interpret. Obviously two different ECGs are displayed simultaneously with different heart rates and frequently different rhythms. The donor heart dominates leads placed over the right side of the chest and the native heart those leads on the left side. The heterotopic donor heart supplies most of the systemic cardiac output, assisting the failing native left ventricle. In patients with pulmonary hypertension, which is one indication for heterotopic heart transplantation, the native right ventricle can often maintain most of the right-sided cardiac output with little help from the transplanted donor heart. These patients may temporarily survive ventricular fibrillation or even asystole of either of the hearts, as long as the other heart functions well enough to sustain life.

LUNG TRANSPLANTATION

Although the first human single-lung transplantation was performed in 1963, this operation has remained experimental and only recently has emerged as a successful procedure. The surgical technique is still being refined, especially to include the bronchial arteries. The lungs are immunologically active organs with a unique position in the circulation, receiving the entire blood flow. Furthermore, they are directly exposed to the environment, rendering them vulnerable to airborne infections. For all these reasons the lungs represent a particular challenge to transplantation surgeons.

Three techniques are used for lung transplantation: single lung, combined heart and lung, and double lung. The indications for these three procedures vary. End-stage pulmonary fibrosis is considered the prime indication for single-lung transplantation, with pulmonary sepsis and lung emphysema as contraindications. These latter conditions are indications for double-lung transplantation as are other end-stage pulmonary diseases, such as bronchiectasis, cystic fibrosis, eosinophilic granuloma, and primary pulmonary hypertension. During the 1980s the most common indications for combined heart and lung transplantation were primary pulmonary hypertension and Eisenmenger's complex. In 1989 one group reported 82% 1-year survival in heart-lung recipients treated with triple drug immunosuppression. Another group has reported 75% survival in a series of 16 double-lung transplants. Single-lung transplantation currently has a lower success rate than combined heart and lung transplantation. Obviously, this field remains in evolution.

The criteria for lung donors are more rigid than with other organs. The pulmonary donor must fulfill the common criteria for cardiac donors as well as the following requirements: age below 45 years; normal chest roentgenogram; normal gas exchange; normal Gram stain of tracheal secretions; normal bronchoscopy findings; no history of primary pulmonary disease or active pulmonary infection; and appropriate size match. Significant aspiration of gastric content is a contraindication to transplantation of one or both lungs from that donor. Unfortunately, aspiration of gastric content is a common occurrence in head-injured patients, who constitute the majority of organ donors. Thus lungs suitable for transplantation are particularly scarce. Cardiopulmonary bypass during procurement facilitates dissection of the mediastinum, obviates the need for close hemodynamic monitoring, and reduces the risk of hemodynamic collapse, including cardiac arrest, in the donor.

More than 1000 transplantations of the heart and lungs en bloc have been performed worldwide. Surprisingly, only three anastomoses are needed for this complex procedure (Fig. 24–4). The first involves the trachea with an end-to-end anastomosis between donor and recipient at a level one or two rings above the carina. Next follows the recipient's right atrium to the right atrium of the donor heart. Since the heart and lungs are transplanted as a single set of organs, the only remaining anastomosis is the ascending aorta, end to end between the donor and the recipient.

For single-lung transplantation, three anastomoses are needed. First the mainstem bronchus is anastomosed end to end. This is followed by the left atrial connection. With use

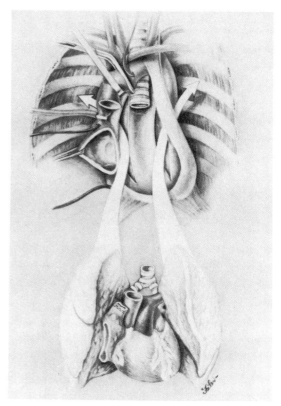

Figure 24–4. Technique for en bloc implantation of heart and lungs. The lungs are inserted behind the phrenic nerve on the left side and behind the venae cavae and the remnant of the posterior wall of the recipient's right atrium on the right side. The anastomoses performed begin with the lower trachea (end to end), followed by the right atrium (side to side), and finally the aorta (end to end). (From Shoemaker WC et al [eds]: Textbook of critical care, ed 2, Philadelphia, 1989, WB Saunders Co.)

of a left atrial cuff, the two donor pulmonary veins are connected to the recipient's left atrium with a single suture line. Finally an end-to-end anastomosis of the main pulmonary artery branch is performed on the involved side of the thorax.

Double-lung transplantation is the most recently developed technique in this field. The lungs are removed from the donor with a posterior left atrial cuff including all four pulmonary venous ostia. The end-to-end tracheal anastomosis, then the left atrial connection, and finally the mainstem pulmonary artery anastomosis are completed.

Only three anastomoses are necessary regardless of the type of lung transplant performed. However, several variations are being evaluated, including separate anastomoses of the two mainstem bronchi instead of the lower trachea in double-lung transplants. The airway anastomosis is the most problematic connection between donor and recipient in lung transplantation. The lower trachea and mainstem bronchi receive their blood supply via the bronchial arteries. These are not normally included in the lung harvest procedure. However, recent efforts have been made to dissect one or two bronchial arteries with a button-shaped cuff of donor thoracic aorta for restoration of at least part of the bronchial arterial blood supply. This technique avoids spontaneous disruption of the tracheal or bronchial anastomoses. Previous efforts to decrease the frequency of this devastating complication include wrapping a stalked flap of the recipient's omentum around the airway anastomosis to stimulate ingrowth of blood vessels and ideally to cover any necrotic perforation in the meantime. This technique has been surprisingly successful both experimentally and clinically.

In addition to the airway problems and subsequent complications, other postoperative complications unique to the lung include pneumonia caused by undiagnosed aspiration in the donor, secretion retention due to absence of mucociliary transport function in the denervated transplanted lung, and unilateral or bilateral phrenic nerve paralysis. The last may be due to stretching of these nerves as the lungs are positioned in the chest, posterior to a pericardial flap containing the phrenic nerve on the left side, and behind the superior and inferior venae cavae, with the phrenic nerve anteriorly, on the right side. This technique is used in en-bloc double-lung and heart-lung transplantations. Injury to the vagal nerves in the posterior mediastinum during dissection in the recipient may lead to paralytic ileus, often serious and prolonged. Finally, bleeding from cardiac and vascular anastomoses and the different cannulation sites is possible. Bleeding from the posterior mediastinum can be difficult to manage, as is bleeding from the chest wall in patients with richly vascularized adhesions characteristic of severe pulmonary hypertension.

LIVER TRANSPLANTATION

Although first performed successfully by Starzl in 1963, liver transplantation did not become a routine procedure until the 1980s when cyclosporine improved postoperative immunosuppression. This drug resulted in successful outcome for the majority, with survival currently exceeding 75% for the first year. More than 1500 liver transplantations are performed each year in the United States.

End-stage liver disease is the main indication for liver transplantation. Primary biliary cirrhosis, postviral necrosis (particularly from hepatitis B), and sclerosing cholangitis are the most common causes of end-stage liver disease. Biliary atresia and inborn errors of metabolism cause most liver failures in children. Malignancy of the liver and liver disease secondary to alcohol abuse are more controversial indications for transplantation.

The surgical technique is well established. The liver is removed from brain-dead donors usually as part of a multiple-organ procurement procedure. Preserved in University of Wisconsin solution, the liver can tolerate up to 24 hours of cold ischemia time and still function well in the recipient. After removal of the native liver in the recipient, the donor liver is implanted orthotopically. Five anastomoses are necessary in this complicated procedure (Fig. 24–5). The donor liver is harvested together with the retrohepatic inferior vena cava. The first anastomosis is a suprahepatic end-to-end anastomosis between the recipient and donor inferior venae cavae. This takes place above the donor hepatic veins, which simplifies the procedure. Next is the infrahepatic end-to-end anastomosis of the donor and recipient inferior venae cavae above the renal veins, after which the portal vein is connected. The fourth anastomosis is of the hepatic artery, usually end to end. At this point the donor liver circulation is carefully flushed through the portal vein (before the suprahepatic clamp is removed and before the infrahepatic inferior vena cava anastomosis is closed) to wash out air bubbles and prevent postreperfusion hyperkalemic cardiac arrest, since the first fluid exiting the liver has a high potassium concentration. Generous irrigation also prevents air embolization.

Unless the gallbladder is used as a conduit in the biliary duct anastomosis, it is removed from the donor liver before implantation, since the denervated gallbladder does not empty well in the recipient and could easily become infected. At the University of Pittsburgh the preferred bile duct anastomosis is either an end-to-end anastomosis over a T tube or an end-to-side choledochojejunostomy on a Roux-en-Y limb of the recipient jejunum. To prevent stenosis of the biliary anastomosis, an internal stent is placed in all choledochojejunostomies. This stent usually exits spontaneously via the intestinal canal during the first few months after surgery. However, the stent may induce obstruction or perforation of the intestinal wall, necessitating surgical removal. Choledochocholedochostomy

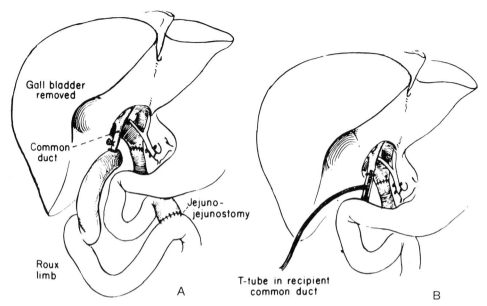

Figure 24–5. After completion of end-to-end anastomoses of the inferior vena cava above and below the liver and of the portal vein and hepatic artery, the biliary tract reconstruction most commonly used is either a choledochojejunostomy using a Roux-en-Y limb over an internal stent *(left)* or a choledochocholedochostomy over a T-tube *(right)*. (From Starz T.E., et al: Orthotopic liver transplantation in ninety-three patients. Surg Gynecol Obstet 142:491, 1976, by permission of *Surgery Gynecology & Obstetrics*.)

over a T-tube has the advantage of permitting continuous external monitoring of bile production. This T-tube is usually clamped and removed after a couple of months. Quantity and quality of bile are important indications of graft function. In a successful transplantation, bile production is observed in the operating room after unclamping of the vascular supply and reperfusion to the allograft.

Hepatic artery anomalies have a reported frequency of 8% to 15%. With the arterial supply of two livers involved, liver transplant surgeons commonly perform various hepatic arterial anastomoses, since it is important that all arteries be reconnected. Postoperative blood flow through the anastomosed vessels is routinely checked by means of ultrasonography. Thrombosis in any of these vessels is deleterious, necessitates another operation, and frequently results in retransplantation. Hepatic artery thrombosis may cause acute sepsis either through necrotic areas and infection of the liver itself or through disruption of the biliary anastomosis, since the arterial supply of the donor choledochus is from the hepatic artery via the hilum of the liver. Bleeding may occur from any of the four vascular anastomoses or from the many small veins divided during removal of the native liver. Postoperative hemorrhage is particularly common in patients with portal hypertension and a rich collateral venous circulation.

Biliary system integrity should be investigated if unexplained fever, leukocytosis, hyperbilirubinemia, or elevated transaminase levels develop. Cholangiography, performed via the T-tube or by a percutaneous transhepatic approach, is required to exclude a disrupted choledochal anastomosis. Emergency operation to repair the anastomosis is necessary if a leak is demonstrated. Because of the many possibilities for surgical complications in liver transplantation, these patients frequently undergo reoperation. Liver transplant patients undergo an average of two operations, and some have three or four procedures. Retransplantation is required in approximately 15% of cases because of primary nonfunction, vascular insufficiency, chronic rejection, or recurrence of the primary disease, particularly reinfection with hepatitis B virus.

PANCREAS TRANSPLANTATION

The first clinical pancreas transplantation was performed in 1966. Recent years have seen a surge in the number of cases and success rate. By January 1989 the International Pancreas Transplant Registry had received reports of 1775 transplantations. The overall recipient 1-year survival was 81%, and 43% of the grafts were functioning well enough to keep therecipients insulin independent. However, prominent transplantation centers now report greater than 90% 1-year patient survival and above 60% 1-year graft survival.

Insulin-dependent diabetes mellitus is a common disorder with at least 100,000 new cases identified worldwide each year. With more and more patients surviving many years of insulin therapy, an increasing number have devastating late complications, such as blindness, peripheral neuropathy, microangiopathic complications, and renal failure. Pancreas transplantation might prevent these complications, but only recently have the results been good enough to indicate that a great increase in the use of this procedure will occur.

Several surgical techniques have been developed for transplantation of the pancreas. The most common method is implantation of the pancreas retroperitoneally into one of the lower abdominal quadrants with a technique similar to that used in kidney transplantation. Even drainage of the pancreatic duct into the bladder is usually arranged through a duodenocystostomy, using the portion of the duodenum directly attached to the pancreatic head and leaving the opening of the pancreatic duct in the duodenum undisturbed (Fig. 24–6). This

surgical technique allows direct monitoring of exocrine functionby measurement of urine amylase concentration, which facilitates the detection of allograft rejection.

Pancreas transplantation has several specific complications. Arterial or venous thrombosis usually necessitates allograft removal. Bleeding anastomoses are caused by technical failures, which may be repaired through reexploration. Leakage of pancreatic juice at the anastomosis with the bladder is less common than when enteric drainage is used. However, its occurrence necessitates immediate reexploration and repair. Postoperative pancreatitis remains a significant problem but is less common than when surgical experience was less extensive.

MULTIPLE-ORGAN TRANSPLANTATION

Double-organ transplantations are not uncommon. They are usually performed as two separate procedures except for the combination of heart and lungs. Another common combination is the implantation of the pancreas and a kidney in diabetic patients with renal failure. Occasionally, the heart and liver, heart and kidney, or liver and kidney have been transplanted to the same recipient. Recently Starzl's group described "cluster" operations in patients with otherwise inoperable malignancies involving the stomach, pancreas, duodenum, bile ducts, or liver. The four organs are removed together from a single donor and implanted en bloc. From an immunologic standpoint, transplanting organs from the same donor should be advantageous. However, that is not always possible, as in the case of asynchronous transplantation of two organs. Interestingly, in multiple-organ transplantation one organ but not the other may be rejected even though they originate from one donor.

The surgical procedure for double-organ transplantation follows the same principles as for single-organ transplantation. The postoperative complications therefore are the same. The originators of cluster operations have presented the procedure in detail. A few patients have had the entire intestinal tract replaced from the esophagus to the sigmoid colon including liver and pancreas, but this is clearly an experimental technique, rarely indicated and beyond the scope of this chapter.

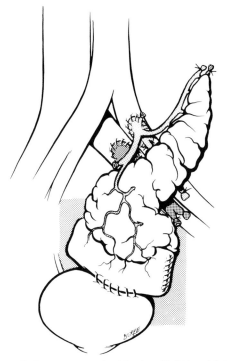

Figure 24–6. Anastomosis of duodenal bubble to bladder. (From Groth CG [ed]: Pancreatic transplantation, Philadelphia, 1988, WB Saunders Co.)

BONE MARROW TRANSPLANTATION

Bone marrow transplantation is not a surgical procedure and is usually performed by hematologists in the United States. Although bone marrow transplantation was attempted in the nineteenth century, the modern era started in 1957 when Thomas and associates infused large amounts of bone marrow intravenously and described transient marrow grafting in humans.

There are three types of bone marrow transplantation depending on the source of marrow cells: autologous transplantation within the same individual; syngeneic transplantation between identical twins; and allogeneic transplantation when the donor is a person other than the recipient's twin. Immunologic problems are anticipated only with the allogeneic bone marrow transplantation. The indications for bone marrow transplantation include all life-threatening forms of leukemia, severe aplastic anemia, some immunodeficiency disorders, certain hemoglobinopathies, and other, less common diseases involving the bone marrow.

Since bone marrow can be stored deep frozen, harvested material can be saved for months and even years before use. After removal from the donor, the marrow is filtered to remove clots and bone fragments. Allogeneic bone marrow is also irradiated to eradicate radiation-sensitive lymphocytes, which might cause graft-versus-host disease (GVHD), especially in an immunocompromised recipient. During transplantation the harvested bone marrow is infused intravenously into the recipient.

Bone marrow transplant recipients do not routinely need intensive care unless complications occur. GVHD is a rare occurrence in solid organ transplantation but relatively common with bone marrow transplantation. This disease may appear within 3 months of transplantation. It particularly affects the skin, liver, and gastrointestinal tract. GVHD is caused by histoincompatibility between the recipient and donor, immunocompetence of the donor cells, and inability of the host to reject the donor cells (that is, the recipient is immunoincompetent).

Another complication in bone marrow transplant recipients is hepatic venoocclusive disease caused by obstruction of small intrahepatic veins, which may lead to fatal liver failure. Interstitial pneumonitis is a common and frequently lethal complication of allogeneic bone marrow transplantation. Infectious complications are also common but not unique to bone marrow transplant recipients. Therefore they are discussed later in the chapter.

INTENSIVE CARE

Kidney transplantations are frequently performed in many medical centers using a well-established, standardized technique. Kidney recipients rarely require postoperative admission to an ICU. Heart transplant patients are routinely admitted to the cardiac surgical ICU, postoperatively, but the majority do well and, in addition to the specific immunosuppressive therapy, need only the ICU management normally applied to post–cardiac surgery patients. However, recipients of liver, lung, and multiple-organ transplants, especially those involving the intestinal tract, frequently need sophisticated intensive care using all currently available resources. When the transplanted organ is in excellent primary condition and the recipient is optimally prepared, has no significant complications beyond the failing replaced organ, and accepts the transplanted organ without rejection, the postoperative period may be smooth. However, if problems develop in the early postoperative phase, the physician must pay close attention and investigate any technical or other postoperative problem without delay, since prompt action is needed to reduce morbidity and prevent death. Even the dreaded multiple–organ system failure (MOSF), which occurs in moribund patients with end-stage liver disease, may be completely resolved by liver grafting, although central nervous system and renal function may return at variable rates.

A detailed description of ICU techniques and treatments necessary for optimal results in transplantation surgery, such as monitoring, pharmacologic support, maintenance of fluid and electrolyte and acid-base balance, antibiotic therapy, and enteral and parenteral nutrition, is beyond the scope of this chapter. These modalities are considered the skills and knowledge of the appropriately trained and experienced critical care physician and are dealt with elsewhere in this book.

IMMUNOSUPPRESSION

Immunosuppressive therapy was not available when solid organ transplantation began almost 40 years ago. The first successful kidney transplantation between identical twins was lifesaving, but in a subsequent series of nine cadaveric kidney transplants without immunosuppression of the recipients, all kidneys were rejected. Medawar and his associates were the first to demonstrate that an immune response causes graft rejection. Obviously, successful organ transplantation required the development of immunosuppressive agents.

Clinical immunosuppression was first based on antiproliferative agents used in chemotherapy for malignancies. *Azathioprine* was synthesized as a purine analog closely related to 6-mercaptopurine to improve its therapeutic efficiency in oncology. This drug, first used in organ transplantation in 1963, has a significant immunosuppressive effect. It is a powerful inhibitor of the primary immune response, not only preventing proliferation of T lymphocytes in standard doses of 2 to 3 mg/kg/d, but also inhibiting formation of all white blood cells. Larger doses produce significant leukopenia, thrombocytopenia, and anemia. Large doses may also be hepatotoxic, another significant drawback with this medication, especially in liver transplantation.

Corticosteroids are important components of immunosuppression protocols. They directly inhibit T cell proliferation by blocking the stimulating action of interleukin-1 (IL-1) on the T cells. Glucocorticoids suppress all forms of inflammation, including those caused by infection. They inhibit recruitment of all types of leukocytes and redistribute lymphocytes to the lymphoid tissues, resulting in lymphocytopenia. Steroids also reverse rejection episodes by preventing the production of interleukin-2 (IL-2), a T cell growth factor.

The major endogenous glucocorticoid is cortisol (hydrocortisone). Prednisone and prednisolone are approximately four times as potent, and methylprednisolone (Solu-Medrol) five times as potent, as hydrocortisone. These are the steroids most commonly used in immunosuppressive therapy for transplant recipients.

The side effects of steroid therapy are well known and involve practically all organ systems. Perhaps of greatest importance in transplantation surgery are decreased wound healing and increased risk of serious infection.

Cyclosporine was incorporated into the immunosuppression armamentarium after its serendipitous discovery. Derived from a fungus (*Tolypocladium inflatum Gams,* formerly designated *Trichoderma polysporum*) detected in common soil, it is a cyclic undacapeptide. Cyclosporine is essentially lymphocyte specific in its action. It blocks both production and action of IL-2, which is necessary for T cell proliferation.

Cyclosporine is administered orally in doses of 10 to 20 mg/kg. Intestinal absorption varies widely depending on the presence or absence of bile, paralytic ileus, diarrhea, and other gastrointestinal conditions. Therefore blood concentrations initially are monitored by daily performance of high-performance liquid chromatography (HPLC) or preferably radioimmunoassay (RIA). Desired concentration in whole blood varies between 400 and 800 ng/ml depending on circumstances and whether double, triple, or even quadruple immunotherapy is used. Much lower doses of cyclosporine are considered adequate for long-term therapy than are needed immediately after transplantation and during rejection.

Because cyclosporine is metabolized by the liver, hepatic dysfunction increases serum levels of both the parent compound and its metabolites, some of which are immunosuppressive or cause side effects, such as neurotoxicity and nephrotoxicity. With the TDx (modified RIA) method, which measures parent compound and metabolites together, we aim for levels of 800 to 1000 ng/ml in the first 2 months and then allow the levels to decrease to between 500 and 600 ng/ml. Cyclosporine levels measured by HPLC are specific for the parent compound, and the final target level is only 250 to 300 ng/ml.

Unfortunately, cyclosporine has significant toxic effects, especially on the kidneys. At least 75% of patients receiving cyclosporine have increased serum creatinine levels. In addition, hypertension develops in the majority of patients treated with cyclosporine. Hepatotoxicity also occurs with cyclosporine but is far less severe than is nephrotoxicity. Myoclonic twitching and even convulsions have been reported in association with this drug. Excessive doses may result in lymphoproliferative disease.

Rabbit, horse, or other heterologous *antiserum against human lymphocytes* has potent immunosuppressive activity. This is available as antilymphocyte globulin or antithymocyte globulin. Both have been used in prophylaxis during the immediate postoperative period and in treatment of rejection episodes. Because of development of host antibodies against these sera and the possibility of subsequent anaphylactic shock, these drugs are limited to treatment periods of 5 to 21 days. The serum is given intramuscularly or intravenously in doses of 5 to 15 mg/kg/d.

Monoclonal antibodies are usually obtained through complicated cloning procedures in mice immunized against human lymphocytes. Antibodies against all maturation stages of the thymocyte are available, but the most commonly used is against T3 thymocytes, although the mouse monoclonal antibody to T3 (OKT3) reacts with all human T cells. After intravenous injection of the first and occasionally the second dose, lysis of T cells may be so rapid and extensive that a septic shock–like state occurs. This may include life-threatening, nonhydrostatic, pulmonary edema. Therefore we keep patients receiving OKT3 in an ICU during the first and second injections.

FK 506 is a macrolide antibiotic produced by *Streptomyces tsukubaensis*. It was discovered in 1984 in Japan and shortly thereafter was demonstrated to be a potent immunosuppressive agent. Initially this drug was reported to produce widespread arteritis, including the heart, in dogs and baboons. Studies of heart, kidney, and liver transplantations performed in Pittsburgh on various animal species supported the safety of a human clinical trial of FK 506. This agent was found to rescue transplanted livers and kidneys in rejection phase when all other drugs failed. Subsequent use of FK 506 as the primary immunosuppressive agent has not led to severe arteritis or other serious side effects in humans. FK 506 is nephrotoxic and neurotoxic, but less so than cyclosporine. Both adverse effects are poorly correlated with the serum level of FK 506. The neurotoxicity may be manifest as tremor, aphasia, confusion, obtundation, and seizures.

FK 506 has effects similar to those of cyclosporine in inhibiting IL-2 stimulation of T lymphocytes. However, FK 506 is approximately 100 times more potent than cyclosporine. Initially this drug was given intravenously in doses of 0.15 mg/kg/h, which provided peak levels of 9 to 20 ng/ml in plasma, but this produced significant toxic effects. Therefore oral doses are started at 0.075 mg/kg every 12 hours and adjusted downward to provide trough levels of less than 3 ng/ml. Plasma concentrations as high as 7 ng/ml have not caused toxicity symptoms.

PRIMARY GRAFT FAILURE

Primary graft failure is usually caused by technical problems. The transplanted organ may have been injured in the donor by hypoxia from hypoperfusion secondary to shock, overzealous use of vasopressors, or resuscitation from cardiac arrest (which, if brief, is not an absolute contraindication to organ transplantation). Hypoxic injury may also occur in the operating room during organ removal, preservation, or transportation involving prolonged cold ischemia before implantation into the recipient.

The symptoms of primary graft failure depend on the organ transplanted. The surgeon suspects this problem if the transplanted organ fails to "pink up" in the operating room when reperfusion begins after declamping of the vessels. Failure of transplanted kidneys, liver, or pancreas to produce urine, bile, or pancreatic juice, respectively, inappropriate contractions of the transplanted heart, or inefficient arterial oxygenation with lung transplantation indicates primary graft injury.

During cold ischemia preservation between donor organ removal and implantation, temperatures even below the freezing point have been noted in experimental work. Such inadvertently low temperatures cause hypothermic cellular injury in the frozen areas of the transplanted organ. These areas appear hard and do not reperfuse well after declamping. Subsequently these organs function poorly and are unusually susceptible to infections. In severe cases of primary organ failure, retransplantation may be necessary.

GRAFT REJECTION

Graft rejection may be hyperacute, acute, or chronic. The most devastating form is hyperacute rejection, which may take place in the operating room. This problem may occur when a high concentration of antibodies against the transplanted organ is already present in the recipient. Extreme narrowing of the endothelium in the transplanted organ's blood vessels has been noted in these situations, which rapidly leads to reduced blood flow with immediate allograft failure. This situation necessitates graft removal and retransplantation or dependence on other means such as an artificial heart, hemodialysis, or return to insulin therapy in the case of heart, kidney, or pancreas transplantation, respectively.

Acute rejection usually occurs after several days or weeks, once recipient antibody production against the transplanted allograft is significant enough to cause rejection. Acute rejection may also occur at any time if immunosuppressive therapy is inadequate. The diagnosis of rejection may be based on clinical observation and laboratory tests but is usually confirmed through biopsy and microscopic examination by an experienced pathologist. The risk of complications is high with allograft biopsies, necessitating meticulous adherence to techniques developed specifically for each organ. Percutaneous biopsy is usually performed if the liver, kidney, or pancreas is being rejected. A transvenous endomyocardial biopsy technique has been developed for the heart. A standardized method of transbronchial biopsy is performed during bronchoscopy of the lungs. Bleeding, organ perforation, and fistula formation are the most obvious complications and carry the risk of subsequent infection.

Once the diagnosis of rejection is made or strongly suspected, immediate action is necessary. If there are no specific contraindications to cyclosporine, the level of the drug is maintained. Methylprednisolone 1 g intravenously is given immediately, followed by 200 mg the next day, and tapering to the previous dose over 1 week, a so-called steroid pulse. This repeats the pattern of steroid administration used in the immediate postoperative period. In addition, monoclonal antibodies or antilymphocyte serum may be administered. As already mentioned, FK 506 is efficient in rescuing organs not responding to other forms of therapy.

If OKT3 is used to treat acute rejection, the cyclosporine blood levels are allowed to drop from between 800 and 1000 ng/ml to between 200 and 300 ng/ml for 7 to 10 days. Thereafter the dose is increased to achieve a level of 800 ng/ml by the last 2 days of OKT3 therapy. Since multiple–organ system failure is common with acute rejection and renal dysfunction is a prominent component of this syndrome, a lower level of cyclosporine may improve recovery of renal function. However, OKT3 is a murine antigen and the patients may develop antimurine antibodies, particularly by the tenth day of OKT3 therapy. A high concentration of antimurine antibodies present at the initiation of a course of OKT3 (that is, from prior exposure) or early resurgence of T lymphocytes (assessed by the CD3 cell level) is associated with poor control of rejection by OKT3.

Chronic rejection necessitates an increase in immunosuppressive medication. Only in its most severe and terminal form is chronic rejection an indication for ICU admission. Therefore it is less of a problem to the intensivist than acute rejection is. Chronic rejection of hepatic allografts is characterized by vanishing bile ducts and arteriopathy. Aggressive immunosuppression at this stage is often used but is rarely successful and usually just results in a high rate of infection. Some patients with chronic rejection have improved after a switch from cyclosporine to FK 506. However, early retransplantation may still be necessary.

INFECTION

The very nature of transplantation procedures, with a vulnerable foreign organ and a heavily immunosuppressed host, leads to a high risk of infection. These infections may be bacterial or viral and may occur at any time. Fungal infections are usually a late occurrence, especially in patients whose organs are functioning poorly or undergoing rejection or in those with severe and prolonged sepsis.

In the early postoperative period the pathogens are usually bacterial, including such organisms as enterococci, staphylococci, *Pseudomonas, Enterobacter, Serratia,* and *Klebsiella.* Anaerobic bacteria may also be present.

Viral pathogens include cytomegalovirus, herpes simplex virus, herpes zoster virus, Epstein-Barr virus, and hepatitis B, C, or non A, non B. Viral infections are primary or reactivated. They occasionally have been transmitted from the donor via the transplanted organ, but current careful screening processes usually eliminate this.

Fungal colonization and superinfection with *Candida, Nocardia,* or *Listeria* have been common in complicated cases, especially in liver and lung transplantation. Invasive *Aspergillus* infection is invariably lethal.

Pneumocystis carinii pneumonia has been common enough in organ transplantation to warrant prophylactic therapy with trimethoprimsulfamethoxazole, which has reduced the frequency of this protozoal infection.

Meticulous sterile technique is indicated for all invasive procedures in immunosuppressed transplantation patients. Cross-contamination between patients usually results from poor handwashing technique and frequency by ICU personnel. Airborne infections are less common, but isolation rooms are preferred for transplantation patients in the immediate postoperative period.

Use of antacids and H_2 blocking agents reduces the frequency of postoperative gastrointestinal bleeding and the formation of ulcers. However, these medications also lead to bacterial invasion of the stomach and secondary colonization of the pharynx. The infection may spread to the respiratory tract through minimal aspiration, which has been shown to occur during mechanical ventilation with endotracheal tubes equipped with large-volume, low-pressure cuffs. These cuffs do not protect against aspiration of small quantities of pharyngeal secretions, which are frequently contaminated with intestinal bacteria. Therefore preoperative intestinal sterilization with antibiotics is being evaluated, especially in liver transplantations.

Systemic antibiotic prophylaxis is provided to most transplantation patients because of their high susceptibility to postoperative infections once immunosuppressive therapy is started. Antibiotic prophylaxis begins in the operating room and continues postoperatively in the ICU with a third-generation cephalosporin and ampicillin for 72 hours. For empiric treatment of sepsis these antibiotics are combined with vancomycin and aminoglycosides while culture results are pending. The principles of antibiotic treatment are the same as for other types of patients, but the volume of distribution of aminoglycosides is larger in patients with end-stage liver disease and a higher loading dose may be required. However, the incidence of aminoglycoside nephrotoxicity is greater in cirrhotic patients.

Fungal infections after transplantation may be devastating, particularly in patients with liver failure. Prophylactic amphotericin B in low doses (0.2 mg/kg/d for 2 weeks) has been used for patients at high risk.

Cytomegalovirus is a significant pathogen in transplantation patients and is frequently present in donor blood. Therefore cytomegalovirus negative blood should be given to cytomegalovirus-negative recipients. Prophylaxis with immunoglobulin or high doses of acyclovir has been used in treatment of these patients.

ETHICAL PROBLEMS AND FUTURE OF TRANSPLANTATION

Efficient medication for immunosuppression has made transplantation surgery far more successful than conventional medical therapy for end-stage disease of vital organs, particularly terminal kidney, heart, or liver failure. The success rate with end-stage pulmonary, pancreatic, or intestinal diseases is not yet equally great. However, because of advances in all aspects of organ transplantation, the explosive growth in transplantation experienced during the 1980s is certain to continue.

Unfortunately, the demand for donor organs outweighs the supply. Three major categories of organ donors can be identified: living donors, brain-dead heart-beating donors, and non-heart-beating cadavers. As the demand for organs increases, various steps are being taken to enlarge the pool of organ donors. These include expanding acceptable age limits of the donors, not excluding organs with mild forms of disease or trauma, and using parts of vital organs removed from living donors, such as the left lobe of the liver for transplantation from a parent into a child. An ongoing debate concerns the relevance of the "whole brain death" concept. Future certification of death might include not only conventional non-heart-beating cadavers and those who are determined brain dead, but also those in persistent vegetative states, and anencephalic babies. However, it is unlikely that the current brain death concept will be expanded in the remainder of this century.

For many years parts of organs with function limited to mechanical support have been replaced with prosthetic devices, such as joints. The first entire organ to be replaced with an artificial device was the heart, but currently available artificial hearts require an external power source with uninterrupted connection to the implanted artificial heart from the outside. So far this has caused unacceptable complications, and artificial heart implantation for permanent use awaits a more sophisticated generation of such devices.

Before acceptable implantable organs can be developed, use of xenografts (organs from other species) for transplantation seems likely. Transplantation of animal organs into human beings has been tried for many years but so far has failed because insurmountable immunologic problems have led to severe rejection in all cases. The most famous of these is the transplantation of a baboon heart into Baby Fae at Loma Linda University in 1985. As better immunosuppressive drugs are developed, these attempts are likely to be repeated with greater success later in this decade.

SUGGESTED READINGS

Alexander JW: The cutting edge. Transplantation 1990; 49:237-240

Auchincloss H Jr: Xenographic transplantation: a review. Transplantation 1988;46:1-20

Bailey LL, Nehlsen-Cannarella SL, Concepcion W, et al: Baboon-to-human cardiac xenotransplantation in a neonate. JAMA 1985;254:3321

Barnard CN: A human cardiac transplant; an interim report of a successful operation at Groote Schuur Hospital in Cape Town. S Afr Med J 1967;41:1271-1274

Beecher H: A definition of irreversible coma: report of the ad hoc committee of the Harvard Medical School to examine the definition of brain death. JAMA 1968; 205:337

Billingham RE, Brent L, Medawar PB: The antigenic stimulus in transplantation immunity. Nature 1956;178:514

Calne RY, Murray JE: Inhibition of the rejection of renal homografts in dogs with Burroughs-Wellcome 322. Surg Forum 1961;12:118

Collins GM, Bravo-Sugarman M, Terasaki PI: Kidney preservation for transportation: initial perfusion and 30 hours' ice storage. Lancet 1969;2:1219

Cooley DA, Bloodwell RD, Hallman GL, et al: Organ transplantation for advanced cardiopulmonary disease. Ann Thorac Surg 1969;8:30-42

DeVries WC: The permanent artificial heart: four case reports. JAMA 1988;259:849-859

Gillis S, Crabtree GR, Smith KA: Glucocorticoid-induced inhibition of T cell growth factor production. II. The effect on the in vitro generation of cytolytic T cells. J Immunol 1979;123:1632

Hardy JD, Webb WR, Dalton ML, et al: Lung homotransplantation in man. JAMA 1963;186:1065-1074

Hume DM, Merrill JP, Miller BF, et al: Experiences with renal homotransplantation in the human: report of nine cases. J Clin Invest 1955;334:327

Kelly WD, Lillehei RC, Merkel FK, et al: Allotransplantation of the pancreas and duodenum along with the kidney in diabetic nephropathy. Surgery 1967;61:827-837

Kusne S, Dummer JS, Singh N, et al: Infection after liver transplantation: an analysis of 101 consecutive cases. Medicine 1988;67:132-143

Lower RR, Shumway NE: Studies in orthotopic homotransplantation of the canine heart. Surg Forum 1960;11:18-19

Lower RR, Stofer RC, Hurley EJ, et al: Complete homograft replacement of the heart and both lungs. Surgery 1961;50:842

Merrill JP, Murray JE, Harrison JH, et al: Successful homotransplantation of the human kidney between identical twins. JAMA 1956;160:277

Mollaret P, Goulon M: Le coma dépassé. Rev Neurol 1959;101:3

President's Commission for the Study of Ethical Problems in Medicine and Biomedical and Behavioral Research: Guidelines for the determination of death: report of the medical consultants on the diagnosis of death. JAMA 1981;246:2184

Reitz BA, Wallwork JL, Hunt SA, et al: Heart-lung transplantation: successful therapy for patients with pulmonary vascular disease. N Engl J Med 1982;306:557-564

Sawada S, Suzuki G, Kawase Y, et al: Novel immunosuppressive agent, FK506: in vitro effects on the cloned T cell activation. J Immunol 1987;139:1797

Starzl TE, Hakala TR, Shaw BW, et al: A flexible procedure for multiple cadaveric organ procurement. Surg Gynecol Obstet 1984;158:223

Starzl TE, Marchiaro TL, Porter KA, et al: The use of heterologous antilymphoid agents in canine renal and liver homotransplantation and in human renal homotransplantation. Surg Gynecol Obstet 1967;124:311

Starzl TE, Marchiaro TL, Von Kaulla K, et al: Homotransplantation of the liver in humans. Surg Gynecol Obstet 1963;117:659

Thomas J, Matthews C, Carroll R, et al: The immunosuppressive action of FK506. Transplantation 1990;49:390-396

Thomas ED, Storb R, Clift RA, et al: Bone marrow transplantation. N Engl J Med 1975;292:832-843

Todo S, Fung JJ, Starzl TE, et al: Liver, kidney, and thoracic organ transplantation under FK 506. Ann Surg (in press)

Wahlberg JA, Southard JH, Belzer FO: Development of a cold storage solution for pancreas preservation. Cryobiology 1986;23:477-482

CRITICAL CARE OF OBSTETRIC PATIENTS

JOY L. HAWKINS, MD, MONICA M. JONES, MD, AND THOMAS H. JOYCE III, MD

The special considerations involved in caring for the seriously ill parturient have rarely been addressed in critical care texts. Since these patients are generally young and in overall good health, many physicians overlook the fact that preexisting maternal medical conditions or peripartum complications can have disastrous consequences. After all, only in the obstetric patient is the potential mortality 200%.

Because both the disease and the therapy employed affect two separate individuals with vastly different physiologies, the critical care physician must balance conflicting maternal and fetal considerations. Knowledge of the normal physiology of pregnancy is a prerequisite to dealing with problems that accompany a complicated pregnancy.

This chapter discusses a number of serious problems that can arise during pregnancy, although it obviously does not address all conditions that may affect a pregnant woman. The goal is to ensure a safe outcome for both mother and child.

PREGNANCY TESTS

When a woman of childbearing age is admitted to the ICU, a pregnancy test should be performed as part of routine admission laboratory work. The presence of a viable intrauterine pregnancy may necessitate changes in pharmacologic or therapeutic maneuvers to prevent teratogenic exposure for the fetus.

All pregnancy tests are based on detection of human chorionic gonadotropin (hCG) produced by placental tissue. Because the alpha subunits of four hormones (follicle-stimulating

hormone, thyrotropin, luteinizing hormone, and hCG) are identical, cross-reactivity to tests for this subunit can occur. The beta subunit for each of these hormones is distinct, however, and detection of an antibody to the beta subunit of hCG in blood or urine is the basis for chemical detection of pregnancy.

The production of hCG begins very early in pregnancy. Radioimmunoassay can show beta hCG by 8 to 9 days after ovulation. The levels of hCG in blood and urine then increase from the time of implantation until they peak at 60 to 70 days' gestation.

Agglutination inhibition is used in most commercially available kits to detect hCG in urine. If no agglutination occurs, the pregnancy test is positive. Radioimmunoassay and the enzyme-linked immunosorbent assay have great sensitivity in measuring small amounts of the hormone.

Commercially available tests using antibody against the beta subunit of hCG are extremely sensitive and specific. False-positive tests are most often caused by cross-reactivity of luteinizing hormone, especially at menopause. The false-negative test most often occurs during the first few days of pregnancy or after the fourth month. With ectopic pregnancies only small amounts of hCG may be produced and not identified by less sensitive tests.

SEPTIC ABORTION

Although serious complications of abortion have decreased since legalization, death from abortion still occurs, and infection is the leading cause. Risk factors for complications are increased by greater length of gestation and technical difficulties in the procedure.

Clinical Manifestations. Infection after abortion is an ascending process involving pathogenic organisms of the bowel or vaginal flora. Although infection is most often confined to the uterus, peritonitis and sepsis sometimes occur, especially with perforation of the uterus or bowel trauma.

Patients usually have fever, chills, abdominal pain, and vaginal bleeding with or without passage of tissue. Pelvic examination may show bleeding, foul odor, and cervical or vaginal lacerations. Bimanual examination reveals uterine tenderness.

Laboratory evaluation should include complete blood count, urinalysis, and chest and abdominal roentgenograms. Samples of blood, urine, and any expelled products of conception should be taken for aerobic and anaerobic cultures, as well as a smear from the cervix for Gram stain. Organisms commonly found in positive blood cultures include anaerobic *Streptococcus* (41%), *Escherichia coli* (14%), group B streptococci (4%), and *Bacteroides* species (9%).

Treatment. Treatment includes replacement of blood and fluids, correction of any coagulopathy, antibiotic therapy, and removal of the infected tissue from the uterus. After culture findings have been obtained, broad-spectrum antibiotic coverage, such as ampicillin, gentamicin, and clindamycin, should be started. Once appropriate monitors have been placed and the patient's condition is stable, the uterus is evacuated and infected products of conception are removed by curettage. Occasionally laparotomy or even hysterectomy is required. Indications include failure to respond to curettage and medical management, perforation of the uterus with suspected bowel injury, pelvic abscess, or clostridial necrotizing myometritis.

Since sepsis can occur during or after curettage, the patient must be monitored carefully in the ICU or recovery room. Further treatment is the same as for septic shock.

INTRACRANIAL ANEURYSMS AND ARTERIOVENOUS MALFORMATIONS

The incidence of subarachnoid hemorrhage (SAH) in the pregnant population has been reported to be 1 in 10,000 with an immediate mortality rate of 43%. Neither incidence nor mortality seems to be increased with pregnancy despite the increases in cardiac output and blood volume. Cerebral aneurysms are generally located in the anterior portion of the circle of Willis, whereas arteriovenous malformations (AVMs) can be anywhere in the cerebral vasculature. The cause is almost always congenital in pregnancy-related cases.

Clinical Manifestations. The most common clinical presentation is sudden onset of severe headache with blurred vision, stiff neck, nausea, focal neurologic signs, or coma. The incidence of SAH associated with aneurysm increases with gestational age; 6% of ruptures occur during the first trimester, 31% in the second, 55% in the third, and 8% after delivery. Surprisingly, rupture is rare during labor. Rupture of an AVM occurs most commonly at 15 to 20 weeks' gestation and during labor and the early postpartum period. The main differential diagnosis is severe pregnancy-induced hypertension with central nervous system involvement. Elevated intracranial pressure resulting from SAH may cause reflex increases in blood pressure. Proteinuria may also occur.

A diagnostic workup should begin with a cerebral computed tomographic scan to find the site of bleeding and determine the presence of hematomas that would require surgical drainage. If computed tomography shows no abnormality, the cerebrospinal fluid should be examined for blood or xanthochromia. Cerebral angiography (with abdominal shielding) should follow to identify any vascular abnormality.

Treatment. Initial treatment is conservative medical management to prevent rebleeding. Measures include bed rest, cautious use of sedatives and analgesics, and stool softeners. Hypertension is thought to be a protective mechanism to preserve cerebral flow, and therefore antihypertensives should be used conservatively. Use of steroids and antifibrinolytic agents is controversial.

The decision to operate depends on the patient's clinical condition, surgical accessibility of the lesion, and the presence of vasospasm. The decision should not be influenced by the fact of the patient's pregnancy, since surgery reduces the mortality rate and the incidence of rebleeding. In general, early surgical intervention is used for conscious patients with no neurologic deficits. Maternal condition is the best predictor of fetal well-being. Fetal and uterine monitoring should be used whenever a pregnant patient undergoes surgery. After 16 weeks of gestation, external Doppler fetal heart rate monitoring can be used to determine fetal well-being, as well as tolerance to techniques used during neurosurgical procedures. Induced hypotension with inhalation agents, nitroprusside (less than 10 μg/kg/min), nitroglycerin, or trimethaphan has been used successfully in pregnant patients, with fetal monitoring to determine adequacy of uterine perfusion. Hypothermia (28° to 32° C) and hyperventilation have also been successful in pregnant patients when indicated. Again, fetal monitoring ensures maintenance of uterine perfusion. Osmotic diuretics, such as mannitol, cross the placenta and cause a net flow of fluid from the fetus to the mother, leading to fetal dehydration. Therefore these drugs should be used cautiously if at all during pregnancy.

Postoperative management of a pregnant neurosurgical patient requires only a few modifications. Because all pregnant patients should be considered as having a full stomach, extubation should be performed only when the patient has intact airway reflexes. A smooth emergence is also important. Left uterine displacement must be maintained at all times to prevent aortocaval compression. Fetal heart rate and uterine contractility should be monitored for at least 24 hours postoperatively, with the aid of a nurse familiar with fetal monitoring if necessary. Use of anesthetic agents and narcotics may eliminate beat-tobeat variability; this does not necessarily indicate fetal distress. Preterm labor is the major cause of fetal morbidity and mortality and therefore must be diagnosed and treated without delay.

Management of delivery after SAH should be based on obstetric indications rather than the maternal condition. Patients with successful surgical treatment of a cerebral aneurysm or AVM need no special management of labor or delivery. A patient with an untreated cerebral aneurysm should have a vaginal delivery under epidural anesthesia. Use of outlet forceps shortens the second stage of labor and avoids the need for Valsalva maneuver associated with the urge to push. The same management may be used for a patient with an uncorrected or surgically inaccessible AVM, but some authorities recommend elective cesarean section because these malformations increase the risk of bleeding or rebleeding during labor. A patient with SAH during the third trimester may require cesarean section, perhaps in conjunction with a repair of the cerebral lesion. If the patient's neurologic status deteriorates after the occurrence of SAH, the obstetrician may have toperform an agonal cesarean section to save the fetus.

MYASTHENIA GRAVIS

Myasthenia gravis (MG) is an autoimmune disorder affecting the postjunctional acetylcholine receptor and most commonly involving the oculomotor, facial, laryngeal, and respiratory muscles. The incidence is 2 to 10 per 100,000, and the disease is twice as common in women. Since the age of onset in women is usually in the third decade, pregnancy is common in myasthenic patients. About one third of patients worsen during pregnancy, most early in gestation or in the postpartum period, whereas two thirds are stable or improve. The maternal mortality rate is about 3%; deaths are due mainly to respiratory complications.

Clinical Manifestations.   MG may first appear in pregnancy as respiratory infection when limited diaphragmatic excursion leads to inability to clear secretions, or patients may suddenly deteriorate with respiratory compromise. Diagnosis is based on a test in which 2 to 10 mg of edrophonium given intravenously rapidly improves symptoms if the patient has MG. This can also help distinguish between myasthenic crisis and cholinergic crisis caused by medication overdose.

Nausea early in pregnancy may lead to inability to retain oral medications, exacerbating MG. Termination of pregnancy is not indicated, since induced abortion has no effect on the course of the disease. A myasthenic crisis may also be precipitated by emotional stress, exertion, or infection (respiratory or urinary infection or chorioamnionitis, for example). A statistically significant number of patients worsen during the postpartum period, with high rates of respiratory failure and maternal mortality. Therefore patients should be monitored for 10 days after delivery.

Treatment.   Medical management of MG includes anticholinesterase drugs (such as neostigmine and pyridostigmine), corticosteroids, and rarely plasmapheresis. Thymectomy is often performed, especially in young patients, as an alternative to long-term steroid use. The incidence of exacerbation seems to be less in obstetric patients who had thymectomy performed before pregnancy.

Since uterine contractility is not affected by MG, vaginal delivery is usually possible, often with epidural analgesia and outlet forceps. Serial assessment of vital capacity allows early detection of respiratory insufficiency resulting from fatigue during labor. Magnesium sulfate is contraindicated in these patients because its effects on the neuromuscular junction decrease acetylcholine release and the sensitivity of the motor end-plate to neurotransmitter.

Regional anesthesia is preferred for vaginal delivery. It decreases the need for systemic medication, prevents maternal fatigue, and provides anesthesia for outlet forceps application at the time of delivery. The ester local anesthetics, such as chloroprocaine, are metabolized by plasma cholinesterase, which is inhibited by anticholinesterase therapy. Therefore their use could produce systemic toxicity. The amide-type local anesthetics are a safer choice. During labor, parenteral anticholinesterase medications should be titrated based on the patient's symptoms and serial vital capacity measurements. Decrement of three serial vital capacity measurements indicates fatigue. The equivalent dosages are one twentieth of the oral dose for intramuscular injection and one thirtieth of the oral dose for intravenous administration.

If cesarean section is required, regional anesthesia can be used, but the benefits must be weighed against the possibility of aspiration or respiratory insufficiency during high blockade. If general anesthesia is used, the endotracheal tube should be left in place until ventilation is adequate and airway control is ensured.

Because of the sedation and respiratory depression associated with the use of parenteral narcotics, epidural narcotics should provide postoperative pain relief for at least 48 hours after delivery. Anticholinesterase requirements vary widely in the postpartum period and must be continually reassessed, since a significant number of patients have worsening of symptoms after delivery. Postpartum exacerbations of MG can be sudden, and a number of maternal deaths, caused chiefly by respiratory failure, have been reported.

Neonatal Myasthenia Gravis. Neonatal MG occurs in 20% to 30% of neonates born to myasthenic mothers because of transplacental passage of maternal acetycholine receptor antibodies. Symptoms appear 12 to 24 hours after birth and include poor sucking, weak cry, expressionless face, and respiratory distress. The syndrome is transient, lasting 10 days to 4 months. Response to medication is usually good.

Anticholinesterase medications in breast milk may cause muscarinic symptoms in the newborn. Since maternal antibodies are also present in breast milk, feeding should be avoided unless the MG is in remission with low antibody titers and no medications.

AMNIOTIC FLUID EMBOLISM

Amniotic fluid embolism (AFE) is a rare obstetric disorder but one that carries a maternal mortality rate as high as 86%. The classic diagnostic triad includes hypotension, hypoxia, and coagulopathy with associated respiratory distress.

Pathophysiology. For AFE to occur, amniotic fluid must have a passage to the maternal circulation. This requires ruptured membranes, an opening in the maternal circulation such as occurs with ruptured uterus, placenta accreta, cesarean section, retained placenta, abruption, or placenta previa. Data from animal studies have indicated that the pathophysiology of AFE involves severe pulmonary hypertension caused by debris occluding the pulmonary vasculature or by vasospastic changes leading to acute failure of the right side of the heart. In contrast, hemodynamic studies in humans have shown only moderate increases in pulmonary pressures but a high pulmonary capillary wedge pressure and evidence of left-sided heart failure based either on a low left ventricular stroke work index or on clinical signs of left ventricular failure. The current theory is that a biphasic hemodynamic response to AFE occurs. The initial response (probably in the first 30 minutes) of the pulmonary vasculature to amniotic fluid and other debris is intense vasospasm leading to pulmonary hypertension and hypoxia with acute cor pulmonale. The secondary phase consists of left-sided heart failure and pulmonary edema caused by the severe hypoxia or a direct myocardial depressant effect of AFE. Residual pulmonary vasospasm may also be present. Coagulopathy occurs in about 40% of patients. The exact cause is unknown, but the thromboplastic effects of trophoblastic material or some other substance contained in amniotic fluid may play a role.

Clinical Manifestations. AFE usually occurs during labor, but it has also occurred during second-trimester abortions, abdominal trauma, amniocentesis, and even after delivery. Predisposing factors include advanced maternal age, multiparity, large baby, short tumultuous labor, pregnancy-induced hypertension, and fetal demise. Given the common use of oxytocin (Pitocin) and the rarity of AFE, an association between this agent and AFE is unlikely.

The clinical presentation is usually one of sudden dyspnea, cyanosis, and hypotension followed shortly by cardiovascular collapse.

Grand mal seizures may occur. Almost half of affected patients die within an hour after symptoms occur. Placement of a pulmonary artery catheter reveals elevated pulmonary capillary wedge pressure (PCWP), depressed left ventricular stroke work index, moderate elevations in pulmonary artery pressure and pulmonary vascular resistance, and a decrease in systemic vascular resistance. Pulmonary edema is often out of proportion to the elevation in PCWP indicating an increase in pulmonary vascular permeability.

In 40% to 50% of patients who survive the initial cardiovascular insult, a consumptive coagulopathy occurs. Bleeding from venipuncture sites and surgical incisions is common. Uterine atony caused either by decreased uterine perfusion with severe systemic hypotension or by a myometrial depressant effect of amniotic fluid often occurs simultaneously. Laboratory abnormalities include evidence of excessive fibrinolysis, such as elevated levels of fibrin split products and decreased fibrinogen concentrations. Prolonged prothrombin time and partial thromboplastin time, as well as thrombocytopenia, are present. The diagnosis of AFE is based primarily on clinical findings. Although the finding of fetal squamous cells in the pulmonary circulation after pulmonary artery catheterization or at autopsy is the classic diagnostic indicator, recent studies have shown that small numbers of fetal squamous cells are almost universally present in the maternal peripheral and pulmonary circulation. The differential diagnosis should include sepsis, aspiration, pulmonary thromboembolism, air embolism, myocardial infarction, and placental abruption with coagulopathy.

Treatment. Treatment is directed at oxygenation, cardiovascular support, and correction of coagulopathy. Cardiopulmonary resuscitation should be initiated if indicated. Patients require intubation and mechanical ventilation with 100% oxygen and positive end-expiratory pressure to maintain arterial oxygen saturation and reduce the massive ventilation/perfusion mismatch. This may help prevent myocardial and cerebral ischemia and reduce pulmonary artery hypertension caused by hypoxia. Insertion of a pulmonary artery catheter allows rapid fluid infusions and rational use of dopamine for cardiac support. Blood should be drawn from the distal port into a heparinized tube to be analyzed for fetal squamous cells; although fetal cells are common, their absence casts doubt on the diagnosis

of AFE. Disseminated intravascular coagulation should be treated as described previously in this text.

COMPLICATIONS OF BETA-MIMETIC THERAPY

Preterm labor complicates approximately 5% of pregnancies and is a major cause of both maternal and fetal morbidity. Beta-sympathomimetic drugs are widely used to inhibit uterine contractions but are associated with a high incidence of maternal complications. Their side effects are often the limiting factor in their use.

Pathophysiology. Although all beta-sympathomimetic drugs are derivatives of epinephrine, drugs in current use, such as terbutaline and ritodrine, have more beta$_2$ selectivity than earlier drugs, such as isoxsuprine. Nevertheless, all compounds have some beta$_1$ activity leading to cardiac effects and lipolysis, as well as the beta$_2$ side effects of vasodilation and glycogenolysis. Maternal side effects can be broadly divided into metabolic and cardiopulmonary complications.

Metabolic side effects are hyperglycemia, hypokalemia, sodium and water retention, and an increase in serum lactate level. Beta stimulation causes gluconeogenesis and glycogenolysis, leading to increased serum levels of glucose and free fatty acids. The serum glucose concentration rises from a baseline of 80 to 90 mg/dl to a peak of 120 to 160 mg/dl within 1 hour. Except in pregnant diabetics the level rarely rises above 200 mg/dl or requires insulin therapy. However, ketoacidosis and fetal death have been reported in an insulin-dependent diabetic patient. Elevated insulin levels are due to direct stimulation of pancreatic beta receptors, as well as a direct response to hyperglycemia. Hypokalemia (average potassium loss of 0.8 mEq/L) is a result of intracellular shift caused by elevated glucose and insulin levels. Because total body potassium is unchanged, serum levels return to normal after discontinuation of therapy, and supplementation is unnecessary. An elevated serum lactate level caused by lipolysis leads to a fall in pH and base excess but is rarely clinically significant.

Plasma renin and vasopressin concentrations are increased during beta-mimetic therapy, causing decreased sodium and water excretion. Renal blood flow and consequently glomerular filtration rate fall, resulting in an increase in plasma volume and extracellular water and a decrease in colloid osmotic pressure and hematocrit value.

The cardiopulmonary complications include hypotension, cerebral ischemia, dysrhythmias, myocardial ischemia, and pulmonary edema. Hypotension with a widened pulse pressure is due to beta-induced vasodilation and may be severe in patients with blood loss (for example, caused by placenta previa). Cerebral ischemia in patients with a history of migraine is thought to result from rebound vasospasm. Sinus tachycardia is common during beta-mimetic therapy, but more serious dysrhythmias, such as supraventricular tachycardia, atrial fibrillation, and premature ventricular contractions, can occur as well. One study found a 2% incidence of unexpected cardiac disease whose symptoms appeared during beta-mimetic therapy; the diseases included Wolff-Parkinson-White and Lown-Ganong-Levine syndromes, atrial septal defect, and hypertrophic cardiomyopathy. All patients should have pretreatment electrocardiography to look for evidence of cardiac disorders.

Myocardial ischemia is usually subendocardial and due to a supply/demand imbalance. Both tachycardia and the increased oxygen consumption of pregnancy increase demand, whereas shortened diastolic filling time, lowered diastolic filling pressure, and the physiologic anemia of pregnancy all decrease supply. Flattened T waves and ST segment depression are common even in asymptomatic women during beta-mimetic therapy and are not associated with cardiac enzyme changes. Again, a pretreatment electrocardiogram is helpful for comparison.

Pulmonary edema is the major cause of maternal morbidity and mortality caused by beta-mimetic therapy. Pulmonary capillary membrane permeability is normal in pregnancy except perhaps in cases of infection, and volume overload with increased capillary hydrostatic pressure is thought to cause beta-mimetic-induced pulmonary edema. A marked fall in urine output associated with sodium and water retention occurs during therapy, and positive fluid balances are common in these patients. Risk factors for pulmonary edema include volume overload (usually iatrogenic), twin gestation, combined therapy with magnesium sulfate, use of corticosteroids, and presence of chorioamnionitis. Hourly intake and output monitoring, use of free water so-

lutions such as 5% dextrose in water or 0.25 normal saline solution, and use of controlled infusion devices for intravenous solutions is recommended.

PREGNANCY-INDUCED HYPERTENSION

Pregnancy-induced hypertension (PIH), which occurs in 5% to 10% of pregnancies, remains a major cause of maternal morbidity and mortality. The diagnosis of PIH requires that two of the following criteria be present: (1) blood pressure greater than 140/90 mm Hg or an increase in systolic blood pressure greater than 30 mm Hg or diastolic blood pressure greater than 15 mm Hg (verified on two readings taken 6 hours apart with the parturient at rest) when compared with baseline blood pressures, (2) urinary protein levels greater than 0.3 g/L in a 24-hour sample period or proteinuria of 1+ or 2+ on two urine samples obtained 6 hours apart, and (3) generalized edema. In some parturients PIH may be superimposed on chronic hypertension.

PIH is defined as severe if any of the following are present: (1) systolic blood pressure greater than 160 mm Hg, (2) diastolic blood pressure greater than 110 mm Hg, (3) urinary protein levels greater than 5 g/24 h, (4) oliguria (less than 400 ml/24 h), (5) central nervous system symptoms (cerebral or visual disturbances), or (6) pulmonary edema. Preeclampsia is redefined as eclampsia when seizures occur.

Pathophysiology and Clinical Manifestations. PIH has the potential for involving almost every organ system. The hypertension results from widespread vasospasm or hyperdynamic cardiac state or both. Pulmonary hypertension is usually not present. Hyperdynamic cardiac function is frequently present with an elevated left ventricular work index and cardiac output. The central venous pressure and PCWP are usually low, indicating a diminished intravascular volume. Some parturients, however, may have depressed cardiac function and pulmonary edema. Pulmonary artery catheterization assists in detecting this subset.

The cause of central nervous system symptoms (scotoma, headache, seizures) is not well defined. Cerebral edema may be visualized on a computed tomographic scan in some patients with central nervous system symptoms, indicating that intracranial pressure may be increased. Seizures associated with PIH occur in approximately 0.1% to 0.2% of parturients. Magnesium sulfate is administered to patients with PIH to decrease the likelihood of seizure occurrence or recurrence. The recurrence of seizures despite therapeutic serum magnesium levels (4 to 6 mg/dl) should lead to a search for other causes, such as a cortical vein thrombosis or a subarachnoid hemorrhage.

The presence of right upper quadrant pain suggests the presence of hepatic involvement. This is detected by findings of increased serum values of liver enzymes. Hepatic subcapsular hemorrhage, which has the potential for liver rupture, occurs rarely but presents a life-threatening situation. Should this occur, the need for large quantities of blood and coagulation replacement products should be anticipated.

HELLP syndrome is a group of signs including hemolysis (H), findings of elevated liver enzymes (EL), and a low platelet count (LP). This triad has been observed in a small group of parturients with PIH and should be sought in any patient exhibiting one of the component signs. If the HELLP syndrome is present, the coagulation abnormalities should be corrected and plans made for imminent delivery. Although hepatic rupture is not considered a part of the triad in HELLP syndrome, it must be considered in a patient with severe hypertension, increased serum values of liver enzymes, and coagulopathy.

PIH may be accompanied by a microangiopathic hemolytic anemia, which can be diagnosed by evaluation of the peripheral blood smear. Thrombocytopenia or a decrease in the fibrinogen level heralds the onset of disseminated intravascular coagulation.

Vasospasm within the renal arteries diminishes renal blood flow and glomerular filtration. Elevations in serum creatinine and blood urea nitrogen (BUN) concentrations with a resultant decrease in creatinine clearance frequently accompany this disease process. The occurrence of oliguria typically reflects severe intravascular volume depletion. Therefore, before the use of diuretics to increase the urine output, intravascular volume should be optimized. The characteristic proteinuria of PIH results in a loss of serum proteins and a further decrease in the colloid osmotic pressure (COP) below the level occurring during a normal pregnancy.

Treatment

LABORATORY EVALUATION. Initial evaluation should include a complete blood count (CBC), coagulation profile (platelet count, fibrinogen level, prothrombin time, partial thromboplastin time), hepatic function tests (alanine aminotransferase, astartate aminotransferase, bilirubin), renal profile (serum creatinine and BUN levels and 24-hour creatinine clearance if time allows, or a 2-hour creatinine clearance may be measured), serum electrolytes and glucose and other tests as indicated (colloid osmotic pressure, arterial blood gas levels, and a chest roentgenogram if eclampsia or respiratory abnormality is present).

MONITORING. ICU monitoring of the parturient with severe PIH should include electrocardiography, blood pressure measurement by intraarterial catheter, pulse oximetry, and a Foley catheter (for strict intake and output records). Several reports have indicated that in the parturient with PIH and severe hypertension the central venous pressure may not correlate with the PCWP as a measure of intravascular volume. Indications for placement of a pulmonary artery catheter in a patient with PIH include severe hypertension unresponsive to conventional antihypertensive therapy, pulmonary edema, persistent oliguria unresponsive to a fluid challenge, or the induction of conduction anesthesia.

MEDICATIONS. Magnesium sulfate is administered to decrease the incidence of seizures in parturients with PIH. A loading dose of 4 to 6 g is given intravenously over 20 minutes followed by an infusion of 2 g/h (until 24 hours after delivery) to maintain a serum magnesium level of 4 to 6 mg/dl. Caution must be exercised with patients who have renal impairment because magnesium is excreted via the kidneys. Magnesium decreases the sensitivity of the end-plate at the neuromuscular junction, as well as the amount of acetylcholine released. If a neuromuscular blocking drug is needed, the neuromuscular junction must be monitored to determine the extent of blockade (less neuromuscular blocker may be needed than in a nonpregnant patient) and the adequacy of reversal. The patient should not be pretreated with a nondepolarizing drug before succinylcholine administration because of these neuromuscular junction effects.

Hydralazine is the antihypertensive most frequently used by obstetricians. Hydralazine acts as a direct vasodilator, decreasing the mean arterial pressure and systemic vascular resistance, but it may increase heart rate and cardiac index. Because of its slow and somewhat unpredictable onset of action, hydralazine is not the ideal drug, although it has increased uterine blood flow in animal studies. Hydralazine is usually titrated in 2.5 to 5 mg intravenous doses with at least 15 minutes between doses.

Nitroprusside is a rapid-acting drug with a short duration of action. Nitroprusside provides excellent, predictable blood pressure control. Concern has been voiced about possible toxic effects of cyanide on the fetus, particularly because ion trapping may occur in an acidotic fetus. However, short-term administration, such as for laryngoscopy, should pose minimal risk to the fetus. Further data are needed before prolonged use in a pregnant woman can be recommended.

Nitroglycerin is primarily a venodilator but in sufficient concentrations may act as an arterial dilator. The effectiveness of nitroglycerin depends on the parturient's volume status. Volume-depleted patients respond at a lower dose, whereas those who are volume overloaded may require a higher dose if they respond at all.

Trimethaphan is a rapid-acting ganglionic blocker. This drug works relatively quickly and is easily titratable in emergency situations. However, tachyphylaxis limits its long-term use. The ganglionic blocking property results in pupillary dilation, which may confuse the interpretation of eye findings when an intracranial disorder is suspected.

Few controlled studies have investigated short-term use of beta blockers in pregnant humans. Concern has been voiced about the side effects of beta blockers (increased uterine tone, impaired fetal glucose homeostasis). However, these problems have not occurred with small doses of propranolol. The use of cardioselective beta blockers, such as metoprolol and labetalol, should further minimize these side effects. These drugs should decrease tachycardia and the systemic vascular resistance in parturients with PIH. Labetalol reduces mean arterial pressure without compromising uteroplacental blood flow. After an initial 5 to 10 mg intravenous dose, the dose is increased at 10-minute intervals until the desired blood pressure is attained. (The maximum recommended dose in the nonpregnant patient is 300 mg. The maximum dose for pregnancy has not been determined.)

Anticonvulsants, such as phenytoin (Dilantin) do not have a role in the routine management of eclampsia unless a specific neurologic problem, such as a tumor or hemorrhage, indicates their use. If therapeutic magnesium levels are present, the occurrence of seizures (eclampsia) should be controlled with pentothal for the short term. A small dose (50 to 100 mg) is commonly effective. If the seizure continues or the airway must be secured, higher doses of pentothal and succinylcholine may be needed. Should seizure activity still continue, benzodiazepines may be administered. Benzodiazepines frequently decrease the fetal heart rate beat-to-beat variability for a prolonged period, interfering with the evaluation of fetal status.

SEIZURES. The seizures associated with PIH are usually short-lived. If they are prolonged, the patient's airway must be secured and oxygenation reestablished. A chest roentgenogram and arterial blood gas measurements should be obtained after the seizure to assess the patient's pulmonary and acid-base status, since pulmonary aspiration is possible. The magnesium level should be determined to ensure that a therapeutic level is present.

The occurrence of a seizure is not in itself an indication for immediate cesarean section. Fetal bradycardia typically occurs during the seizure when the mother is hypoxic. However, the fetal status should improve and the bradycardia resolve as the mother's oxygenation is restored. If this improvement is not seen, other causes for the fetal distress (such as abruption) may be present and could necessitate an emergency cesarean section.

Other causes of seizures (such as intracranial hemorrhage or cortical vein thrombosis) should be kept in mind, especially if a therapeutic magnesium level is maintained. Deterioration of the patient's mental status or the development of focal signs should be investigated with computed tomography.

HYPERTENSION. Hypertension may be treated with the antihypertensives previously discussed. The choice of antihypertensive depends on the patient's hemodynamic status. For example, the presence of tachycardia may indicate the need for a beta blocker, especially if hydralazine is used, because this drug may further increase the heart rate. The use of nitroglycerin or nitroprusside for prolonged periods before delivery may cause fetal methemoglobinemia or cyanide intoxication. Nitroglycerin or nitroprusside can be safely used in most parturients for blood pressure control during short periods of anesthesia induction and endotracheal intubation.

OLIGURIA. If oliguria occurs, a fluid bolus (500 to 1000 ml of a balanced salt solution) may be administered to observe if the urine output increases. If no improvement occurs, a pulmonary artery catheter should be inserted to optimize intravascular volume. If the PCWP is less than 15 mm Hg, a balanced salt solution or a colloid-containing solution should be given to increase the PCWP to 15 mm Hg. In addition, the cardiac output should be optimized and manipulated pharmacologically if needed to ensure optimal renal blood flow. Should the PCWP increase to greater than 18 mm Hg without an increase in urine output, the use of a diuretic (such as furosemide) or low-dose dopamine (1 to 3 μg/kg/min) improves urine output unless further intrinsic renal disease prevents renal function.

PULMONARY EDEMA. The presence of pulmonary edema may be due to volume overload, cardiac failure secondary to the increased afterload, or in a few patients an imbalance in the COP/PCWP gradient.

If a parturient has PIH, strict intake and output records should be maintained. Pulmonary edema should be treated by the customary methods (oxygen, diuretics, fluid restriction, treatment of the precipitating cause).

The presence of a low (less than 4 mm Hg) or negative COP/PCWP gradient has been documented in some parturients with severe PIH complicated by pulmonary edema. The COP normally decreases during pregnancy from 22 to 18 mm Hg and decreases further in the parturient with PIH because the kidneys excrete protein. This lower COP may contribute to PIH, especially in the postpartum period. During that time the COP further decreases as extravascular fluid is mobilized. An increase in intravascular volume and PCWP subsequently occurs during this mobilization period. Increases in the PCWP above 22 mm Hg may be treated empirically with diuretics and fluid restriction to minimize elevation and hopefully prevent the onset of acute pulmonary edema. In parturients with a low or negative COP/PCWP gradient, decreasing the PCWP and increasing the COP assists treatment.

MAGNESIUM OVERDOSE. As the magnesium level rises, the first sign of magnesium overdose is the loss of peripheral reflexes, which occurs at a serum magnesium level of approximately 10 mg/dl. This is followed by respiratory arrest (at 15 to 20 mg/dl) and cardiac arrest (at 20 to 30 mg/dl). Therefore peripheral reflexes should be monitored periodically when a patient is receiving a magnesium infusion.

If respiratory impairment or cardiac arrest occurs, calcium chloride 1 g intravenously should be given in addition to standard cardiopulmonary resuscitation.

OTHER DRUGS USED IN THE INTENSIVE CARE UNIT AND THEIR IMPLICATIONS IN PREGNANCY

Many drugs may be needed in the ICU to provide optimal care for a critically ill parturient. The first- and second-trimester fetus is at highest risk for drug-induced malformations. Therefore great caution should be exercised in the selection of drugs used during this period. Near the time of delivery the major concern of drug administration is usually neonatal effects.

Antibiotics

The penicillin antibiotics have been available for many years. Ampicillin and penicillin do not cause major or minor malformations when administered during pregnancy.

The aminoglycoside antibiotics (amikacin, gentamicin, neomycin, kanamycin, streptomycin) have not been linked to congenital defects. Drugs in this class, when administered to neonates, may be ototoxic. However, reports have appeared of neonatal ototoxicity after administration of kanamycin or streptomycin to mothers while the infant was still in utero. Therefore these two drugs should not be administered to the parturient.

Several cephalosporin antibiotics are available. At present no controlled studies are available on their use in pregnancy. No association with fetal abnormalities has been noted. Drugs in this class are widely used for prophylaxis before cesarean section.

Erythromycin and clindamycin have not been associated with any major or minor fetal malformations and can be safely administered to the parturient if indicated.

The tetracycline class of drugs poses several risks during pregnancy. The administration of tetracycline to a pregnant patient may discolor deciduous teeth and inhibit fibula growth in her infant if born prematurely. Also, tetracycline may have adverse effects on the mother's liver. Unlike acute fatty liver of pregnancy, hepatotoxic effects from tetracycline use do not improve with termination of the pregnancy. Several studies of tetracycline use have found no major malformations associated with the drug. Three possible associations were identified: hypospadias, inguinal hernia, and hypoplasia of a limb or part thereof. The risks associated with administration of drugs in this class indicates that they should be used with caution, if at all, during pregnancy.

Rarely, the parturient may need an antifungal antibiotic. Amphotericin B has not been associated with any congenital defects and can be used during pregnancy if needed. Griseofulvin is embryotoxic and teratogenic in some animal species. Based on these data, some suggest that griseofulvin should not be administered during pregnancy.

Antipyretics

Acetaminophen is commonly administered during pregnancy to relieve pain and lower elevated body temperature. This drug has not been associated with fetal malformations. Its occasional, short-term use appears safe during pregnancy.

Aspirin, although frequently taken during pregnancy, should probably be avoided, especially in long-term or high-dose regimens. Because of aspirin's effects on platelet function, it increases the risk of both maternal and fetal hemorrhage. An increased perinatal mortality rate and intrauterine growth retardation have been related to high-dose administration of aspirin. Therefore the use of aspirin during pregnancy is not recommended.

Nonsteroidal antiinflammatory agents (ibuprofen and indomethacin) have not been associated with any specific congenital defects. Theoretically these prostaglandin synthetase inhibitors could cause ductus arteriosus constriction in utero, leading to persistent pulmonary hypertension in the newborn. At present the manufacturer recommends that ibuprofen not be used during pregnancy. The same consideration seems to apply to indomethacin.

H$_2$ Blockers

No reports have linked cimetidine or ranitidine with congenital defects. They appear safe to use during later pregnancy when indicated (data are lacking on use during the first trimester).

Narcotics

Narcotics administered during labor may result in a dose- and time-dependent neonatal respiratory depression and a decrease in the beat-to-beat variability. The therapeutic use of fentanyl and morphine has not been associated with major congenital malformations.

Methadone, which is used almost exclusively for the treatment of heroin addiction, has not been associated with specific congenital defects, although the infants of methadone addicts have increased rates of neonatal mortality, sudden infant death syndrome, jaundice, and thrombocytosis.

No major or minor malformations have been related to meperidine administration, although a possible association with inguinal hernia has been identified.

Codeine is found in many combination drugs. Its use has been linked to major malformations. Associations have been suggested between codeine administration during pregnancy and the occurrence of respiratory and genitourinary malformations, Down's syndrome, umbilical and inguinal hernia, hydrocephaly, and pyloric stenosis.

All drugs in the narcotic category have the potential for causing respiratory depression and addiction, leading to withdrawal syndrome in the mother and fetus.

Sedatives

Secobarbital has not been associated with congenital defects, although barbiturate withdrawal and hemorrhagic disease of the newborn may theoretically occur.

Diazepam freely crosses the placenta and exhibits a prolonged half-life in the newborn because of a decreased clearance rate. Various congenital defects have been reported. Ingestion during the first trimester has been associated with cleft lip and palate, inguinal hernia, cardiac defects, and pyloric stenosis. Administration during the second trimester has been associated with hemangiomas and circulatory and cardiac defects. Infants of mothers who have been on long-term diazepam regimens may have a withdrawal syndrome characterized by intrauterine growth retardation, tremors, irritability, hypertonicity, diarrhea, vomiting, and vigorous sucking. Diazepam has also been associated with "floppy infant syndrome," which consists of hypotonia, lethargy, and sucking difficulties. In addition, alterations of thermogenesis, loss of beat-to-beat variability in the fetal heart rate pattern, and decreased fetal movement may be seen. The risk/benefit ratio should be considered before administration of diazepam to the parturient.

No information is available on midazolam in relation to congenital defects.

First-trimester ingestion of chlordiazepoxide, a benzodiazepine, has been associated with mental deficiency, spastic diplegia, deafness, microcephaly, duodenal atresia, and Meckel's diverticulum, although a definitive relationship has not been established. Neonatal withdrawal may occur if long-term administration has occurred during pregnancy.

No reports have associated chloral hydrate with congenital defects. It has been administered during labor and does cross the placenta. Neonatal sedative effects from administration during labor have not been studied.

RADIOLOGY AND PREGNANCY

Irradiation during pregnancy is undesirable because it increases the risk of fetal anomalies. This risk is increased by 1% to 3% when a woman receives more than 5 rads to the pelvis during the first trimester. A chest roentgenogram exposes the fetus to only 36 mrads, and this is further decreased by abdominal shielding with a lead apron. Therefore a chest roentgenogram should be obtained only if needed for diagnosis.

ASTHMA AND PREGNANCY

Approximately one third of parturients with preexisting asthma will have deteriorating pulmonary status during pregnancy, necessitating medication changes.

Theophylline has not been associated with any congenital malformations and if needed should be continued during the pregnancy. It does cross the placenta, and neonatal toxic reactions can occur just as they do in the mother, especially because of the increased fetal sensitivity to and slower fetal elimination of theophylline. Dosage calculations should be based on maternal lean body weight with close monitoring of maternal serum levels (preferably maintaining serum theophylline levels no higher than 14 µg/ml).

Beta-agonist drugs have been used during pregnancy without causing harmful fetal effects. These drugs, in addition to causing bronchodilation, inhibit uterine contractility and delay the onset of labor. Beta-mimetic drugs should probably be discontinued as the fetus nears term if the parturient's clinical state allows. Postpartum uterine atony and hemorrhage are a risk in parturients receiving beta agonists. Long-term administration of epinephrine-containing solutions should probably be avoided, since an increased incidence of fetal malformations has been reported when these

drugs were used during the first 4 months of pregnancy. Corticosteroid therapy with prednisone is considered safe during pregnancy if needed to control asthma. The fetal risk of uncontrolled maternal asthma (increased perinatal mortality) is greater than the risk of prednisone administration.

EPILEPSY AND PREGNANCY

Of parturients with a preexisting seizure disorder, 45% to 50% have increased seizure frequency. This is probably due to the decrease in plasma anticonvulsant levels, which results from the expanded plasma volume, increased hepatic metabolism, and increased renal clearance. Therefore anticonvulsant levels should be closely monitored in the parturient.

Phenytoin (hydantoin), the most commonly used anticonvulsant, has been associated with a "fetal hydantoin syndrome" characterized by hypoplasia of the distal phalanges, rudimentary nails, growth deficiency, mental retardation, and characteristic facial abnormalities. Because of these problems an attempt is usually made, after discussion with the patient's neurologist, to substitute phenobarbital for phenytoin if her disease is controllable with this drug. If phenytoin administration must continue, the lowest effective dose should be used, and folic acid supplementation (1 mg/d) is administered.

Neonates of mothers receiving phenytoin or phenobarbital may be deficient in vitamin K–dependent clotting factors despite normal maternal levels. Therefore vitamin K should be administered to the newborn prophylactically.

Status epilepticus is treated as in a nonpregnant woman. If the patient was not a known epileptic, other causes of seizures (such as eclampsia, intracranial tumor or bleeding, or hypoglycemia) must be sought. Special attention must be paid to the airway, since the parturient is at increased risk of aspiration and prolonged hypoxia and may damage the fetus at any gestational age.

SUGGESTED READINGS

Briggs GG, Freeman RK, Yaffe SJ: Drugs in pregnancy and lactation, 2nd ed. Baltimore, 1986, Williams & Wilkins

Clark SL: Amniotic fluid embolism. Clin Perinatol 1986; 13:801-811

Clark SL, Cotton DB: Clinical indications for pulmonary artery catheterization in the patient with severe preeclampsia. Am J Obstet Gynecol 1988;158:453-458

Cotton DB, Gonik B, Dorman K, Harrist R: Cardiovascular

alterations in severe pregnancy-induced hypertension: relationship of central venous pressure to pulmonary capillary wedge pressure. Am J Obstet Gynecol 1985; 151:762-764

Cruikshank DP: Neurologic disease. In Danforth DN, Scott JR (eds): Obstetrics and gynecology, 5th ed. Philadelphia, 1986, JB Lippincott Co

Gonik B, Allen SJ: Intracranial hemorrhage in pregnancy. In Clark SL, Phelan JP, Cotton DB (eds): Critical care obstetrics. Oradell, NJ, 1987, Medical Economics Books

Inglis MD, Morgan M: Management of the patient with amniotic fluid embolism. Clin Anaesthesiol 1986;4: 359-371

James FM III: Pregnancy-induced hypertension. In James FM III, Wheeler AS, Dewan DM (eds): Obstetric anesthesia: the complicated patient, 2nd ed. Philadelphia, 1988, FA Davis Co

Jouppila P, Kirkinen P, Koivula H, Ylikorkala P: Labetalol does not alter the placental and fetal blood flow or maternal prostanoids in preeclampsia. Br J Obstet Gynaecol 1986;93:543-547

Niederman MS, Matthay RA: Asthma and other severe respiratory diseases during pregnancy. In Berkowitz RL (ed): Critical care of the obstetric patient. New York, 1983, Churchill Livingstone

Plaunche' WC: Myasthenia gravis. Clin Obstet Gynecol 1983;26:592-604

Pritchard JA, MacDonald PC, Gant NF: Williams obstetrics. Norwalk, Conn, 1985, Appleton-Century-Crofts, pp. 484-488

Rolbin SH, Levinson G, Shnider SM, Wright RG: Anesthetic considerations for myasthenia gravis and pregnancy. Anesth Analg 1978;57:441-447

Rosen MA: Cerebrovascular lesions and tumors in the pregnant patient. In Newfield P and Cottrell JE (eds): Handbook of neuroanesthesia: clinical and physiologic essentials. Boston, 1983, Little, Brown

Sweet RL, Gibbs RS: Infectious diseases of the female genital tract. Baltimore, 1985, Williams & Wilkins, pp 142-144

Tuttelman R, Gleicher N: Central nervous system hemorrhage complicating pregnancy. Obstet Gynecol 1981; 58:651

ACQUIRED IMMUNODEFICIENCY SYNDROME IN THE INTENSIVE CARE UNIT

A. JOSEPH LAYON, MD, ELOISE M. HARMAN, MD, AND
ROBERT A. KILROY, PharmD

The total number of new cases of acquired immunodeficiency syndrome (AIDS) reported in 1988 was 30,847; in 1989 35,238 cases were reported, an increase of 14%. Each week, the number of cases reported to the Centers for Disease Control (CDC) ranges from 280 to 900. As of late October 1990, 33,498 cases had been reported to the CDC. The World Health Organization estimates that approximately 150,000 cases of AIDS have occurred worldwide. Homosexuality or bisexuality and intravenous drug abuse (among heterosexuals), account for 65% and 17%, respectively, of AIDS cases in the United States. Heterosexual transmission (no intravenous drug use) accounts for only 4% of U.S. cases but is one of the fastest growing categories. In 1988, 317 cases were reported in children under 13, an increase of 64% over the previous year. Approximately 77% of these children were infected perinatally, probably before birth.

The U.S. Public Health Service estimates that, in 1986, 1 to 1.5 million persons in the United States were infected with human immunodeficiency virus (HIV); within 5 years 20% to 30% of these persons will likely have clinical AIDS. Barring changes in the infection rate, in 1992 more than 80,000 new cases will be diagnosed, 172,000 persons with AIDS will seek medical care, 66,000 will die, and the cumulative incidence of and deaths from AIDS will be approximately 365,000 and 263,000 cases, respectively. The model by which these estimates are derived may underestimate the morbidity

and mortality of the syndrome by as much as 20%. The lifetime cost of medical care per patient ranges from $80,000 to $140,000. Thus the cumulative medical costs for the above-mentioned 365,000 cases are between $29 and $51 billion, the wide range relating to the cost differential between outpatient and inpatient care. The greatest cost to our economy, however, will be in terms of lost productivity. The estimated loss per patient ranges from $490,000 to $623,000, with cumulative indirect costs to the economy ranging from $179 to $227 billion.

Based on available data, we believe that the number of patients with AIDS admitted to ICUs will increase in the next few years. As this occurs, physicians, nurses, and administrators, each in his or her own manner, will be forced to deal with the attendant medical and ethical dilemmas.

ETHICAL CONSIDERATIONS FOR ADMISSION TO THE INTENSIVE CARE UNIT

Some health workers have privately questioned allocating health resources to the terminally ill, especially the appropriateness of ICU care for AIDS patients. The implication is that because AIDS has no long-term therapy nor expectation of survival, consumption of scarce resources by AIDS patients is wasteful. This attitude could affect clinical judgment. Many non-AIDS patients admitted to ICUs have no guarantee of either return to a productive life or recovery. Furthermore, short-term outcome for AIDS patients may not be as poor as has been thought. For example, the mortality rate of *Pneumocystis carinii* pneumonia (PCP) requiring endotracheal intubation and mechanical ventilation can be as low as 60% in contrast to the 85% mortality rate previously reported. Recent data from a placebo-controlled trial of zidovudine in HIV-infected persons who were asymptomatic or mildly symptomatic suggest that it has a prophylactic effect. In these two studies, investigators found that subjects whose T4 cell count was less than 500/mm³ who were receiving zidovudine, 500 mg/d in one protocol and 1200 mg/d in the second, had roughly half the rate of progression to AIDS or severe AIDS-related complex of those who received placebo. Despite this improvement in short-term survival, the mortality rate from AIDS is nearly 100% over a period of several years. Although society may mandate the development of ICU admission criteria, based on resource rationing, that exclude the terminally ill, at present clinical judgment is the primary tool for admission decisions.

The basic conflict surrounding the concept of rationing ICU care is that of the physician as gatekeeper. If physicians accept the concept of "ethic of agency," that their responsibility to patients is to obtain every possible necessary service for those persons, they can rationalize keeping necessary care from their patients only by using the most convoluted logic. A key concept is embodied in the term "necessary." No conflict exists when a physician does not arrange for an ICU bed for a healthy outpatient. When the situation is less clear, as in the preceding example with PCP, the conflict is evident. What is the appropriate response of a physician caring for a patient with PCP? As the patient's agent, the physician is justified, indeed mandated, to obtain every necessary resource for that person. Could a physician perform this function if, at the same time, he or she were forced as an agent of society to conserve scarce resources? We think not. However, the patient's agent is not required to make use of all available resources, only those the patient and physician deem necessary. Aggressive treatment does not denote unintelligent or uncompassionate care.

AIDS patients have considered these issues. When 118 male outpatients with AIDS were questioned regarding their desire for life-sustaining treatment, 95% said they would opt for hospitalization and antibiotic therapy for PCP,

55% for ICU care and mechanical ventilation, and 46% for cardiopulmonary resuscitation (CPR) were that required. However, when questioned about PCP and concomitant severe memory loss, only 19% and 17% wanted ICU therapy including mechanical ventilation and CPR, respectively. Although 73% wanted to discuss this matter with their primary care physician, only 33% had done so.

Thus, if an AIDS patient desires full supportive therapy and understands its consequences, no reason exists to refuse such a request. If during the course of an illness the patient clearly deteriorates and further therapy is not indicated, and the physician discussed this possibility with the patient at the time of diagnosis or admission to hospital, aggressive support can be stopped. Each patient with AIDS should be encouraged to give durable power of attorney to someone trusted so that therapy can be changed even if the patient is too ill to approve the alteration. AIDS patients, who must be given the same considerations as any other critically ill patient, should be consulted and informed about ICU care, endotracheal intubation, and CPR, should any or all of these become necessary. Most important, we must make it abundantly clear to the humans we care for that they will not be abandoned, even if therapy is to be withdrawn.

ASSESSMENT OF PATIENTS WITH ACQUIRED IMMUNODEFICIENCY SYNDROME AND SUSPECTED OPPORTUNISTIC INFECTION

Known Pathophysiology

The causative agent of AIDS, HIV, is known to be transmitted sexually and parenterally. When HIV infection occurs, 50% to 90% of persons who have undergone seroconversion relate symptoms of an acute viral illness. This is characterized as "mononucleosis-like" with attendant symptoms; persons who have seroconverted, compared with those who remain HIV negative, have a greater incidence of lymphadenopathy, truncal rash, depression, and irritability. HIV has a selective tropism for the helper lymphocyte. The cellular selectivity of HIV is related to viral use of the CD4 molecule (one of the morphological designates of a T lymphocyte that makes it a helper cell) as its receptor-attachment site. After cell entry the virus is uncoated, its genomic RNA is transcribed to

DNA via the enzyme reverse transcriptase (RT), and a portion of the proviral DNA is integrated into the host cell's chromosomal genetic material. Although the virus, after integration with host cell DNA, may enter a latent phase, HIV ultimately induces progressive destruction of the T4 helper lymphocyte. This results in a marked suppression of cellular immunity and a predisposition to opportunistic infections in which cellular immune mechanisms are important. Because HIV also affects macrophages and monocytes (the antigen pre-senting and processing cells), the immunosuppression is profound.

With identification of the viral agent the classification scheme for HIV infection has become more detailed (Table 26–1). A patient may not be reclassified into a preceding group if clinical symptoms resolve. No evidence suggests that clinical improvement reflects a change in the severity of underlying disease; rather, data suggest that when seropositive persons become seronegative, they remain latently infected with HIV.

TABLE 26–1. Classification System for Human Immunodeficiency Virus Infection

GROUP	TYPE OF ILLNESS	DESCRIPTION OF ILLNESS
I	Acute infection	Mononucleosis-like syndrome and seroconversion to HIV with or without aseptic meningitis
II	Asymptomatic infection	No signs or symptoms of HIV infection; no signs or symptoms in past that would have led to classification in group III or IV; patients may be subclassified by laboratory studies (complete blood count with differential, platelet count, T-helper and T-suppressor counts)
III	Persistent generalized lymphadenopathy*	Lymph node enlargement ≥1 cm at two or more extrainguinal sites lasting >3 mo without reason other than HIV infection
IV		
Subgroup A	Constitutional disease	One or more of following: fever lasting >1 mo, involuntary weight loss >10% of baseline, diarrhea lasting >1 mo, absence of any reason for findings other than HIV infection
Subgroup B	Neurologic disease	One or more of following: dementia, myelopathy, peripheral neuropathy, absence of any reason for findings other than HIV infection
Subgroup C	Secondary infections	
C-1	Listed by Centers for Disease Control in surveillance definition of acquired immunodeficiency syndrome	One or more of following: *Pneumocystis carinii* pneumonia, chronic cryptosporidiosis, toxoplasmosis, extraintestinal strongyloidiasis, isosporiasis, candidiasis (esophageal, bronchial, pulmonary), cryptococcosis, histoplasmosis, *Mycobacterium avium-intracellulare*, cytomegalovirus, chronic mucocutaneous or disseminated herpesvirus infection, progressive multifocal leukoencephalopathy
C-2	Other	Symptomatic or invasive disease caused by one of following: oral hairy leukoplakia, multidermatomal herpes zoster, recurrent *Salmonella* bacteremia, nocardiosis, tuberculosis, oral candidiasis
Subgroup D	Secondary cancers	Kaposi's sarcoma, non-Hodgkin's lymphoma (small noncleaved lymphoma, immunoblastic sarcoma), primary lymphoma of the brain; clinical presentation must fulfill definition of acquired immunodeficiency syndrome
Subgroup E	Other conditions	Findings or diseases not listed in other categories that may be attributable to HIV, e.g., chronic lymphoid interstitial pneumonitis

Modified from Centers for Disease Control: Classification system for human T-lymphotropic virus type III/lymphadenopathy-associated virus infections. Reproduced with permission from Ann Intern Med 1986;105:234-237.
*Patients in group III may be subclassified on the basis of a laboratory evaluation as noted in group II.

Assessment

These six important principles should be considered in the approach to HIV-associated opportunistic infections:

- Fungal, viral, and bacterial infections in AIDS are rarely cured and may require long-term suppressive therapy.
- Most HIV infections represent endogenous reactivation.
- A poor response to treatment may result from a second concurrent infection rather than treatment failure.
- The incidence of certain fungal and parasitic infections reflects the incidence of asymptomatic infection in the local population of a given geographic area (place of origin and travel history are important).
- Bacterial infections, such as pneumonia, are associated with HIV infection.
- HIV-associated infections are often disseminated and severe when diagnosed.

Diagnosis of opportunistic infection is often delayed because of subtle or unusual symptoms, difficulty of diagnosing a new infection in a chronically ill, debilitated patient; fatalistic attitudes of patient and physician; and inadequate knowledge. A febrile HIV-positive patient requires a careful physical examination that includes the following:

- Inspection of the entire skin for raised purple lesions (Kaposi's sarcoma) and other skin lesions, which could indicate disseminated opportunistic infections
- Inspection of mucous membranes for evidence of candidiasis or herpetic lesions
- Funduscopic examination for evidence of retinal involvement by opportunistic pathogens
- Complete neurologic examination, including evaluation of mental status
- Routine cultures, including blood and stool cultures for *Mycobacterium avium-intracellulare* in patients with lymphadenopathy or hepatosplenomegaly

Although diarrhea in AIDS may be caused by common enteric pathogens, unusual organisms such as cytomegalovirus or *Cryptosporidium* may cause debilitating diarrhea. If a patient has diarrhea, the stool should be examined for white blood cells, ova, and protozoa and cultured for bacterial, fungal, and mycobacterial pathogens.

COMPLICATIONS

Pneumonia

Pneumonia is the most common HIV-associated infection. PCP is the initial opportunistic infection in 60% of AIDS patients and occurs eventually in an additional 20%. The differential diagnosis of pneumonia in patients with HIV (Table 26–2) includes pyogenic bacterial infections, tuberculosis, parasitic and fungal infections, and nonspecific and lymphocytic interstitial pneumonitis. In autopsy series of AIDS patients, cytomegalovirus disease and pneumocystosis were the cause of death in more than 50%; cryptococcosis and toxoplasmosis accounted for an additional 25%.

The onset of PCP may be acute with fever, tachycardia, dyspnea, and an unproductive cough or more subtle with the insidious onset of dyspnea and cough associated with a normal or minimally abnormal chest roentgenogram. Since prompt, early diagnosis and treatment of PCP may improve outcome, aggressive evaluation of pulmonary symptoms is warranted.

The differential diagnosis of pneumonia in AIDS patients is broad; thus empiric therapy during the attempt to establish a diagnosis

TABLE 26–2. Pulmonary Complications of Human Immunodeficiency Virus

RELATION TO HIV INFECTION	COMPLICATION
Opportunistic infections diagnostic of acquired immunodeficiency syndrome	Candidiasis
	Cryptococcosis
	Cytomegalovirus infection
	Herpes simplex infection
	Histoplasmosis
	Mycobacterium avium-intracellulare infection
	Pneumocystis carinii pneumonia
	Pulmonary strongyloidiasis
	Toxoplasmosis
HIV-related infections	*Mycobacterium tuberculosis* infection
	Nocardiosis
Presumed HIV-related disorders	Lymphocytic interstitial pneumonitis
	Nonspecific interstitial pneumonitis
	Pyogenic bacterial pneumonia
AIDS-related pulmonary neoplasia	Kaposi's sarcoma
	Non-Hodgkin's lymphoma

Modified from Friedman BF, Edwards D, Kirkpatrick CH: *Mycobacterium avium-intracellulare*—cutaneous presentations of disseminated disease. Am J Med 1988;85: 257-264.
HIV = human immunodeficiency virus.

is recommended only for very ill patients. Such therapy should include broad-spectrum antibiotics and trimethoprim-sulfamethoxazole (TMP-SMX) and generally should be limited to 48 hours.

In nonintubated patients the diagnosis of PCP may be made by silver stain of sputum induced by inhalation of hypertonic saline solution from an ultrasonic nebulizer. When the test is done carefully, induced sputum is positive for *Pneumocystis* in about 50% of patients proven bronchoscopically to harbor the organism. If sputum smears are negative, fiberoptic bronchoscopy is indicated. In intubated patients, nonbronchoscopic lavage with modified suction catheters may be an alternative.

When *Pneumocystis* is present, the use of fiberoptic bronchoscopy with bronchoalveolar lavage and transbronchial lung biopsy yields the diagnosis in 90% of cases. Bronchoalveolar lavage is performed by wedging the bronchoscope into a segmental bronchus, instilling 20 to 40 ml aliquots of nonbacteriostatic normal saline solution to a total of about 100 to 150 ml, and then suctioning it back into a sterile container. The specimen is sent for viral, bacteriologic, fungal, and mycobacterial culture and stains and for cytologic examination with silver stain for *Pneumocystis*. Bronchial brushings are less sensitive and need not be done in conjunction with bronchoalveolar lavage. Transbronchial biopsy should be performed on all patients unless contraindicated by coagulopathy or need for mechanical ventilation. If bronchoscopy does not establish a diagnosis and the patient's condition is deteriorating, repeat bronchoscopy should be considered. Open lung biopsy is unlikely to yield a treatable diagnosis missed by fiberoptic bronchoscopy.

With early diagnosis and treatment the survival rate for a first episode of PCP may exceed 90%. Mild hypoxemia with an alveolar-arterial oxygen gradient ($[\text{A-a}]D_{O_2}$) of less than 30 mm Hg and mild radiographic abnormalities suggest a good prognosis for a first episode. The two drugs considered standard for PCP are TMP-SMX and pentamidine. The response rate to these drugs is 60% to 80%; the relapse rate is about 35% by 6 months and up to 60% by 12 months. TMP-SMX is probably the agent of first choice because the response rate is greater, the survival rate is higher, and toxic reactions are less frequent than with pentamidine. For both agents, the response to treatment is relatively slow. Patients require 6 to 9 days to become afebrile and 7 to 15 days for the $(\text{A-a})D_{O_2}$ to improve by at least 10 mm Hg. Both drugs have

a high incidence of side effects (50% to 100% in most series), including rash and anemia with TMP-SMX and nephrotoxicity, hypotension, and hypoglycemia with pentamidine. Pentamidine in rare cases is associated with cardiac toxicity and multifocal ventricular tachycardia (torsades de pointes).

TMP-SMX is given intravenously, TMP 20 mg/kg/d and SMX 100 mg/kg/d, in four equally divided doses. Serum levels of TMP (if they can be monitored) should be maintained at 5 to 8 μg/ml by dosage adjustment. Pentamidine is given intravenously at a dose of 4 mg/kg/d, infused slowly over 60 minutes. If serum creatinine concentration rises with this therapy, the dose should be reduced by 30% to 50%, although the effect of such dosage reduction on the development of nephrotoxic reactions is uncertain. Patients frequently have persistent cysts of the organism present in sputum after 2 weeks of therapy, so treatment should be continued for 21 days. Presence of *Pneumocystis* in sputum after 3 weeks of therapy correlates with a poor long-term prognosis. Probably no additional benefit is derived from the simultaneous use of TMP-SMX and pentamidine; patients who fail to respond to the former are not likely to benefit from a switch to the latter.

In patients with PCP who require intubation and mechanical ventilation because of respiratory failure, prognosis for survival ranges from 15% to 37%. Expiratory airway pressure (positive end-expiratory pressure, continuous positive airway pressure) may improve oxygenation and can be administered by mask to selected patients. Methylprednisolone 40 to 60 mg intravenously every 6 hours has been associated with improvement in some desperately ill patients with PCP, although a controlled trial has not been carried out. Caution is advised when considering use of steroids for AIDS patients. Patients successfully treated for PCP should receive long-term prophylactic therapy with either oral TMP (5 mg/kg) and SMX or inhaled pentamidine to prevent recurrence. The recommended dose of aerosolized pentamidine for PCP prophylaxis is 300 mg every 4 weeks, administered through the Respigard II nebulizer.

Several experimental therapies are being studied for the treatment of PCP: inhaled pentamidine, oral dapsone-trimethoprim, oral or intravenous trimetrexate and leucovorin, and intravenous or oral difluoromethylornithine. Inhaled pentamidine offers the advantage of less toxicity. Pentamidine administered by nebulizer once a day at a dose of 4 mg/kg or 600 mg has a high degree of success. However, deviation from the precise delivery systems used in the validating study may alter success rates, and this therapy must be considered experimental. Furthermore, anecdotal reports of disseminated *Pneumocystis* suggest that, for PCP, systemic therapy is preferable to local therapy.

Central Nervous System Complications

The central nervous system (CNS) is a common site of involvement in patients with AIDS, as a result of both HIV infection of the CNS and opportunistic infection with *Toxoplasma gondii, Cryptococcus, Mycobacterium avium-intracellulare,* cytomegalovirus, and other pathogens. Neurologic symptoms occur in approximately 60% of patients, and up to 90% of patients have neuropathologic abnormalities at autopsy. The four major neurologic manifestations of HIV infection are aseptic meningitis; encephalopathy, resulting in a dementia in up to 50% of patients with AIDS; myelopathy with ataxia and incontinence; and peripheral neuropathy. Lymphoma or autoimmune phenomena, such as Guillain-Barré syndrome, may also affect the CNS. An AIDS patient with abnormal mental status or focal neurologic abnormalities should undergo testing that includes a computed tomographic (CT) scan of the head and, if not contraindicated, lumbar puncture. Focal abnormalities on CT scan should be evaluated aggressively, in most instances by biopsy. Treatment of AIDS-related neurologic diseases is often frustrating and unsuccessful.

T. gondii, an obligate intracellular parasite, is the most common cause of focal encephalitis in patients with AIDS. Toxoplasmosis has occurred in 3.5% of AIDS cases reported to the CDC. CNS toxoplasmosis is most likely to be found at autopsy and is considered the primary cause of death in 15% of those with AIDS.

CNS toxoplasmosis is more common in Haitians than in other groups of AIDS patients, consistent with the high prevalence of toxoplasmosis in tropical regions. A wide variety of causes of CNS dysfunction are noted in non-Haitian patients: viral syndromes (subacute encephalitis, atypical aseptic meningitis, herpes simplex encephalitis, multifocal leukoencephalopathy), mycobacterial and fungal infections, neurosyphilis, and neoplasms (lymphoma, metastatic Kaposi's sarcoma), among others.

CNS toxoplasmosis usually has a subacute onset with fever, headaches, and neurologic symptoms developing over 1 to 2 weeks. In 90% of patients the neurologic symptoms are focal, most commonly a mild hemiparesis. Signs of brainstem and cerebellar involvement are common but usually occur in conjunction with other findings. A diffuse encephalopathy is characterized by confusion and lethargy in about 63% of patients, with both focal signs and encephalopathy in slightly more than half. Because toxoplasmosis is considered to represent reactivation of previous infection, a high proportion of patients have anti-*Toxoplasma* immunoglobulin G (IgG) although the titer may be low and IgG is occasionally absent in biopsy-proven infections. Anti-*Toxoplasma* immunoglobulin M antibody is not helpful because a titer increase is uncommon. The most useful test for diagnosis is the CT scan, which usually shows multiple hypodense lesions with ring enhancement on contrast administration. CT of the head with a double dose of contrast and magnetic resonance imaging (MRI) may be the most sensitive diagnostic tests. Examination of cerebrospinal fluid (CSF) from patients with *Toxoplasma* encephalitis usually shows an elevated protein concentration, but mononuclear pleocytosis occurs in less than 50%.

In an AIDS patient with multiple ring-enhanced lesions on head CT and a positive IgG titer for *Toxoplasma,* some authors advocate 2 weeks of empiric treatment for toxoplasmosis with brain biopsy reserved for nonresponders. Others recommend biopsy because of the numerous other possible causes for focal brain lesions. Empiric therapy is probably warranted in Haitians with AIDS and in patients whose lesion is in an unfavorable location; in the remainder, either open or stereotaxic needle biopsy should be performed.

Even with treatment the mortality rate of *Toxoplasma* encephalitis is about 80%, with a median survival of 4 months. Therapy is a combination of pyrimethamine (25 mg/d) and sulfadiazine (100 mg/kg/d) administered with leucovorin. An initial loading dose of pyrimethamine (50 mg/d orally for 3 days) should be given. If a clinical response is not seen in 1 to 2 weeks, pyrimethamine and sulfadiazine doses can be titrated up to 75 mg/d and 8 g/d, respectively. Persons alert at the initiation of therapy have a better prognosis than obtunded patients. Toxic responses to treatment occur in 60% and are most commonly manifest as leukopenia, rash, and thrombocytopenia. Therapy is usually continued for 2 to 6 months for the acute infection, but since relapse occurs in about 50%, chronic suppressive therapy with pyrimethamine 25 mg/d is indicated. If sulfadiazine causes profound leukopenia, clindamycin 900 mg every 6 hours may be administered with pyrimethamine. The use of dexamethasone to treat edema surrounding toxoplasmal lesions is controversial. Caution is advised because of the potential worsening of immunosuppression. Other therapies that show promise for toxoplasmosis in vitro and in animal studies include TMP-SMX, spiromycin, and clindamycin.

Cytomegalovirus (CMV), a member of the herpesvirus family, infects virtually all AIDS patients and can cause fever, leukopenia, diffuse interstitial pneumonia, ulcerative gastrointestinal lesions, retinitis, hepatitis, maculopapular rash, thrombocytopenic purpura, and encephalitis. Disseminated CMV infections have been treated with intravenous ganciclovir 7.5 to 15 mg/kg/d administered as a once-daily infusion 5 days a week. Interruption of therapy reactivates the disease, so treatment must be lifelong. Neutropenia is the most common toxic manifestation of ganciclovir. Patients should not be treated with ganciclovir and zidovudine concurrently because severe granulocytopenia may develop. Controlled trials evaluating foscarnet for the treatment of CMV retinitis and disseminated CMV disease are under way.

Cryptococcal meningitis occurs in approximately 11% of patients with HIV infection. Although the CSF glucose and protein concentrations and the cell count are frequently normal, the antigen titer, fungal culture, and India ink stain are almost always positive for *Cryptococcus.* Treatment consists of intravenous amphotericin B 0.4 to 0.7 mg/kg/d as tolerated for a total dose of 1.5 to 2 g. If the patient has a normal white blood cell count, enteral flucytosine 100 to 150 mg/kg/d may be added for a total of 6 weeks. The combination of amphotericin B and flucytosine may allow a reduction in the dose and duration of amphotericin B. In non-AIDS patients the combination may be associated with a decreased mortality rate, clinical improvement, more rapid sterilization of CSF, and less nephrotoxicity. This finding, however, is controversial and needs further study. Nonrandomized studies of small numbers of AIDS patients suggest no benefit from combination therapy. Relapses occur in more than half the patients treated with amphotericin B for cryptococcal meningitis. Maintenance therapy with intravenous amphotericin B 100 mg once a week may prevent relapse in some patients.

Encephalitis caused by herpes simplex or herpes zoster is a common and severe neurologic complication in AIDS patients. Treatment consists of intravenous acyclovir, 10 mg/kg every 8 hours for 10 days. Acyclovir should be infused over at least 1 hour, and adequate hydration maintained throughout the course of therapy. Obstructive nephropathy caused by drug precipitation and crystallization in the collecting ducts of the distal nephrons can elevate the serum creatinine concentration if the patient is not adequately hydrated. The dosage of acyclovir may require adjustment if renal failure develops.

Disseminated *Mycobacterium avium-intracellulare* complex (MAC) infection is reported as the index diagnosis in about 3% to 4% of AIDS cases and is present in 25% to 30% of patients with AIDS at the time of death. The proportion of disseminated MAC infections has remained constant over several years of reporting, which suggests that this organism is derived from a common environmental source, probably water, rather than from reactivation or contagion. The primary site of entry is most likely the gastrointestinal system.

Disseminated MAC infections present several different syndromes including a wasting illness characterized by fever, diaphoresis, and weight loss; generalized lymphadenopathy; abdominal symptoms associated with hepatosplenomegaly and retroperitoneal lymphadenopathy; and chronic diarrhea associated with infiltration of the bowel with acid-fast organisms. In disseminated MAC the organism is characteristically found in large numbers in multiple organs, including blood, bone marrow, liver, spleen, adrenal glands, gastrointestinal tract, brain, and lungs, in association with slight inflammatory response and poor granuloma formation. MAC may be merely a marker of endstage AIDS or may itself cause death.

Disseminated MAC infection is usually diagnosed by means of culture of blood and stool; acid-fast stains of stool are often positive. Accurate, rapid diagnosis can be made by blood culture systems that employ lysis and centrifugation.

Until recently no satisfactory therapy was available for disseminated MAC infection in AIDS. Two experimental agents, rifabutin (ansamycin) and clofazimine, exerted considerable action against MAC in vitro, but this combination has had disappointing results in AIDS patients. In September 1990 a study evaluating combination drug therapy for disseminated

MAC infection was published. A regimen of amikacin, ethambutol, rifampin, and ciprofloxacin decreased mycobacterial load and systemic symptoms in AIDS patients.

Other Neurologic Diseases Caused by Human Immunodeficiency Virus

The HIV may enter the CNS early in the course of infection, even before seroconversion. Therefore neurologic symptoms may be evident at the time of diagnosis. In one study HIV was recovered from 30 of 48 CSF specimens from seropositive persons with and without neurologic symptoms. However, the presence of HIV in the CSF did not necessarily correlate with the recovery of HIV from the serum. HIV may thus replicate in the brain of some patients but not cause immediate neurologic symptoms.

The most commonly occurring CNS manifestation in AIDS is a subacute encephalopathy, with dementia as a dominant feature. This progressive neurologic deterioration, known as AIDS-related dementia (ARD) or the AIDS-dementia complex, occurs in up to two thirds of AIDS patients. Early clinical symptoms, frequently mistaken for depression, include mental slowing, apathy, and impaired concentration. Progressive deterioration can result in memory loss, slowing of speech, gait disturbances, hyperreflexia, delirium, and general disability.

Diagnostic tests for AIDS-related neurologic abnormalities include a complete neurologic examination, CT and MRI scans of the head, and a lumbar puncture if possible. Metabolic or drug-induced encephalopathy, intracranial mass lesions, and other infectious diseases, such as cryptococcal meningitis, neurosyphilis, and cerebral toxoplasmosis, must be ruled out. Neuroimaging studies are often helpful in confirming the diagnosis of AIDS-related CNS disease. CT scans demonstrate cortical atrophy in 64% of patients with early ARD and 77% of patients with late ARD. The degree of cerebral atrophy often parallels the patient's clinical deterioration. MRI may provide superior resolution and sensitivity, particularly for white matter lesions, and has detected abnormalities in one third of AIDS patients with normal CT scans.

Infections thought to be due to the HIV virus itself — such as ARD — may respond to specific antiretroviral agents that cross the blood-brain barrier. Zidovudine, ribavirin, and foscarnet achieve adequate anti-HIV concentrations in CSF after intravenous administration, although only zidovudine has been beneficial for this syndrome. One study demonstrated neurologic improvement in six of seven AIDS patients with neurologic disease during therapy with zidovudine. Before this treatment can be recommended, however, more data are needed to assess the efficacy of these agents in reversing progressive dementia. Ribavirin and zidovudine, antagonistic in vitro, should not be administered together.

Bacterial and Non–Central Nervous System Viral Infections

Several bacterial infections, thought to be associated with abnormalities in B cell function, occur frequently in patients with HIV disease. Pulmonary infections are often caused by *Streptococcus pneumoniae* and *Haemophilus influenzae*. The incidence of pneumococcal pneumonia in AIDS patients is 17.9:1000 persons compared with 2.6:1000 persons in the general population. TMP-SMX acts against both organisms, as well as the more common offender *P. carinii*, so this agent is a good choice if empiric therapy for a community-acquired pneumonia is needed. Routine use of pneumococcal vaccine and parenteral gamma globulin remains controversial.

Bacteremia caused by *Salmonella typhimurium* and *Shigella* species may be associated with HIV disease. *S. typhimurium* enteritis occurs 20 times more frequently in AIDS patients than in the general population, possibly because of gastrointestinal tract abnormalities or mucosal defects. Bacteremia caused by *Listeria monocytogenes* and *Pseudomonas aeruginosa* remains rare.

Treponema pallidum infection (syphilis) can follow a severe, protracted course in patients with AIDS, and standard therapy may be inadequate. Treatment for neurosyphilis in an AIDS patient should be intravenous aqueous penicillin G 2.4 million units/d for 8 to 10 days. Benzathine penicillin should not be used, since an adequate CNS concentration is not achieved.

Mucocutaneous herpes simplex infections, common in patients with HIV disease, can cause severe, progressive perianal and rectal ulcers. Less severe mucocutaneous herpes simplex infection is treated with oral acyclovir 200 to 400 mg five times a day. However, severe disease requires intravenous acyclovir 15 mg/kg/d. Suppressive maintenance therapy with oral acyclovir 200 mg three times daily is necessary to prevent recurrence.

Patients in whom severe herpes zoster infections (shingles) develop should receive intravenous acyclovir 30 mg/kg/d for at least 5 days.

THERAPY AGAINST HUMAN IMMUNODEFICIENCY VIRUS

Research is under way to develop therapies that can inhibit or kill HIV. Current approaches include antiviral agents, immunomodulators, and vaccines.

Antiviral Agents

Antiviral agents may effectively block HIV replication at several different target sites. Most of the agents thus far developed possess at least some activity against reverse transcriptase (RT), which is essential for HIV replication. Since RT is not essential for mammalian cell function, these agents should act selectively against retroviruses. Drugs that inhibit RT include zidovudine, foscarnet, suramin, HPA-23, dideoxycytidine (ddC), α-interferon, rifabutin, and inosine pranobex. Compounds such as Peptide T and AL-721 prevent viral attachment to the cell. Interferon appears to impair viral release from infected cells. The antiviral mechanism of ribavirin is thought to involve alterations in the intracellular guanosine pool and the guanylation step required for a 5′-capping of viral messenger RNA. Dextran sulfate and rCD4 may inhibit viral binding. Potential target sites for new anti-HIV drugs include intracellular uncoating of the virus, viral DNA integration into the host cell genome, posttranscription processing of viral messenger RNA, and assembly and release of virus from the host cell.

Zidovudine

Of the antiretroviral agents developed thus far, the only one approved by the Food and Drug Administration and clinically effective is zidovudine. It is a thymidine analog converted by cellular enzymes to triphosphate form and subsequently incorporated into the HIV DNA chain by HIV RT. This incorporation terminates HIV DNA synthesis. Zidovudine reduces the frequency and severity of opportunistic infections, improves T cell function, doubles or triples the number of T cells, improves ARD, reverses skin test anergy, prolongs survival, and decreases mortality. It is therefore indicated to treat adults with symptomatic HIV infection who have a history of confirmed PCP

or an absolute T4 lymphocyte count less than 200/mm^3. As mentioned earlier, prophylaxis with zidovudine may also be indicated in asymptomatic or mildly symptomatic HIV-positive persons with a T4 lymphocyte count less than 500/mm^3. For the former group the dose should be 100 mg every 4 hours while the patient is awake (or 500 mg/d), and for the latter, 200 mg every 4 hours (or 1200 mg/d). Adverse effects of this drug, primarily bone marrow toxicity, limit its usefulness. The most common of these, granulocytopenia and anemia, are directly related to dosage and duration of therapy. The anemia results from impaired erythrocyte maturation, evidenced by increases in mean cellular volume. Other adverse effects include headache, fever, malaise, nausea, vomiting, myalgias, rashes, pruritus, and mild confusion.

Zidovudine therapy is initiated at 200 mg orally every 4 hours around the clock. Because zidovudine in the intracellular phosphorylated form has a longer half-life than in plasma, some advocate administering the drug every 8 hours. Monitoring of hematologic indexes every 2 weeks is necessary because anemia may become significant 2 to 4 weeks after therapy starts; granulocytopenia may be seen after 6 weeks of therapy. Dose reduction or discontinuation is indicated if the hemoglobin level becomes less than 7.5 g/dl or the granulocyte count is less than 750/mm^3. Continuous intravenous infusion of zidovudine, when available clinically, may decrease its toxicity. Lithium may reverse zidovudine-induced neutropenia.

Zidovudine may interact with other agents used in AIDS patients. Use of drugs that competitively inhibit hepatic glucuronidation (acetaminophen, rifampin, cimetidine, ranitidine, indomethacin, and others) should be carefully considered because zidovudine is metabolized via the same pathway. Additive toxicity may develop with concurrent ganciclovir, flucytosine, dapsone, ribavirin, amphotericin B, pentamidine, or interferon therapy. Synergy between zidovudine and acyclovir has been demonstrated.

Other strategies to combat HIV infection include immunomodulators and vaccine development. Immunotherapy is aimed at correcting the immunodeficiency in AIDS. Specific immunomodulator therapy includes α-interferon, interleukin-2, immune reconstitution with lymphocyte transfusions and bone marrow transplantation, transfer factor, granulocyte-macrophage colony–stimulating factor, inosine pranobex, and naltrexone. These therapies, especially in combination with antiviral agents, require further study. Vaccine development is ongoing, but widespread clinical use remains years away.

PREVENTION OF HUMAN IMMUNODEFICIENCY VIRUS TRANSMISSION TO HEALTH CARE WORKERS

Studies involving more than 5000 health care workers suggest that the risk of HIV seroconversion after a puncture wound with a blood- or secretion-contaminated instrument is less than 1%. Furthermore, data reported by the CDC do not indicate an excess prevalence of AIDS in health care workers. Exposure to HIV is usually preventable by adequate precautions. However, depending on geography and age, a pool of HIV-positive persons, ranging from 16% to 18% of the populations studied, are apparently asymptomatic.

Precautions should be taken to prevent transmission of HIV (Table 26–3). The universal precautions recommended by the CDC should be taken with all patients because HIV-infected persons frequently cannot be identified by history and physical examination.

These precautions are particularly important in emergency care settings, where exposure to blood or body fluids is likely and infectious status of patients is unknown. In addition to universal precautions, invasive precautions should be taken when any invasive procedure is performed. Laboratory precautions, in addition to universal precautions, are recommended during work in clinical laboratories. The CDC defines an invasive procedure as surgical entry into tissues, cavities, or an organ or any repair of traumatically induced lesions, including lesions treated in a physician's office or the emergency room. Cardiac catheterization and other angiographic procedures, vaginal or cesarean delivery, and dental surgical procedures are considered invasive. Blood and body fluids from all patients must be considered infectious. HIV transmission in the health care setting will be eliminated only if the recommended precautions are consistently and carefully followed.

Although many therapeutic approaches to HIV infection are possible, a curative therapy or vaccine is unlikely in the near future. To date the only effective treatment is prevention. Therefore the entire medical community, including intensive care physicians, must educate patients and the general public about AIDS

TABLE 26–3. Precautions for Health Care Workers to Prevent Contamination with Human Immunodeficiency Virus

TYPE OF PRECAUTION	BARRIER TO CONTAMINATION				SPECIAL CONSIDERATIONS
	CLOTHES	DECONTAMINATION	FLUIDS AND TISSUES	EQUIPMENT	
Precautions to Use with All Patients					
Universal	Wear gloves and masks, eyewear (as appropriate)	Wash hands	Dermatologic precautions: with exudative lesions, use gloves and wash hands	Do not bend, break, or resheath needles Use ventilation device for resuscitation	Pregnant health care workers take extra care
Precautions in Addition to Universal Precautions					
Invasive*	Wear gowns Check gloves frequently for tears	Use routine surgical procedure			
Laboratory	Remove contaminated clothing	Wash work surface after spills	For samples, use well-constructed containers with tops For droplets, use biologic safety cabinets	*Only use needles if no other alternative; use caution* Use mechanical pipettes Decontaminate/ clean equipment before transport/ repair	Use caution in disposal of waste No mouth pipetting

*Refers to surgical procedures and diagnostic procedures such as angiography.
Based on information from Centers for Disease Control: Recommendations for prevention of HIV transmission in health-care settings. MMWR 36(suppl 25):35–185, 1987.

prevention by talking about sex and drugs frankly, a very different manner from that to which we are accustomed.

SUGGESTED READINGS

Brenner M, Ognibene FP, Lack EE, et al: Prognostic factors and life expectancy of patients with acquired immunodeficiency syndrome and *Pneumocystis carinii* pneumonia. Am Rev Respir Dis 1987;136:1199-1206

Centers for Disease Control: Human immunodeficiency virus infection in the United States—a review of current knowledge. MMWR 1987;36(suppl S-6):1-48

Centers for Disease Control: Recommendations for prevention of HIV transmission in health-care settings. MMWR 1987;36(suppl 2-S):3S-18S

Chiu J, Nussbaum J, Bozzette S, et al: Treatment of disseminated *Mycobacterium avium* complex infection in AIDS with amikacin, ethambutol, rifampin, and ciprofloxacin. Ann Intern Med 1990;113:358-361

Devita VT, Broder S, Fauci AS, et al: Developmental therapeutics and the acquired immunodeficiency syndrome. Ann Intern Med 1987;106:568-581

Farzadegan H, Polis MA, Wolinsky SM, et al: Loss of human immunodeficiency virus type 1 (HIV-1) antibodies with evidence of viral infection in asymptomatic homosexual men. Ann Intern Med 1988;108:785-790

Fauci AS: The human immunodeficiency virus—infectivity and mechanisms of pathogenesis. Science 1988;239:617-622

Fischl MA, Richman DD, Hansen N, et al: The safety and efficacy of zidovudine (AZT) in the treatment of subjects with mildly symptomatic human immunodeficiency virus type 1 (HIV) infection. Ann Intern Med 1990;112:727-737

Friedman Y, Franklin C, Rackow EC, et al: Improved survival in patients with AIDS, *Pneumocystis carinii* pneumonia, and respiratory failure. Chest 1989;96:862-866

John DR, Tierney M, Felsenstein D: Alteration in the natural history of neurosyphilis by concurrent infection with the human immunodeficiency virus. N Engl J Med 1987;316:1569-1572

Kaplan LD, Wofsy CB, Volberding PA: Treatment of patients with acquired immunodeficiency syndrome and associated manifestations. JAMA 1987;257:1367-1374

McArthur JC: Neurologic manifestations of AIDS. Medicine 1987;66:407-437

Murray JF, Garay SM, Hopewell PC, et al: Pulmonary complications of the acquired immunodeficiency syndrome—an update. Am Rev Respir Dis 1987;135:504-509

Piot P, Plummer FA, Mhalu FS, et al: AIDS—an international perspective. Science 1988;239:573-579

Purdy BD, Plaisance KI: Current concepts in clinical therapeutics: immunologic treatment of human immunodeficiency virus infections. Clin Pharm 1987;6:851-865

Sandstrom EG, Kaplan JC: Antiviral therapy in AIDS—clinical pharmacological properties and therapeutic experience to date. Drugs 1987;34:372-390

Shilts R: And the band played on—politics, people, and the AIDS epidemic, New York, 1988, Viking Penguin

Steinbrook R, Lo B, Moulton J, et al: Preferences of homosexual men with AIDS for life-sustaining treatment. N Engl J Med 1986;314:457-460

Tartaglione TA, Collier AC: Development of antiviral agents for the treatment of human immunodeficiency virus infection. Clin Pharm 1987;6:927-940

Volberding PA, Lagakos SW, Koch MA, et al: Zidovudine in asymptomatic human immunodeficiency virus infection. N Engl J Med 1990;322:941-949

Wachter RM, Luce JM, Turner J, et al: Intensive care of patients with the acquired immunodeficiency syndrome—outcome and changing patterns of utilization. Am Rev Respir Dis 1986;134:891-896

Witt DJ, Craven DE, McCabe WR: Bacterial infections in adult patients with the acquired immune deficiency syndrome (AIDS) and AIDS-related complex. Am J Med 1987;82:900-906

27

NUTRITIONAL SUPPORT IN THE CRITICALLY ILL

MICHAEL J. MURRAY, MD, PhD

The exceptional needs of critically ill patients extend to the area of nutrition, and nutritional intervention is an integral part of treatment for any ICU patient. The management of nutrition in the ICU has two steps. First, an accurate assessment must be made of the patient's nutritional status. Second, a rational program must be formulated to meet the patient's unique nutritional needs, recognizing the stress affecting these patients.

ASSESSMENT OF NUTRITIONAL STATUS

Nutritional assessment has two aims. The first is to assess the patient's energy stores. Most energy is stored in the body as either fat or protein. (Glycogen and carbohydrate account for a very small amount of the body's energy stores. In addition, there are no true protein reserves; the protein used as an energy source has been serving vital functions elsewhere, and its use as an energy source threatens normal organ function.)

The body can be divided into three compartments: the adipose tissue compartment, which contains the body's fat stores; the body cell mass, which includes the body's protein stores; and the extracellular mass, which is composed primarily of water and electrolytes and contributes little to the body's energy stores.

Assessment of energy reserves is important because ICU patients who have decreased energy stores may be at risk for increased morbidity and death. The clinician must differentiate healthy individuals, such as athletes who have a low ideal body weight, were well nourished before their ICU admission, and are not at increased risk because of their nutritional status, from individuals who enter the ICU with depleted adipose and protein stores and whose nutritional status indeed places them at increased risk.

The second aim of nutritional assessment is to determine whether a patient is in positive energy-nitrogen balance. Patients in negative balance require more specialized support. Energy balance should be distinguished from protein balance. Patients in negative energy balance have marasmus, an adaptation to semistarvation in which caloric intake is insufficient for the body's requirements. Such individuals are likely to have maximized the body's ability to conserve protein stores (Table 27–1).

Patients in negative protein balance, described classically as kwashiorkor and more recently as hypoalbuminemic malnutrition, are undergoing a metabolic response to the stress of illness or injury (Table 27–1). This response, mediated via the hypothalamic-pituitary-adrenal axis and by a variety of peptide and monokine mediators, is a fundamental mechanism for the maintenance of homeostasis. Inability to control the response by endogenous mechanisms or by such interventions as nutritional support increases the risk of morbidity and mortality. The assessment of nutritional status, including the quantification of energy reserves and the determination of energy and protein balance, is the first step in planning nutrition support.

History

Assessment begins with a review of the medical record and interviews with the patient and family members. The goal is to identify

477

TABLE 27–1. Comparison of Marasmus and Hypoalbuminemic Malnutrition

CAUSE	MARASMUS	HYPOALBUMINEMIC MALNUTRITION
	Insufficient energy intake	Metabolic response to injury
Hormonal and metabolic alterations	Depression in metabolic rate; hypoinsulinemia	Counterregulatory hormones (aldosterone, antidiuretichormone); insulin resistance; monokine response
Visceral protein stores	Normal serum albumin; no acute-phase protein response; diminished in liver and gut	Low serum albumin; acute-phase protein response; increased in liver but diminished in gut
Immune function	Intact unless body weight <85% of ideal	Impaired if injury response prolonged
Clinical presentation and anthropometric measurements	Weight loss; low AMC	Markers of stress (fever, leukocytosis with increase in band forms, hypoalbuminemia, elevated catabolic index); normal or low AMC
Anticipated response to appropriate nutritional therapy	Restoration of lean tissue; positive nitrogen balance	Restoration of lean tissue may or may not occur; persistent hypoalbuminemia; return of immunocompetence
Prototypic disease states	Starvation; anorexia nervosa; cardiac cachexia; malabsorption; esophageal cancer	Sepsis; head injury; burns; multiple trauma; selected cancers

AMC = arm muscle circumference.
From McMahon M, Bistrian BR: Anthropometric assessment of nutritional status in hospitalized patients. In McMahon M, Bistrian BR (eds): Anthropometric assessment of nutritional status. New York, 1988, Allen R Liss, Inc.

high-risk conditions that may accompany, or predispose a patient to, malnutrition. Interviews should include questions about the nature and duration of any underlying illnesses, usual eating habits, the intake of medications and alcohol, and the presence of weight loss or gain.

In a busy ICU with limited resources, the history of a 10-pound weight loss over the preceding 3 to 6 months is the single most important indicator of increased risk for morbidity and mortality. An individual with such a weight loss should have a thorough nutritional assessment with plans made for early nutritional support.

Anthropometric Measurements

Such measurements as height, weight, triceps skinfold (TSF), and arm muscle circumference (AMC), a measure of the body's skeletal muscle mass, have been the traditional tools of nutritional assessment and are useful in characterizing populations of patients. The problem with these techniques is that they have wide confidence intervals and are difficult to apply to individual patients. For the TSF, which provides an estimate of adipose stores, in addition to the problem of wide confidence limits, individuals vary widely in how their bodies store adipose tissue. Furthermore, subcutaneous edema, present in many ICU patients because of congestive heart failure, low

colloid oncotic pressure, or massive fluid resuscitation, alters TSF measurement. Indexes incorporating several body fold measurements are cumbersome and time consuming to apply to ICU patients.

Despite these limitations, certain anthropometric measurements are valuable, especially the AMC, an index of the body's protein stores. It correlates reasonably well with more sophisticated techniques of assessing skeletal muscle mass (which comprises approximately 50% of protein stores) and also with both serum albumin level and percentage of weight loss. The technique is easy to use and requires no specialized equipment (Fig. 27–1).

Laboratory Determinations

The loss of skeletal muscle mass, although important in terms of loss of function, such as decreased diaphragmatic contractility, is critical because it correlates with a decrease in visceral protein stores. The catabolism of visceral protein is manifest as a loss of cellular integrity, altered immune function, and decreased enzymatic function, all of which contribute to a poor outcome.

Several laboratory markers, including serum albumin, transferrin, prealbumin, and retinol-binding proteins, reflect visceral protein stores. A decrease in the serum levels of these proteins is due to both an increase

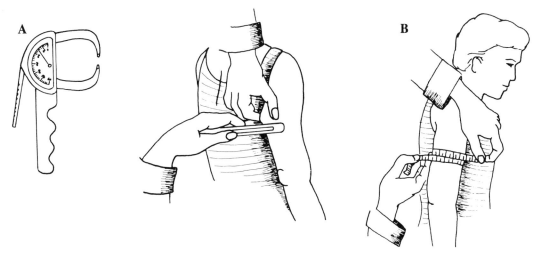

Figure 27–1. Technique for measurement of arm muscle circumference. **A,** Technique for measuring triceps skinfold at the midpoint of the upper arm with the subject's arm relaxed. **B,** At the same point the circumference of the upper arm is measured. Arm muscle circumference = Upper arm circumference − (π × Triceps skinfold). Nomograms for arm muscle circumference can be found in standard texts or in Frisoncho A: Am J Clin Nutr 1981;34:2540.   (From Grant A, DeHoog S [eds]: Nutritional assessment and support, ed. 3. Seattle, 1985, p 13.)

in protein catabolism and decreased protein synthesis in stressed and malnourished patients.

Serum albumin is a readily available marker. If levels are between 2.8 and 3.2 g/dl, the prognosis is poor, and the patient might benefit from aggressive intervention. However, serum albumin is as much a marker of injury response as of nutritional status. The level may remain low despite adequate nutritional support because of a marked stress response. Furthermore, it is less useful than other protein markers as an indicator of positive nitrogen balance and the anabolic state.

Therefore, although a low serum albumin level indicates the need for more aggressive intervention, a second marker, such as serum prealbumin or somatomedin-C, is a better indicator of positive nitrogen balance and should be measured at baseline and at least weekly thereafter to monitor the adequacy of nutritional intervention.

Other laboratory tests that should be part of a nutritional assessment are measurements of serum glucose and serum electrolytes, including sodium, potassium, magnesium, calcium, and phosphorus. Some patients have vitamin or trace element deficiencies, either because of the underlying disease process or because of the duration and nature of the nutritional state. These situations must be assessed individually. Awareness of the possibility of vitamin deficits is the most important factor in identifying patients whose vitamin or trace element levels should be measured.

Skin Antigen Testing

Skin antigens have been less commonly tested in nutritional assessment in recent years. Although the loss of reactivity to commonly employed skin tests (mumps, *Candida, Trichophyton,* streptokinase/streptodornase) correlates with malnutrition, the test results correlate no better with outcome than do visceral protein markers. A more important reason for the declining use of these tests has been recognition that many nonnutritional elements, such as technical and patient factors, the presence of benign or malignant disease, immune alterations, and iatrogenic factors, can influence the reactivity rate. Skin antigen testing is therefore not recommended for routine nutritional assessment.

Nitrogen Balance

Increasing protein synthesis to equal or exceed the rate of protein catabolism is the most fundamental goal of nutritional support, contributing in a vital way to a positive outcome. Nitrogen balance studies are an integral part of nutritional assessment and can be used to calculate the degree of protein breakdown, estimate the magnitude of the stress response as reflected in the catabolic rate, and assess the efficiency of nutritional interventions.

A balance measurement defines whether a patient is in positive or negative nitrogen balance. This is done by measuring the patient's daily protein intake and, since dietary protein has an average nitrogen content of 16%, dividing the protein intake by 6.25 to calculate the amount of nitrogen given. The amount of nitrogen lost is subtracted from the amount given to calculate whether the patient is in positive or negative balance.

The body loses nitrogen (N_2) via the skin and feces and in the urine as urea, creatinine, and ammonia. Typically a 24-hour urine specimen is collected, and the total amount of nitrogen in the urine (Kjeldhal technique) or in urea (the major source) is measured. The small amount lost in the gastrointestinal tract or skin is assumed to be about 2 g/d, and if only urine urea is measured, an additional 2 g/d as nonurea nitrogen is assumed to be lost. Therefore,

$$N_2 \text{ balance} = N_2 \text{ in} - N_2 \text{ out}$$
$$(N_2 \text{ out} = \text{Urine urea } N_2 + 4 \text{ g or} \qquad \text{(Eq. 1)}$$
$$\text{Total urine } N_2 + 2 \text{ g})$$

Nitrogen balance information can also be used to estimate the patient's level of metabolic stress. One such measure is the catabolic index, in which total urea excretion is divided into that arising from exogenous protein administration and that arising from gluconeogenesis (glucose-alanine cycle). The catabolic index (CI) is equal to the difference between measured and predicted urine urea nitrogen:

$$\text{CI} = 24 \text{ Hour urine } N_2 - (0.5 \times N_2 \text{ intake} + 3 \text{ g}) \quad \text{(Eq. 2)}$$

A CI of less than zero indicates minimal, zero to 5 indicates moderate, and greater than 5 indicates severe stress.

Nitrogen balance studies should be performed at baseline and after 3 to 7 days of nutritional support to document efficacy of the nutrition regimen.

Indirect Calorimetry

It is also possible to measure energy balance:

$$\text{Energy balance} = \text{Caloric intake} - \qquad \text{(Eq. 3)}$$
$$\text{Caloric expenditure}$$

Patients with positive or slightly negative energy balance have a better outcome than those with a severe negative balance.

Caloric intake is easier to measure than caloric expenditure, but the latter must be known to calculate energy balance. Direct calorimet-

ers that measure heat production exist, but mainly in research laboratories. The preferred clinical technique for measuring energy expenditure is by indirect calorimetry, which is based on oxygen consumption and carbon dioxide production in the metabolism of food substrates. By measuring oxygen consumption and carbon dioxide production, the clinician can calculate energy expenditure. The small amount of protein metabolized by nonoxidative processes can be taken into account in calculating energy expenditure, although it comprises less than 2% of daily energy expenditure. Several commercial machines are available for measuring energy expenditure, but all have limitations. They must be run by experienced personnel, must be carefully calibrated, and are difficult to use for certain groups of patients, such as patients with endotracheal tubes and mechanical ventilation who require a fraction of inspired oxygen greater than 0.5. In addition, the sicker the patient, the less accurate the measurement.

Given the proclivity to overfeed ICU patients, indirect calorimetry does have a role in establishing a reasonable level of caloric support. However, certain admonitions must be kept in mind. In these stressed patients the examiner measures a resting metabolic rate (RMR) and documents that rate for an extended period (10 to 30 minutes). Evidence suggests that the true metabolic rate of an ICU patient over a 24-hour period is 10% to 30% higher than the RMR. In some institutions, indirect calorimetry is performed at baseline and periodically thereafter; in others, caloric needs are estimated, alimentation is begun, and the initial measurement is done 48 to 72 hours later.

Nomograms

The clinician can use several nomograms to estimate patients' energy and protein requirements. The Harris-Benedict equation is a widely used estimate of energy requirement. Probably it overestimates true energy consumption by 5% to 10%, but this is an acceptable range and no other test has replaced it.

For males: RMR = 66.4 + 13.8 W +
5 H − 6.8 A
For females: RMR = 65.5 + 9.6 W +   (Eq. 4)
1.8 H − 4.7 A

Where:

W = weight (kg)
H = height (cm)
A = age (y)

Assessment Technique

Clinical skills and acumen are important in assessing an ICU patient's nutritional status. Following the recommendations outlined, the clinician should begin with a brief history and examination, obtain AMC and serum albumin measurements, and assess the patient's energy balance. If the patient is in negative balance (that is, has an inadequate intake) and is expected to remain so for several days, further steps should be taken. A nitrogen balance study should be ordered and indirect calorimetry performed. Plans should then be made for alimentation via the routes and with one of the formulations discussed later in the chapter.

For example, a 71-year-old woman with dementia is brought to the ICU with sepsis after a cholecystectomy. She has lost 10 pounds over the previous year. Her adipose stores are depleted, her AMC is less than 70% of the predicted circumference, and her serum albumin level is 2.9 g/dl. This patient is malnourished and at a high stress level. The clinician should plan alimentation and order nitrogen balance and indirect calorimetry studies.

MANAGEMENT OF STRESS RESPONSE AND STARVATION

Having made a nutritional assessment, the clinician must design a nutrition regimen that meets the patient's individual needs. Central to alimentation of critically ill patients is an understanding of the stress response, a unique response dissimilar to that seen during starvation. During starvation the body has a number of adaptive processes to conserve protein stores. During even a brief fast the majority of tissues utilize fatty acids to meet their caloric needs, although cells in the nervous system and some other cells continue to utilize glucose. During a brief fast the brain consumes approximately 85% of the glucose produced by the liver. With more prolonged fasting even the brain is able to utilize fatty acid metabolites, ketone bodies, to meet its energy requirements. During a prolonged fast, lipids meet 75% to 80% of the body's energy requirements, which spares protein and preserves its important cellular functions.

Unlike starvation, in stress states an almost obligatory degradation of muscle and visceral protein occurs. The released amino acids are available for energy production by gluconeogenesis and oxidation. They also serve as substrates in the liver for the synthesis of proteins involved in the acute-phase response, proteins essential to immunologic defense and wound healing. Prolonged and uncompensated mobilization of protein leads to devastating muscle weakness, loss of structural components of cells with deterioration of cellular integrity, and a decrease in cellular enzymes and thus enzymatic activity.

In stressed patients a variety of interventions have been studied, such as glucose, insulin, anabolic steroids, fats, and branched-chain amino acids, but none has consistently inhibited this protein breakdown. The catabolic state is probably caused by an endogenous monokine, such as tumor necrosis factor, and the restoration of protein synthesis requires a diminution of this monokine's activity and supplementation with the proper nutritional substrates.

Principles

Assessment should give the clinician sufficient information to determine whether the patient is malnourished, the type of malnutrition, and the degree of stress. The greater the malnutrition or stress, the earlier and more aggressive the intervention needed. Malnourished patients should not remain on "nothing by mouth" (NPO) status for more than 5 days; no patient, regardless of preexisting nutritional status or disease state, should be allowed to remain NPO for more than 10 days. Having decided to intervene, the clinician must determine how to meet the individual patient's nutritional requirements.

Calories

How many calories ICU patients should be fed, and how these calories should be provided, is a matter of debate. Work in the 1970s indicated that critically ill patients are markedly hypermetabolic with energy requirements 50% to 100% above their baseline RMR. More recent studies have refuted this. Faced with the choice between overfeeding a patient, with the attendant risks of a fatty liver, hyperosmolality, increased carbon dioxide production, and respiratory failure, and underfeeding a patient by 5% to 10% of the RMR, many nutritionists would opt for the latter course. Ideally, however, patients should receive 10% to 30% above their RMR whether this is calculated from the Harris-Benedict equation, or by multiplying the body weight (in kilograms) by 24 to give the number of kilocalories required per 24 hours, or by measuring the RMR with an indirect calorimeter.

A second controversy is the proportions of carbohydrate and fat in the calorie intake. Before the introduction of lipid emulsions into routine clinical practice, all nonprotein calories came from carbohydrate. However, critically ill patients can metabolize only a limited amount of glucose; large amounts lead to hyperglycemia with its attendant problems.

The addition of insulin to the regimen may drive glucose into the cells but does nothing to promote glucose oxidation. High intracellular levels of glucose may be detrimental in areas of reduced perfusion and hypoxia.

Many physicians have advocated lipids as an energy source to replace glucose in parenteral and enteral nutrition formulations. However, large lipid loads may alter pulmonary and immune function, perhaps mediated by arachidonic acid metabolites. Therefore, although lipids and carbohydrates are both considered appropriate nutrients for critically ill patients, large amounts of either substrate may be harmful.

Carbohydrate

Glucose is the carbohydrate most commonly used to meet patients' caloric requirements because it is inexpensive and physiologic. The activity of pyruvate dehydrogenase, the rate-limiting step for the oxidation of pyruvate and glucose, is depressed in many ICU patients. The excess pyruvate is released from cells, returns to the liver, and serves as a substrate for gluconeogenesis. In patients with regional hypoxemia the pyruvate may be a substrate for lactic acid production and worsen ischemic insults. Thus stressed individuals should probably receive no more than twice the amount of glucose that can be completely oxidized.

In ICU patients the total glucose load should be limited to 5 g/kg/d. No more than 3.5 g/kg/d should be given to patients with more severe stress (Table 27–2) as determined by protein balance studies, the catabolic index, the RMR, and other indicators.

Fructose and glycerol can be used as caloric sources, but each has its limitations and the practitioner should be familiar with these compounds before adding them to a patient's regimen.

Lipid

Since critically ill patients can metabolize only a limited amount of glucose, lipid can be

TABLE 27–2. Glucose Administration via Total Parenteral Nutrition* in Critically Ill Patients

	STRESS LEVEL		
	SEVERE	MODERATE	MILD
Glucose (g)	200-300	300-400	400-500
D20 Amount (L)	1.0-1.5	1.5-2.0	2.0-2.5
kcal	680-1020	1020-1360	1360-1700

*For a 70 kg patient.

used as an alternative energy source with limitations. Traditionally lipids have been incorporated into patients' diets to avoid the sequelae of essential fatty acid deficiency. Over the past decade increasing amounts of lipid have been used as a caloric source because of the ease of administration, the lack of toxicity if given properly, and the effect of decreasing carbon dioxide production, which may be beneficial for patients with respiratory failure who cannot handle large carbon dioxide loads.

Dietary lipids can be expensive if given intravenously and are not without risk. Whereas healthy volunteers may be able to metabolize up to 4 g of lipids/kg/d, critically ill patients should be limited to between 1 and 1.5 g/kg/d. Like glucose metabolism, lipid metabolism is altered by stress. Cells are unable to effectively metabolize exogenous lipid, which leads to elevated plasma triglyceride and fatty acid levels. Increased hepatic deposition of these fatty acids can cause a fatty liver. Elevated fatty acid levels may alter immune function directly by inactivating membrane receptors on the surface of antigen-sensitive leukocytes, or more likely by increasing the concentration and availability of arachidonic acid, the precursor for prostaglandins, thromboxanes, and leukotrienes, important immune modulators. The current recommendation is to limit lipids to 1 to 1.5 g/kg/d.

Protein

All nutrition regimens should contain enough protein to supply the necessary amino acids for endogenous protein synthesis, but the amount and type of protein are controversial.

Stressed patients have increased protein catabolism. The released amino acids serve as substrates for gluconeogenesis and for synthesis of acute-phase reactants, which with a decrease in protein synthesis leads to negative nitrogen balance. No therapeutic regimen yet found consistently and completely inhibits this negative nitrogen balance. Negative nitrogen balance appears to be an almost obligatory response to an injury. It lasts for hours to days, depending on injury severity, and may continue unabated if the disease process is not controlled and the appropriate nutrients are not provided. Any nutrition regimen must therefore have adequate protein, as well as calories.

The daily protein requirement for a healthy adult is 0.5 to 0.6 g/kg/d. For ICU patients this requirement is probably 1 to 1.4 g/kg/d, although some authorities advocate regimens containing more than 2 g/kg/d. Such regimens are expensive and carry some risk, since they may increase blood urea and ammonia levels and unnecessarily stimulate respiratory drive.

The current recommendation is to start protein administration with 1 to 1.4 g/kg/d and base subsequent decision making on nitrogen balance studies. The goal is not necessarily positive nitrogen balance, but at least nitrogen parity or a zero protein balance in which the amounts in and out are equal.

The ideal composition of exogenous protein is also unknown. Whereas there is agreement that essential and nonessential amino acids should be supplied, the ratios of individual amino acids are not established. Since branched-chain amino acids appear to be preferentially metabolized in stress states, probably 50% of the amino acids supplied to moderately or severely stressed patients should be the branched-chain type. Evidence is still insufficient to make this a definitive recommendation, however.

Vitamins

The majority of ICU patients' vitamin requirements can be met with commercially available preparations. The preparations should be administered daily. Their omission, as occurred during a recent national shortage of intravenous vitamins, can lead to death, probably from thiamine deficiency.

The standard adult intravenous vitamin preparations contain the recommended daily allowances of all vitamins except vitamin K. The Food and Drug Administration, when originally approving vitamin preparations, removed vitamin K because of the large number of patients who receive anticoagulants, such as warfarin. Therefore vitamin K supplements are needed if weekly measurement of prothrombin time indicates a deficit. Supplementation can be given orally if tolerated or parenterally. If the parenteral route is used, injections can be intramuscular or intravenous, although many practitioners think the risk of anaphylaxis is less with intramuscular injections.

Patients with gastrointestinal disease and fat malabsorption may have vitamin deficits that require specialized supplementation of the fat-soluble vitamins (A, D, E, and K).

Alcoholics or others with thiamine deficits require additional amounts of thiamine, since only 10 mg/d is included in the standard vitamin preparation.

Minerals and Trace Elements

Parenteral and enteral nutrition regimens contain various combinations of sodium, potassium, calcium, magnesium, chloride, phosphorus, and acetate, which sometimes can be altered to suit the needs of individual patients.

In malnourished patients receiving adequate nutrition who have a net synthesis of protein, hypophosphatemia may develop because phosphorus is incorporated into the newly formed protein. Hypophosphatemia can lead to a wide variety of syndromes, including muscle weakness and respiratory failure. Current regimens usually contain adequate phosphorus, but levels must be checked periodically and the electrolyte combination adjusted accordingly.

Hyperchloremia was common in the early days of parenteral nutrition support. Current parenteral nutrition regimens include less chloride, but if an ICU patient has metabolic acidosis, the parenteral nutrition formula can be altered by decreasing the amount of chloride and increasing the acetate, and vice versa for a patient with alkalosis.

Many ICU patients who have a forced or spontaneous diuresis, as well as patients with heart disease, require monitoring and adjustment of serum calcium, magnesium, potassium, and sodium levels.

Whereas the electrolytes just described can be assessed and manipulated daily, the guidelines for the trace elements are less firm. Most of the many trace elements (Table 27–3) are difficult to measure, the exact "normal" value for each is unknown, and the recommended daily allowance for critically ill patients is not established. Guidelines will be established only when more accurate methods are developed for assessing and monitoring trace element status in ICU patients. It does seem clear that critically ill patients require additional zinc and copper. Therefore the current recommendations for trace elements are 4 mg zinc, 0.8 mg copper, 0.4 mg manganese, and 8 µg chromium per day.

TABLE 27–3.   Trace Element Requirements in Total Parenteral Nutrition

TRACE ELEMENT	BIOCHEMICAL FUNCTIONS	EFFECTS OF DEFICIENCY	LABORATORY TESTS	RECOMMENDED INTAKE
Zinc	Over 100 metalloenzymes; especially nucleic acid and protein synthesis	Skin lesions; alopecia; impaired wound healing; impaired T lymphocyte function; mental depression/apathy	Plasma zinc (ref. range 12-18 μmol/L; 80-120 μg/dl); 24-h urine zinc; leukocyte zinc; alkaline phosphatase	50-100 μmol/d (3.0-6.5 mg/d)
Copper	Metalloenzymes (e.g., lysyl oxidase, superoxide dismutase, ceruloplasmin)	Hypochromic anemia; neutropenia; demineralization of bone; vascular aneurysms	Serum copper (ref. range 15-25 μmol/L; 100-150 μg/dl); serum ceruloplasmin	8-24 μmol/d (0.5-1.5 mg/d)
Iron	Hemoglobin; myoglobin; cytochromes	Anemia	Serum ferritin; transferrin saturation; hemoglobin	20-50 μmol/d (1.0-2.5 mg/d)
Selenium	Glutathione peroxidase	Cardiomyopathy; skeletal muscle myopathy; hair and nail changes	Plasma selenium (ref. range 0.8-2.0 μmol/L; 6-15 μg/dl); red blood cell glutathione peroxidase	0.4-2.5 μmol/day (30-200 μg/d)
Chromium	Glucose tolerance factor	Glucose intolerance; peripheral neuropathy; hyperlipidemia	Serum chromium (ref. range < 10 nmol/L; 0.04-0.35 μg/L); urine chromium after glucose load	200-300 nmol/d (10-15 μg/d)
Manganese	Mucopolysaccharide synthesis; many enzymes (e.g., superoxide, dismutase)	Not clear	Serum manganese (ref. range 7-29 nmol/L; 40-180 ng/dl)	3-13 μmol (0.15-0.8 mg)
Molybdenum	Xanthine oxidase; sulfite oxidase	Amino acid intolerance	Urine sulfate; xanthine; uric acid; urine molybdenum	200 nmol/d (−20 μg/d)
Magnesium*	Neuromuscular activity	Neuromuscular irritation—tetany	Serum magnesium (ref. range 0.7-1.0 nmol/L; 1.7-2.4 mg/dl)	5-10 mmol (120-240 mg)
Phosphorus*	Intermediary metabolism	Muscle weakness; red cell rigidity; reduced oxygen release from hemoglobin	Serum phosphate (0.8-1.4 mmol/L 2.5-4.3 mg/dl)	15-30 mmol (465-930 mg)

*These are not trace elements but are included here for completeness.
From Shenkin A: Intensive Crit Care Dig 1988; 7:20-23.

Selenium deficiencies, which may lead to arthritis or myocardiopathy, are rare, but common practice is to include a small amount of selenium (20 to 80 μg) in the diet every day.

Because of the risk of anaphylaxis with parenteral iron administration, parenteral nutrition products do not contain iron. Patients receiving long-term parenteral nutrition support may require iron supplementation.

Monitoring is an important aspect of nutritional support. The serum calcium, potassium, sodium, chloride, and bicarbonate concentrations should be monitored daily initially and weekly thereafter (Table 27–4). The copper, iron, magnesium, and zinc levels should be checked at baseline and weekly thereafter. The selenium level can be checked only monthly after the initial evaluation unless circumstances dictate otherwise.

Specific Disease States

Renal Failure

Patients in renal failure, whether undergoing dialysis or not, commonly require alteration in their nutritional support. Patients who cannot excrete a normal volume of urine should receive as little free water in their diets as possible to

TABLE 27–4. Guidelines for Laboratory Monitoring in Total Parenteral Nutrition

		DAY OF THERAPY								
	BASELINE*	2	3	4	7	14	21	28	35	42
Electrolyte panel†	X	X	X	X	X	X	X	X	X	X
Chemistry panel‡	X				X	X	X	X	X	X
Complete blood count	X							X		
Triglycerides§	X									
Prothrombin time	X				X	X	X	X	X	
Trace elements screen‖	X				X	X	X	X		
Selenium	X							X		

*Baseline tests preceding initiation of parenteral nutrition.
†To include sodium, potassium, chloride, bicarbonate, glucose, and blood urea nitrogen.
‡To include albumin, phosphorus, calcium, magnesium, alkaline phosphatase, asparate aminotransferase, and bilirubin.
§Repeat level prior to the start of the second bottle of fat emulsion.
‖To include copper, zinc, and iron.

decrease the chance for volume overload. Frequently the amount of protein in the diet must be changed. Although these patients were once thought to require alteration in the type of protein as well, most outcome studies have not shown any benefit with diets that contain only essential amino acids. Furthermore, whereas the majority of patients with chronic renal failure do well with a diet restricted in protein (less than 0.4 g protein/kg/d), ICU patients have altered protein requirements as already discussed. Protein kinetic studies are difficult to perform in patients undergoing dialysis but are one way to assess protein requirements. As empiric treatment, however, critically ill patients with renal failure may receive up to 1 g protein/kg/d, and patients undergoing dialysis may benefit from up to 1.2 g protein/kg/d. Decisions on protein dosage should be further guided by assessing the importance of positive nitrogen balance and its influence on wound healing, strength, and cellular integrity; the need for and frequency of dialysis; and blood urea and creatinine levels.

Tubular defects, along with the defect in clearance of free water, may also lead to electrolyte abnormalities. Although these must be assessed individually, treatment is commonly a decrease in the amounts of potassium, phosphorus and magnesium and an increase in the amount of acetate these patients receive in parenteral alimentation to combat the metabolic acidosis seen in renal failure.

Respiratory Failure

Nutritional status can affect the pulmonary system in a number of ways. Protein malnutrition can lead to emphysematous changes in the lung, loss of diaphragm mass and strength, and increased susceptibility to infection owing to altered immune status. Nutrition replenishment has several potentially adverse side effects. Too many calories increases oxygen consumption and carbon dioxide production, and large amounts of intravenous amino acids increase respiratory drive, none of which may be tolerated in patients with marginal respiratory reserve. Large amounts of intravenous fat emulsions may alter thromboxane/prostaglandin ratios, impairing lung perfusion, ventilation, and possibly immune function.

The goal in patients with respiratory failure is to supply adequate but not excessive amounts of protein (1 to 1.4 g protein/kg/d) and calories (10% to 30% above RMR). The caloric composition is controversial. Some authorities believe that patients with respiratory failure should receive a large proportion (30% to 70%) of their calories from dietary lipids. Oxidation of lipid decreases carbon dioxide production, which may benefit patients with marginal alveolar ventilation. However, evidence suggests that providing sufficient calories without overfeeding is the most important determinant of carbon dioxide production and that a high-fat diet has little effect on carbon dioxide production. Therefore nutritional management should be possible without resorting to expensive enteral or parenteral products designed to lower carbon dioxide production and the respiratory quotient.

Hepatic Failure

Up to 65% of patients receiving parenteral nutrition have altered liver function (as indicated by increased aspartate aminotransferase and alkaline phosphatase levels). Some ICU patients have hepatic steatosis or fatty infiltration of the liver because of overfeeding. Therefore all ICU patients receiving nutritional support need liver function monitoring.

For patients with preexisting liver disease, nutrition regimens may need further modification. Patients receiving enteral antibiotics or lactulose tolerate tube feedings poorly. Depending on the extent of disease, water, sodium, and protein restriction may be needed as well.

Hepatic encephalopathy is associated with elevated levels of the aromatic amino acids and decreased amounts of branched-chain amino acids. Nutrition products have been formulated with elevated levels of branched-chain amino acids and decreased levels of methionine and aromatic amino acids. However, since hepatic encephalopathy has a number of causes, not all patients benefit from such regimens.

In summary, the recommendation for patients with liver disease is not to overfeed; to restrict water, sodium, and protein (0.8 to 1.2 g protein/kg/d) as necessary; to give mineral and vitamin supplements; and to use specialized formulas *only* for patients who have hepatic encephalopathy and show benefit. If hepatic encephalopathy does not improve, the expense of specialized formulas is difficult to justify, since they do not have salutary effects on liver function itself.

Postoperative Treatment

Postoperative patients undergo an obligatory catabolic period, and many clinicians believe this period cannot be shortened by intervention. Therefore many patients receive no nutrition intervention during the perioperative period and begin dietary intake postoperatively only when they request it. That these patients do well is testament to their preoperative nutritional status and perhaps relatively minor surgical stress. For a significant number of surgical patients, however, including those who are malnourished preoperatively and those with a significant stress response in the perioperative period, the catabolic period is indefinite and continues unabated with an increased risk of complications, including sepsis and multiple–organ system failure. Although it is true that an obligatory catabolic period follows surgery, effective interventions can limit its duration. Studies have found that perioperative nutritional support can improve wound healing, decrease perioperative complications, and decrease hospital stay and cost. However, such nutrition is only supportive; it does not replace but complements standard perioperative interventions designed to decrease complications.

Paramount in nutritional support is the preoperative recognition of malnourished patients. They should receive nutritional support before surgery in all but emergency situations. Well-nourished and moderately well-nourished patients must be assessed 3 to 5 days postoperatively. If they have not begun or cannot begin consuming an adequate diet, intervention should be planned. No patient should be allowed to remain NPO for greater than 10 days without commencing alimentation either parenterally or enterally.

The preceding discussion of nutrition assessment and the composition of the diet is germane to treatment of the perioperative patient, but particular emphasis must be given to the protein content of the nutrition regimen. Supplying adequate protein (1 to 1.4 g/kg/d) is the most important means of shortening the catabolic period and putting the patient in positive nitrogen balance. Studies in which branched-chain amino acids were administered to postoperative patients have shown that they improve nitrogen balance without improving survival; their role in postoperative management is yet to be defined.

Tube Feeding

Once having decided to intervene, the clinician should make all efforts to use the enteral route to supply nutrients. Not only is enteral nutrition less expensive and more like normal body function, but it may decrease the incidence of stress-related gastric ulceration, bacteremia, and sepsis. If nutrients are supplied parenterally, the intestines atrophy; this atrophy coupled with a depletion in the body's glutamine stores may break down the intestine's mucosal brush border and impair an important defense against acid in the stomach and bacterial invasion in the intestine.

Indications and Contraindications

Supplemental or total enteral nutrition should be considered whenever a patient has inadequate oral nutrition for 5 days or when the patient's intake is less than 50% of desired for the previous 7 to 10 days. Malnourished patients should begin receiving enteral nutrition sooner. Patients with dysphagia, those who are unable or unwilling to eat, anorectic burn patients, patients with small bowel resections (who need nutrition to stimulate anabolism in the remaining intestine), and patients with enterocutaneous fistulas (fed distal to the fistula if the fistula is proximal and vice versa) should all be considered candidates for enteral nutrition by whichever route works best.

The contraindications to enteral nutrition include complete mechanical obstruction, ileus, severe diarrhea, high-output fistulas, severe pancreatitis, and shock. It should not be used when aggressive nutritional support is unwarranted or refused by the patient.

Routes

The nasal route is preferred for ICU patients who have an intact and functioning gastrointestinal tract but are unable to eat (for example, because of an endotracheal tube, stroke, coma, or oral surgery). A small-bore Silastic nasogastric tube, usually with a weighted radiopaque tip, can be inserted with relative ease, is well tolerated, and is easy to maintain. After placement but before use, the tube's location must be confirmed by roentgenogram. These catheters have been mistakenly placed in the trachea with catastrophic consequences.

Gastric residuals must be checked periodically, depending on the patient's status, because large stomach residuals lead to an increased risk of aspiration. For a patient receiving a continuous infusion of enteral products, gastric residuals of greater than twice the hourly rate for patients receiving up to 50 ml/h, or 150% of the hourly rate for patients receiving more than 50 ml/h, necessitate stopping the infusion. For patients receiving bolus infusions, the residuals should be less than 100 ml before the next feeding. If the residual is excessive, it is rechecked in 1 hour. If it is still excessive, the patient should be evaluated for complicating factors, such as a developing ileus. However, if the residual has decreased, the feedings can be reinstituted but at a lower rate or volume. If problems persist and an intestinal disorder can be ruled out, the clinician should consider passing the feeding tube past the pylorus into the duodenum and small intestine.

For patients at risk of aspiration, access to the duodenum and jejunum is possible with long, weighted tubes. Occasionally these tubes pass into the jejunum on their own. If not, placing the patient in a modified right lateral decubitus position and administering metoclopramide 10 mg intravenously may increase gastric motility and cause the tube to pass beyond the pylorus. If this is not successful, the tube may be manipulated under fluoroscopic guidance in the radiology department.

Gastrotomy. Enterostomies are indicated when long-term feeding is anticipated or when nasal or esophageal obstruction eliminates the nasal route from consideration. Several surgical techniques can be used to create a gastrotomy, but despite its relative simplicity, the use of this technique in critically ill patients may lead to serious complications in 15% to 25% of patients and even death. Percutaneous endoscopic gastrotomy is becoming the preferred technique; it can be performed at the bedside with little or no sedation, and the rare complications are usually related to infection or dislodgment of the gastrotomy tube. Previous abdominal surgery or any condition that makes it impossible to oppose the anterior gastric wall to the abdominal wall is a contraindication to this technique, as is disease of the gastric wall, obstruction of the gastrointestinal tract, or a fistula in the stomach or proximal small bowel.

In patients with significant risk of aspiration, jejunal tubes may be placed surgically or endoscopically at the time of the gastrotomy.

Jejunostomy. Needle catheter jejunostomy is gaining acceptance as an alimentation route in patients undergoing laparotomy for other reasons. Indications include malnutrition, planned postoperative nutritional support, limited vascular access, and the need to deliver medications that might otherwise require a central venous catheter. At the time of surgery the catheter is tunneled for about 6 cm in the jejunal wall before being inserted into the jejunal lumen for 30 to 45 cm.

Complications are rare and include intestinal obstruction at the entrance site, infection, intraabdominal leakage of enteral feedings, and problems, such as diarrhea, that are related to the nutrition regimen. Catheter occlusion can be managed with forceful flushing or if necessary by passing a guidewire through the catheter. The needle catheter jejunostomy and the percutaneous placement of gastrotomy tubes obviate the need for formal feeding jejunostomies.

Formulations

A wide variety of enteral formulations are available, including modular diets in which the amount of each component (carbohydrate,

TABLE 27–5. Some Currently Available Enteral Nutrition Products

FORMULA	CALORIC DENSITY (kcal/ml)	NUTRIENTS PER 1000 CALORIES		
		PROTEIN (g) [% kcal]	FAT (g) [% kcal]	CARBOHYDRATE (g) [% kcal]
Modular Nutrient Support*				
Carbohydrate				
Polycose (Ross)	2.00 (4 kcal/g)			500 ml (250 g) [100%]
Moducal (Mead Johnson)	2.00 (4 kcal/g)			500 (250 g) [100%]
Fat				
MCT Oil (Mead Johnson)	7.70 (8.3 kcal/g)		130 ml [100%]	
Microlipid (Cheseborough-Ponds)	4.50		222 ml [100%]	
Protein				
Casec (Mead Johnson)	(4.0 kcal/g)	238 [95]	5 [5%]	0 [0%]
Pro Mod (Ross)	(4.2 kcal/g)	129 [71]	21.4 [19]	24 [10]
Blended Foodstuffs†				
Complete (Sandoz)	1.07	43 [16]	43 [36]	128 [48]
Complete-Modified (Sandoz)	1.07	43 [16]	37 [30]	141 [54]
Lactose Containing‡				
CIB (Carnation)	1.10	60 [21]	36 [29]	136 [50]
Meritene Liquid (Sandoz)	0.96	58 [24]	32 [30]	110 [46]
Sustacal Powder (Mead Johnson)	1.33	77 [24]	34 [22]	180 [54]
Lactose Free§				
Hypercaloric				
Sustacal HC (Mead Johnson)	1.50	61 [16]	58 [34]	190 [50]
Travasorb MCT (Travenol)	1.50	74 [20]	50 [30]	185 [50]
Ensure Plus (Ross)	1.50	55 [15]	53 [32]	200 [53]
Twocal HN (Ross)	2.00	83 [17]	90 [40]	216 [43]
Normocaloric				
Osmolite (Ross)	1.06	37 [14]	38 [31]	145 [55]
Isocal (Mead Johnson)	1.06	34 [13]	44 [37]	132 [50]
Precision Isotonic (Sandoz)	1.00	29 [12]	30 [28]	144 [60]
Travasorb Liquid (Travenol)	1.06	34 [14]	35 [32]	136 [55]
Ensure HN (Ross)	1.06	44 [17]	36 [30]	141 [53]
Sustacal Liquid (Mead Johnson)	1.00	61 [24]	23 [21]	140 [55]
Monomeric (Elemental) Formulation‖				
Vivonex Std (Norwich Eaton)	1.00	20 [8]	1.5 [1]	23 [91]
Vital HN (Ross)	1.00	42 [17]	10 [9]	185 [74]
Criticare HN (Mead Johnson)	1.06	37.5[14]	3.3 [3]	222 [83]
Travasorb HN (Travenol)	1.00	45 [18]	13 [12]	175 [70]

*Specific nutrients to be added; not nutritionally complete; contents per 1000 ml unless otherwise specified.

†Contain nondigestible residue; may or may not contain lactose; require intact bowel function; protein fat, carbohydrate based on blended mix of food; not intended for oral use.

‡Moderate to low residue; milk base; protein intact; semipurified isolates; high molecular weight; carbohydrate — lactose, sucrose, corn syrup solids; hyperosmolar; palatable; designed as oral supplement.

§Moderate to low residue; protein intact; semipurified isolates; high molecular weight; derived from casein salts or egg white solids; carbohydrate — starches, maltodextrins; glucose oligosaccharides, corn syrup solids; fat contributes greater percentage of calories; fat as corn oil, soy oil, MCT; isomolar as well as hyperosmolar; palatable.

‖Minimal residue; lactose free; assimilated readily with little or no digestion; protein predigested (hydrolyzed protein, dipeptides and tripeptides, or crystalline amino acids); fat — small amount of essential fatty acids with or without medium-chain triglycerides; hyperosmolar; poor palatability; designed primarily for tube feeding.

protein, fat, minerals, vitamins, and water) can be varied to meet the patient's exact calculated needs. Such diets are expensive and time consuming to prepare; for most patients a complete or prepackaged formula is adequate (Table 27–5). Complete diets can be divided into polymeric and monomeric formulas.

Polymeric products are composed of whole protein, fat, polysaccharides, and disaccharides. They have a high molecular weight and low osmolality. They tend to be less expensive than monomeric formulas but require an intact gastrointestinal tract for digestion and absorption of nutrients. Formulas may contain lactose or be lactose free and may be hypercaloric or normocaloric. Normocaloric formulas can be further divided into isosmotic and hyperosmotic formulas and those with higher or lower nitrogen

NON-PROTEIN NITROGEN: kcal	NUTRIENTS PER 1000 CALORIES			VOLUME (ml) TO MEET VITAMIN REQUIREMENTS
	OSMOLALITY (mOsm/kg)	SODIUM (mg/mEq)	POTASSIUM (mg/mEq)	
	850	29/1.1	10/0.26	
	725	18/0.6	10/0.3	
		410/18	27/0.7	
		460/21	2300/59	
1:131	405	1300/56	1400/36	1500
1:131	300	670/29	1400/36	1500
1:92	677-715	966/42	2808/72	1373
1:79	505+	880/38	1600/41	1250
1:80	700-1010	1200/54	3400/87	800
1:134	650	840/37	1480/38	1200
1:100	488	524/23	1480/38	
1:146	600	1141/50	2113/54	1600
1:126	740	1052/46	2316/59	950
1:153	300	634/28	1014/26	1887
1:167	300	530/23	1320/34	1887
1:183	300	770/34	960/25	1560
1:154	488	738/32	1266/33	1896
1:125	470	930/40	1564/40	1320
1:79	625	941/41	2085/53	1080
1:281	550	468/20.4	1172/30.0	1800
1:125	460	467/20.3	1333/34.1	1500
1:148	650	634/27.6	1323/33.8	1892
1:126	560	920/40.0	1170/30.0	2000

content. The exact composition of the protein is less critical, but some products contain high concentrations of branched-chain amino acids (advocated for severely stressed patients) or essential amino acids (for renal failure patients). Unless clear indications exist for these products, most patients' needs can be met with polymeric compounds containing whole protein.

Monomeric or elemental formulas are made up of compounds requiring little digestive and absorptive capability. They contain free amino acids or short-chain peptides, oligosaccharides, and medium-chain triglycerides with small amounts of essential fatty acids. They tend to have high osmolality because of the low molec-ular weight of their constituents, are expensive, and are not very palatable, so they are usually given by tube feeding.

Selection of an appropriate formula thus rests on cost factors and on the patient, including the status of the gastrointestinal tract, the extent of malnutrition, the presence or absence of enzyme deficiencies, the degree of stress, and the presence or absence of extenuating factors, such as diarrhea, ileus, and specific disease states (for example, respiratory, hepatic, or renal failure).

Osmolality. The greater the osmolality of the infused nutrients, the higher the incidence of gastrointestinal side effects, such as distention, bloating, cramps, and diarrhea. In general the elemental diets are more hyperosmolar than the polymeric ones, but any hyperosmolar formula may require dilution to a physiologic osmolality before being fed to the patient. Although diluting formulas to make them hypoosmotic is common practice, there is little physiologic justification for this maneuver.

Calories. Caloric requirements in an enteral feeding regimen are calculated based on the patient's individual needs. The majority of commercially available enteral formulas contain 1 kcal/ml of product; a few products with 1.5 to 2 kcal/ml are designed for patients who are volume restricted or have unusually high caloric requirements. Animals fed enterally after an injury have a slower metabolic response to injury; therefore in an ICU patient fed enterally the RMR should be checked periodically to match the caloric load to the patient's needs.

Protein. Since the amount of enteral formula a patient receives is usually dictated by caloric and fluid requirements, and the protein content of the complete products is fixed (usually at a kilocalorie/nitrogen ratio of 150:1, range 100:1 to 200:1), not all patients receive the amount of protein they require. Protein replacement should be guided by nitrogen balance studies. Patients' requirements should be met by adjustment of the quantity of product administered if possible, a change to a product with a different protein density, or the addition of protein to the formula.

Fat. The fat sources for enteral products have traditionally received little attention except in the elemental diets, in which medium-chain triglycerides and small amounts of essential fatty acids are supplied. For the complete products milk or vegetable oil is used as the fat. Enteral products with increased fat content have been advocated for patients with pulmonary disease, but no study has convincingly demonstrated their usefulness.

Vitamins, Minerals, and Trace Elements. The majority of formulas supply 100% of the RDAs for vitamins, minerals, and trace elements if administered in sufficient quantity (1500 to 1800 ml/d). If less than the required amount of formula is administered or deficiencies are detected, vitamin and mineral supplements are needed.

Water. The amount of free water in enteral products varies. Since the free water requirement of an adult is approximately 1 ml/kcal provided, the amount of water that must be supplemented can be calculated if the amount of free water in the product is known. Dehydration is seldom a problem in ICU patients receiving enteral products.

Complications

The majority of complications related to enteral nutrition have to do with tube placement and the composition and rate of the feeding (Table 27–6). Tube placement should be checked by radiologic techniques when possible. Since hyperosmotic formulas are associated with distention, ileus, or diarrhea, formulas can be diluted to an isosmotic concentration. ICU patients tolerate continuous feedings better than bolus feedings, but no method is perfect. If the gastric route is used, the solution is started at 25 ml/h and the osmolality of the solution is increased to the maximum before the rate of formula administration is advanced (usually by 25 ml/h every 12 to 24 hours). If the feeding is administered into the small intestine, the necessary volume should be achieved first, advancing by 25 ml/h per day, before the osmolality of the formula is increased. Rate and concentration should not be varied simultaneously.

The most dreaded complication of enteral feeding is aspiration leading to pneumonitis. In critically ill patients and those receiving mechanical ventilation, the risk of aspiration is sometimes considered to outweigh the benefits of enteral nutrition. However, if guidelines are followed and enteral tubes are placed in the duodenum and jejunum when indicated, enteral

TABLE 27–6. Common Tube Feeding Problems and Their Causes

Vomiting

Improper tube placement
Tube too large
Rate of feeding too fast
Residual volume from previous feeding too great
Osmolality of feeding too high
Medications given with feeding

Diarrhea

Rate of feeding too high
Osmolality of feeding too high
Intolerance to formula ingredients (e.g., lactose)
Medications (e.g., antibiotics)
Severe protein-calorie malnutrition
Malabsorption
Bacterial overgrowth

Constipation

Lack of bulk in diet
Inadequate fluid
Lack of activity

nutrition has a role even if a patient is intubated and is being mechanically ventilated.

Other means of averting pulmonary and gastrointestinal complications include elevating the head of the patient's bed to a 30-degree angle and checking gastric residuals every shift or more often if indicated for continuous infusions or before each feeding for bolus infusions. If residuals are excessive or distention is a problem, reduction in osmolality or in the rate of administration may be indicated. Metoclopramide may be indicated for patients with delayed gastric emptying.

Diarrhea is a common problem with enteral nutrition. Not only do the osmolality and volume contribute to diarrhea, but it is also associated with lactase deficiencies, widespectrum antibiotic use, bacterial overgrowth, and hypoalbuminemia. A majority of patients can tolerate enteral feedings if the osmolality and rate are decreased and time is allowed for adaptation. If these changes do not work, switching products or adding an antidiarrheal agent should be considered.

Patients receiving enteral nutrition are at the same risk for metabolic sequelae, including hyponatremia, hyperkalemia, hypophosphatemia, and hyperglycemia, as patients receiving parenteral nutrition. These conditions can be readily treated, but they underscore the importance of routine monitoring.

Techniques

Before a patient can be given enteral alimentation, a feeding tube must be inserted. Based on the nutritional assessment, a formula is chosen that meets the patient's caloric, nitrogen, water, and other requirements. The majority of patients can be fed enterally with one of the less expensive formulas such as Osmolite or Isocal. A lactose-free product is used in critically ill patients because of the high probability of a transient lactase deficiency. Some nutrition experts advocate elemental diets such as Vivonex or Vital for patients with gastrointestinal dysfunction or those who have not been allowed oral intake for extended periods; if these are tolerated, they are replaced with a less expensive product. Patients with fluid restrictions can be given Magnacal or Polycose, which have high caloric densities. Patients with specific diseases might benefit from specialized formulas, such as Hepatic-aid or Travasorb Hepatic for patients with liver failure. Initiation of the feedings should follow a standardized or systematic approach. The solution should be isosmotic and started at an infusion rate of 25 ml/h. Residuals should be checked frequently; if symptoms develop or the residual is greater than the amount given in the preceding hour, the rate should be decreased. As already mentioned, the rate (for jejunal feedings) or osmolality (for gastric feedings) is increased every 12 to 24 hours until the desired rate or osmolality is achieved. Once a given rate or osmolality is reached, the other component is increased each day as tolerated until the desired rate or concentration is achieved.

Bolus gastric feedings can be given by the enteral route but carry a higher risk of aspiration. A rate of 30 ml/min and a volume of less than 350 ml per feeding appear to be the maximum patients can tolerate.

Parenteral Nutrition

Indications and Contraindications

In parenteral nutrition a patient's required nutrients are delivered intravenously. Parenteral nutrition can meet partial or complete needs and can supply enough substrate to either maintain nutritional status or replete a malnourished patient. Both the American College of Physicians and the American Society for Parenteral and Enteral Nutrition have recently published guidelines for the use of this important clinical therapy.

Parenteral nutrition should be administered to patients unable to absorb nutrients from the gastrointestinal tract; those with malignancy undergoing intensive treatment, such as bone marrow transplantation, chemotherapy or radiotherapy, which renders them unable to eat, digest, or absorb adequate nutrients; patients with severe acute pancreatitis; malnourished patients whose gastrointestinal tract will be nonfunctional for 5 to 7 days (if the patient is significantly stressed, earlier intervention is required); and severely catabolic patients with or without malnutrition if the gastrointestinal tract is not considered usable within 5 to 7 days.

Parenteral nutrition may also be useful in the following situations: well-nourished patients undergoing major surgery who are not expected to be able to resume an oral diet within 7 to 10 days; patients with moderate stress who cannot resume an oral diet within 7 to 10 days; patients with enterocutaneous fistulas; patients with inflammatory bowel disease unresponsive to

TABLE 27–7. Complications of Parenteral Therapy

COMPLICATION	CAUSE	SIGNS AND SYMPTOMS	TREATMENT	PREVENTION
Major Technical Complications				
Catheter insertion				
Pneumothorax	Subclavian venipuncture; unusual anatomy	Dsypnea; chest pain; cyanosis	Observation if small Chest tube if large or progressive	Use internal jugular vein for high-risk patients
	Improper training			Trained/approved by physician
	Multiple punctures			Stop after several attempts and get help
	Failure to remove positive pressure ventilation			Stop ventilating during thrust of needle
Malposition	Anatomic	Pain or tingling in ear or neck	Reposition with fluoroscopy or new puncture; catheter removal	Proper position if possible
Arterial puncture	Incorrect insertion	Hematoma; may lead to tracheal obstruction	Pressure to puncture site; close patient observation	Strict adherence to technique
Catheter embolism	Shearing off of catheter	Cardiac irritability	Radiologic or surgical removal	Never pull back catheter through needle
Air embolism	During catheter threading	Dsypnea; chest pain; cardiac arrest; etc.	Aspiration from heart; left side down in Trendelenburg position	Trendelenburg position; keep hub covered at all times
Catheter maintenance				
Air embolism	Tubing disconnection	Dsypnea; chest pain; cardiac arrest	As above; reconnect tubing	Tape connections; Luer-Loks
	Patent tract after removal of catheter	Dsypnea; chest pain; cardiac arrest		Ointment and/or occlusive dressing for 12-24 hours
Catheter obstruction	Mechanical (pump) failure; kink in catheter	Solutions stop running; occlusion alarm	Adjust pump; flush catheter	Hourly monitoring of solution
Thrombosis	Mechanical irritation; patient's hypercoagulable state	Distended veins and edema	Catheter removal; intravenous heparin; venogram	Not always possible; heparin in TPN solution; do not start TPN if low antithrombin III
Major Septic Complications				
Catheter-related sepsis	Inadequate asepsis; immunosuppression	Infected site; fever; increased white blood cells; septic shock	Remove catheter; cultures; blood culture; fluid; antibiotics	Rigid adherence to specific policies and procedures; inspection of catheter site for each dressing change procedure
Septic thrombosis	Untreated catheter sepsis; bacteremic seeding from unknown/other source	Above plus unilateral pain and swelling in arm, shoulder, and neck	Venogram; remove catheter and culture tip; intravenous heparin; antimicrobial therapy	Immediate response to suspected sepsis; periodic changes of catheter (i.e., new puncture or over guidewire) when other septic source known

TPN = total parenteral nutrition, IV = intravenous, IM = intramuscular.

TABLE 27-7. Complications of Parenteral Therapy—cont'd

COMPLICATION	CAUSE	SIGNS AND SYMPTOMS	TREATMENT	PREVENTION
		Major Metabolic Complications		
Hyperglycemia	Diabetes mellitus	Elevated blood glucose; glycosuria	Regular insulin subcutaneously	Coordinate initiation and insulin requirement
	Too rapid initiation		Slow rate	Start slow with step increments (i.e., 1 L on day 1, 2 L on day 2, etc.)
	Infection/sepsis		Addition of regular insulin; slow rate until blood glucose stable	
	Drug related (i.e., steroids)		(may increase fat source for calories)	Advance more slowly
	Stress from major surgery		Slow rate or stop infusion	Decrease infusion rate during surgery
Hyperglycemic; hyperosmolar, nonketotic dehydration	Uncontrolled hyperglycemia	Elevated blood glucose level (500-1000 mg/dl or higher); coma; death	Stop hypertonic solution; hydration with free water; judicious doses of IV insulin and potassium; close monitoring	Immediate and proper control of blood glucose levels >200 mg/dl
Hypoglycemia	Sudden decrease or stop of infusion due to mechanical problem	Blood glucose in range of 40 mg/dl; lethargy	Bolus dextrose infusion; monitor serum glucose	Accurate administration with hourly patient monitoring
Hyperkalemia	Inability to utilize administered potassium; renal failure; shock	Cardia arrhythmias; bounding or diminished pulses	Stop infusion; change to low potassium solution	Close metabolic monitoring
Hypokalemia	Increased requirement with anabolism; excessive losses	Cardia arrhythmias; muscle weakness; impaired respiratory function	Increase potassium in solution; measure and replace losses	Close metabolic monitoring
Hypophosphatemia	Lack of phosphate supplementation; excessive use of phosphate binders (i.e., antacids); increased demand during anabolism	Lethargy; altered speech; peripheral paresthesias; increased respirations; coma	Add phosphate to solution; may require peripheral repletion; adjust amount per patient	Close metabolic monitoring; standard solutions
Hypocalcemia	Lack of or insufficient supplementation	Paresthesia; twitching; positive Chvostek's sign	Add or adjust calcium in solution	Close metabolic monitoring
Hypomagnesemia	Lack of or insufficient amounts of magnesium in solution	Tingling sensation around mouth; paresthesia; dizziness; disorientation	Add or adjust magnesium in solution	Standardized solutions; close metabolic monitoring
Essential fatty acid deficiency	Lack of fat supplement	Dry, scaly skin; hair loss	IV administration of 10% or 20% fat emulsion	Routinely include infusion each week
Vitamin K deficiency	Deficient oral intake; jaundice; antibiotics	Bleeding; purpura; increased prothrombin time	Weekly administration orally or IM of vitamin K	Monitoring prothrombin level
Iron deficiency	Excessive blood loss	Pallor; fatigue; listlessness; exertional dyspnea	IM iron (Dextran) or whole blood	Serial determination of hemoglobin and serum iron
Zinc deficiency	Chronic illness; catabolic states	Diarrhea, central nervous system disturbances, skin lesions, poor wound healing	Refeed and treat skin illness; addition of zinc to solution	Serial determination of serum zinc

medical therapy; patients with hyperemesis gravidarum of more than 5 to 7 days' duration; and patients in whom enteral nutrition cannot be established within 7 to 10 days.

Parenteral nutrition is of limited value in well-nourished patients with minimal stress or in the postoperative period of the gastrointestinal tract is functional within 10 days.

Parenteral nutrition should not be used if the patient has a functional gastrointestinal tract or is anticipated to require parenteral nutrition less than 5 days. Urgently needed surgery should not be delayed in favor of parenteral nutrition, nor should parenteral nutrition be used if the patient refuses, the prognosis does not warrant aggressive support, or the risks are judged to exceed the benefits.

Routes

Parenteral nutrition is administered by two routes: central and peripheral. If the patient's total nutrient needs are to be met parenterally, the osmolalities of the concentrated dextrose and amino acid formulas necessitate administration into a large-bore central vein such as the jugular or subclavian. Patients who can tolerate enteral nutrition, but not enough to meet their full requirements, may receive supplemental parenteral nutrition via a peripheral intravenous route. Lipid emulsions, which are all isosmotic, can be given peripherally, as can dilute glucose (5% to 10%) and amino acid (2% to 4%) solutions. Although the entire amount of nutrients could be given peripherally, the volume load would be prohibitively excessive. The complication rate is lower with peripheral parenteral alimentation, but for patients who need central alimentation its benefits outweigh the risks.

Formulations

Parenteral nutrition formulas are relatively unstable and are ideal media for bacteria. Therefore they are prepared in hospital pharmacies just before use. The most common practice is to compound the amino acid, glucose, vitamins, minerals, and trace elements into one formulation, which is given centrally, and then to give the lipid emulsions either peripherally or piggy-backed into the central line. In the increasingly popular 3-in-1 formulations, all the components are combined in one container that is infused over 24 hours. The preparation of such a solution requires special equipment and additional time in the pharmacy.

Carbohydrate. Dextrose monohydrate solutions of 70% concentration are used in parenteral nutrition formulas and are usually diluted to the desired concentration with amino acids. Since the glucose is hydrated, it supplies 3.4 kcal/g of glucose, and this figure should be used in calculating caloric content. In the United States other caloric sources, such as fructose and glycerol, are seldom used.

Lipids. Intravenous emulsions are given both as a source of calories and to avoid the sequelae of essential fatty acid deficiency. They are usually soybean or soybean-safflower blends that contain both omega-6 and omega-3 essential fatty acids. To avoid essential fatty acid deficiency these emulsions should be given once or twice a week; because lipid is used as a calorie source, it is more frequently given on a daily basis. Complications of intravenous lipid administration are less likely if the infusion is administered over 12 to 24 hours. As noted previously, all the available formulas are isosmotic and may be given peripherally.

Amino Acids. The amino acid solutions currently used in the United States are composed of synthetic crystalline amino acids. Although some institutions are able to adjust the proportions of the individual amino acids, the majority of hospitals use prepared amino acid formulas of varying concentration (9% to 15%).

Specialized formulas contain only essential amino acids for renal disease, branched-chain amino acids for moderately to severely stressed patients, or branched-chain amino acids with decreased aromatic amino acids for patients with hepatic disease. Such should be used only when benefit can be demonstrated.

Electrolytes. Electrolytes are part of some amino acid products. Since calcium is not contained in amino acid preparations and patients' needs vary, additional electrolytes must be added when the final product is mixed.

Vitamins. Several manufacturers offer standardized vitamin preparations that can be added to parenteral formulas for daily administration. The reports of several deaths during a recent national shortage of these preparations underscore their importance.

Trace Elements. See the previous discussion.

Complications

Parenteral nutrition can lead to a number of complications, the majority of which are associated with central alimentation. Complications can be related to mechanical problems associated with catheter placement and use, infection, and metabolic abnormalities (Table 27–7).

Having experienced personnel place and manage central lines is the critical determinant in decreasing the incidence of mechanical complications. The use of strict aseptic technique and a single dedicated central line that is not violated are the best measures to decrease the risk of infection. The use of silver-impregnated catheters for parenteral nutrition has not been explored. Judicious monitoring of the patient and laboratory values detects metabolic complications quickly (Table 27–4).

Techniques

Once having decided to use parenteral nutrition, the clinician must choose between central and peripheral therapy. If total parenteral nutrition (TPN) is chosen, a central line must be placed, preferably by personnel experienced with central lines and TPN. After roentgenographic confirmation of the catheter tip location in the vena cava, the TPN solution may be started.

As discussed previously, the formula should provide 10% to 30% more kilocalories than the RMR, 1 to 1.4 g protein/kg/d, 60% to 80% of nonprotein calories as glucose (3 to 5 g/kg/d), and 20% to 40% of nonprotein calories as lipid (1 to 1.5 g/kg/d). Vitamins, electrolytes, and trace elements must be added according to the patient's needs. Most TPN solutions do not contain the large amounts of glucose that were once used, but it is still prudent to start the formula slowly and advance it to the target rate over 24 to 48 hours. Although hypoglycemia following abrupt termination of TPN is less a problem than in the past, TPN should also be discontinued gradually, usually by substitution of 10% dextrose for the TPN solution.

SUGGESTED READINGS

Abbott WC, Echenique MM, Bistrian BR, et al: Nutritional care of the trauma patient. Surg Gynecol Obstet 1983;157:585-597

Anderson CF, Loosbrock LM, Moxness KE: Nutrient intake in critically ill patients: too many or too few calories? Mayo Clin Proc 1986;61:853-858

ASPEN Board of Directors: Guidelines for use of total parenteral nutrition in the hospitalized adult patient. J Parenter Enter Nutr 1986;10:441-445

ASPEN Board of Directors: Guidelines for the use of enteral nutrition in the adult patient. J Parenter Enter Nutr 1987;11:435-439

Bursztein S, Elwin DH, Askanazi J, Kinney JM (eds): Energy metabolism, indirect calorimetry and nutrition. Baltimore, 1989, Williams & Wilkins

Cuthbertson DP, Fell GS, Smith CM, Tilstone WJ: Nutrition in the post-traumatic period. Nutr Metabol 1972; 14(suppl):92-109

Jeejeebhoy KN: Micronutrients—state of the art. In New aspects of clinical nutrition. Basel, 1983, Karger, pp 1-24

Kinney JM, Jeejeebhoy KN, Hill GL, Owen OE (eds): Nutrition and metabolism in patient care. Philadelphia, 1988, WB Saunders Co

Lang CE (Ed): Nutritional support in critical care. Rockville, Md, 1987, Aspen Publishers

Long CL, Crosby F, Geiger JW, Kinney JM: Parenteral nutrition in the septic patient: nitrogen balance, limiting plasma amino acids, and calorie to nitrogen ratios. Am J Clin Nutr 1976;29:380-391

Marvin JA: Nutritional support of the critically injured patient. Crit Care Nurs Q 1988;11:21-34

Negro F, and Cerra FB: Nutritional monitoring in the ICU: rational and practical application. Crit Care Clin 1988; 4:559-572

Pomposelli JJ, Flores EA, Bistrian BR: Role of biochemical mediators in clinical nutrition and surgical metabolism. J Parenter Enter Nutr 1988;12:212-218

Report of the 1988 ASPEN Research Workshop: the role of lipids in nutrition and disease. J Parenter Enter Nutr 1988;12:35S-138S

28

PAIN MANAGEMENT IN THE INTENSIVE CARE UNIT

ROBIN J. HAMILL, MD

Modalities to conquer pain have been sought for many centuries. In the last century advances have been dramatic, but much is left to be done. Delay in applying developments to patient care accounts for a great deal of this problem. Critical care medicine, on the other hand, is a relatively new field. Only lately has the significance of good pain management in critically ill patients been appreciated. Because of recent advances in technology, understanding of physiology, and the pharmacologic armamentarium, critical care physicians have become capable of more safely and effectively tailoring analgesic and anesthetic modalities to severely ill patients.

Pain or fear of pain is the most common complaint of ICU patients. Pain is stressful, and stress can be detrimental. The metabolic response to stress is well documented (Table 28–1). Although these physiologic changes are vital as part of the fight-or-flight response, under other circumstances, such as postoperative or posttraumatic pain, the hormonal, metabolic, cardiovascular, respiratory, and psychologic responses are not functional and can be deleterious. For example, an association exists between operative stress, as measured by intraoperative epinephrine and norepinephrine levels, and postoperative complications, such as congestive heart failure and renal insufficiency. The presumed mechanism is a catecholamine-induced increase in myocardial work and the diversion of blood flow from the gut, liver, and kidney.

Pain produces anxiety, disturbs sleep, and can cause confusion, delirium, and paranoia. Pain may cause muscle spasm after thoracotomy, laparotomy, or chest trauma. The results are

TABLE 28–1. Metabolic Stress Response

Endocrine

Increased adrenocorticotropic hormone, cortisol
Increased catecholamines
Increased growth hormone
Increased renin, angiotensin II, aldosterone, antidiuretic hormone
Net result: catabolic metabolism

Fluid-Electrolyte Balance

Water and sodium retention
Magnesium loss
Potassium loss
Net result: increased volume, hypokalemia, hypomagnesemia

Metabolic

Hyperglycemia from insulin resistance, gluconeogensis, glycogenolysis
Muscle and fat breakdown
Net result: over time, depletion of energy stores, muscle wasting and weakness, hypoproteinemia

Cardiovascular

Arteriole constriction (increased systemic vascular resistance, hypertension)
Venoconstriction (decreased venous capacitance)
Tachycardia
Increased myocardial contractility
Net result: increased myocardial oxygen consumption

Respiratory

Increased oxygen requirements
Increased ventilation-perfusion mismatch, hypoxia
Increased carbon dioxide production
Net result: increased work of breathing

Psychologic

Fear, anxiety, agitation
Net result: further increase in metabolic demand

From Wilson PR: Probl Anesth 1988;2(3):312-320. Adapted from Kehlet H: Pain relief and modification of the stress response. In Cousins MJ, Phillips GD (eds): Acute pain management. New York, 1986, Churchill Livingstone, p 49.

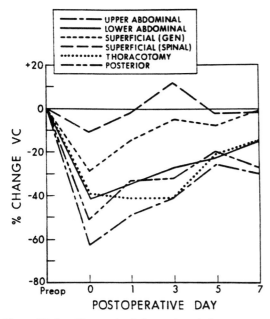

Figure 28–1. Changes in vital capacity relative to preoperative values for several surgical sites. Upper abdominal incisions show the most marked decrease in vital capacity. All sites other than superficial or spinal still show diminished vital capacities 1 week postoperatively. (From Ali J, Weisel RD, Laung AB, et al: Am J Surg 1974;128:376.)

decreased pulmonary volumes (Fig. 28–1), atelectasis, and poor clearance of secretions, all of which can lead to pneumonia. Studies have shown that good pain control improves pulmonary function as measured by objective findings and subjective patient reports. If poorly controlled, pain can cause tachycardia, hypertension, arrhythmias, and a subsequent increase in myocardial work and oxygen consumption. In a critically ill patient any one of these effects can be devastating and at least increases the risk of complications, prolongs ICU and hospital stay, and hence adversely affects outcome and increases expense. Control of pain by morphine administration to critically ill patients has been shown to decrease resting energy expenditures by 6% to 20% from premedication levels.

MECHANISMS OF PAIN

An understanding of pain physiology can be helpful in selecting optimal analgesic therapy. Acute pain is a protective mechanism, mediated by nociceptors, that warns of tissue injury. Nociceptors, found in many body tissues, including skin, blood vessels, subcutaneous tissue, muscle, fascia, periosteum, and joints, respond to thermal, chemical, or mechanical stimuli.

The noxious stimulus is carried by A-delta (larger, thinly myelinated) and C (unmyelinated, slow-conducting) afferent nerve fibers. Other nerve fiber classes, such as A-alpha, A-beta, and B fibers, are not involved in pain transmission. Visceral pain is carried by C fibers, which follow sympathetic afferents to the dorsal root ganglia. A-delta and C fibers carry somatic pain to the dorsal horns. Their cell bodies lie in the spinal ganglia. The fibers enter the dorsal horn posteriorly and synapse in the dorsal horn laminae I and V and the substantia gelatinosa (laminae II and III). From there fibers may synapse with autonomic preganglionic neurons or somatic neurons or ascend to the thalamus and subsequently other brain segments. These various synapses account for the multifaceted nature of pain and help to integrate the somatic, emotional, and hemodynamic responses to a painful stimulus.

Two spinal tracts transmit pain: the neospinothalamic and the paleospinothalamic. Impulses that account for sharp, well-defined, well-localized pain are carried by the neospinothalamic tract by way of the ventrolateral and posterior thalamus and subsequently terminate in the somatosensory cortex. The more primitive paleospinothalamic or spinoreticular tract has fibers projecting to the reticular formation, medulla, midbrain, periaqueductal gray matter, hypothalamus, and medial thalamus. These projections give rise to perceptions of burning, aching, dull, and poorly localized pain and also integrate the emotional perception of pain.

Pain is mediated by a number of vasoactive amines and neurotransmitters. Locally serotonin, bradykinin, histamine, prostaglandins (especially E_1 and E_2), and potassium ion released from damaged cells contribute to nociception. Vasoactive substances in the dorsal horn, especially lamina I and the substantia gelatinosa, modulate pain transmission. Substance P, released from unmyelinated fibers in the dorsal horn, stimulates nociceptive nerve endings, whereas somatostatin, released from different cells in the dorsal horn, is thought to be inhibitory.

Endogenous opioid peptides include endorphins, enkephalins, and dynorphin. Beta endorphin is active in the upper thalamus and midbrain periaqueductal gray matter. Evidence suggests that transcutaneous electrical nerve stimulation (TENS) and acupuncture act by stimulating beta endorphin release. Enkephalins and dynorphin are present in the spinal cord, midbrain, and hypothalamus. Input from the cortex, amygdala, hypothalamus, and brainstem goes to the periaqueductal gray matter. Efferent fibers descend from the periaqueductal gray matter by way of the medulla to the spinal cord. These neurons can inhibit nociception.

Four types of opioid receptors have been described: mu, delta, kappa, and sigma. The mu receptor can be activated by morphine, beta endorphin or met-enkephalin, causing profound analgesia to thermal, chemical, and pressure stimuli. Leu-enkephalin, met-enkephalin, and beta endorphin act at the delta receptor, but the delta receptor is a less potent mediator of antinociception than the mu receptor. Another type of receptor, the kappa receptor, acts much like the mu receptor but is ineffective against thermal stimuli. Pentazocine predominantly affects the kappa receptor. The sigma receptor is responsible for dysphoric and hallucinogenic characteristics of various narcotics, such as pentazocine, but is not known to have analgesic qualities. Table 28–2 summarizes the effects of the opiate receptors and their agonists and antagonists. Subclasses of each receptor type may be defined with further research.

In 1965 Melzack and Wall devised the gate control theory of pain. This postulates that stimulation of large, nonnociceptive fibers that enter laminae II and III adjacent to small nociceptive fibers modifies pain transmission. These large fibers inhibit the smaller fiber cells in the substantia gelatinosa. Fibers from the cortex of the brain to the dorsal horn further control the "gate" and hence the transmission of pain. For example, the reticulospinal pathway has inhibitory input into lamina V of the dorsal horn. This is thought to be mediated by serotonin, a major pain-inhibiting neurotransmitter.

TABLE 28–2. Opioid Substances and Their Interaction with Opiate Receptors

	MU	DELTA	KAPPA	SIGMA
Morphine	+		+	0
Beta endorphin	+	+		
Met-enkephalin	+	+		
Leu-enkephalin		+		
Pentazocine	−		+	+
Butorphanol	0		+	+
Nalbuphine	−		(+)	(+)
Buprenorphine	(+)			0
Naloxone	−	−	−	(−)

+ = agonist, − = antagonist, (+) = partial agonist,
(−) = partial antagonist, 0 = no significant action.
  Modified from Jaffee JH, Martin WR: Opioid analgesics and antagonists. In Gilman AG, Goodman LS, Rall TW, Murad F (eds): The pharmacological basis of therapeutics, ed 7. New York, 1985, Macmillan, Inc.

The perception and interpretation of pain depend on many factors, including environmental influences, emotional state, social expectations, fatigue, and secondary gain issues. The reticular activating system and limbic structures mediate these motivational and affective inputs. It is by way of these pathways that concentration and hypnosis can inhibit pain.

When treating acute pain in the ICU, the caregiver must be sensitive to aspects of pain perception much more complex than the location and size of incision. Fatigue, fear, and anxiety are significant components of pain in most critically ill patients. Appropriate explanations, psychologic support, sedatives, and sleep medications help relieve the patient's distress.

PATIENT ASSESSMENT

Much of the pain in critical care units results from trauma, surgery, or immobility. Proper treatment of pain requires an assessment of its severity, a task at which clinicians are notoriously poor. No scientific or mathematical means of measuring pain exist. Furthermore, ICU patients have difficulty expressing the source and severity of their pain because of endotracheal tubes, sedatives, restraints, neuromuscular blockade, and the like. Numerous studies have shown a significant discrepancy between the health care provider's perception of the patient's pain and the patient's perception. In a study of 93 U.S. burn centers, 70% of the health care providers assessed adult patients' pain during "tanking" for debridement as "moderate," although the meperidine doses varied from 25 to 375 mg for this procedure. The patients, in contrast, tended to rate the pain as "excruciating," "severe," and "the worst pain ever experienced." The review found that narcotic administration to burned children was even less consistent. Those providing therapy assessed the pain as less severe than the patients did, and narcotics were frequently not given at all, despite burns of comparable severity to those in the adults.

When assessing pain in critically ill patients, what does the practitioner look for? Verbal complaints are helpful but frequently not possible. Three possible responses to painful stimuli are avoidance, autonomic response, and higher level perception, interpretation, and modification. Critical care physicians modify and inhibit expression of these responses. The primary concerns in the ICU tend to be treatment of segmental and suprasegmental reflexes, including muscle spasm, hyperventilation, and automonic and endocrine responses, since these complicate treatment of an unstable, critically ill patient. Yet, physicians also have an obligation to address the higher level integrative responses, such as psychologic trauma, fear, helplessness, and sleep deprivation that ICU interventions inflict on patients. Confusion, paranoia, delirium, and agitation are common manifestations of inadequate pain control. All of these can significantly increase sympathetic nervous system activity.

Another possible reaction to pain, most notably seen in injured animals, is a primitive response of depression, withdrawal, and immobility to facilitate healing. The clinician cannot assume that absence of overt pain expression rules out the presence of significant pain. Children often use this coping mechanism and also frequently lack the verbal skills to express their pain or fear. Probably 95% of the patients in a general ICU have significant pain. Even an elderly patient with severe chronic obstructive pulmonary disease (COPD) and respiratory failure has substantial discomfort from the endotracheal tube and the immobility imposed by long-standing osteoarthritis. Perhaps the question intensivists should ask themselves is, "Why should we *not* treat this patient for pain?", rather than the reverse.

When determining a mode of pain control, the physician must consider a number of issues. Patients' needs and abilities vary. A 21-year-old man with a flail chest and fractured femur has needs very different from a 48-year-old woman with intraabdominal sepsis, multisystem organ failure including adult respiratory distress syndrome, and a minute ventilation of 20 L, or from a 70-year-old man with an exacerbation of COPD and respiratory failure. Each patient is unique and can be treated for pain in a number of ways.

Several questions may help direct the caregivers. Is the patient alert and mentally capable of self-administering therapy? Is sedation desirable? What is the source of the pain: somatic or visceral, discrete or diffuse? Is respiratory depression a concern (that is, is the patient receiving mechanical ventilation or not, being weaned or not weanable)? Is analgesia required for an extended period (hours to days) or briefly as during a procedure? Will underlying sepsis, hepatic or renal dysfunction, or cardiovascular instability influence therapy? In general, if the clinical situation is suitable, regional techniques are preferable to systemic, an alert and cooperative patient is more desirable than an obtunded one, and patient involvement in therapy is preferable to that based on the caregiver's interpretation of pain behavior.

MEDICATIONS

Parenteral Analgesia

The analgesic drugs used in the ICU include narcotic agonists, narcotic partial agonists (buprenorphine [Buprenex]), agonist-antagonists (butorphanol [Stadol] and nalbuphine [Nubain]), and ketamine.

The characteristics of a desirable analgesic in the critically ill patient are good analgesia without cardiorespiratory depression and pharmacodynamics uninfluenced by underlying renal or hepatic disease. The drug should have rapid onset and a short half-life, making it easy to titrate in an unstable patient (Table 28–3). Ideally the drug allows the patient to remain awake but relaxed, calm, and capable of voluntary motion. The patient can move spontaneously in physical therapy, which decreases the incidence of thrombophlebitis, stasis ulcers, and muscle wasting. Sedative medication is used as a supplement to maintain a near-normal wake-sleep cycle.

Morphine and fentanyl are the narcotic agonists most frequently used in the ICU. Morphine is inexpensive and has excellent analgesic qualities and some sedative effect. Its half-life is relatively short, although longer than those of the newer synthetic narcotics. Regardless of the route of administration, it may cause nausea and vomiting, increased smooth muscle tone and sphincter spasm, decreased gastrointestinal motility, and pruritus. Morphine also causes histamine release, which can result in hypotension and bronchospasm. Fentanyl, another excellent analgesic, causes less cardiovascular lability than morphine, although its vagotonic effects can decrease heart rate. It is well tolerated when given by bolus or infusion, but it is more expensive than morphine. Fentanyl and sufentanil both decrease cerebral metabolism and intracranial pressure, although sufentanil offers less cardiovascular lability and better brain relaxation for neurosurgical procedures. Sufentanil does not otherwise add significantly to the benefits of fentanyl.

Alfentanil administered as an infusion is finding increasing use. Alfentanil has a short elimination half-life (100 minutes), and therefore its action, particularly its respiratory depression, is rapidly reversed. In a study of

TABLE 28–3. Narcotic-Type Analgesics for Moderate to Severe Pain

NAME	ROUTE(S)	EQUIANALGESIC DOSE (mg)*	DURATION (h)	PLASMA HALF-LIFE (h)	PRECAUTIONS
		Morphinelike Agonists			
Morphine sulfate (MS)	IM/SC	10	4-6	2-3.5	Use with caution in patients with bronchial asthma, impaired ventilation, increased intracranial pressure with hypoventilation, or liver failure; lower doses for older patients
	PO	60†	4-7		
	IV	10‡			
	IT	¹⁄₆₀ of the 24-hour dose of MS (IM)			
	ED	⅒ of the 24-hour dose of MS (IM)			
	PR	60‡			
Meperidine (Demerol)	IM	75	4-5	3-4 (Plasma half-life of normeperidine is 12-16 hours)	Normeperidine accumulates with chronic use causing central nervous system excitation and seizures; do not use in patients with impaired renal function or who are receiving monoamine oxidase inhibitors; like morphine
	PO	300	4-6		
	IV	75‡			
Methadone (Dolophine)	IM/SC	10	1-6	15-30	May accumulate with chronic use causing excessive sedation and other side effects; same as morphine; requires careful titration in initial dosage to avoid accumulation
	PO	20			
	IV	10‡			
Levorphanol (Levodromoran)	IM/SC	2	4-6	12-16	Same as methadone
	PO	4	4-7		
	IV	2‡			
Hydromorphone (Dilaudid)	IM/SC	1.5	4-5	2-3	Same as morphine
	PO	7.5	4-6		
	IV	1.5‡			
	PR	7.5‡			
Oxymorphone (Numorphan)	IM	1	4-6	2-3	Same as morphine
	PR	10			
Codeine	IM	130	4-6	3	Same as morphine
	PO	200			
		Mixed Agonist-Antagonists			
Pentazocine (Talwin)	IM	60	4-6	2-3	Psychotomimetic effects; may precipitate withdrawal in physically dependent patients
	PO	180	4-7		
Nalbuphine (Nubain)	IM	10	4-6	5	Like pentazocine; fewer psychomimetic effects; may precipitate withdrawal in physically dependent patients
	IV	10‡			
Butorphanol (Stadol)	IM	2	4-6	2.5-3.5	Like pentazocine
	IV				
		Partial Agonists			
Buprenorphine (Temgesic)	IM	0.4	4-6	Unknown	May precipitate withdrawal in physically dependent patients
	SL	0.8	5-6		

*E quianalgesic dose based on single-dose studies when the patient was experiencing moderate to severe pain.

†With repetitive doses when the patient is medicated before the onset of moderate to severe pain, the equianalgesic dose, based on clinical experience, is 1:3 not 1:6.

‡Estimated equianalgesic dose based on clinical practice nct on controlled studies.

Ab: IM = intramuscular, SC = subcutaneous, PO = orally, ED = epidural, IT = intrathecal, PR = rectally, SL = sublingual.

Modified from Coyle N: Nurs Clin North Am 1987;22(3):734-735.

postoperative cardiac patients an initial bolus of alfentanil 1 mg followed by an infusion of 0.25 µg/kg/min for up to 19 hours resulted in good ventilator tolerance and adequate analgesia. Within 4 hours of discontinuation of infusion, all patients were extubated and showed no evidence of respiratory depression. This may be due in part to development of tolerance to the respiratory depressant effects after prolonged infusion.

Meperidine can cause tachycardia and is a much more potent myocardial depressant than morphine. Its use in a long-term infusion is not recommended because of the potential for neuropsychiatric effects. The accumulation of normeperidine, the *N*-demethylated metabolite of meperidine, causes progressive neuronal excitation. Delirium, hallucinations, paranoia, myoclonus, and seizures occur. Toxic reactions may be evident as early as the first day of infusion and with blood levels as low as 128 ng/ml. Seizures occur at blood levels greater than 400 ng/ml. Because renal dysfunction decreases clearance of both meperidine and normeperidine, patients with renal failure are much more likely to exhibit toxic reactions.

Use of levorphanol and hydromorphone has not been extensively studied in critically ill patients, but these agents offer little benefit over morphine or fentanyl.

Buprenorphine (Buprenex) is a morphinelike narcotic partial agonist. Its analgesic action is similar to morphine's but without psychomimetic effects. It is reputed to have a plateau effect in terms of respiratory depression, a characteristic that may make it useful in patients not receiving mechanical ventilation. Buprenorphine can cause orthostatic hypotension and can also cause withdrawal when administered to patients physically dependent on narcotics.

Butorphanol (Stadol) and nalbuphine (Nubain) are nalorphine-like narcotic agonist-antagonists. Butorphanol probably has little use in the ICU. It causes significant sedation, but is a less potent analgesic than morphinelike medications. It commonly causes disorientation and dysphoria and, like buprenorphine, can initiate narcotic withdrawal. Nalbuphine is a less potent analgesic than morphine, but its analgesic effects are additive to those of narcotic agonists. Several characteristics make nalbuphine unique. In low doses, it partially reverses the respiratory depression occurring with narcotic overdosage. It has been known to reverse sphincter spasm and narcotic-induced biliary pain without reversing the analgesic and sedative effects of the narcotics. It has little or no cardiovascular or psychotropic effect. Pentazocine (Talwin) is another agonist-antagonist drug. Like butorphanol it causes dysphoria and hallucinations. Therefore, it has *no* place in the ICU.

Ketamine, a nonbarbiturate dissociative anesthetic related to phencyclidine, produces profound analgesia. Because ketamine stimulates the sympathetic nervous system, it maintains blood pressure in critically ill patients better than do other analgesics. It must be used with care, however, because it can cause significant tachycardia and hypertension or can produce direct myocardial depression. In patients who have a maximally stimulated sympathetic nervous system, whose central sympathetic system is not intact, or who have insufficient catecholamine, myocardial decompression may predominate. Large, rapidly given doses can cause respiratory depression. This effect may also occur with smaller doses if narcotics or barbiturates have been administered. Hallucinations sometimes occur but can be countered by concomitant benzodiazepine administration. Ketamine is contraindicated in patients with severe hypertension, myocardial disease, or increased intracranial pressure. However, its superb analgesia, amnesia, and sympathetic stimulation make it an excellent drug for painful interventions such as burn debridement, dressing changes, or abdominal irrigations. Ketamine's bronchodilatory and sedative properties also make it useful to assist mechanical ventilation in critically ill patients when other modes of sedation fail.

Regional Anesthesia

Drugs in a number of classes have been used to provide regional anesthesia. Obviously, these include local anesthetics. Narcotics, narcotic agonist-antagonists, partial agonists, ketamine, and clonidine have been added to paraspinal blocks. The choice of medication is determined by many factors, including location of block, desirability of sympathetic blockade with peridural blocks, need for muscle relaxation, and desired degree of mobility.

Of the local anesthetics, the esters are rapidly metabolized and hence are of little use in pain management. Of the amides, the longer-acting drugs (etidocaine and bupivacaine) are more useful and, because of lower cumulative dose, are less likely to have toxic effects. Since bupivacaine offers a less profound motor blockade, it has become the most frequently used local anesthetic. Addition of epinephrine 1:200,000 (5 μg/ml) increases bupivacaine's duration of action and decreases systemic absorption, limiting both the cumulative dose and the likelihood of toxicity. Depending on the severity and location of pain, bupivacaine concentrations as low as 0.125% can give excellent pain relief with minimal motor blockade. Shorter-acting local anesthetics, such as lidocaine or procaine, should be used for infiltration before any invasive monitoring or intravenous access.

With peridural anesthesia even low concentrations of local anesthetics cause sympathectomy. Other concerns about local anesthetics involve their toxicity with accumulation or intravascular injection. Seizures, usually seen before cardiac toxicity, tend to be short lived and self-limited. More profound central nervous system toxicity leads to coma. Treatment includes discontinuation of drug administration, airway management with oxygen delivery, and small doses of barbiturates or benzodiazepines. Myocardial toxicity from inhibition of sodium and potassium conductance in the myocardium leads to depression, slowed conduction, and increased PR interval and QRS duration. Bupivicaine binds strongly to the cell membrane, making myocardial toxicity resistant to therapy.

Epidural and spinal narcotics provide excellent analgesia through action on opiate receptors in the dorsal horn. Spread is determined by the lipid solubility of the drug chosen. The more lipid-soluble drugs, such as hydromorphone, meperidine, methadone, and fentanyl, produce a more limited block because the drugs rapidly penetrate the spinal cord. More water-soluble drugs, such as morphine, remain in the cerebrospinal fluid longer, allowing greater cephalad distribution. As a result, morphine more commonly causes respiratory depression. Addition of epinephrine 1:200,000 to the narcotic, as with local anesthetics, decreases vascular uptake but increases cephalad spread. In some institutions patients are monitored for delayed respiratory depression for 24 hours after the last dose of epidural morphine. The side effects of epidural narcotics can be treated with intravenous naloxone infusion in very low doses (Table 28–4) or intravenous nalbuphine infusion. Because the more lipid-soluble narcotics give a more predictable block with less risk of delayed respiratory depression, these drugs may be preferable for patients breathing room air. Morphine, however, can be readily used in patients receiving mechanical ventilation.

TABLE 28–4. Protocol for Peridural Narcotics Administration

1. Have head of bed elevated at least 20 degrees at all times.
2. Keep ampule of naloxone (Narcan) and syringe at bedside at all times when peridural narcotics are in use and for 24 hours after last dose of peridural narcotic.
3. Naloxone dosage is 0.08 mg (i.e., 0.2 ml of 0.4 mg/ml naloxone) intravenously every minute as needed while respiratory rate is less than 8 breaths/min.
4. If patient requires naloxone bolus more than twice in 30 minutes, start naloxone drip: 1 mg naloxone in 250 ml of D5W (i.e., 4 μg/ml) via infusion pump. Start at 5 μg/kg/h and titrate to maintain respiratory rate at 12 to 16 breaths/min.
5. Nalbuphine (Nubain) 10 to 20 mg intravenously every 2 hours as needed for pain.
6. Diphenhydramine (Benadryl) 25 mg intravenously every 30 minutes to maximum of 50 mg in 4 hours as needed for itching.
7. Droperidol 0.5 mg intravenously every 30 min to maximum of 1.5 mg in 4 hours as needed for nausea.
8. Naloxone drip: 1 mg naloxone in 250 ml D5W (4 μg/ml) via infusion pump at 2 μg/kg/h as needed for nausea or pruritus not relieved by the above medications. Titrate until nausea and itching are controlled (maximum dose 10 μg/kg/h).
9. All additional analgesics will be ordered by an anesthesiologist while the peridural catheter is in place.
10. Vital signs as ordered, except check respiratory rate every 10 minutes for 30 minutes immediately after each top-off dose, then every 30 minutes while catheter in place and for 24 hours after last dose of peridural narcotic.
11. Call anesthesia service for questions of respiratory depression, inadequate pain control, persistent nausea, or pruritus.

Fentanyl is also commonly used in paraspinal analgesia. Rapid onset makes fentanyl easier to titrate, and limited spread means less risk of respiratory depression. In addition, fentanyl's short duration makes it particularly useful for administration by infusion. For example, epidural infusion of fentanyl provides excellent analgesia in patients with postoperative abdominal aneurysm. Sufentanil has been used similarly. However, it has a tendency toward systemic accumulation. Compared with morphine, fentanyl and alfentanil cause similar rates of nausea, pruritus, and urinary retention but more significant sedation, obviating the need for supplemental sedatives. Other drugs, including hydromorphone, meperidine, methadone, butorphanol, calcitonin, and clonidine, have been used epidurally, but little research has been done on these agents. They probably offer little advantage over fentanyl and morphine in the ICU.

MODES OF DELIVERY

Intramuscular Injections

Intramuscular injections are seldom necessary in critically ill patients. Such injections are commonly given every 3 to 4 hours, requiring larger doses and resulting in higher peak blood levels than with infusion or patient-controlled analgesia. Sedation occurs in up to 45% of patients. Addition of promethazine or hydroxyzine increases the incidence of sedation. Generally the plasma concentrations fall to subanalgesic levels some time before the next dose is due (Fig. 28–2). This leaves the patient vacillating between uncontrolled pain and significant sedation. After intramuscular injection of meperidine 100 mg, blood levels remain above minimum analgesic concentration less than 40% of a 4-hour dose interval. Pain at the injection site, risk of hematoma formation or infection, and, particularly, unpredictable absorption of the drug administered, especially in patients with sepsis or myocardial compromise, make intramuscular injection less than desirable. Most ICU patients have some type of intravenous access because so many require parenteral medications. Intramuscular injection may be necessary only for confused, combative patients who have managed to extricate themselves from the intravenous apparatus and require emergency sedation before they harm themselves or ICU personnel.

Intravenous Injections

Intravenous injections are much more commonly used than intramuscular ones. They permit administration of medication on an as needed (PRN) basis, as a regularly scheduled bolus, or by infusion. Because health care professionals tend to underestimate the severity of pain, a strictly PRN regimen is likely to undertreat the patient. It should be reserved for analgesia related to painful procedures, such as line placement, physical therapy, and dressing changes. Regularly scheduled intravenous administration of analgesics tends to be somewhat better because it helps eliminate the cycle of request-wait-anticipate-anxiety associated with PRN regimens. However, the patient has a significant peak-trough alteration of drug blood level and a comparable variation in pain severity.

Intravenous Infusions

The administration-related variation in pain is largely eliminated by intravenous infusion. Intravenous infusion allows titration of analgesics to a steady-state plasma level that is adequate for baseline pain yet minimizes the respiratory depressant and sedative effects caused by PRN boluses. For painful procedures, PRN boluses commonly are needed in addition to infusion. In the event that sedation is needed to help control ventilation, an infusion can be readily titrated to the desired effect without the hemodynamic consequences of intravenous bolus administration. The most frequent limitations of this regimen in the ventilated patient are a relative overdose caused by accumulation, which, for example, inhibits neurologic examination, and the continuous need for an intravenous line, which can be difficult in patients requiring multiple infusions. In an ICU patient not receiving mechanical ventilation, respiratory depression is also a concern.

Patient-Controlled Analgesia

The concept of patient-controlled analgesia (PCA) was introduced in 1968 by Sechzer who used a nurse as the PCA device. The first

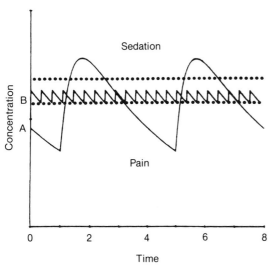

Figure 28–2. Hypothetical plasma concentrations of a narcotic analgesic. Curves were computer simulated with identical clearances and dosage rates but differing administration routes and doses per administration. Solid line *A* represents conventional intramuscular doses every 4 hours. Solid line *B* shows the smaller variations of patient-controlled analgesia, which notably lies above subanalgesic plasma levels of narcotic but below sedative levels. (Modified from and reproduced with permission from: Graves DA, Foster TS, Batenhorst, RL, et al: Ann Intern Med 1983;99:361.)

commercially produced pump, the Cardiff Palliator, became available in 1972. Subsequently, technologic advances led to the development of many computerized pumping systems (Table 28–5).

Most pumps now permit basal rate infusion, as well as intermittent bolus doses. A lockout period between bolus doses and the maximal dose per hour can also be chosen. Devices have various memory capabilities, providing a practitioner with information regarding the number of attempts made, number of doses given, and total dose received over a period of time. This information can show whether the patient is using the pump appropriately and getting an adequate dose. Also, the stored data can be readily accessed for research purposes. Printers are available, allowing permanent records of machine usage and drug delivery.

PCA can be used with intravenous or subcutaneous narcotics, as well as peridural narcotics or local anesthetics. Peridural administration is addressed later in the chapter. The effectiveness of PCA depends on the patient's ability to titrate the medication to his or her unique need. This requires the psychomotor capability of pushing the button for administration and adequate comprehension of how to use the pump and set it for dose delivery. Patients may have many misconceptions, such as "pushing the button a little gives a small dose," a technique frequently used by patients concerned about overdosage. Reassurance and repeated explanations usually remedy these problems. Mental retardation and youth are not contraindications to PCA, as long as the practitioner selects the patient carefully and offers adequate instruction and reinforcement.

Postoperative patients frequently report incomplete and inadequate pain relief when medication is administered by PRN intramuscular injection. Caregivers routinely underestimate analgesic requirements, particularly during the first 48 hours postoperatively. Health professionals tend to overestimate the risk of addiction. With demand analgesia patients can maintain a stable plasma level of analgesia for hours with good pain control and minimal respiratory depression (Fig. 28–2). Compared with intramuscular administration, PCA interferes less with normal sleep pattern, spontaneous activity, and deep breathing. Again, in comparison with PRN intramuscular injection, patients receiving PCA use comparable amounts of narcotic during the first 48 hours, but they tend to self-administer significantly more during the first 12 to 24 hours and less during the second 24 hours and then require significantly less narcotics after 48 hours. In the total postoperative period they use significantly less narcotic, but their level of comfort is generally more satisfactory than with intramuscular injection.

Advantages of PCA, when compared with more conventional modes of narcotic therapy, include more stable plasma concentrations and consequently better pain control with less medication, less sedation, and a shorter delay between the onset of discomfort and relief (Table 28–6). As a result patients have less anxiety, more satisfaction, and a better outlook. In addition, adequate pain control improves pulmonary function and general mobility, decreasing postoperative complications. In the ICU population, this could mean decreased requirements for mechanical ventilation, a

TABLE 28–5. Comparative Evaluation of Four Commercially Available Patient-Controlled Analgesia Systems

FEATURE	ABBOTT LIFE CARE PCA	BARD HARVARD PCA	GROSEBY CARDIFF PALLIATOR	PHARMACIA PROMINJECT
Drug concentration	Fixed	Variable	Variable	Variable
Incremental dose	0.1–5.0 ml	0.1–10.0 ml	1–999 mg	0.1–20.0 ml
Delivery rate (bolus)	4 ml/min	2.5 ml/min	Variable	Variable
Lockout/delay interval	5–99 min	3–60 min	1–99 min	5–999 min
Continuous infusion	No	Yes	No	Yes
Maximum dose limit	Yes	No	No	No
Cumulative dose	Yes	Yes	Yes	Yes
Demand signal	Single press	Single press	2 presses/sec	2 presses/sec
Memory/printer	No	Memory	No	Printer
Battery	>8 h	>3 h	No	>3 h
Alarms/safety	Yes	Yes	Limited	Yes
Security	Door, pump	Door, pump	Door only	Door only
Weight	7 kg	4 kg	8 kg	6 kg

From White PF: Semin Anesth 1985;4(3):259.

TABLE 28–6. Advantages of Patient-Controlled Analgesia over Conventional Parenteral Narcotic Therapy

Superior pain relief with less medication
Less sedation during daytime hours
Decreased delay between request for analgesic and relief
Minimized inappropriate "screening"
Improved pulmonary function tests
Fewer pulmonary complications postoperatively
Accommodation for diurnal changes in drug requirement and a wider range of analgesic requirements
Lower potential for overdosage when small doses per activation are prescribed
Improved continuous incremental titration

Reproduced with permission from Graves DA, Foster TS, Batenhorst RL, et al: Ann Intern Med 1983;99:362.

lower incidence of pulmonary emboli, and shorter ICU stays.

Problems with PCA are listed in Table 28–7. Complications are rare. More common complaints include drowsiness, dizziness, dry mouth, itching, and nausea. Respiratory depression is unlikely if basal rates and boluses are adjusted appropriately for age, size, and current narcotic and sedative experience; however, acute respiratory depression as evidenced by elevated arterial carbon dioxide tension has been reported in two patients. Both were hypovolemic at the onset of respiratory depression. One episode was treated with naloxone,

TABLE 28–7. Problems Occurring with Patient-Controlled Analgesia

Operator Errors

Misprogramming PCA device
Failure to clamp or unclamp tubing
Improperly loading syringe or cartridge
Inability to respond to safety alarms
Inappropriate silencing of safety alarms
Inappropriate dose order
Delay in availability of replacement syringe from pharmacy
Misplacing PCA pump key

Patient Errors

Failure to understand PCA therapy
Inability to effectively depress dosage button
Misunderstanding of PCA pump device
Confusion or short-term memory dysfunction
Intentional analgesic abuse

Mechanical Problems

Failure to deliver on demand
Cracked drug vials or syringes
Defective one-way valve at Y connector
Faulty alarm systems
Infiltrated intravenous catheter
Malfunctions (e.g., lock)

Modified from White PF: Anesthesiology 1987;66(1):82
PCA = patient-controlled analgesia.

and the other resolved with fluid resuscitation alone. I have also witnessed a single episode of respiratory depression and near respiratory arrest in a 20-year-old woman with Crohn's disease. Intraabdominal sepsis developed postoperatively and led to fulminant adult respiratory distress syndrome. While the patient was using PCA morphine to treat her progressive hypoxia and respiratory distress, severe carbon dioxide retention developed. Although respiratory depression is rare in postoperative patients, the margin of safety may be narrower in severely ill patients. Nursing observation and monitoring in the ICU should identify a potential problem before the consequences become significant. Because of the risk of respiratory depression, a standing order for naloxone administration should be available. Use of naloxone requires special care to avoid precipitating narcotic withdrawal, severe hypertension, or tachycardia.

Many narcotics are useful in parenteral PCA. Table 28–8 summarizes the more commonly used narcotics and suggests guidelines for dosage and lockout period. Preferred drugs have a rapid onset and a relatively short half-life, facilitating titration of plasma level to the optimal effect. Long-acting narcotics, such as methadone, are less suitable for acute pain.

An initial titrated loading dose can be given to quickly establish an adequate plasma level of narcotics. Subsequently a basal rate is set, and bolus doses and lockout interval are determined. For example, the average postlap-

TABLE 28–8. Guidelines for Bolus Dosages and Lockout Periods for Parenteral Analgesics Commonly Used with Patient-Controlled Analgesia

DRUG	BOLUS DOSE	LOCKOUT INTERVAL (min)
Agonists		
Morphine	0.5-3.0 mg	5-20
Hydromorphone	01.-0.5 mg	5-15
Meperidine	5-30 mg	5-15
Fentanyl	15-75 μg	3-10
Sufentanil	2-10 μg	3-10
Alfentanil	50-200 μg	3-10*
Partial Agonist		
Buprenorphine	0.03-0.2 mg	5-20
Agonist-Antagonist		
Nalbuphine	1-5 mg	5-15

Modified from White PF: Semin Anesth 1985;4(3)261.
*Data from Janssen P: The development of new synthetic narcotics. In Estafanous FG (ed): Opioids in anesthesia, Boston, 1984, Butterworth, p 41.

arotomy patient who has not been treated with opiates previously does well with morphine at a basal rate of 1 mg/h and a 1 mg bolus with a lockout period of 6 to 10 minutes. With this regimen patients frequently use only one to three self-administered doses per hour for the first 24 hours and then taper administration. In patients who are ill, elderly, or hypovolemic, a lower basal rate, smaller bolus, or longer lockout period may be necessary. If the patient's tolerance is unknown, a lower basal rate, very low bolus doses, and shorter lockout interval allow the patient to self-administer more doses per hour if needed. In reviewing the history, the practitioner can note the number of attempts, number of doses administered, and patient's assessment of pain control to adjust parameters accordingly. If narcotic tolerance has developed, particularly in patients with cancer pain, a basal rate of 15 mg or more of morphine per hour is not uncommon. The rule of thumb is to begin at the lower end of the dosage range expected to make the patient comfortable and titrate upward as needed. The size of the initial loading dose is also useful in estimating the initial delivery parameters.

If intractable nausea and vomiting develop after administration of the bolus dose, changing narcotics may alleviate this problem. Caution must be used in administering antiemetics, such as droperidol, promethazine, or hydroxyzine, because they increase sedation. When beginning a narcotic infusion of any kind in a spontaneously breathing patient, the practitioner must give specific orders for monitoring the patient's respiratory rate. A person experienced in airway management must be immediately available. An order for naloxone should be present, and a naloxone ampule should be taped to the infusion device or head of the patient's bed at all times (Table 28–9).

Subcutaneous Infusion

Subcutaneous infusion of narcotics, a less commonly used modality, can be useful when patients require parenteral analgesics but have poor intravenous access. Postoperative analgesia with subcutaneous hydromorphone self-administered with a PCA device has been found as effective as intravenous administration. Total number of doses (Fig. 28–3, *A*) and amounts (Fig. 28–3, *B*) over 48 hours were higher in the subcutaneous group, probably because of incomplete absorption from the subcutaneous site.

TABLE 28–9. Protocol for Patient-Controlled Analgesia

1. Order drug (e.g., prefilled syringe of morphine 1 mg/ml).
2. Select mode:
   a. PCA
   b. PCA and continuous
   c. Continuous
3. Order loading dose (e.g., morphine 2 to 4 mg intravenously every 10 minutes as needed [maximum 10 mg]) while patient is in recovery room.
4. Order bolus dose (e.g., morphine 1 mg).
5. Lockout period: _____ minutes (e.g., 6 minutes).
6. Basal rate: _____ ml/h (e.g., morphine, 2 mg/h).
7. _____ hour limit: _____ ml/ _____ hours (_____ mg/h).
8. Medication for nausea and vomiting: e.g., droperidol 0.5 mg intravenously every 30 minutes to a maximum of 1.5 mg in 4 hours.
9. Naloxone 0.1 mg intravenously stat for respiratory rate less than 8 breaths/min. Repeat every minute for 3 minutes. Page anesthesia service stat.
10. No systemic narcotics (intravenous, oral, or intramuscular) while PCA is in place unless approved by anesthesia service.
11. Resume oral, intramuscular, or intravenous narcotics per attending service after PCA is discontinued.
12. Monitor and record respiratory rate, sedation, and analgesic level every 2 hours for 12 hours, then every 4 hours.
13. Page anesthesia service stat for respiratory rate less than 8 breaths/min.
14. Seek consultation with acute pain specialist for nonurgent problems.
15. Keep ampule of naloxone (0.4 mg/ml) and syringe attached to PCA pump at all times.

PCA = patient-controlled analgesia.

Nausea and sedation occur less often with subcutaneous morphine infusion than with intermittent intramuscular doses.

A 25- or 27-gauge butterfly needle can be inserted into the subcutaneous tissue of the extremities, thigh, abdomen, or chest wall and can be changed as infrequently as once a week depending on infusion rate and local irritation. Medications that work well with this modality include morphine, levorphanol, and hydromorphone. The infusion rate can be determined by the total requirement over 24 hours given intermittently divided by 24 to give a rate per hour. This rate can then be titrated to the optimal effect.

Regional Techniques

Peridural Anesthesia and Analgesia

The peridural approach to pain management in the critically ill patient may be underused. Epidural and intrathecal administration

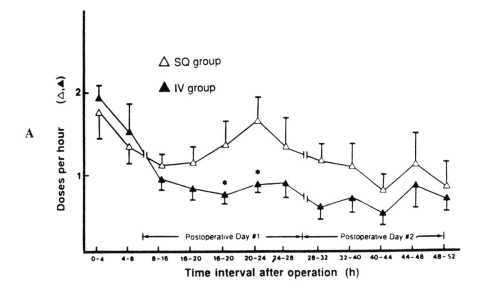

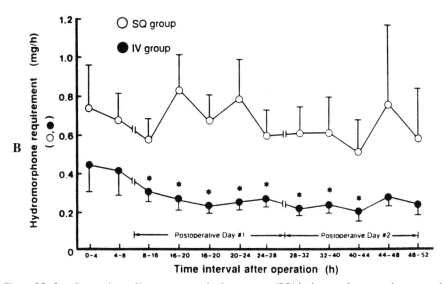

Figure 28–3. Comparison of intravenous and subcutaneous (SQ) hydromorphone requirements administered to postoperative patients by patient-controlled analgesia pump shows higher narcotic dosage in the SQ group (**A**) but similar decline in requirements over 48 hours in both groups (**B**). The higher hydromorphone requirement in the SQ group may indicate incomplete absorption from this site. Data points represent hourly requirements (**B**) and self-administered doses per hour (**A**) averaged for each 4-hour observation period. *Significant difference between treatment groups, $p < 0.05$. (From Urquhart ML, Klapp K, White PF: Anesthesiology 1988;69[3]:428-432.)

of narcotics or local anesthetics can control pain caused by thoracotomy, pelvic or lower extremity orthopedic trauma, flail chest, and laparotomy, while producing an alert, cooperative, and comfortable patient.

The physiologic effects of epidural anesthesia may or may not be desirable. Hypotension is common with paraspinal anesthesia because of sympathetic blockade from local anes-

thetics. Onset of hypotension tends to be more rapid with spinal than with epidural anesthesia. Fluid loading counteracts both to some extent, but ephedrine or even phenylephrine infusion may be required. In some cases, however, this vasodilatory effect is beneficial. Decreased preload and afterload reduce myocardial oxygen demand to a greater extent than myocardial oxygen supply is compromised.

Epidural anesthesiathesia improves regional wall motion and increases ejection fraction in patients with coronary artery disease. Patients can tolerate even sympathetic blockade of the cardiac accelerator fibers (T1-4) if an adequate mean blood pressure is maintained.

Respiratory effects are limited to decreased lung volumes, particularly functional residual capacity and vital capacity, because of respiratory muscle blockade from high, dense local anesthetic blocks. Peridural analgesia to relieve abdominal or thoracic pain improves respiratory volumes. Although vital capacity may increase, however, hypoxemia and functional residual capacity do not improve in patients with both parenchymal damage and chest wall trauma. A patient who has a significant pulmonary lesion with increased venous admixture and subsequent hypoxemia needs mechanical ventilation regardless of the mode of analgesic therapy.

Sympathetic blockade increases gastrointestinal motility, which causes nausea and vomiting. Increased peristalis can lead to bowel perforation in patients with bowel obstruction. As long as marked hypotension is avoided, changes in renal or cerebral blood flow are minimal. Paraspinal anesthesia improves the peripheral arterial inflow and venous emptying rates, thereby decreasing the incidence of thromboemboli. Similar advantages are likely when peridural anesthesia is used for bedridden, critically ill patients, a group commonly found to have pulmonary embolism at autopsy.

Peridural narcotics eliminate the problems associated with sympathectomy and motor blockade while providing excellent analgesia. Problems with this technique include pruritus, nausea, and urinary retention. More significantly, delayed respiratory depression can occur, particularly with the water-soluble narcotics, such as morphine. These side effects can be managed with nalbuphine or naloxone, by bolus or infusion, as detailed in Table 28–4.

In addition to problems related to the medication, infection is a significant concern with the peridural approach. Although an infrequent complication, its effects can be catastrophic. Strict aseptic technique in placement and care of the catheter is paramount. Filters are thought to decrease the incidence of catheter contamination. Although subcutaneous-tunneled catheters can be left in for months, the high incidence of sepsis in ICU patients makes it unlikely that a catheter will be left for more than 4 to 7 days at a time. Epidural catheters should be treated like any other invasive line. With the advent of sepsis the catheter must be removed.

Intercostal Block

Intercostal nerve block is a useful anesthetic technique for postthoracotomy pain, rib fractures, and upper abdominal incisions. Bupivacaine with epinephrine 1:200,000 is the most commonly used drug because of its prolonged duration. The epinephrine significantly decreases plasma bupivacaine levels after injection. This mode of analgesia improves pulmonary function and makes chest physiotherapy easier. Injection should include at least the intercostal nerves to the fractured segments and one rib higher. Pneumothorax is possible, but injection with a small needle (23-gauge) minimizes that risk. Infection, bleeding, nerve damage, and drug toxicity are also potential complications.

Intrapleural Blocks

Because of the risk of pneumothorax and the discomfort associated with repeated administration of intercostal blocks, placement of an intrapleural catheter has been advocated. Onset of anesthesia with bupivacaine 0.5% is approximately 15 minutes, and duration is 9 to 13 hours. This technique facilitates nursing care and decreases pulmonary complications. It is also effective for upper abdominal incisions, such as for cholecystectomy. In a patient with an indwelling chest tube with scant drainage and minimal to no air leak, the local anesthetic can be injected through the chest tube and the chest tube occluded for 5 to 10 minutes while the patient is placed so that the painful area is dependent. Concerns with this technique include infection and inadvertent failure to open the chest tube to drainage.

ADJUVANT THERAPY

Benzodiazepines

Diazepam, midazolam, and lorazepam are frequently used as sedatives and amnesics in the ICU. They are generally administered as an intravenous bolus, but midazolam particularly can also be given with a patient-controlled pump. In therapeutic doses benzodiazepines cause little or no hemodynamic change. When used in combination with narcotics, however, they significantly decrease mean arterial pressure and systemic vascular resistance. The exact mechanism of this potentiation is unknown. Benzodiazepines may augment the respiratory depression caused by narcotics. Generally the sedative effects of narcotics and benzodiazepines are additive. When a muscle relaxant is administered, concomitant use of an amnesic should be routine, as either a regularly scheduled dose or an infusion. Narcotics alone do not guarantee lack of awareness, and PRN scheduling of amnesics leaves too much room for error.

Barbiturates

Barbiturates have three main uses in the ICU: as short-acting anesthetics for such procedures as endotracheal intubations, as anticonvulsants, and in some institutions for treatment of elevated intracranial pressure. Barbiturates are not analgesics. They can cause hypothermia and hypotension by histamine release and by central hypothalamic stimulation. Since they produce respiratory depression, mechanical ventilation is required under most circumstances. Patients placed in pentobarbital coma for control of intracranial pressure have high incidence of sepsis and hypotension. Although barbiturates do help control intracranial pressure, their impact on ultimate outcome is the subject of debate.

Etomidate

During the late 1970s and early 1980s, etomidate infusions were used as sedative supplements to narcotic analgesia in ICUs. This practice stopped when a significant increase in the mortality rate was noted in patient groups receiving etomidate, despite injury severity scores comparable to those of group not given etomidate. In one study the mortality rate was 28% in mechanically ventilated patients given morphine with or without benzodiazepine and 77% in a group receiving etomidate plus morphine. After discontinuation of the use of etomidate the mortality rate fell to 25%. Etomidate infusions interfere with the stress response by inhibiting cortisol and aldosterone production in the adrenal cortex. In the preceding study patients died of sepsis and multiple–organ system failure rather than overt adrenal insufficiency, probably because of the attention paid to maintaining fluid and electrolyte balance. In addition, the etomidate group required inotropic support more frequently and had a higher incidence of renal failure than the group not receiving etomidate.

Methotrimeprazine

Methotrimeprazine (Levoprome) is a phenothiazide that also has significant analgesic effects. Morphine 10 mg is equianalgesic with methotrimeprazine 15 mg. Methotrimeprazine has antiemetic effects but can also cause sedation and hypotension. Its use in critically ill patients has not been studied.

Transcutaneous Electrical Nerve Stimulation

Transcutaneous electrical nerve stimulation (TENS) uses low-intensity, high-frequency or high-intensity, low-frequency electrical stimulation to produce analgesia. The former is more commonly used. The exact mechanism of action is unclear, but evidence suggests that high-intensity, low-frequency stimulation is at least partially mediated by the endogenous opioid system. In contrast, low-intensity, high-frequency stimulation produces analgesia that is not reversible with naloxone. The sensation generated by low-intensity, high-frequency stimulation is that of vibration or buzzing below the pain threshold. Therefore the effect of TENS may be mediated by altered neuronal input into the dorsal horn gating mechanism.

TENS has been widely used to manage chronic pain, but its use for acute pain has been limited. It has been used to treat the pain of flail chest with good results. The technique could also be applied to abdominal or chest pain from incisions, pain from orthopedic injuries, and low back pain caused by immobility. The great advantage of this technique is the paucity of side effects, the most common of which is a local skin reaction to the adhesive of the skin electrodes.

Acupuncture

The effect of acupuncture, whether by pressure, needle, or electrical stimulator, is thought to be modulated by endogenous opioid activity. Acupuncture can be useful in the treatment of pain syndromes, but a well-trained acupuncturist is required. This is not a technique for the unsupervised novice, and certification standards vary widely from state to state.

Hypnosis

Hypnosis, contrary to its popular stage image, is a state of intense concentration in which the subject is only peripherally aware of his or her surroundings and has a distorted time perception. This phenomenon occurs naturally for many people and is not unlike day-dreaming. Self-hypnosis is a learned skill that accentuates the depth of achievable concentration.

Hypnotic suggestability varies among people but also for a single individual, depending on the circumstances. A person who is stressed, in pain, or afraid is more receptive to hypnosis. In fact, patients in emergency rooms, operating rooms, and ICUs are often very suggestible without any formal hypnotic induction. Under hypnosis a person interprets verbal information literally and concretely. Therefore the wording of statements can have significant impact. For example, "I'm going to give you some medicine in your IV that is going to make you [to force you to] go to sleep [as in putting an old dog to sleep]" is very different in meaning from, "I'm going to give you some medicine in the IV to help you feel more relaxed and comfortable," although the intent of the statements is the same.

Hypnosis is excellent for pain management in the ICU, particularly during painful procedures. In addition to helping patients focus on more pleasant imagery, it affords patients some sense of control over situations and procedures that are imposed on them.

Formal hypnosis should not be used if a patient is psychologically unstable. Suggestions given during hypnosis are taken literally and thus must be well thought out and presented. Frequently the health care worker can assist the patient in refocusing attention from the painful source and can reassure the patient by being calming and soothing. For example, the practitioner can ask a patient to think of a favorite place or experience, then to close his or her eyes, take slow, deep breaths, and try to envision that setting. The patient should refocus on details—colors, sounds, smells—while exhaling and allowing the muscles to relax. Children can be asked about favorite television shows or stories, then asked to close their eyes, relax, and imagine the television screen. For many people a soothing voice and the redirection of attention to more positive thoughts help decrease fear, anxiety, and pain. Some patients who require repeated procedures (such as tubbing for debridement of burns) can be formally trained in self-hypnosis, which they can ultimately use at will and without assistance from nursing or medical staff.

CONCLUSION

With the evolution of ICUs has come the introduction of many invasive and painful procedures. ICU clinicians place tubes in every available orifice, disrupt normal sleep-wake cycles, overload patients with sensory stimulation, and strip away any sense of control patients might have of themselves or their environment. Sadly, much of this inhumanity is necessary to provide the kind of thorough care critically ill patients require. However, by being sensitive to what is being asked of patients, minimizing intrusion into their diurnal biocycles, helping them to control pain, and providing appropriate levels of sedation and good explanations of treatment, perhaps physicians can improve the quality of care and the overall experience for patients. Equally important is the mission to decrease complications and improve the functional outcome for these extremely ill patients.

Research is needed concerning the impact of pain control on complication rate, patient experience, and overall outcome. In this day of increasing financial pressures, strong evidence that appropriate pain control decreases ICU stay, total hospital stay, and thus hospital bills would make hospital administrators more likely to approve capital expenditures for sufficient numbers of infusion pumps, the more expensive PCA pumps, and additional anesthesia personnel to staff a regional anesthesia service for acute pain. If ICU physicians are to offer patients the best care, they must provide compassion, understanding, and humanity, along with ventilators, antibiotics, monitors, and invasive procedures.

SUGGESTED READINGS

Basbaum EI, Fields HL: Endogenous pain control systems: brainstem spinal pathways and endorphin circuitry. Ann Rev Neurosci 1984;7:309-338

Berre J: Relief of pain in intensive care patients. Resuscitation 1984;11:157-164

Bromage PR et al: Epidural narcotics for postoperative analgesia. Anesth Analg 1980;59:473-480

Cohen AT et al: Assessment of alfentanyl by intravenous infusion as long-term sedation in intensive care. Anaesthesia 1987;42:545-548

Coriat P et al: Lumbar epidural anesthesia improves ejection fraction in patients with poor left ventricular function. Anesthesiology 1987;67(3A):A259

Fagerhaugh SY: Pain expression and control on a burn care unit. Nursing Outlook 1974;22(10):645-650

Goudie TA et al: Continuous subcutaneous infusion of morphine for postoperative pain relief. Anaesthesia 1985;40:1089

Ibanez J et al: Thoracic epidural analgesia and chest trauma. Intensive Care Med 1987;13:297

Mackersie RC et al: Continuous epidural fentanyl analgesia: ventilatory function improvement with routine use in treatment of blunt chest injury. J Trauma 1987;27(11):1207-1212

Parko RF et al: Analgesia and mood effect of heroin and morphine in cancer patients with postoperative pain. N Engl J Med 1961;305:1501-1505

Perry Samuel et al: Management of pain during debridement: a survey of US burn units. Pain 1982;13:275

Pflug AE et al: Effects of postoperative peridural analgesia on pulmonary therapy and pulmonary complications. Anesthesiology 1974;41(1):8-17

Saada M et al: Segmental wall motion in coronary artery disease: patients evaluated by two-dimensional echocardiography after lumbar epidural anesthesia. Anesthesiology 1987;67(3A):A270

Shocket RB, Murray GB: Neuropsychiatric toxicity of meperidine. J Intensive Care Med 1988;3:246-252

Shulman M et al: Post-thoracotomy pain and pulmonary function following epidural and systemic morphine. Anesthesiology 1984;61(5):569-575

Swinamer DL et al: Effect of routine administration of analgesia on energy expenditure in critically ill patients. Chest 1988; 92(1):4-10.

Urquhart ML, Klapp K, White PF: Patient-controlled analgesia: a comparison of intravenous vs subcutaneous hydromorphone. Anesthesiology 1988;69(3):428-432.

Watt I, Ladingham I: Mortality amongst multiple trauma patients admitted to intensive therapy units. Anaesthesia 1984;39:973-981

Yate PM et al: Alfentanil infusion for sedation and analgesia for intensive care. Lancet 1984;18:396-397

29

LEGAL AND ETHICAL ISSUES IN THE INTENSIVE CARE UNIT

V. RANDOLPH GLEASON, JD, AND
LIN C. WEEKS, DrPH, RN

Technologic advances in medicine have resulted in an imbalance between its capacity to prolong life and its capacity to relieve suffering. Extraordinary medical treatments, such as mechanical ventilation and dialysis, can sustain vital functions without reversing the underlying disease processes. The resulting legal and ethical problems became evident as early as 1958 when an anesthesiologist wrote to Pope Pius XII asking for help with a ventilator-dependent comatose patient. "On what grounds," asked the physician, "should doctors, patients, families and society reach judgments when issues of suffering versus maintaining life functions are raised?" The pope responded by discussing the moral grounds for the application of ordinary versus extraordinary means and demonstrated a concept of humanity that would prove invaluable in the context of medical technology: human life must be distinguished from the simple life of organs.

Technology and the problems with its use are common in the ICU. This chapter is intended as a simple guide to assist the practitioner in approaching the more common legal and ethical issues. It is not intended as legal advice. When in doubt, the practitioner should consult a hospital attorney or institutional ethics committee. The role of ethics committees is discussed in the last section of this chapter.

BRAIN DEATH

Brain death now is recognized under ordinary medical standards to be an acceptable criterion for a diagnosis of death. This is true even in states that have not recognized brain death by judicial or legislative action. Most states passed brain death legislation in response to pressure brought about by new technology, the organ transplant movement, and fear of liability. The use of brain death as a diagnostic criterion has become so widespread that it is virtually a national standard. This may represent the first broad consensus on a bioethical issue in the United States. Thus, as long as physicians have not been negligent, that is, ordinary medical standards and procedures have been followed, there is no reason to fear liability.

Even so, when practicing in a state that has a brain death statute, the physician should be aware of its requirements and act accordingly. The brain death standard is usually expressed as irreversible cessation of total brain function or similar language. From there, state statutes vary, and the physician should note the appropriate requirements. Some states, such as Iowa, require diagnostic confirmation by a second physician. Others, such as Virginia, require the involvement of certain medical specialists in the diagnosis.

Texas and several other states require pronouncement of death before removal of artificial means of support. Some states, such as Louisiana, prohibit the involvement of a physician who is also the physician of a proposed organ recipient. Others, such as Connecticut, specifically state that pronouncement must occur before organ retrieval can begin. It is good practice to observe all of these rules even in the absence of a specific requirement in the relevant brain death statute. Arguably, it may be more important to follow all such guidelines in states without brain death legislation.

The most common problem associated with brain death is not in making the diagnosis, but rather in presenting the death to the patient's family. It is not uncommon for a hospital's legal counsel or medical ethics committee chairman to be telephoned by the perplexed attending physician of a brain-dead patient whose family is protesting against the withdrawal of the ventilator. This situation can arise if the physician fails to understand that when brain death occurs, a ventilator may be removed without the consent of the family. The same physician who would not hesitate to remove a ventilator from a patient who has been pronounced dead because of cessation of cardiopulmonary function will ask a brain-dead patient's family for consent to remove a ventilator. Not only is this legally unnecessary, it also is an injustice to families because it makes them believe that a life-or-death decision is theirs to make. The best practice is to pronounce the patient dead, remove the ventilator and other support devices, and then advise the family that the patient has died. If institutional policy permits family visitation of the body before its removal, those arrangements should be made as soon as possible. The brain-dead patient should not be treated differently in this respect from the patient whose death resulted from cardiopulmonary arrest.

The possibility of organ donation may prevent this course from being followed exactly. In such cases the protocol stated above should be followed except that the family must be advised that the ventilator and other support devices are being continued temporarily pending their decision about organ donation. Sometimes families can be approached about organ donation before death is pronounced. Although this approach may make family members feel that the staff's concern is not for the patient, but rather for retrievable organs, making this decision early has many advantages and is done frequently. The timing of consent for organ donation and the decision about who may obtain it may be affected by state law and institutional policy, and physicians should be aware of both.

DO-NOT-RESUSCITATE ORDERS

Although some consider *do-not-resuscitate* (DNR) orders to be part of the broader subject of withholding life-sustaining treatment, for several reasons they are discussed separately in this chapter. First, cardiopulmonary resuscitation (CPR) in the hospital setting is unique among life-sustaining interventions because, rather than being provided only on a physician's order, CPR is provided automatically unless there is an order directing that it be withheld. Second, although an argument can be made that withholding CPR suggests that other technologic interventions should be withheld as well, for many patients aggressive technologic support is appropriate but CPR is not indicated when it becomes apparent that aggressive treatment is not going to save a patient's life. Third, the Joint Commission on Accreditation of Healthcare Organizations (JCAHO) has elected, implicitly at least, to separate the DNR issue from the broader issue. JCAHO now requires hospitals to have written guidelines concerning the withholding of resuscitation, while not yet requiring written guidelines for withholding life-sustaining treatment. Last, one can argue that CPR is not so much a life-sustaining treatment as a death-reversing one, for it is called into play only as a last resort and under circumstances in which, before its development and availability, clinical assessment would qualify the patient for a pronouncement of death.

CPR was developed to prevent unexpected death. Its utility is in transforming what otherwise would be a lethal cardiac or respiratory episode into a transient one. Although survival rates within the community range as high as 80%, the effectiveness of CPR in hospitalized patients is poor. Most studies report a survival rate of less than 15%. In a study of 294 patients initially responding to CPR, no patient with cancer, acute stroke, sepsis, or pneumonia survived. Clearly survival following CPR relates to the underlying illness. This is why CPR is not indicated, and need not be offered, when it will not improve the patient's chances of being discharged from the hospital. Therefore, although physicians are wise to seek appropriate consultations to verify their medical judgments, the purely medical appropriateness of DNR orders is rarely at issue.

To be valid and supportable, a DNR order should be written in the patient's chart on the order sheet as would any other order. Now that the JCAHO requires hospitals to have written guidelines concerning the withholding of resuscitation, the physician is more likely to have a definitive hospital policy for a guide. Physicians should familiarize themselves with the policy at each hospital where they practice. Such policies may allow only certain physicians to write DNR orders (for example, attending or admitting physicians), or they may provide that DNR orders written by house staff are valid for only a limited time (for example, 24 hours) unless countersigned. A DNR policy should state that such an order in and of itself does not mean that nursing care will be reduced. Physicians should assure themselves of this and, if they have any doubt, clearly communicate their intentions to the nursing staff, both orally and in the patient's chart.

One last issue concerns patient or family consent to DNR orders. Patients have a right of self-determination, and the DNR issue should be discussed with them when possible. Unfortunately, this is possible only infrequently for patients in ICUs because of their condition. When institutional policy requires documented family consent, there is little choice; where the policy does not, the physician must choose either to inform the family of the DNR order and obtain their understanding or to make only a recommendation and let the family's wishes control. The latter approach has two drawbacks. First, because of psychologic denial, feelings of guilt, or poor communication, the family may not make the choice that is in the patient's best interests. Because the physician is obligated to do what is in the patient's best interests, an immediate conflict can result. Second, this situation allows laypersons to make what essentially is a medical decision about what interventions and what level of technology shall be applied. Still, obtaining family consent probably is the more common approach and is seldom a problem if the physician takes the time to explain what resuscitation involves and why it will not benefit the patient. If vigorous and unreasonable family opposition is encountered, the physician may wish to consult with the hospital's institutional ethics committee (IEC). An IEC can provide an excellent forum for resolving such issues as the DNR order.

INFORMED CONSENT

The doctrine that patient consent to medical treatment must be based on an informed choice is well established in medical jurisprudence and is inculcated in medical students throughout the United States. A thorough review of this legal doctrine and its many implications is beyond the scope of this chapter. Therefore we have chosen to provide only a brief but important update on the trend in this area and then to move on to a discussion of some consent-related problems that complicate ICU practice.

Early in its formulation and application by the courts, informed consent was based on what has come to be called the "objective" standard.

Under this standard, physicians were required to disclose to their patients only the risks that ordinarily were disclosed by physicians practicing within the particular specialty. This standard of disclosure was measured from the physician's point of view. Although many physicians have yet to realize it, the current trend, and now the law in most jurisdictions, is what is called the "subjective" standard. Under this standard the scope of the physician's communications to the patient is measured by the patient's need to know rather than by what the physician would suppose is material to an informed patient decision. State statutes that establish this standard ordinarily provide that the physician must disclose risks that could influence "a reasonable person" or "a reasonable patient" or similar language.

Physicians must realize that the patient-oriented standard is more stringent and that it probably will be a lay jury that evaluates, in the bright illumination of hindsight, the adequacy of disclosure. Ordinarily informed consent withstands legal attack if the physician has disclosed, preferably in writing, the risks and potential benefits of the proposed procedure, the risks and potential benefits of any alternative procedures, and the risks of forgoing treatment altogether.

Several issues related to consent to treatment seem to surface repeatedly in ICUs. The first concerns the refusal, on religious grounds, to consent to lifesaving transfusion of blood or related components. The law recognizes the right of competent adults to refuse treatment even when such refusal will lead to death. Physicians are most likely to encounter such a refusal in connection with patients who are members of the Jehovah's Witness sect. The physician must ensure that the patient's refusal is an informed choice made after the patient is advised of the serious consequences of forgoing blood transfusions. However, once the patient's decision is made and documented, it should be respected even though the patient may later become incompetent owing to progression of the disease. To do otherwise is unethical and exposes the physician to civil liability for battery.

A different situation is presented when the patient (for example, a child) is incompetent for purposes of consent because of physical or mental impairment or legal disability and consent to transfusion is withheld by surrogate decision makers. When the patient is a child, the law does not recognize a parent's right to refuse lifesaving transfusion.

In the absence of a hospital policy that provides clear direction in such matters, the physician should contact the hospital's attorney or administrator to obtain a court order. This is also the course to follow for an incompetent adult when surrogate decision makers are refusing blood and the patient never expressed a fully conscious decision to refuse blood. The outcome of such situations depends on the amount and weight of evidence that demonstrates what the patient would decide if competent. This evidence is better judged by the court or IEC.

Another thorny situation is presented when parents refuse major medical interventions in the care of their child. Some jurisdictions, such as Texas, allow parents to make such decisions in concert with the attending physician when the child has a terminal illness. In the absence of such narrow circumstances, the physician should consult the hospital attorney or IEC. This is particularly important when the patient is an infant because hospital policy and therefore hospital intervention may be influenced by the controversial Baby Doe Guidelines promulgated by the Department of Health and Human Services. This influence on hospital policy and neonatal medical practice continues even though these guidelines, when finalized, applied to state child protective agencies and not directly to hospitals and physicians. The guidelines require that agencies, to receive federal grant money, have a mechanism in place for investigating allegations of medical neglect. Several states have chosen to forfeit federal funding to avoid the guidelines altogether.

Most states, by statutes often referred to as "natural death acts," have sanctioned the use of a document most often called a "directive to physician," commonly known as a living will. The living will constitutes a patient's advance directive that life-sustaining treatments not be used if the patient has a terminal condition. In a sense a living will withdraws consent for such treatments, and physicians should treat it as doing just that. Ordinarily the state statute provides both civil and criminal immunity for the physician and all members of the health care team in connection with abiding by the patient's wishes to withdraw or withhold life-sustaining treatment.

Several myths about living wills need to be dispelled. First, a living will applies to all terminal conditions, including those caused by an injury (for example, trauma). Second, a living will does not become invalid when the patient becomes incompetent; such a result would defeat the living will's purpose. Last, family members cannot cancel or override a patient's living will. Only the patient can revoke it. In the case of a competent patient the physician should discuss with the patient whether the patient has had a change of heart about the living will. In all cases the physician should verify that a patient's living will conforms with state law. When the patient has not made a decision on withdrawal or withholding of treatment and no longer can do so, it is up to the physician and, when appropriate, surrogate decision makers.

WITHHOLDING OR WITHDRAWING TREATMENT

Much has been written about withdrawing or withholding treatment from the gravely ill patient. A medical school education oriented toward supporting life, a fear of litigation, and the specter of failure because a patient died create a psychologic block or aversion to approaching this issue. For some physicians, withdrawal of treatment may be psychologically equated to killing the patient, whereas not starting it at all is more acceptable. Understanding one's own beliefs and feelings and working to gain a more enlightened view of the legitimate aims of the practice of medicine are crucial to the physician's ability to deal with both the logical and the emotional aspects of this subject.

Physicians have no legal or moral obligation to initiate or continue treatment that will not benefit the patient. Treatments that provide little or no benefit may be withheld or withdrawn. However, in the acute situations within an ICU, particularly within hours or days of admission, withholding technologic support may be inappropriate because of uncertainty about prognosis and response to treatment. When the medical outcome is uncertain, time-limited trials can determine the appropriate level of care. The physician can implement specific life-sustaining treatments that can be reevaluated after a designated period. Moreover, trial periods can help patients, their families, and the health care team by providing a realistic approach to terminal or incapacitating illness without extinguishing hope for recovery.

Physicians need not feel that they alone must resolve these issues. IECs offer experience and advice for resolution of such issues.

INSTITUTIONAL ETHICS COMMITTEES

The recent proliferation of IECs has many reasons, but the issues addressed earlier in this chapter attest to the complexity and ambiguity of the questions surrounding the use of technology in the care of critically ill or dying patients. Although most states have conferred "right-to-die" decision-making power on the individual patient, few patients are able to actualize this decision-making power. Thus physicians frequently find themselves in the driver's seat for difficult decisions about extraordinary measures. Furthermore, the patient and family usually are strangers to the physician in a tertiary-care teaching hospital. Worse still, the medical decision maker may change from month to month because of schedule rotations. Obviously many physicians appreciate assistance in this decision making.

IECs received legal sanction when, in the Karen Ann Quinlan case of 1976, the New Jersey Supreme Court suggested that IECs were the proper vehicle for resolving ethical dilemmas in hospitals. In 1978 less than 1% of American hospitals had IECs. Now, an estimated 60% to 70% of hospitals have them. Although the size of the committees varies, membership tends to be multidisciplinary, with representatives from the lay community and from such professions as law, medicine, nursing, social work, and the clergy. IECs now perform a variety of important functions, including policy development, education, and case consultation.

For purposes of case consultation, IECs develop one or more sets of operating guidelines that vary as widely as does membership. Such guidelines usually are available for inspection by anyone considering a consultation. Physicians should acquaint themselves with the guidelines, as well as with hospital policies and medical staff bylaws that pertain to the roles of the IECs within their hospitals. One important reason for familiarity with such policies is the difference among IEC models. Many hospitals have an optional/optional model, wherein resorting to an IEC consultation is optional and following the IEC's recommendations is also optional. But some employ optional-mandatory and mandatory-mandatory models. Furthermore, access to the committee may be restricted to the attending physician, or anyone involved in the patient's care, including family members, may be allowed to request an IEC consultation. Clearly, then, the physician must know both what to expect from the committee and what may be expected of the physician.

The need for and effectiveness of IECs remains a critical question in the increasingly bureaucratic environment of health care. Some physicians believe that IECs are a form of medicine by committee. Some think that "ethical" issues are merely problems in communication and that involvement of a committee exacerbates the problem. For that reason some hospitals have found success in using informal ethics consultations.

Originating as a case-screening mechanism, the informal consultation consists of one or more discussions about the case with the IEC chairperson. These conversations may include the hospital attorney or chief of staff when appropriate. With their knowledge of institutional policy and experience with case consultation, these individuals initiate communication and mediate among the patient, the family, and the health care team to move toward agreement on a course of action.

Physicians may find that after one or two experiences with an IEC, further case consultations are unnecessary. By virtue of this educational component of the IEC, the physician becomes better able to distinguish the medical realities of a case from its ethical issues. Once this distinction is clear in the physician's mind, the physician can help the patient or surrogate decision makers do the same.

SUGGESTED READINGS

Bedell W, Pelle D, Maher PL, Clearly PD: Do not resuscitate orders for critically ill patients in the hospital. JAMA 1986;256:233-237

Blackhall L: Sounding board: must we always use CPR? N Engl J Med 1988;117(20):1281-1284

Doudera A, Peters J: Legal and ethical aspects of treating critically and terminally ill patients. Ann Arbor, Mich, 1982, AUPHA Press

Gleason V: Legal and ethical considerations in withholding resuscitation. In Weeks L (ed): Advanced cardiovascular nursing. Boston, 1986, Blackwell

Joint Commission on Accreditation of Healthcare Organizations: Accreditation manual for hospitals. Chicago, 1988, The Commission

Reiser SJ, Dyck AJ, Curran WJ: Ethics in medicine: historical perspectives and contemporary concerns. Cambridge, Mass, 1977, MIT Press

Rozovsky FA: Consent to treatment — a practical guide. Boston, 1984, Little, Brown

Society for the Right to Die: Handbook of living will laws. New York, 1987, The Society

Thomlinson T, Brody H: Ethics and communication in do-not-resuscitate orders. N Engl J Med 1988;318:43-46

Zimmerman JE, Knaus WA, Sharpe SM, et al: The use and implications of do-not-resuscitate orders in intensive care units. JAMA 1986;255:351-356

ADMINISTRATION OF THE INTENSIVE CARE UNIT

GRAZIANO C. CARLON, MD, I. ALAN FEIN, MD, AND DONALD CHALFIN, MD

DEFINITIONS

Many different terms are used to identify the hospital areas where patients with special, and usually life-threatening, problems receive more attentive care and are more closely monitored than elsewhere in the same institution. For convenience, in this chapter we refer to all of them as intensive care units (ICUs). The body of knowledge required to provide optimal care to patients in ICUs is defined here as critical care medicine.

PHYSICAL PLANT OF THE INTENSIVE CARE UNIT

Planning to Meet Needs

A major responsibility of an ICU administrator is to determine the number and types of patients who require critical care support. With this information the administrator can determine objectively how many critical care beds are needed in a hospital and whether specialized or general purpose medical-surgical ICUs are required to accommodate all the patients needing care.

Unfortunately, this comprehensive approach to planning is rare. In the real world, politics and economics determine ICU size and patient composition in each institution. Despite the numerous and often remarkable investigations on severity of illness in the last 15 years, no universally accepted standards of care define which patients and which morbid conditions benefit from ICU management. Local biases, as well as the medical, nursing, and support staff available outside the ICU, significantly influence decisions on ICU use. The only organization attempting to set national standards, the Joint Commission for Accreditation of Healthcare Organizations (formerly the Joint Commission for Accreditation of Hospitals), a voluntary body whose suggestions have all the force of law, has chosen not to address these issues. JCAHO requirements mandate that hospitals identify conditions for admission to or discharge from their ICUs and provide alternative plans of care when demand exceeds availability. As is the case for most JCAHO regulations, however, each hospital is free to define its own criteria for ICU admission and will not be faulted as long as it remains consistent with its self-imposed standards.

The absence of regional or national data on ICU use also makes difficult ICU planning. This problem was recently highlighted when the Department of Health of the State of New York discovered that although hospitals were required to collect many items of information, none allowed retrospective identification of ICU admission diagnoses. Thus even a crude evaluation of the outcome of patients with similar complications, treated in or outside the ICU, proved impossible. The federal government fares little better; in a highly publicized and politicized move, mortality by admission diagnosis for different hospitals is now made public by the Department of Health and Human Services and often used as a score card for adequacy of performance. These reports, however, do not classify patients by severity of illness or by modality of support and are therefore of questionable value. For example, a hospital in which unnecessary cardiac surgery was performed on relatively healthy patients could report exemplary mortality rates; a different institution in which similar patients had surgery but did not receive adequate postoperative ICU care might have "average" mortality rates, whereas much lower values should have been expected if meaningful indicators had been used. A prospective, randomized, multicenter investigation, with rigid ICU admission criteria, standardized plans of management, and strict supervision of protocol implementation could perhaps objectively identify patients and clinical conditions that should be treated in ICUs. Such a project is unlikely in the foreseeable future. Even assuming that parochialism and prejudice could be overcome and that enough hospitals with sufficiently representative patient populations agreed to use standardized ICU admission criteria and management protocols, the necessity of obtaining informed consent from patients would probably preclude meaningful data collection. The national trial of azidothymidine for the treatment of AIDS showed that people cannot be persuaded to enter a prospective study when there is already an overwhelming bias in favor of one of the treatment modalities. Even though no research has been conducted on the subject, it is difficult to imagine that many people are unaware of the existence of ICUs or have not been conditioned to believe that only there can life-threatening illnesses be successfully treated. Alternatively, some patients may have equal, and equally unscientific, objections to receiving extraordinary means of life support. In both cases a true randomization would be impossible to enforce.

Since patients who should be admitted to the ICU cannot be positively identified, classification of ICU types is blurred. Again, the guidelines of JCAHO offer little assistance; their manual identifies, for descriptive purposes, many different types of ICUs (Table 30–1) but does not endorse any definition, nor does it clearly specify which types of patients should be exclusively or preferentially admitted to each ICU.

In conclusion, strategic planning of ICU type and size based on objective data does not seem possible at present. ICU administrators must therefore rely on their judgment and their perception of local conditions. Similar problems with planning occur in other countries, from the developing nations to the highly structured and

TABLE 30–1. Special Care Units Identified in the 1989 JCAHO *Accreditation Manual of Hospitals*

UNIT NAME	PATIENT POPULATION
Special care unit	Any patient requiring continuous and concentrated care
Specific care unit	
Burn unit	Burn patients
Intensive care unit (cardiac, cardiovascular surgery, respiratory, neonatal)	Acute care of patients designated by the name of the unit
Renal unit	Renal dialysis patients

nationalized health care organizations of Switzerland, Germany, and Italy.

Designing or Renovating the Intensive Care Unit

The absence of hard data about ICU use does not relieve ICU administrators from the frequent obligation to reconsider the ICU's physical plant. Government agencies and the JCAHO regularly revise ICU code requirements and often mandate structural modifications. In rare circumstances ICU designers are able to start from the blueprints of a new hospital. The location of the unit or units may then be decided strictly on the basis of functional requirements, without consideration for existing structures or activities that may not be easily reconfigured or moved. Far more commonly, however, existing ICUs must be modernized within economic and spatial constraints. Three basic concepts should guide the planning team: ICUs should be functional, accessible, and easy to modernize.

To improve ICU functionality, designers should reduce the efforts required to perform each activity, especially those directly involving patient care. The design of bedside stations, or cubicles, should allow unimpeded movement of equipment and the simultaneous presence of several health professionals to deal with emergencies. In each cubicle, wall outlets for compressed gases, suction devices, and electrical sockets should be placed in similar locations. Indeed, this consideration should be extended to all supplies needed for routine care (Fig. 30–1). Since ICU activities are unpredictable and complications may develop at any time, the number of variables with which the staff must contend should be minimized. Frantic

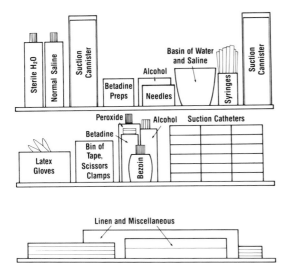

Figure 30–1. Standard supplies required in an intensive care unit cubicle.

searches for equipment or drugs are distracting during emergency situations and can jeopardize patients' safety. Most ICUs have a large transient staff; the youngest and least experienced physicians and nurses are often assigned to night and weekend shifts, when stock room attendants may not be on duty. JCAHO sensibly requires that a list of all supplies in the ICU be maintained, with clear information on their location; the list should be kept in an easily accessible and widely known site. In general, cubicle design and placement of supplies should be guided by the Latin proverb: "Order is not a substitute for intelligence, but its indispensable complement."

Patients in ICUs are among the largest users of other hospital services, especially the laboratory and radiology departments. Frequently they must be transported to and from the operating rooms or other specialized areas. Certainly many diagnostic tests and surgical procedures can be performed at the bedside, and indeed portable equipment is becoming smaller and more sophisticated. For instance, echocardiograms and Doppler flow measurements are now as reliable and informative when obtained at the bedside as they are in a cardiology suite. Other important interventions, however, may be necessary to fully evaluate or treat critically ill patients. Pulmonary ventilation-perfusion scanning, gated radionuclide cineangiocardiography, cardiac catheterization, computed tomography, magnetic resonance imaging, positron emission tomography, and radiation therapy are all part of the common practice of medicine. Most of these procedures are ineffi-

cient, impractical, or impossible to perform at the bedside. Thus the location of each ICU in relation to the facilities that provide specialized functions can determine the availability of those services to critically ill patients. Transporting a patient who is receiving mechanical ventilation and requires the continuous infusion of one or more drugs to maintain cardiovascular function is clearly a complex undertaking. If the patient must be moved in and out of elevators, the task may be so daunting that it is postponed or avoided altogether. When possible, therefore, acute care facilities should be on the same floor as the service structures their patients frequently use. ICUs primarily or exclusively for surgical patients should be adjacent to operating rooms. Interestingly, although the advantages of physical proximity appear self-evident, neither government agencies nor JCAHO has stipulated the relative locations of ICUs within the hospital.

Monitoring and data management equipment is continually being improved; new devices are developed to maintain the function of failing organs; new drugs are introduced to control or reverse the course of life-threatening disease. At times structural changes to the ICU are necessary to provide the benefits of these discoveries to ICU patients. Typically, monitoring and data management systems require cables connecting bedside terminals to central stations. Placement of those cables within dropped ceilings covered by removable tiles is possible, but over the course of the years new installations overlap older systems until an unrecognizable mass of intertwining cables, some functioning and some obsolete, crisscrosses the ceiling of the ICU. Furthermore, enclosed ceilings usually harbor opportunistic microorganisms, especially *Aspergillus fumigatus, Candida albicans,* and other fungi. These are released into the environment when the tiles are opened to advance new cables. Immunocompromised patients may be contaminated, with potentially disastrous consequences. Although environmental surveys can identify the problem, prevention is difficult. Microwave-operated wireless bedside stations minimize construction, but cost considerations and the risk of interference from other equipment operating on similar wavelengths have limited the appeal of this option. When the physical plant allows it, a grid may be placed underneath the ICU floor, with pods opening in each cubicle (Figs. 30–2 and 30–3). New equipment can then be installed without

Physical Plan — Special Care Unit

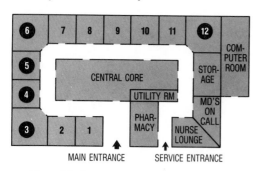

Connecting-Grid Underneath S.C.U.

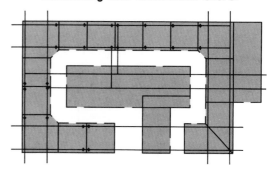

Figure 30–2. Schematic representation of the intensive care unit of Memorial Sloan-Kettering Cancer Center in New York. In addition to patient care and supply areas, the plan demonstrates the grid underneath the floor of the unit. Through the grid, cables can be advanced from one location to another without the necessity for opening the ceilings or disrupting the function of the unit beyond the areas directly affected.

much disruption of the ICU and with less risk of contamination. Furthermore, a grid structure can facilitate the separation of the many different wires and cables required by additional monitoring equipment.

ICU designers must remember that most innovations introduced in the ICU operate on electrical power. Many drugs must be administered in precise and constant amounts for best effect and therefore require volumetric infusion pumps. Indeed, nursing time has become too precious to waste on manual adjustment of intravenous infusions. Accordingly, the design of ICU cubicles should include numerous electrical power sources. Furthermore, the location of the sockets should eliminate or minimize obstacles presented by multiple electrical cords.

PERSONNEL IN THE INTENSIVE CARE UNIT

Physician-Director

A well-designed, functional, and modern ICU is only the shell within which patient care takes place. The most important organizational task is to provide the continuous presence of trained physicians, nurses, and other health professionals, who prevent problems when possible or immediately respond if they develop. JCAHO has not taken an official position on medical staffing in the ICU. JCAHO mandates only that each ICU have a physician-director, who implements hospital policies in regard to patient care in the ICU, is responsible for quality assurance, and supervises educational programs for residents and other health professionals who prac-

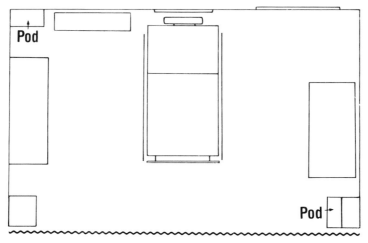

Figure 30–3. Schematic representation of a patient cubicle in the intensive care unit of Memorial Sloan-Kettering Cancer Center in New York. The pods that open to the underground grid are identified.

tice in the unit. The regulations do not define the degree of autonomy that the physician-director must have and do not even require formal training in critical care medicine. Thus the director's responsibilities and authority can range from those of a figurehead, who rubber-stamps policies formulated elsewhere, to those of a division chief or department chairman, charged with supervising all aspects of care for critically ill patients and entrusted with considerable autonomy in allocating staff and other resources to the ICU.

Not every hospital can afford, or needs, a full-time ICU staff or even a full-time physician-director. However, certain organizational issues must be addressed regardless of the size of the hospital or the number or type of patients admitted to the ICU. Although some problems can be resolved without the contribution of a competent and dedicated director, logically any effort will be better directed by a committed administrator.

House Staff

In a busy ICU, with many critically ill patients, a single shift staffed by inadequately trained personnel can negate the efforts of all other professionals no matter how well qualified. Despite this, the assignment of physicians to ICU duties does not always reflect a recognition of the changes in critical care medicine and the level of competence required to operate effectively in ICUs. When ICUs were created in the late 1950s, they were specially staffed observation areas where a few patients received mechanical ventilation or had continuous electrocardiographic or arterial blood pressure monitoring. The equipment used, including mechanical ventilators, could perform only relatively rudimentary functions. Drugs to treat most life-threatening conditions were few and of modest efficacy. A brief review of the evolution of technology and pharmacology in the last 20 years (Table 30–2) provides unquestionable evidence of the knowledge that must be mastered to provide minimum standards of care to ICU patients. These demanding requirements contrast starkly with the reality of medical school and postgraduate training in critical care medicine. An informal review of the curricula of medical schools in the Northeast, from Washington, D.C., to Boston, indicated that none had mandatory courses in critical care medicine. Only one school required attendance at a 1-hour class on mechanical ventilation, and a few pro-

TABLE 30–2. Advances in Technology and Pharmacology in the Intensive Care Unit

INTERVENTION	YEAR
Before 1969	
Intermittent positive-pressure ventilation	
Epinephrine	
Norepinephrine	
Isoproterenol	
Aminoglycosides	
First-generation cephalosporins	
After 1969	
Positive end-expiratory pressure	1969
Flow-directed pulmonary artery catheters	1970
Thermodilution cardiac output	1972
Intermittent mandatory ventilation	1973
Portable radionuclide cineangiography	1978
Percutaneous oxygen monitoring	1983
Portable capnography	1985
Two-dimensional echocardiography with Doppler flow	1985
Dopamine	1971
Dobutamine	1974
Amrinone	1979
Calcium channel blockers	1975/1980
Angiotensin-converting enzyme inhibitors (intravenous)	1983
Semi-synthetic penicillins	1969
Second-, third-, fourth-generation cephalosporins	1970/?
Carbapenems	1985
Monobactams	1985
Quinolones	1985

This brief list mentions only some of the most common additions to ICU practice. More sophisticated equipment (mass spectrometry, computerized data management systems, etc.) is available but not indispensable to meet minimum standards of care.

vided a brief review of monitoring equipment during the surgical clerkship. None had tutorials on risks, indications, and interactions of vasoactive and antiarrhythmic drugs in critically ill patients. Unfortunately, students generally have little awareness of their limitations.

Although clearly ill prepared for serving in ICUs, new graduates are nonetheless assigned there without formal training. Even in major academic centers, the only physicians present in the ICU at night or on weekends may be in their first or second year of residency. At times the only support available is represented by pulmonary or cardiology fellows, living off campus or with responsibilities limited to specific procedures. Although in some institutions more experienced staff members are readily available for backup, they can intervene only if alerted that complications are developing. Recognition of such developing problems requires experience and maturity.

Scheduling
Medical Coverage

At present, few guidelines, and no mandatory regulations, are available at the national or local level to indicate the number and minimum training of physicians who should staff ICUs. Preparing a schedule to provide continuous medical coverage in the ICU may not even be the responsibility of the physician-director. In large academic centers and in hospitals with house staff, this task may be assigned to the chief medical or chief surgical resident, who must balance the ICU's needs with those of other areas. Other institutions may have no ICU medical staff but may rely on private physicians to manage the care of their patients. Whenever possible, the ICU physician-director should insist on some minimum standards to ensure patients' safety:

- If the institution has a house staff and some of its members are assigned to the ICU, a physician with sufficient experience to recognize serious complications, if not necessarily to treat them, should always be present in the unit. The concept that continuity of care is best provided by assigning responsibility for ICU patients to the same house officers who cared for them before admission to the ICU should be strenuously opposed. ICU admission is usually prompted by a substantial change in the patient's condition, representing almost a new disease. Also, the patient requires attentive and continuous care, which cannot be provided by a harried house officer whose primary area of activity is distant from the ICU.

- If the ICU staff is not trained, or not allowed, to perform invasive procedures or manage mechanical ventilators, they should be able to obtain immediate assistance from physicians who have those privileges.

- The ICU staff should be allowed to intervene immediately when sudden life-threatening events develop, performing the necessary procedure or administering the appropriate drugs. Delays resulting from failure to establish communication with the team that has maintained primary responsibility for patient care are not acceptable if they expose patients to unnecessary risks.

- In hospitals without an ICU house staff, there should be a functional and reliable mechanism for obtaining emergency care when unexpected complications develop. If the patient's physician-of-record is not immediately available, other qualified professionals should be allowed to perform the necessary interventions. Similar arrangements operate successfully in other practices, such as obstetrics, in which unexpected complications develop with the same urgency as in the ICU. Relying on occasional consultation with pulmonary medicine and cardiology specialists, and on skilled nursing care only at all other times, may not prevent serious complications and enormous liability.

- The physician-director should have the right to recommend and even request consultations by appropriate specialists when complications develop that clearly lie outside the expertise of the physician-of-record. The opinion of highly competent physicians should always be available to severely ill patients if the highest standard of care is to be maintained.

Limitation of Working Hours

To complicate the already difficult task of providing continuous, high-quality medical care in the ICU, a movement to restrict working hours of health care professionals is developing. In New York State, for example, new regulations limit the working hours of house staff to 80 per week, averaged over 4 weeks, and to no more than 24 consecutive hours. These restrictions apply not only to the time spent in direct patient care, but also to educational activities. The regulations require credentialing of house officers before they can perform invasive procedures, and they mandate that physicians who are at least in their last year of training be present in the hospital; however, they make no specific reference to ICU coverage.

Many of the requirements adopted by New York State are being considered by other legislatures and may be included in the training requirements for critical care medicine fellows proposed by the Society of Critical Care Medicine. Thus they may soon be a concern for ICU physician-directors all over the country. Incredibly, these new regulations have been issued without any objective evidence that they will improve standards of care. The few studies of the effects of fatigue on judgment and performance of house officers have shown contradictory and inconclusive results. Nonetheless, a system that has operated for several generations and is providing perhaps the best medical care in the world is being changed on the basis of anecdotal evidence and political furor, without even a trial period. To paraphrase Aldous Huxley, any statement without factual basis can become an absolute truth, if repeated often enough.

Generalizations about the impact of these regulations are impossible, since the effects depend on the size of the house staff, the level of training of house officers who have ICU responsibilities, and the availability and responsibilities of fellows in critical care medicine, cardiology, or pulmonary medicine. However, some problems should concern all ICU administrators:

- A schedule that prohibits more than 24 consecutive hours of work prevents ICU physicians from providing continuity of care. Plans of therapy must inevitably be passed from one team to another, with little time for in-depth discussion. Even if the staff assigned to the ICU is large enough to provide "daytime only" physicians, who receive information from the outgoing team in the morning and transfer it to the incoming physicians in the evening, the approach to management will acquire some aspects of assembly-line work. Patients and families will be hard pressed to establish a relationship with one physician, and the essential element of individual trust, which facilitates patient care and prevents negligence suits, will be lost. The concept that the physician-of-record can maintain the continuity of care needed by patients and families is at best naive. Depending on their primary specialty and professional obligations, physicians-of-record may be unfamiliar with the nature and evolution of the critical illness, or may have to be absent themselves for many hours at a time while serious and frightening events unexpectedly take place and must be dealt with immediately by the ICU staff.

- The solution of using nighttime only staff may make preparing a schedule easier but can only widen the gulf between patients and physicians. Furthermore, night workers may have considerable difficulty adapting to changes in circadian rhythm. Fatigue, irritability, lack of concentration, and depression (the very complications the new regulations should theoretically avoid) usually resolve only after 4 to 6 weeks on the new schedule. Trainees cannot be assigned to several consecutive months of nighttime only work, since most educational aspects of residency take place during the day.

- In most hospitals the number of house officers is unlikely to increase and indeed may be reduced under the pressure of government agencies and third party payers. The same department of health that mandated the reduction in working hours for house staff in New York State has also recommended that the number of residency positions be decreased by nearly 33% over the next few years. To accommodate these regulations, the medical staff present in the hospital at any time must be reduced. However, the new mandates, theoretically designed to increase patient safety, can be followed to the letter by assigning new graduates to cover the ICU while arranging for the presence, within the hospital, of a senior physician who would intervene when necessary. Thus the new rules will not reduce the risk that inexperienced house officers will fail to identify serious problems.

Education of the Medical Staff

The United States has fewer than 100 training programs in adult critical care medicine. Since the number of ICUs in the country exceeds 7000, most physicians will care for critically ill patients at some time in their career and will have to be taught the concepts and procedures of critical care outside a formal training program in that subspecialty. Thus ICU physician-directors should not only maintain standards of care that will ensure patients' safety, but also provide residents, who will not continue in the practice of critical care medicine, with basic principles that may assist them through the remainder of their professional life. Considering the rapid evolution of technology and pharmacology, practicing physicians will not have the time or interest to keep abreast of innovations in critical care medicine unless they require that knowledge in their daily activities. Therefore, less emphasis should be placed on teaching residents manual skills in invasive procedures or on empiric management of mechanical ventilation, since those techniques will become obsolete within a few years. The physician-director should instead help trainees understand that a patient cannot be divided into separate components, each with problems amenable to independent treatment. Education should emphasize that most critical illnesses sequentially involve many organ systems even when they originate from discrete, recognizable primary insults. Thus treatment plans should consider the peripheral effects of each intervention. Residents who have learned these concepts are better prepared to accept future innovations with which they are not personally familiar.

Interaction Among Health Professionals

The ICU is a complex organization that operates properly only if all cooperating elements interact harmoniously. JCAHO requires that each hospital establish a multidisciplinary committee to maintain standards of care in the ICU. Although the composition of the committee is left largely to the discretion of each institution, the physician-director and head nurse of the ICU must be included. Thus JCAHO indirectly recognizes what appears self-evident: quality and continuity of care in the ICU depend primarily on committed critical care physicians and dedicated, specialized critical care nurses.

Critical Care Nurses

ICUs can and do operate without trained critical care physicians and at times without any identifiable medical staff. Although these conditions are hardly ideal, they do not prohibit patient care. No ICU, however, can exist without critical care nurses. The nursing profession has found one of its most successful expressions in the practice of critical care medicine. Nurses' traditional concern for the well-being and personal integrity of patients and families has been seamlessly engrafted in the sophisticated technology and advanced pharmacology used in ICUs. Furthermore, nurses have developed a far more comprehensive concept of ICU organization than physicians and have established and validated standards of practice. As the literature proves, the vast body of knowledge on ICU management developed by nurses has no counterpart in the medical profession. Many of the statements in this chapter regarding scheduling or assignment of responsibilities to physicians are simply our opinions, based on personal experience. Objective evidence to support most of them is limited. The nursing literature, however, abounds with excellent studies that analyze in detail all aspects of ICU administration, from the responsibilities of different staff members, to their personal problems, to the cooperation with other health professionals and the interaction with patients and families.

The contribution of nurses to critical care medicine, both as organizers and as providers of care, is vitally important. The diminishing number of nurses interested in a long-term career in critical care nursing is nothing short of catastrophic. The present practice and future evolution of critical care medicine are seriously threatened by the potential shortage of trained nurses. Unfortunately, even though the indispensable role of nurses is widely recognized both inside and outside the medical system, little is being done to address the problem of nurses' growing dissatisfaction.

Recruitment of nurses is the responsibility of the department or division of nursing, and direct physician involvement is neither required nor appropriate. The medical staff, however, should assist with the recruitment efforts in every possible way, primarily by creating an atmosphere of professional cooperation and mutual respect within which all health care providers may thrive. Critical care specialists should feel particularly compelled to assist with these efforts because in the ICU the cooperation between nurses and physicians reaches levels unparalleled in any other area of the hospital, except perhaps the operating room. Indeed, the relationship of nurse anesthetists and anesthesiologists closely parallels that of critical care nurses and critical care physicians. In both cases special competence can be recognized by certifying boards and there is a large area of common responsibility, with nurses and physicians performing essentially identical therapeutic interventions. Examples include adjusting mechanical ventilators on the basis of physiologic measurements and administering vasoactive, sedative, and analgesic drugs on the basis of clinical requirements.

Critical care physicians and critical care nurses have a vested interest in supporting each other, since neither can practice effectively without the other. In an environment without trained and committed critical care physicians, nurses may not be able to express the full latitude of their competence, since the responsible physicians may be unreceptive to innovations with which they themselves are not familiar. For their part, critical care physicians who have had the unfortunate experience of practicing in ICUs where the nursing staff is inadequately trained and has little professional interest in the practice of critical care medicine know that their efforts would be far more rewarding if their therapeutic plans were developed with and implemented by experienced nurses.

Even though physicians and nurses participate in the same national and regional societies, many aspects of joint practice have not been fully defined. In many ICUs a highly functional system has been developed to everyone's benefit, but issues that significantly affect the interaction of ICU physicians and nurses are seldom formally discussed. An important omission is the participation of critical care nurses in the economic aspects of joint practice, as is the case for nurse anesthetists. Many ICU interventions for which physicians bill patients are performed at least in part by nurses or require their close cooperation. This interaction goes well beyond functions classically associated with the nursing profession, since critical care nurses routinely perform independent therapeutic interventions. The monetary rewards of critical care nurses should reflect these specialized functions and should have some relationship to the overall professional income of the ICU.

Although money alone cannot procure qualified individuals in the absence of professional gratification, it is a powerful incentive. Moral satisfaction will not be sufficient to attract and retain more than a million nurses, despite the prospect of a lifetime of inadequate remuneration. Unfortunately, many people still view nurses as idealized, selfless caregivers who draw their entire motivation from nurturing the infirm. This attitude is shortsighted, patronizing, or self-serving, depending on those who espouse it. Nurses are one of the largest professional groups in the country. They have the same goals as physicians or lawyers: job satisfaction, respect, empowerment, and income. As long as these realities are ignored, numbers of nurses, and of more immediate concern here, critical care nurses, will continue to decrease, seriously jeopardizing both medical care and medical practice in the hospital.

Although most of these problems require global solutions and legislative interventions, steps can be taken at the local level to retain the irreplaceable human resource represented by a qualified nursing staff. ICU administrators should propose policies that will reduce the stress of critical care nurses while increasing their professional identification with the ICU. Issues to be considered include automatic mechanisms to adjust the ICU census to the size of the nursing staff and assuring critical care nurses that they will not have to practice outside the ICU even when the patient census transiently decreases. Also, all ICU policies should be developed with the close cooperation

(and not just a cosmetic "consultation") of critical care nurses. ICU nurses have specialized theoretical and practical knowledge of pathophysiology, pharmacology, and technology as they apply to critically ill patients. Thus nurses should be involved in the formulation of management protocols, as well as admission and discharge decisions. A full partnership in all aspects of ICU practice and management is a difficult but necessary goal toward which physicians and nurses should strive together.

Other Health Professionals

Although the relationship of critical care physicians and nurses is uniquely privileged, a modern ICU draws on the support of many other health professionals. The responsibilities of these individuals are usually more circumscribed, dealing with specific organ functions or instruments rather than with all aspects of patient management. However, they are indispensable for the safe and efficient operation of the ICU.

Respiratory Therapists

For a number of inappropriate reasons, usually based on political expediency, many states, including highly regulated ones such as New York, have no formal licensing process for respiratory therapists. As a consequence, their responsibilities vary widely, depending on the hospital and on the involvement of the medical director. An almost universal function of respiratory therapists is the maintenance and operation of mechanical ventilators in the ICU and in the hospital at large. There are numerous reasons to assign this responsibility to trained respiratory therapists. The technical sophistication of respiratory therapy equipment has been steadily increasing. The computer-controlled, programmable, expandable, multifunction mechanical ventilators of today bear little resemblance to the devices of 20 years ago. With the new potential, however, has come greater complexity, necessitating specially trained and experienced staff who can use all features to the patient's best advantage.

The increasing need for professionally committed respiratory therapists is creating a serious discrepancy between demand and availability, which threatens quality of care in the ICU almost as much as the shortage of nurses. This profession must be made more appealing, with the necessary combination of official recognition, empowerment, and income.

The functions of respiratory therapists are not limited to operating mechanical ventilators. Such a restriction would seriously underutilize skilled technologists, who are fully competent to recognize the indications for, and supervise the administration of, pharmacologic and physical means of pulmonary therapy. In many hospitals respiratory therapists administer oxygen, maintain monitoring equipment and other instruments, and calibrate transducers for vascular pressures. JCAHO regulations mandate that respiratory therapists be supervised by a medical director, who is often a pulmonary physician or an anesthesiologist. It could be argued, however, that with the development of critical care as a separate subspecialty, respiratory therapy services should be supervised by physicians with training in critical care medicine. The ICU is one of most significant users of mechanical ventilators, monitoring equipment, and other life support devices. Also, outside the ICU, respiratory therapists often treat patients with serious lung disease, who are highly susceptible to complications that may eventually require ICU admission. Early identification of developing problems and more timely interventions might be possible if respiratory therapists could refer these patients to experienced ICU physicians. Prompt therapy and expeditious ICU admission, when indicated, can reduce morbidity and mortality.

In conclusion, an excellent respiratory therapy service is indispensable for the proper function of a busy ICU, and the cooperation between critical care physicians and respiratory therapists could be usefully extended outside the ICU.

Biomedical Technologists

ICUs are increasingly dependent on advanced technology. The functions and complexity of monitoring equipment are steadily growing. However, there are conflicting recommendations, based on clinical, ethical, and economic considerations, for and against the continual introduction of new devices in the ICU. The debate is beyond the scope of this chapter. However, on one point there is universal agreement: all instruments necessary for good patient care must operate flawlessly. Once having accepted this basic premise, ICU administrators must carefully consider its numerous ramifications. With some devices proper function is evident or can be independently verified with ease. For instance, direct observation

can ascertain the accuracy of a volumetric infusion pump or a drop counter. A continuous electrocardiographic monitor must produce recognizable and meaningful waveforms; the experienced eye recognizes artifacts with little difficulty. Other instruments, however, report values that cannot be validated by observation alone, although they can be confirmed by a second device that operates on a different principle. Invasive catheterization, Doppler monitoring, and sphygmomanometry can all be used to measure systemic blood pressure. Although some of these techniques are more accurate, especially when pressure values are low, together they verify one another. As instruments become more complex, however, validation of the results they provide is increasingly elaborate and requires considerable technical expertise. Furthermore, as instrument monitoring and support become indispensable in clinical practice, the sudden failure of any commonly used device can severely affect the ability to provide acceptable care. Even the most astute clinician would be seriously challenged if required to manage, without invasive monitoring of systemic and pulmonary artery pressure, cardiac output measurements, and blood gas determinations, the treatment of a patient receiving mechanical ventilation for respiratory compromise and several different vasoactive drugs for cardiac failure. Before these monitoring aids were introduced in clinical practice, complex cardiac support therapy with multiple drugs was simply unavailable. Thus ICU clinicians must be certain that their instruments perform accurately, reliably, and continuously. Such requirements have led to the addition of biomedical engineers to the support staff of the ICU. These individuals are primarily electronics experts but also have enough knowledge of physiology and pathophysiology to understand the medical purpose of the devices used. Bioengineers bring to the multidisciplinary ICU team the perspective of a rigorous, mechanically oriented discipline, which is indispensable for the safe use of increasingly powerful but exactingly complex devices.

Dietitians

Dietitians play an important role in the ICU. Critically ill patients, and indeed most patients with significant organ dysfunction, cannot receive unrestricted alimentation. In many cases the oral route is unavailable and patients must receive gastric or jejunal feedings. Often,

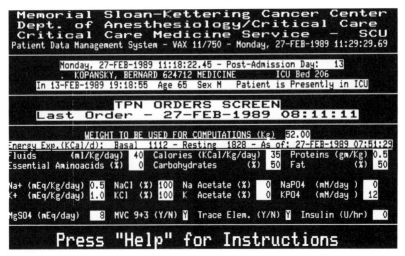

Figure 30–4. Computerized order for total parenteral nutrition, as it appears on a terminal screen. The ordering physician can adjust each nutritional component on the basis of the patient's physiologic requirements.

too, intestinal function does not allow enteral alimentation, and intravenous nutrition is required. Professional dietitians can be invaluable in determining the patients' energy and nutrient requirements. Computer-controlled total parenteral nutrition mixing systems permit the preparation of intravenous solutions tailored to the needs of any patient (Figs. 30–4 and 30–5). Thus the role of dietitians in the ICU will presumably continue to expand.

Physical Therapists

Physical therapists provide indispensable assistance to patients confined to bed for long periods. The therapeutic goals for ICU patients

extend beyond the immediate recovery of failing organs. Full recuperation should be attempted when possible. Painful or crippling muscle contractions should therefore be prevented through proper use of physical therapy.

Computer Specialists

Many ICUs make substantial use of data management equipment, from simple instruments that measure physiologic variables to sophisticated minicomputers with dozens of terminals. As with any other type of electronic instrumentation, once the ICU staff begins to rely on computers for clinical information, they would perform less well if these devices failed.

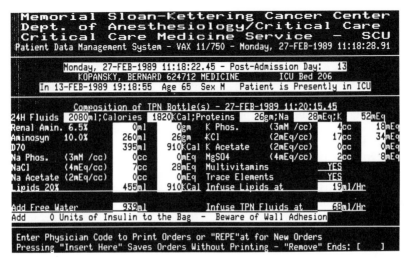

Figure 30–5. The computer performs all necessary calculations and generates a complete order for total parenteral nutrition.

Competent technical support should be readily available at all times. Thus systems managers and even systems analysts will become increasingly common components of the multidisciplinary ICU team as computer equipment becomes a standard element of clinical medicine.

Pharmacists

The ever-expanding variety of drugs available for the treatment of the critically ill has increased the importance of pharmacists as members of the ICU team. Pharmacists not only are qualified to prepare drugs, but also have in-depth knowledge of dosages, routes of administration and elimination, and adverse reactions and interactions. They can be invaluable resource persons when new substances with unknown side effects are introduced into a clinical protocol.

Attending Staff

We have discussed the roles of the house staff and of the many nonmedical professionals who practice in the ICU. Ultimately, however, the responsibility for planning and supervising the care of patients resides with the attending staff. This is required by custom, by law, and most significantly by the patients, who expect that their care will be provided by competent physicians. Thus an important aspect of the administrative structure of the ICU is the definition of the composition, privileges, and functions of the attending staff.

In larger hospitals the entire medical practice of the ICU director and of many other critical care specialists takes place in the ICU. The benefits of this arrangement are obvious. The full-time staff can continuously supervise patients whose conditions change often and unpredictably. The demands of continuing education in a field as varied and complex as critical care rarely permit the maintenance of adequate skills in other specialties. The pharmacology and technology that critical care physicians must master have exponentially increased in the last 20 years (Table 30–2). They must select appropriate and cost-efficient drugs, devices, monitors, and instruments, and each decision may significantly influence ICU costs and quality of care for years to come.

The literature provides objective evidence that a full-time ICU staff improves care, especially when the only variable truly relevant to patients, survival, is considered. Of course, smaller hospitals or very specialized ICUs may be unable to afford one or more physicians who have only ICU obligations. However, since the requirement for continuing education in critical care cannot be sacrificed without compromising patient care, even a part-time ICU physician-director should have a schedule that gives priority to ICU activities.

ADMISSION AND DISCHARGE POLICIES

The authority of the ICU director should include meaningful control over admissions and discharges. JCAHO regulations require only that the ICU director enforce the hospital admission and discharge policies, a subtle but significant distinction. Indeed, when the position of ICU director exists only on paper or is assigned to a junior staff member, effective supervision is unrealistic. ICU admissions and discharges may then depend on factors other than patients' needs. More senior physicians may be able to obtain preferential allocation of beds, a simple queueing system (first come, first served) may operate, or by default junior staff members may be in a position to make decisions affecting the well-being of patients in the ICU and elsewhere in the hospital. None of these situations is consistent with an efficient allocation of ICU resources.

If a harmonious atmosphere can be developed, however, it should be possible to define the criteria that qualify patients for ICU admission or indicate they are ready to be discharged. Furthermore, the ICU should have a clear triage policy when requests for admission exceed availability. A constructive interaction between ICU physicians, who control bed allocation, and admitting physicians can be developed if confidence and mutual respect exist. To achieve these goals, the ICU administrator should widely circulate the guidelines for admission and discharge and should obtain the approval of all relevant department heads. The cooperation of the more senior physicians of all services should be enlisted, and they should strictly refrain from requesting waivers of the regulations for their own patients. The hospital administration should unequivocally support the ICU staff when veiled or open threats follow an admission or discharge decision that complies with all existing policies. A committee of respected members of the medical staff should periodically review the reasons for, and consequences of, rejecting admissions or forcing discharges and should recommend policy changes if indicated.

When these conditions apply, none of the staff physicians should fear that ICU care is arbitrarily and unjustly denied to their patients; ICU physicians should be protected from uncomfortable and unfair pressures; and hospital administrators should be satisfied that costly ICU care is allocated to patients who can most benefit from it. Consensus, of course, is far easier to recommend than to achieve. Simple recommendations that can be applied to all institutions do not exist. Agreements must be locally forged and enforced. However, the benefits in terms of ICU staff morale, general perception of fairness, and interaction with patients and families should justify even herculean efforts.

RESPONSIBILITY FOR PATIENT MANAGEMENT

If the task of allocating critical care resources is daunting, defining who has final responsibility for medical decisions affecting ICU patients is even more difficult. Essentially three parties are involved with each ICU patient: the physician-of-record, the ICU staff, and the patient with family and friends. The interactions among them are complex, stressful, and affected by the continuous awareness of a possibly lethal illness. Each group may fall into inappropriate or self-defeating behavior; therefore all individuals involved, especially medical staff members, must try to minimize conflict and concentrate on the patient's best interest.

The physician-of-record, who often has little if any critical care training, may have strong biases regarding patient management. The physician's judgment may be clouded by feelings of guilt and denial, which are inevitable when patients have complications requiring ICU admission.

ICU physicians may display a detachment that the primary physician interprets as intolerable callousness, especially if the latter has developed a deep emotional involvement with the patient over the course of a long and difficult illness. Critical care physicians must avoid any attitude that implies a judgment of their colleagues' professional actions. Complications are often unpredictable or unavoidable, even when treatment is in the most experienced hands; even if negligence or poor judgment is obvious, accusations and recriminations exchanged while attempting to resolve the patient's urgent problems do not improve therapy or prognosis.

Thorough reviews of the complications that resulted in an unexpected ICU admission and recommendations aimed at preventing their recurrence should be left to the quality assurance process of the primary service. Critical care physicians must also resist any tendency to retire into an ivory tower of high technology. The obligation to explain to patients, in intelligible terms, all aspects of proposed care must be extended also to colleagues, whose grasp of sophisticated technology and advanced pharmacology may be extensive.

Family members, who usually have not met the critical care physician before the complication developed, become angry, frightened, and confused when they perceive differences of opinion regarding patient management between the primary team and ICU physicians. The inevitable tendency to side with one medical team creates further animosity and more confrontations, which can only worsen patient care.

ICU patients who are conscious and aware of their surroundings, a condition that may occur more often than is believed, are severely disturbed by even the slightest signs of disagreement or animosity among the physicians providing their care.

Most physicians would agree that the purpose of their profession is to restore health, or at least to provide comfort and pain relief to patients. Thus any type of behavior that may negatively affect care, including open conflicts among health professionals, must be avoided. The best way to obtain this result is to define clearly the responsibilities and the boundaries of autonomous decisions by critical care and primary physicians. When this goal is satisfactorily achieved within an ICU, territorial controversies and personal feuds can be removed from the immediate area of patient care and resolved within the policymaking structure of the hospital.

CRITICAL CARE PHYSICIANS AS EXCLUSIVE CARE PROVIDERS

The critical care team may have full responsibility for all aspects of patient care. This arrangement is common only in specialized ICUs, such as coronary care units or cardiovascular surgery units, where the physician-of-record and the ICU physician may even be the same person and therefore have no reason for conflict. In general medical or surgical ICUs where most critical care physicians practice, however, the distinction between physicians responsible for the ICU and those whose patients are admitted there is often definite. Under those circumstances a complete renunciation of responsibility on the part of the physician-of-record is rare and generally undesirable. It is justified, perhaps, only when the complication requiring ICU admission is unrelated to the primary disease and the role of the physician-of-record in caring for the patient has been completed. For instance, respiratory failure, secondary to pulmonary embolism, may develop in a young woman after a breast biopsy. The surgeon would have little to offer in management of the complication, and the patient would have no further need of surgical assistance. Except for this or similar unusual and well-defined circumstances, however, the physician-of-record should maintain a continuing involvement with the patient's care, even after admission to the ICU.

CRITICAL CARE PHYSICIANS AS PRIMARY CARE PROVIDERS

Patients admitted to the ICU may be treated by the critical care team for all aspects of the problems that require ICU care, while the physician-of-record retains responsibility for management of the underlying disease and is informed of all care the patient receives. Such cooperation can provide the best possible medical care to patients, drawing on the expertise of all physicians involved. For instance, a patient with a systemic malignancy, in whom sepsis and respiratory failure develop, should continue to receive specialized treatment for the primary disease, a function for which the physician-of-record is best suited. On the other hand, failure to understand and treat the acute complications of the disease is as inexorably fatal as an uncontrolled progression of the primary disease. The critical care staff, who are continuously present in the ICU, can formulate comprehensive plans of care, taking into consideration all requirements of the patient, including fluids, nutrition, antibiotic therapy, hemodynamic support, and ventilatory assistance, without interfering with the functions of the physician-of-record. This distribution of responsibilities is also useful in dealing with another source of problems in the ICU, the interaction with the families of critically ill patients. The transition from other areas of the hospital to the ICU is almost always traumatic for patients and families. The family perceives, often correctly, that the patient's illness

has become more severe; the new environment is noisy, confusing, and hostile; the visiting hours are restricted, adding separation to the many other sources of anguish; and the ICU staff is unfamiliar, engaged in activities that may appear alien and forbidding. In this tense atmosphere, nothing may trouble families more than receiving contradictory information. The physician-of-record, concentrating on the primary disease, may interpret improvements in that aspect of the clinical picture as a sign of iminent recovery and transmit this optimistic perception to the family. Their temporary relief may be negated by a far more pessimistic report on the evolution of organ system failures treated by the ICU staff. Confusion is painful to families and diminishes their confidence in all physicians caring for the patient. Physicians' mutual respect for one another's expertise and responsibilities can minimize or prevent conflicts. Patients and their families usually understand that many different specialists may be needed to provide optimal care; they readily accept that one physician cannot be conversant with all aspects of medicine and therefore must defer to colleagues to treat, and discuss with patients and families, some aspects of the disease. Identifying the ICU physician as the provider of care and the liaison with the family for the morbid condition that required ICU admission does not diminish or interrupt the family's vital relationship with the physician-of-record.

CRITICAL CARE PHYSICIANS AS CONSULTANTS

The theoretical and practical benefits of a full-time critical care team are clear. However, in major university hospitals with many medical and surgical residencies, as well as in small hospitals without house staff, the role of critical care physicians is commonly restricted to that of consultants or to performance of very specific functions, such as mechanical ventilator management. As previously mentioned, a number of studies suggest that outcome may improve when patient care is supervised by physicians with special training and full-time commitment to critical care. Although evidence that ICU practice should be restricted to, or at least supervised by, critical care physicians may be impossible to obtain, any policy that ignores the basic nature of critical illness as a disease process that affects all parts of the organism should be strongly opposed. Parceling the patient to satisfy the parochial requirements of each service or department is simply bad medicine. It may be convenient to believe that adequate care can be rendered if a pulmonary specialist is responsible for the lungs, a cardiologist for the heart, a nephrologist for fluids and electrolytes, and so on. In reality, each therapeutic intervention significantly affects the function of other organs and therefore must be integrated in a total management plan. Critical care physicians, when they operate as consultants, should express their opinion on the aggregate plan of care, coordinating suggestions and recommendations from other specialists to avoid potentially conflicting treatments. They should not assume responsibility for single aspects of a patient's management, such as mechanical ventilation, outside the context of the entire therapy plan. Attempts to divide the patient are the antithesis of the principles of critical care medicine.

INTENSIVE CARE UNIT BUDGET

ICUs use approximately 20% of in-patient health care resources, or 1% of the gross national product. The absolute expenditure for ICU care is $40 billion dollars per year, exceeding, for instance, the total cost of the Apollo Project that put a man on the moon. These figures are staggering, and this uncontrolled consumption cannot continue. Despite the restrictions that third party payers are now placing on medical expenditures, the process of budgetary reconciliation in the ICU remains haphazard. These problems are related to poor definition of the ICU administrative structure. The departmental assignment of ICUs varies from hospital to hospital. In some institutions the nominal responsibility for ICU expenditures rests with the chairman of one department but the physicians responsible for patient care belong to a different specialty. In others the ICU is administered by a large, multidisciplinary committee, and therefore no department has a vested interest in the ICU infrastructure and quality of medical care. Commonly the responsibility for disposable supplies, a significant share of total ICU expenditures, is assigned to the department of nursing, although actual costs depend on medical decisions, such as the frequency of use of pulmonary artery catheters, over which the nursing department has no control.

To set the fiscal house in order, administrators should strictly apply the principles of direct accountability and cost-effectiveness to ICUs and for that matter to all services of the hospital.

Direct Accountability

The individuals who generate costs should also be responsible for the budget. This may appear self-evident, a corollary of the basic principle "No taxation without representation." As the previous examples indicate, however, it has often not applied to ICUs. The consequence is cost overrun, if the budget is expanded to accommodate the requests of those who generate the expenditures, or random rationing, if the availability of supplies is restricted by budgetary decisions made without consulting care providers.

The physician-director, the head nurse of the ICU, and possibly other experienced ICU staff members should be intimately involved in the budget process. They should assess patients' clinical needs as objectively as possible and requisition the resources required to meet those needs. They should also develop a rational priority system to accommodate economic constraints, regularly review the adherence of the expenditures to the budget, and carefully examine clinical practices if the estimates are not respected.

Cost-Effectiveness

A basic principle of budgeting is to minimize wasteful expenditures. Although physicians are notoriously resistant to allowing cost considerations to determine their practice, in the ICU a sound fiscal policy is also good medicine. If costly supplies and expensive instruments were used only when a clear benefit to the patient could be proved, the budgetary problems of many hospitals would be solved. In the ICU this concept can be extended to almost all aspects of medical practice, from the routine administration of expensive new antibiotics when older, less expensive ones would be as effective, to the use of pulmonary artery catheters when the clinical indications are doubtful.

Cost-effectiveness should especially be considered when new technology is introduced in the ICU. Although safety and efficiency are important reasons for innovations, they cannot be the sole justification; new systems should be introduced only when they provide a measurable improvement over previous ones. This concept should not be interpreted as regressive or inimical to scientific discoveries; on the contrary, the requirement to obtain objective verification of each hypothesis is the essence of science. Of course, cost-effectiveness cannot be measured exclusively in direct monetary terms; more abstract considerations, such as patient safety or staff comfort, must also apply. However, new monitoring devices or drugs should never be introduced in the ICU just because they are available, without a clear understanding of how they will improve patient care.

Cost-conscious management in the ICU requires a dedicated and possibly full-time medical staff. Waste can be eliminated only through policies restricting the unnecessary use of drugs and supplies. Monitoring such policies is time consuming and requires considerable expertise. Once approved, policies must be continually reiterated and enforced, especially in areas where many different professionals operate, often as transients with little vested interest in the operation of the ICU. Clearly responsibility for cost control must be assigned to a senior staff member with proven competence and continuing interest in critical care medicine.

QUALITY ASSURANCE AND UTILIZATION REVIEW

The delivery of the highest quality of care has always been the implicit goal of American medicine. However, explicit standards of quality assurance were not developed until the 1960s, when Medicare and Medicaid legislation was enacted and the nation began to notice the alarming rise in the cost of health care. At the same time the comfortable conviction that medical care was constantly improving the health of the population was challenged. It was suggested that the system favored unnecessary surgery and hospitalization at the expense of preventive care, and that despite rising costs, the level of health remained the same or even declined for a significant segment of the population. Pressured by Congress and by public opinion, the medical community began to develop techniques to define and measure the quality of medical care. The adoption of the prospective reimbursement system and diagnosis related groups (DRGs) further increased the importance of critical reviews of care to control costs without sacrificing standards. Unlike the previous method of retrospective payments based on historical costs, DRGs encourage institutions to shorten length of stay and to curtail or even eliminate high-cost, low-yield activities. DRGs have a variable im-

pact on different clinical specialties but are exceedingly significant for ICU services. As Smith (1987) writes, "The field of critical care is particularly vulnerable to many of the negative aspects of prospective, end-product oriented reimbursement." Thus delineation of patterns of use of ICUs, as well as measurement and assessment of quality of care, will assume increasing importance.

Quality Assurance

To ensure that hospitals and other health care facilities abide by established norms and standards, the methods of care and results obtained must be carefully monitored. Although the precise definition of "quality" continues to elude the experts, a general consensus about its meaning exists. In medicine, quality measures the degree to which individual physicians and institutions adhere to accepted clinical practices and the extent to which the expected outcome is achieved for a given set of clinical circumstances. This definition assumes that constant "means" attain predictable "ends." Valid quality assurance standards must also precisely define the concept of "health." The health status of each individual depends on many factors, not only the presence or absence of a morbid condition. Thus measuring tools must be standard and uniform for proper interpretation of quality assurance results.

History

The concept of quality assurance dates to the early 1900s, when standards of care were first proposed by the American College of Surgeons. However, formal programs have been developed only in the last two decades. JCAHO, a voluntary but extremely powerful organization, has assumed jurisdiction for nationwide quality assurance programs and has introduced uniform minimal standards of care. A major impetus to the development of standards has come from the growing demand, felt across the nation, that expanded health care services be made available to all sectors of the population; at the same time the shift of costs of medical care to the government or to large private insurance companies has obligated hospitals to be more accountable for the services they deliver.

Throughout the 1970s JCAHO continually revised the standards, eventually creating a framework for objective and systematic review.

In 1979 JCAHO approved radically new quality assurance standards, based on a less rigid approach. Previously the emphasis had been on formal audits, which often represented only exercises in data collection and did not measurably affect the care rendered. The revised standards mandated that hospitals (and later other health care institutions) develop programs to monitor their activities and to prevent or correct any deficiencies in patient care. Under these guidelines, quality assurance has become increasingly concerned with economic issues and strategic planning. Evidence now exists that strict application of the JCAHO standards can improve care. Thus JCAHO accreditation, although theoretically voluntary, has become essential to the operation of any health care facility.

Multidisciplinary Approach

Current JCAHO standards state that hospitals must have "an ongoing quality assurance program designed to objectively and systematically monitor and evaluate the quality and appropriateness of patient care, pursue opportunities to improve patient care, and resolve identified problems." These standards define the concept of quality assurance and specify minimum conditions that each clinical service must provide to gain accreditation. Furthermore, each service, whether clinical or nonclinical, must develop an explicit program for continuing evaluation and monitoring of the quality of care. The programs must ensure adequate measurement, interpretation, continuity, and feedback and include the following steps:

- Assignment of responsibility to an identifiable individual
- Elaboration of the scope or mission
- Identification of the pertinent aspects of service
- Exact stipulation of the dimensions and indicators of services
- Identification of objective and predetermined criteria
- Data collection and processing
- Identification, analysis, and resolution of problems
- Follow-up and assessment
- Sharing of information with the overall institutional quality assurance program

Quality Assurance in the Intensive Care Unit

ICUs, like any other department or division within a hospital, must develop valid quality assurance programs, although the required procedural steps are not always easy to follow in the ICU. ICU patients have a broad range of clinical disorders; thus classification into well-defined groups, whose expected outcome can be established, is difficult. The development of severity of illness measures, such as the Acute Physiology and Chronic Health Evaluation (APACHE), Mortality Prediction Model (MPM), and Therapeutic Intervention Scoring System (TISS), has reduced but not eliminated the problem of interpatient variability. Thus definition of goals against which standards of care may be measured is more readily subject to dispute for ICU patients than for other services. For example, if ICU discharge is used as an endpoint for quality assurance programs, an inherent bias remains, since discharged patients may die elsewhere in the hospital, leave the hospital alive, or return to the ICU for further care. These very different outcomes may have been influenced by factors that preceded the discharge. Furthermore, the documentation of care delivered in the ICU may not meet quality assurance standards, since the critical nature of the disease and the rapid change in clinical status may result in suboptimal charting of procedures and techniques. At the same time ICUs, more than most other services, require effective quality assurance programs, since recent changes in health care financing have ominous implications for poor ICU practices. Since the 1960s, ICU use has grown considerably and, as previously mentioned, now accounts for a significant proportion of all hospital expenditures and even of the gross national product. Hence the appropriateness and benefits of the care provided must be strictly accounted for and deficiencies must be quickly corrected. The rapid growth of medical technology and the unabated proliferation of negligence litigation add to the importance and urgency of reliable ICU quality assurance.

In the ICU, and elsewhere, good quality assurance demands close cooperation among all individuals responsible for the provision of services. Ultimate authority and responsibility should rest with an individual closely identified with the ICU, in most cases the physician-director. The chain of command must then flow both laterally and vertically. In particular, the medical and nursing staffs must freely and frequently interact as a well-coordinated team. As an example of a quality assurance program that can be developed in an intensive care setting, the ICU at Memorial Sloan-Kettering Cancer Center in New York explicitly states the procedures and services it provides and specifically defines its ultimate clinical goals. To ensure adherence to this policy and to detect and correct deviations from accepted norms, nurses and physicians maintain an objective, computer-based assessment of all patients under their care. Periodically a retrospective review is performed to identify unexpected outcomes and correct resultant deficiencies through the recommendations of a multidisciplinary committee. This approach fully adheres to JCAHO requirements.

Utilization Review

Definition and History

Utilization review and quality assurance overlap, but the substantial differences between the two must be recognized. Quality assurance is the process through which standards of care are established and compliance with those standards is monitored. Utilization review refers to the frequency with which a specific aspect of medical care is delivered by a practitioner or institution and how it conforms to the expected frequency of occurrence, according to local or national patterns. As with quality assurance, the impetus for utilization review programs originated with the passage of Medicare and Medicaid legislation. Further pressure came from the federal mandate to establish professional services review organizations (PSROs) in the early 1970s. The major push toward organized utilization review, however, came in 1977 when JCAHO published specific guidelines defining its goals. The current *Accreditation Manual for Hospitals* states that:

The hospital shall demonstrate appropriate allocation of its resources through the conduct of an effective utilization review program. The results of the utilization review activity shall be contributory to the quality of patient care and shall be reflected in the other quality-protective functions of the hospital and the medical staff.

Current Framework

Initial utilization review efforts were directed toward profile analysis, in which crude data, such as length of stay, were analyzed retrospectively. The current guidelines emphasize a more introspective approach to the issue of resource utilization. For instance, whereas trends of length of stay were previously monitored, today the actual necessity for a particular admission and for the services rendered to the patient during hospitalization is scrutinized. Prospective reimbursement and DRGs have greatly increased the importance of formal, comprehensive utilization review. Furthermore, Medicare now delineates specific activities that must be included in review programs. Most notably, any institution receiving Medicare payments for in-patient care must contract with a qualified external peer review organization (PRO) to obtain independent audits. Although PROs are the logical extensions of the PSROs, the stipulation for "peer" input into the review process is new and the official mandate and the power to enforce a recommendation through denial of payment are much stronger.

Basic Components

Admission Review.   All admissions to a hospital or to a particular service must be appropriately justified. Associated with this requirement is a program to monitor the specific patterns of admission and to analyze whether patients may be as well cared for in less expensive settings (such as outpatient clinics). Institutions must also identify patients who may be prematurely and inappropriately discharged.

Outlier Analysis.   Under DRGs, provisions for additional reimbursement exist for patients who may require longer or more expensive care than allowed by a given DRG. Utilization review should be directed toward the analysis of these patients to document and validate the added use of resources.

Specific Diagnosis Related Group Assignment. To prevent a phenomenon termed DRG creep, the assignment of patients to inappropriate DRGs to procure greater reimbursement, utilization review should match each patient with the correct DRG.

Overall Quality Review.   Utilization review and quality assurance and assessment are invariably linked, since they share the goal of delivering appropriate care and guaranteeing adherence to standards of practice. Hence a review must include analysis of alternative modalities of care that may achieve identical results. Cost-benefit and cost-effectiveness analysis are implicit in the evaluation of alternative services for a clinical condition.

Utilization Review in the Intensive Care Unit

The analysis of trends and patterns of resource utilization is more important in ICUs than in most other areas of the hospital. ICUs use a large amount of health care resources, but the current framework of DRGs does not adequately represent the diagnoses or the patients who require ICU admission. Thus considerable disparity exists between costs and payments. The outcomes of ICU treatment are also the subject of growing debate, since studies have shown that the patients who generate the highest costs are often those who do not survive. With the availability of methods, such as APACHE, TISS, and MPM, that objectively measure the severity of illness and the use of resources, utilization review should address the efficient use of ICU resources, precisely define the outcome of intensive care for different clinical conditions, and describe the process through which these outcomes are achieved. Despite the reluctance of physicians to allow cost-effectiveness to guide therapy, it is impossible to continue expanding the share of common wealth allocated to postponing death of patients who have gone beyond the limits of medical science. Utilization review and quality assurance techniques can provide an objective framework for reasonable and nondiscriminatory decisions about who will receive care. Attempts to avoid hard decisions, however, will only enforce the limitations of care based on arbitrary rather than scientific criteria, increasing the risk of conflict, animosity, resentment, and litigation.

SUGGESTED READINGS

Carlon GC, Fein AI: Current activities of physicians trained in critical care medicine. Crit Care Med 1988;16:401

Cullen DJ, Keene R, Waternaux C, et al: Results, charges and benefits of intensive care for critically ill patients: update 1983. Crit Care Med 1984;12:102-106

Dunbar S: Should CCRN nurses receive a salary differential? Dimens Crit Care Nurs 1985;4:361-367

Fields WL, Loveridge C: Critical thinking and fatigue: how do nurses on 8 and 12 hour shifts compare? Nurs Econ 1988;6:189-195

Graham NO: Historical perspective and regulations regarding quality assessment. In Graham NO (ed): Quality assurance in hospitals. Rockville, Md, 1982, Aspen Publishers.

Grimaldi PL, Micheletti JA: Utilization and quality review under the prospective payment system. Qual Rev Bull 1984;12:30-37

Hilberman M: The evolution of intensive care units. Crit Care Med 1975;3:159-165

Joint Commission on Accreditation of Healthcare Organizations: Accreditation manual for hospitals. Chicago, 1989, The Commission

Kahn KL, Brook RH, Draper D, et al: Interpreting hospital mortality data: how can we proceed? JAMA 1988;260:3625-3628

Knaus WA, Draper EA, Wagner DP, et al: APACHE II: a severity of disease classification system for acutely ill patients. Crit Care Med 1985;13:818-822

Kuhn RC, Canobbio MM, Alspach JA, et al: Education standards for critical care nursing: conceptual framework. Heart Lung 1985;14:149-155

Lemeshow S, Teres D, Avrunin JS, Pastides H: A comparison of methods to predict mortality of intensive care patients. Crit Care Med 1987;15:715-722

Munoz E, Chalfin D, Calabro S, et al: Costs of pulmonary medicine and DRGs: access and quality of care for the future. Am Rev Respir Dis 1988;137(4):964-968

Opal SM, Asp AA, Cannady PB Jr, et al: Efficacy of infection control measures during a nosocomial outbreak of disseminated aspergillosis associated with hospital construction. J Infect Dis 1986;153(3):634-637

Parker MM, Schubert W, Shelhamer JH, Parrillo JE: Perceptions of a critically ill patient experiencing therapeutic paralysis in an ICU. Crit Care Med 1984;12:69-71

Rhee KJ, Donabedian A, Burney RE: Assessing the quality of care in a hospital emergency unit: a framework and its applications. Qual Rev Bull 1987;15:4-16

Roberts JS, Coale JG: A history of the Joint Commission on Accreditation of Hospitals. JAMA 1987;258:936-940

Ryan DW, Copeland PF, Miller J, Freeman R: Replanning of an intensive therapy unit. Br Med J 1982;285:1634-1637

Sanford S. CCRN validation: a milestone for AACN. Focus Crit Care 1984;11:65-66

Smith CM: The impact of prospective, end-product-oriented reimbursement on critical care units. In Fein AI, Strosberg MA (eds): Managing the critical care unit. Rockville, Md, 1987, Aspen Publishers

Staff of the Division of Education and the Division of Accreditation, Joint Commission on Accreditation of Hospitals: Monitoring and evaluation of the quality and appropriateness of care: a hospital example. Qual Rev Bull 1986;14:326-330

Teres D, Brown RB, Lemeshow S, Parsells JL: A comparison of mortality and charges in two differently staffed intensive care units. Inquiry 1983;20:282-289

Turnbull A, Paggioli J, Carlon GC, Groeger JS: ICU readmission of surgical patients. Crit Care Med 1988;16:411

31

TRANSPORT

RONALD G. PEARL, MD, PhD, AND ALVIN HACKEL, MD

Medical transport had its beginnings in warfare. Napoleon's colleague Baron Larrey arranged "for the speedy evacuation of battle casualties by dedicated horse-drawn vehicles." In 1870, during the Siege of Paris, 160 civilians were airlifted by hot-air balloon. In the American Civil War railroad cars were used for medical transport. During World War I airplanes were used for medical evacuation by the Serbian army and later by the French and American armies. The German air force used aeromedical evacuation in the Spanish Civil War in 1936 and in Poland in 1940.

The first American military "elective" aeromedical evacuation occurred in 1943 when five patients were transferred from Karachi, India, to Washington, D.C., in a DC3. The trip took 7 days. Care in transit was provided by a U.S. Army nurse with no transport or flight experience. She was so tired on her arrival at the receiving hospital that she could not remember her name. The present sophistication of military aeromedical transport was reached as a result of developments in rapid medical transport during the military actions in Korea and Vietnam.

The civilian development of critical care transport began in neonatal intensive care. In the early 1900s premature infants were transferred for long-term care to regional centers in specially marked horse-drawn carriages. In the 1960s Usher and others developed new modalities for the treatment of the infant respiratory distress syndrome. These modalities (cardioactive drugs, aggressive fluid management, supplemental oxygenation, and assisted ventilation) could be performed only in regional intensive care facilities by personnel specially trained in neonatal intensive care. A significant difference in outcome was demonstrated between critically ill infants born in community hospitals who were transported to regional neonatal intensive care facilities and those who were not. As a result, regional networks were established around central neonatal intensive care nurseries, with hospital-based critical care transport programs an important component. These networks are a standard part of modern neonatal intensive care. They have fostered similar systems for high-risk maternity and critically ill pediatric patients.

Hospital-based systems of critical care transport were initiated in the civilian sector in Europe in the 1950s, when intensive care teams led by anesthesiologists transferred polio patients requiring ventilatory support to regional care centers. In the 1960s a system of intercontinental "repatriation" of civilians by specialized medical teams covered by prepaid medical travel health insurance was instituted. Today almost any type of patient requiring medical care can be transported successfully, even over long distances.

The term "critical care transport" was coined in 1970 to describe a concept of medical transport newly introduced in the United States. Medical transport teams composed of personnel from the ICUs of regional medical centers provided care during transport as an extension of the critical care provided in their ICUs (neonatal, pediatric, or adult). The goal of this critical care transport was to extend the capabilities of ICUs to patients in community hospitals. In trauma and emergency care the success of the military trauma prehospital transport program developed during the Korean War led to similar programs in the civilian sector. The definition of critical care transport was thus extended to include critically ill patients requiring emergency triage transported from out-of-hospital scenes to a nearby hospital and then to a regional center. More than 200 programs for transporting patients to or between hospitals exist in the United States today. These programs extend intensive care capabilities to optimize the care of critically ill patients.

Critical care transport programs are multidisciplinary. They are usually based in regional medical centers. The organizational format of a program depends on the types of patients to be transferred. The basic concept is to bring together the personnel with the specialized skills and experience needed to practice transport medicine.

Hospital-based critical care transport programs have the same medical and administrative base as other types of hospital patient care units. Transport programs are responsible for the same standards as in-hospital care units and should have the same mechanism for reporting to the hospital's chief-of-staff and medical board. Nevertheless, each medical transport program has its own personality, based on the type of hospital to which it belongs and the transport patient population.

A medical director must be responsible for the medical care provided en route and shares administrative responsibility for the safety and proper use of the transport program. This responsibility includes the formation and operation of a medical control plan for the individual transports, the development of a readily available pool of appropriately trained physicians, nurses, and other health care personnel, the establishment of medical criteria for transport, the creation of quality assurance and utilization review programs, and participation in regular safety programs for all aspects of medical transport.

Each transport should be managed by a medical control physician. This is a staff physician experienced in transport medicine. He or she organizes the transport with the referring physician, recommends the care to be administered during the remaining period before transport, and is responsible for the medical activities of the transport team. The medical control physician must be knowledgeable in the concepts of medical transport, as a basis for both the medical care to be delivered en route and the decisions on team composition and carrier selection.

The medical control physician responsible for a case selects the transport team. Team members should be part of the trained transport team personnel pool. They should be chosen for the pool after being recognized by their peers as competent and experienced in critical care. For most neonatal and pediatric critical care transport programs, the personnel are chosen from

ICUs. For adult programs they are chosen from intensive care, anesthesia, or emergency medicine units. The number of team members is limited by the size and configuration of the vehicle. Surface ambulances can carry three or four team members, helicopters two to five, and air ambulances two to four, depending on the particular vehicle.

Team personnel must understand the unique aspects of transport medicine and be knowledgeable in the operations of the program. They should be trained in the management of patients in aircraft and surface ambulances. If possible the training should be conducted by one person, a senior member of the program experienced in transport and skilled in teaching. The curriculum should include technical and psychologic aspects of transport, management of clinical problems, and physiologic effects of transport on the patient and the team. Medical guidelines for team participation are needed to avoid factors that limit the ability to function optimally in air or surface transport.

An emergency medical communications system is needed to handle requests efficiently and to ensure that interactions between the vehicles are as smooth as possible, for both medical and legal reasons. The communications system should be able to connect the referring physician or hospital, the medical transport team, the dispatcher, the medical control physician, and the surface or air ambulance carriers. The dispatchers for the communications system must be skilled in handling transport requests under stress. Medical transport should be their primary duty; they should not be nurses with patient care responsibilities. They should be trained by the program's senior staff members, who provide backup at all times.

Life support medical equipment must be portable, lightweight, battery powered, reliable, and safe for medical use. Recent advances in transport equipment include the pulse oximeter and capnometer.

In general, the transport process is initiated by physician-to-physician referral. On receipt of the call, the medical control physician of the transport program evaluates the patient's clinical condition by telephone with the referring physician and determines whether transport is appropriate. Special consideration must be given to problems of respiratory failure and altered cardiac output or cerebral blood flow, as well as the patient's ability to withstand the fatigue and the psychologic stress of long-distance transport. If the patient is deemed suitable for transport, the transport team composition, equipment, and type of air carrier are determined.

A knowledge of aircraft characteristics, including cabin pressurization and environment, is necessary. Since transported patients often require intensive care, special medical equipment (such as an intraaortic balloon pump) may be required. The equipment must be compatible with the electronic and other operational systems of the air carriers.

The modern concept of interhospital critical care transport involves maintaining care at a level equivalent to that of the ICU throughout the transport. In addition to selection of team and equipment, adequate patient stabilization before transport is critical for achieving this goal. Transport can adversely affect patients because of psychologic stress, activation of the autonomic nervous system, acceleration and deceleration, alterations in barometric pressure caused by altitude, and changes in patient position. The impact of these changes can be seen in the example of a patient with myocardial infarction complicated by mitral regurgitation, cardiogenic shock, and pulmonary edema. In such a patient, systemic vasoconstriction caused by anxiety increases preload and afterload, exacerbating mitral regurgitation and pulmonary edema; tachycardia caused by anxiety exacerbates myocardial ischemia; positional changes and acceleration and deceleration may exacerbate pulmonary edema or hypotension; decreases in barometric pressure proportionately reduce inspired oxygen tension and arterial oxygen tension. Such a patient may appear to be compensated before transport but undergo fulminant cardiopulmonary failure during transport. Treatment of such problems during transport is complicated by limited access to the patient, limited equipment, and limited personnel. Therefore successful transport involves anticipating intratransport problems and correcting them before transport. This process begins with a brief but comprehensive problem-oriented review of the medical record, supplemented by additional history and physical examination. Invasive hemodynamic monitoring is considered for assessment of cardiovascular and pulmonary pathophysiology. The potential for complications should be assessed with particular reference to hemodynamic, pulmonary, and central nervous system deterioration. Based on this assessment and a knowledge of the stresses of transport, consideration should be given to further interventions, such as intubation and mechanical ventilation for a patient with pulmonary or central nervous system problems or placement of an intraaortic balloon pump for a patient with cardiogenic shock. Although the need for such interventions varies with the individual patient and the duration of transport, only rarely is it appropriate to transport a patient who is potentially unstable (for example, a patient with aortic dissection). Almost all patients can be adequately stabilized before transport.

The efficacy of critical care transport continues to be debated. In part, this debate reflects the differences among programs, including patients, staff, vehicles, quality of care by the referring institution, transport distances, transport team philosophies, and budget. Patient categories may include trauma patients transported from the scene to the trauma center, trauma patients stabilized at a local hospital emergency room and then transported to the trauma center, nontrauma patients with acute problems transported from an emergency room at one hospital to a tertiary care hospital, patients with acute or chronic medical or surgical conditions transported from the ICU of one hospital to the ICU of a tertiary care hospital, patients with acute myocardial infarction, high-risk obstetric patients, pediatric patients, and neonates. The reasons for transport may similarly include regionalization of care (trauma, pediatric, neonatal), need for special expertise (intensive care), or access to surgery (for example, cardiac surgery) or other procedures (such as angioplasty, cardiac catheterization, or hemodialysis) not available at the referring institution. In addition, the quality of care before transport for a patient with chronic disease and the adequacy of stabilization for a patient with acute disease may vary widely. Since the purpose of critical care transport is to provide a higher level of care than can be provided at the referring institution, these variables are major factors in determining whether transport will improve patient outcome.

In addition to the preceding variables related to patient populations and referring institutions, transport programs differ in their approach to critical care transport. Program philosophies vary from "scoop and run" without stabilization to prolonged stabilization at the referring institution. The personnel responsible for transport include various combinations of physicians, nurses, paramedics, and respiratory therapists, who may or may not have specific transport training and experience. The mode of transport may be ambulance, mobile critical care unit, airplane, helicopter, or a combination. Transport distances range from several miles to worldwide. Finally, budgetary constraints may affect an operation's equipment, personnel, vehicles, and hours of operation. In general, each program combines these variables to produce optimal transport for the patient population it serves.

Since the net value of transporting the critically ill patient depends on a balance between the benefits of improved care and the risks of transport, studies differ in their assessment of the value of transport. The risk of transport is small in most well-organized programs. Therefore the major consideration is improvement in patient care. Such improvement may occur from consultation between the referring physician and the transport team or accepting physician before transport, from diagnostic and therapeutic interventions by the transport team before or during transport, and from more sophisticated patient care by the accepting institution after transport. Thus transport is most likely to benefit patients when the referring institution cannot provide definitive care. The current concept of regionalization of care suggests that transport is of value in selected groups of patients, including neonates, children, women with high-risk pregnancies, trauma victims, and patients with acute myocardial infarction.

Several aspects of the transport of trauma patients remain controversial. A review of the early experience of the Maryland Institute of Emergency Medical Service (MIEMS) demonstrated a low mortality rate among severely injured patients who were rapidly transported from the scene. A multicenter study found a 21% reduction in the expected mortality rate when helicopter transport was used, and an earlier study demonstrated that the mortality rate was reduced by helicopter versus ambulance transport. A similar study compared helicopter and ambulance transport of trauma patients who were stabilized at a local hospital before transport. Helicopter transport increased survival (89% versus 61%), particularly in patients with moderately severe injuries (trauma score 5 to 10). The improved outcome appeared to be related to an increased number of interventions (such as blood transfusions and intubation) by the helicopter team. These interventions appeared to greatly reduce hemodynamic instability (none versus 43%) during transport. Similar survival advantages with helicopter transport have been observed in some but not all other studies.

The ideal team composition varies with the specific program. The use of the mobile coronary care unit appeared to reduce deaths by rapidly bringing a trained team to the patient. In one study of interhospital transport the flight physician's skill or judgment made an important contribution in 22% of transports. Another study compared flight nurse–paramedic crews with flight nurse–physician crews for the transport of trauma patients. Among patients who survived there were 19 procedural problems (including six failed intubations and two unrecognized esophageal intubations) with the flight nurse–paramedic crew and only two complications with the flight nurse–physician team. Similarly, among patients who died there were nine procedural problems (including three intubations) with the nurse-paramedic crew and no procedural problems with the nurse-physician crew. Still another study demonstrated that the ability to perform a mock resuscitation during helicopter transport was extremely poor among personnel without extensive helicopter transport experience. Overall, these studies of trauma patients show how variability among transport programs can alter the optimal vehicle and team composition. Reduction in deaths is related primarily to more rapid delivery of sophisticated care, either by rapidly bringing the patient to a trauma center or by bringing a skilled medical team to the patient.

In summary, transport of critically ill patients can greatly improve patient outcome by delivering a higher quality of care. The transport team should be adequately trained so that this level of care begins with or before the team's arrival at the referring facility. The team's initial goal is adequate stabilization of the patient to minimize the physiologic and psychologic effects of transport and avert additional morbidity. Except in specific circumstances the quality, training, and experience of the medical personnel are the major determinants of transport outcome. The variability in objectives among transport programs suggests that no one model is sufficient for all programs.

SUGGESTED READINGS

Barger J: Strategic aeromedical evacuation: the inaugural flight. Aviat Space Environ Med 1986;57:613-616

Baxt WG, Moody P: The impact of a rotorcraft aeromedical emergency care service on trauma mortality. JAMA 1983;249:3047-3051

Baxt WG, Moody P: The impact of a physician as part of the aeromedical prehospital team in patients with blunt trauma. JAMA 1987;257:3246-3250

Baxt WG, Moody P, Cleveland HC, et al: Hospital-based rotorcraft aeromedical emergency care services and trauma mortality: a multicenter study. Ann Emerg Med 1985;14:859-864

Boyd CR, Corse KM, Campbell RC: Emergency interhospital transport of the major trauma patient: air versus ground. J Trauma 1989;29:789-793

Harris BH: Performance of aeromedical crew members: training or experience? Am J Emerg Med 1986;4:409-411

Jones DR: Aeromedical transportation of psychiatric patients: historical review and present management. Aviat Space Environ Med 1980;51:709-716

Lachenmyer J: Physiological aspects of transport. Int Anesthesiol Clin 1987;25:15-41

Mackenzie CF, Shin B, Fisher R, Cowley RA: Two-year mortality in 760 patients transported by helicopter direct from the road accident scene. Am Surg 1979;45:101-108

Moylan JA, Fitzpatrick KT, Beyer J, Georgiade GS: Factors improving survival in multisystem trauma patients. Ann Surg 1988;207:679-683

Pearl RG, Mihm FG, Rosenthal MH: Care of the adult patient during transport. Int Anesthiol Clin 1987;25:43-75

Rhee KJ, Strozeski M, Burney RE, et al: Is the flight physician needed for helicopter emergency medical services? Ann Emerg Med 1986;15:174-177

Schiller WR, Knox R, Zinnecker H, et al: J Trauma 1988;28:1127-1134

Usher RH: The role of the neonatologist. Pediatr Clin North Am 1970;17:199-202

Index

Page numbers in *italics* refer to figures. Page numbers
followed by a "t" refer to tables.